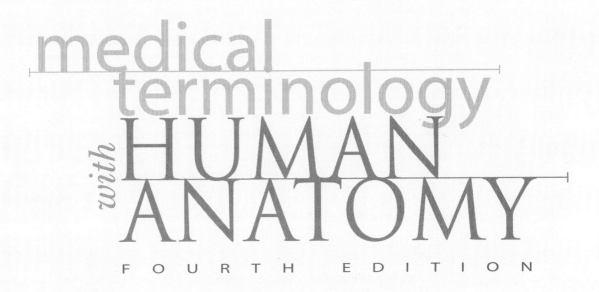

medical terminology *with* HUMAN ANATOMY

FOURTH EDITION

Jane Rice, RN, CMA-C
Medical Assisting Program Director
Coosa Valley Technical Institute
Rome, Georgia

Spanish Language Consultant
Adie DeLaGuardia, AS, CMA-C
Broward Community College
Ft. Lauderdale, Florida

APPLETON & LANGE
Stamford, CT

Copyright © 1999 by Appleton & Lange
A Simon & Schuster Company
Copyright © 1995, 1991 by Appleton & Lange
Copyright © 1986 by Appleton-Century-Crofts

www.appletonlange.com

99 00 01 02 03 / 10 9 8 7 6 5 4 3 2 1

Prentice Hall International (UK) Limited, *London*
Prentice Hall of Australia Pty. Limited, *Sydney*
Prentice Hall Canada, Inc., *Toronto*
Prentice Hall Hispanoamericana, S.A., *Mexico*
Prentice Hall of India Private Limited, *New Delhi*
Prentice Hall of Japan, Inc., *Tokyo*
Simon & Schuster Asia Pte. Ltd., *Singapore*
Editora Prentice Hall do Brasil Ltda., *Rio de Janeiro*
Prentice Hall, *Upper Saddle River, New Jersey*

Library of Congress Cataloging-in-Publication Data
Rice, Jane.
    Medical terminology with human anatomy / Jane Rice ; Spanish
language consultant, Adie DeLaGuardia. — 4th ed.
        p.   cm.
    Includes indexes.
    ISBN 0-8385-6274-4 (pbk. : alk. paper)
    1. Medicine—Terminology.   2. Human anatomy—Terminology.
I. Title.
    [DNLM: 1. Nomenclature.   2. Anatomy terminology.   W 15 R496m
1998]
R123.R523 1998
610'.1'4—dc21
DNLM/DLC
for Library of Congress   98-15836

Editor-in-Chief: Cheryl Mehalik
Acquisitions Editor: Kimberly Davies
Development Editor: Elena Mauceri
Production Editor: Lisa M. Guidone
Art Coordinator: Eve Siegel
Illustrator: Barbara Cousins
Designer: Mary Skudlarek

Printed in the United States of America

0-8385-6274-4

9 780838 562741

90000

Dedicated with love and appreciation to Larry Rice, my best friend and love, to our daughter, Melissa Rice-Noble, son-in-law Doug, and grandchildren Zachary, Benjamin, and Jacob. You are the flowers in my life.

In special memory of my parents, Warren Galileo and Elizabeth Styles Justice.

CONTENTS IN BRIEF

CONTENTS

PREFACE

Medical Terminology With Human Anatomy, fourth edition, is a comprehensive, self-instructional, write-in text with a built-in dictionary. It is written for any person who needs to acquire and use medical terminology. It is arranged by body systems and speciality areas. By using the body-systems approach one may master the component parts of medical words as they are directly related to the topic of the chapter.

▶ THREE-DIMENSIONAL TEXT

This text may be used in a traditional classroom setting, as a programmed text, and/or as a self-instructional workbook.

▶ WORD-BUILDING TECHNIQUE

Prefixes and suffixes are repeated throughout the text, while word roots and combining forms are presented according to the system or specialty area to which they relate. Once the material in Chapters 1 and 2 has been mastered, you should know 30 prefixes, 39 roots/combining forms, and 45 suffixes. To build a medical vocabulary, all you have to do is recall the word parts that you have learned and link them with the new component parts presented in the chapter. This word-building technique, while not complicated, is different from other terminology texts that have students learn prefixes, roots, combining forms, and suffixes as separate entities, generally not related to the terminology of a body system. It is much easier and better to learn component parts directly associated with a body system or specialty area. This is the key to the classic design of *Medical Terminology With Human Anatomy.*

▶ ORGANIZATION AND CLASSIC DESIGN

The fourth edition has been updated with new information, full-color art, photographs of diseases, disorders, and/or conditions, x-ray pictures, and tables. Its classic design has been maintained, and throughout the text, vibrant use of full color strengthens the presentation. The Anatomy and Physiology Overviews are at the beginning of the chapters, so that you may acquire an appreciation of the basic structure and function of the body before proceeding to the terminology, vocabulary, and other sections of the chapter. Each chapter is organized in the same manner, thereby allowing you to participate in a systematic learning experience in which medical terminology becomes a new, easily learned, and interesting part of your vocabulary.

▶ NEW FEATURES

- **Chapter Outlines and Objectives** appear at the beginning of each chapter. The outlines identify the organizational content of the chapter. The objectives state the learning concepts that should be obtained by the learner from studying the chapter.

- To provide the learner with a visual reference of diseases, disorders, and/or conditions, **108 color photographs and many x-ray pictures** are strategically placed throughout the text.

- **New full color illustrations** for Anatomy and Physiology give you access to essential diagrams of the human body. This is a perfect complement to the discussion of the anatomy and physiology overview in Chapters 2 to 16.

- **Life Span Considerations** presents interesting facts about the human body as it relates to the child and the older adult.

- **Terminology Spotlight** focuses on a term that relates to a particular disease, disorder, and/or condition. Current findings in medicine and/or interesting facts about the term are provided.

- **Word Parts Study Sheets** provides you with the opportunity to write in the correct answers for the most commonly used word parts that are related to the subject of the chapter.

- **Critical Thinking Activities** are presented in a case-study format that highlights a disease, disorder, and/or condition that relates to the subject of the chapter. A synopsis of a patient's visit to a physician is presented with present history, signs and symptoms, diagnosis, treatment, and prevention. Critical thinking questions follow the synopsis and provide the learner with an opportunity to develop and apply essential thinking skills.

▶ FEATURES FROM PREVIOUS EDITION

- **Anatomy and Physiology Overview** (Chapters 2 to 16). Comprehensive coverage of the structure and function of the body with new art and tables.

- **Terminology With Surgical Procedures & Pathology.** Each term has a pronunciation guide directly under it, word parts are identified and defined, and then the general meaning of the term is provided. Each term is presented in alphabetical order for easy reference.

- **Vocabulary Words.** Common words or specialized terms associated with the subject of the chapter are provided to enhance your medical vocabulary. Each word is presented in alphabetical order with a pronunciation guide.

- **Abbreviations.** Selected abbreviations with their meanings are included in each chapter. These abbreviations are in current use and directly associated with the subject of the chapter.

- **Drug Highlights** presents essential drug information that relates to the subject of the chapter.

- **Communication Enrichment: English/Spanish.** This feature provides you with the opportunity to learn English and/or Spanish for selected general terms and medical terms associated with the subject of the chapter.

- **Diagnostic and Laboratory Tests** provides you with currently used tests and procedures used in the physical assessment and diagnosis of certain conditions/diseases that are related to the subject of the chapter.

- **Learning Exercises** provides you with the opportunity to write in the correct answers for questions that relate to the anatomy and physiology. The Word Parts section is arranged in alphabetical order and includes all of the word parts presented in the chapter. This is an excellent method for learning the component parts that are used to build medical words. Identifying Medical Terms allows you to build medical words, and the Spelling Section allows you to test your spelling skills.

- **Review Questions** includes matching and fill-in-the-blank. These questions are based upon the vocabulary words, abbreviations, and diagnostic and laboratory tests.

- **Appendix I: Answer Key** for the learning exercises and review questions. All answers are provided so that you may easily check your work.

- **Appendix II: Answers** to the Critical Thinking Activities are provided.

- **Appendix III: Glossary of Component Parts** includes 89 prefixes, 640 roots and combining forms, and 160 suffixes with their meanings. Also includes 10 suffixes that mean "pertaining to" and 7 suffixes that mean "condition of." When you have completed *Medical Terminology With Human Anatomy* you will know 889 component parts and be able to use these component parts to understand the technical language of medicine.

- **Flash cards**

- **English/Spanish Index** includes over 4500 words.

▶ ANCILLARIES FOR THE INSTRUCTOR

- **Instructor's Manual/Test Bank.** Contains a course Syllabus, Progress Sheet, Test Schedule, Answer Sheet for Post Test A and Post Test B, two tests for each chapter. Form A and Form B, two final exams, over 2000 questions and all answers are provided. Also includes answers to the Word Parts Study Sheets. Several transparency masters are included for every chapter!

- Also included with the Instructor's Manual is a **Computerized Test Bank** (IBM compatible). A DOS computer program designed to create examinations, it consists of *the same* test items included in the *Instructor's Manual/Test Bank*, but provides the instructor with maximum flexibility due to the computerization of the material.

► STUDY AIDS FOR THE STUDENT

The following learning tools are available:

- **Computerized Study Guide for Students.** Over 1000 questions are provided in a multiple choice, true/false, fill-in-the-blank format. The learner is tested on material in a given chapter with the correct answer explained, as well as referenced by page number. A study plan is then generated from questions that were answered incorrectly. Study plans may be viewed directly on the computer screen or printed.

- **A three-tape set** (45 minutes each side) of all the terms listed in the terminology sections is available as an aid to pronunciation and understanding of the terms. Each term is pronounced and broken into its component parts; the definition of the part is given and then the term is pronounced again. By learning the component parts that are used to build medical words, one may easily acquire a working knowledge of medical terminology. The tape set is available by contacting Appleton & Lange customer service at 1-800-423-1359.

ACKNOWLEDGMENTS

It does not seem possible, but *Medical Terminology With Human Anatomy,* my "dream" text, is 13 years old. During these 13 years so many people have stood by my side, guided me, and helped me in so many ways. A special thank you to all the Medical Assisting, Radiologic Technology, Respiratory Therapy, Nursing, and Business and Office Technology students that I have had the privilege to teach. With this new edition, I have kept you at the forefront of my thoughts.

The added photographs, used to enhance the visual effects of this edition, were made possible by Jason L. Smith, MD, Northwest Georgia Dermatology and Skin Surgery Center, and his professional staff: Missy Litton, Sally Dean, DeAnn Richardson, Christy Hart, Holly Siniard, and Kristie Eubanks. I am so thankful and grateful to you for allowing me to come into your office and for helping me to select appropriate pictures of diseases, disorders, and/or conditions for my text. I also thank Missy West and Teresa Resch, Radiologic Technology Program Director at Coosa Valley Technical Institute, for assisting me and providing me with x-ray pictures for this edition.

There are many special people who help me in all that I do and I extend to each of you my warmest appreciation and gratitude:

Charles Larry Rice
Melissa Rice-Noble
Doug, Zachary, Benjamin, and Jacob Noble
Sue and Gordon Nelson
Cheryl Mehalik
Kimberly Davies
Elena Mauceri
Eve Siegel
Barbara Cousins
Fran Levine
Fred Velardi
Pete Tourtellot
Lisa M. Guidone
Mary Skudlarek
Susan Hunter
Nicole Cooper

I would like to express my appreciation to the following reviewers for their valuable input:

Anne Bello
Academic Coordinator of Clinical Education
Southwestern Community College
Sylva, North Carolina

Sherri Cooper
Program Director, Medical Assisting
Concorde Career Institute
Denver, Colorado

Diane Garcia
Instructor, Diagnostic Medical Imaging Department
City College of San Francisco
San Francisco, California

Earl Goldberg
Chair, Nursing & Allied Health Programs
Gloucester Community College
Mount Laurel, New Jersey

Rita Haggard
Allied Health Core Curriculum Coordinator
Kentucky Tech Central Campus
Lexington, Kentucky

Trudi James-Parks
Clinical Coordinator, Radiologic Technology
Lorain County Community College
Elyria, Ohio

Trudi Kenny
Program Director
Baker College
Muskegon, Michigan

Maryagnes Luczak
Director of Training
Career Training Academy
Monroeville, Pennsylvania

Molly Savage
Instructor, Health Sciences Department
Central Piedmont Community College
Charlotte, North Carolina

Kyle Thornton
Instructor, Diagnostic Medical Imaging Department
City College of San Francisco
San Francisco, California

Jane Rice

NOTE TO THE STUDENT

Don't be afraid of the long, strange-looking and -sounding medical terms included in this text. Medical terms are made up of prefixes, roots, combining forms, and suffixes. By learning the various word parts included in each chapter, you will soon know the component parts used to build medical words. Next, you will be able to relate their definitions to the meanings of the terms and be able to analyze almost any medical word that you encounter in your studies.

To assist you in learning to speak the language of medicine, a pronunciation guide is provided for each medical term, vocabulary word, and the diagnostic and laboratory tests. With this edition audiotapes are again available, and can be ordered through Appleton & Lange customer service at 1-800-423-1359, so that you may listen to the word and then pronounce the word.

Enhance your medical vocabulary by learning the words included in the vocabulary section. This section has been expanded to include the most current words used in the field of medicine.

Further expand your knowledge of medicine by studying the abbreviations included in each chapter. Abbreviations are usually capitalized and periods are not generally used. Exceptions to this general rule are the abbreviations used for medications and prescriptions. Many of these are in lower case and do use periods. Since most abbreviations have more than one meaning, you will need to be careful with their use.

This text is not just about words and their meanings. Integrated within each chapter is information on diagnostic and laboratory tests, and the amazing human body. By studying these sections, you will be surprised at how much they can help you.

You can test yourself by using the learning exercises and review questions at the end of each chapter. An answer key, located in Appendix I at the back of the text, is provided for use in checking your progress. Further suggestions for studying medical terminology are:

1. Use a building process to learn medical terminology. Take the first 10 terms in the chapter and learn their word parts and definitions. Then, relate this information to the meanings of the terms. Take the next 10 terms and do the same thing. Review what you have learned and then continue with this same process.
2. You may wish to make additional flash cards with the word part on one side and the definition and an example term on the other side. This can be a helpful technique as you begin to learn word parts. Finally, check with your instructor to see if the accompanying audiotapes are available at your school. These audiotapes will help you correctly pronounce the words that are included in the Medical Terminology sections.

Thank you for choosing this text, and may you gain a "world of knowledge" that will help you in all that you do.

Jane Rice

GUIDE TO KEY FEATURES

CHAPTER OUTLINE
Familiarizes you with the key sections and overall organization of the chapter.

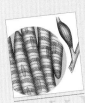

5

THE MUSCULAR SYSTEM

OUTLINE

OBJECTIVES

- Anatomy and Physiology Overview
- Types of Muscle Tissue
- Functions of Muscles
- Life Span Considerations
- Terminology with Surgical Procedures & Pathology
- Vocabulary Words
- Abbreviations
- Drug Highlights
- Diagnostic and Laboratory Tests
- Communication Enrichment
- Study and Review Section
  - Learning Exercises
  - Word Parts Study Sheet
  - Review Questions
  - Critical Thinking Activity

On completion of this chapter, you should be able to:

- Describe the muscular system.
- Describe types of muscle tissue.
- Provide the functions of muscles.
- Describe muscular differences of the child and the older adult.
- Analyze, build, spell, and pronounce medical words that relate to surgical procedures and pathology.
- Identify and give the meaning of selected vocabulary words.
- Identify and define selected abbreviations.
- Review Drug Highlights presented in this chapter.
- Provide the description of diagnostic and laboratory tests related to the muscular system.
- Successfully complete the study and review section.

CHAPTER OBJECTIVES
Lists the essential learning concepts in each chapter.

---

144 Chapter 5

▶ ANATOMY AND PHYSIOLOGY

The muscular system is composed of muscles and ... scribe the three basic types of muscles and ... primary tissues of the system. They make up appro... weight and are composed of long, slender cells known as ... ferent lengths and shapes and vary in color from white to deep red. ... sists of a group of fibers held together by connective tissue and enclosed in a ... sheath or *fascia*. See Figure 5–1. Each fiber within a muscle receives its own nerve im... pulses and has its own stored supply of glycogen, which it uses as fuel for energy. Mus... cle has to be supplied with proper nutrition and oxygen to perform properly; therefore, ... blood and lymphatic vessels permeate its tissues.

▶ TYPES OF MUSCLE TISSUE

Skeletal muscle, smooth muscle, and *cardiac muscle* are the three basic types of muscle tissue classed according to their functions and appearance (Fig. 5–2).

SKELETAL MUSCLE

Also known as *voluntary* or *striated* muscles, *skeletal muscles* are controlled by the con... scious part of the brain and attach to the bones. There are 600 skeletal muscles that ... through contractility, extensibility, and elasticity, are responsible for the movement of ... the body. These muscles have a cross-striped appearance and thus are known as striated ... muscles. They vary in size, shape, arrangement of fibers, and means of attachment to ... bones. Selected skeletal muscles are listed with their functions in Tables 5–1 and 5–2 ... and shown in Figures 5–3 and 5–4.

Skeletal muscles have two or more attachments. The more fixed attachment is known as the *origin*, and the point of attachment of a muscle to the part that it moves is the *in-section*. The means of attachment is called a *tendon*, which can vary in length from less than 1 inch to more than 1 foot. A wide, thin, sheet-like tendon is known as an *aponeuro-sis*.

A muscle has three distinguishable parts: the *body* or main portion, an *origin*, and an ...

THE MUSCULAR SYSTEM

ORGAN/STRUCTURE	PRIMARY FUNCTIONS
Muscles	Responsible for movement, help to maintain posture, and produce heat
Skeletal	Through contractility, extensibility, and elasticity, are responsible for the movement of the body
Smooth	Produce relatively slow contraction with greater degree of extensibility in the internal organs, especially organs of the digestive, respiratory, and urinary tract, plus certain muscles of the eye and skin, and walls of blood vessels
Cardiac	Muscle of the heart, controlled by the autonomic nervous system and specialized neuromuscular tissue located within the right atrium that is capable of causing cardiac muscle to contract rhythmically. The neuromuscular tissue of the heart comprises the sinoatrial node, the atrioventricular node, and the atrioventricular bundle
Tendons	A band of connective tissue serving for the attachment of muscles to bones

ANATOMY AND PHYSIOLOGY OVERVIEW
Provides at the beginning of each chapter a concise overview of the body system to which terminology relates.

The Muscular System 145

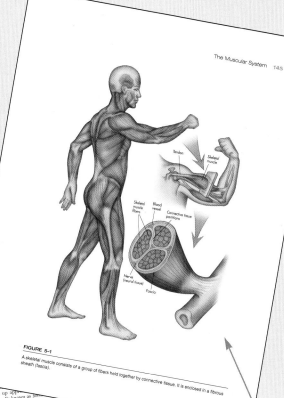

FIGURE 5–1
A skeletal muscle consists of a group of fibers held together by connective tissue. It is enclosed in a fibrous sheath (fascia).

A FULL-COLOR ART PROGRAM
Provides a visual reference of illustrations of the human body and selected diseases, disorders, and conditions. Includes both illustrations and photos.

LIFE SPAN CONSIDERATIONS

▶ THE CHILD

At about 6 weeks the size of the embryo is 12 mm (0.5 inch). The limb buds are extending and the skeletal and muscular systems are developing. At about 7 weeks the **diaphragm**, a partition of muscles and membranes that separates the chest cavity and the abdominal cavity, is completely developed. At the end of 8 weeks, the embryo is now known as the **fetus**. Fetal growth proceeds from head to tail (**cephalo** to **caudal**), with the head being larger in comparison to the rest of the body.

During fetal development the bones and muscles continue growing and developing. At about 32 weeks the developed skeletal system is soft and flexible. Muscle and fat accumulate and the fetus weighs approximately 2000 g (4 lb, 7 oz). At about 40 weeks the fetus is ready for birth and extrauterine life.

The movements of the newborn are uncoordinated and random. Muscular development proceeds from head to foot and from the center of the body to the periphery. Head and neck muscles are the first ones that can be controlled by the baby. A baby can hold his head up before he can sit erect. The baby needs freedom of movement. The bath is an excellent time for the newborn to exercise.

▶ THE OLDER ADULT

With aging changes related to mobility are most significant. There is a decrease in muscle strength, endurance, range of motion, coordination and elasticity, and flexibility of connective tissue. There is an actual loss in the number of muscle fibers due to **myofibril atrophy** with fibrous tissue replacement, which begins in the fourth decade of life.

To prevent loss of strength, muscles need to be exercised. Regular exercise strengthens muscles and keeps joints, tendons, and ligaments more flexible, allowing active people to move freely and carry out routine activities easily. Exercises such as aerobic dance, brisk walking, and bicycling improve muscle tone and heart and lung function. To maintain aerobic fitness one needs to participate in such activities for 20 minutes or more at least three times a week and work at one's target heart rate. The target range declines with age and the following table shows the correct range during exercise for women between 45 and 65 years old.

AGE	TARGET HEART RATE (BEATS PER MINUTE)
45 years old	108 to 135
50 years old	102 to 127
55 years old	99 to 123
60 years old	96 to 120
65 years old	93 to 116

VOCABULARY WORDS

Vocabulary words are terms that have not been divided into component parts. They are common words or specialized terms associated with the subject of this chapter. These words are provided to enhance your medical vocabulary.

WORD	DEFINITION
amputation (ăm″ pū-tā′ shŭn)	Surgical excision of a limb, part, or other appendage
contracture (kŏn-trăk′ chūr)	A condition in which a muscle shortens and renders the muscle resistant to the normal stretching process
degeneration (dē-gĕn″ ĕ-rā′ shŭn)	The process of deteriorating; to change from a higher to a lower form
dermatomyositis (dĕr″ mă-tō-mī″ ō-sī′ tĭs)	Inflammation of the muscles and the skin; a connective tissue disease characterized by edema, dermatitis, and inflammation of the muscles. See Figure 5–6.
diathermy (dī′ ă-thĕr″ mē)	Treatment using high-frequency current to produce heat within a part of the body; used to increase blood flow and should not be used in acute stage of recovery from trauma. Types: **Microwave.** Electromagnetic radiation is directed to specified tissues **Short-wave.** High-frequency electric current (wavelength of 3–30 m) is directed to specified tissues **Ultrasound.** High-frequency sound waves (20,000–10 billion cycles/sec) are directed to specified tissues
Dupuytren's contracture (dū-pwē-tranz′ kŏn-trăk′ chūr)	A slow, progressive contracture of the palmar fascia causing the ring and little fingers to bend into the palm so that they cannot be extended. See Figure 5–7.
dystrophin (dĭs-trŏf′ ĭn)	A protein found in muscle cells; when the gene that is responsible for this protein is defective and sufficient dystrophin is not produced, muscle wasting occurs
exercise (ĕk′ sĕr-sīz)	Performed activity of the muscles for improvement of health or correction of deformity. Types: **Active.** The patient contracts and relaxes his or her muscles **Assistive.** The patient contracts and relaxes his or her muscles with the assistance of a therapist **Isometric.** Active muscular contraction performed against stable resistance, thereby not shortening the muscle length **Passive.** Exercise is performed by another individual without the assistance of the patient

---

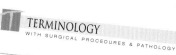

TERMINOLOGY
WITH SURGICAL PROCEDURES & PATHOLOGY

TERM	WORD PARTS			DEFINITION
abductor (ăb-dŭk′ tŏr)	ab duct or	P R S	away from to lead a doer	A muscle that, on contraction, draws away from the middle
adductor (ă-dŭk′ tŏr)	ad duct or	P R S	toward to lead a doer	A muscle that draws a part toward the middle
antagonist (ăn-tăg′ ō-nĭst)	ant agon ist	P R S	against agony, a contest agent	A muscle that counteracts the action of another muscle
aponeurorrhaphy (ăp″ ō-nū-ror′ ă-fē)	apo neuro rrhaphy	P CF CF	separation nerve suture	Suture of an aponeurosis
aponeurosis (ăp″ ō-nū-rō′ sĭs)	apo neur osis	P R S	separation nerve condition of	A fibrous sheet of connective tissue that serves to attach muscle to bone or to other tissues
ataxia (ă-tăks′ ĭ-ă)	a taxia	P S	lack of order	A lack of muscular coordination
atonic (ă-tŏn′ ĭk)	a ton ic	P R S	lack of tone, tension pertaining to	Pertaining to a lack of normal tone or tension
atrophy (ăt′ rō-fē)	a trophy	P S	lack of nourishment, development	A lack of nourishment; a wasting of muscular tissue that may be caused by lack of use

☼ **TERMINOLOGY SPOTLIGHT**

Atrophy occurs with the disuse of muscles over a long period of time. Bedrest and immobility can cause loss of muscle mass and strength. When immobility is due to a treatment mode, such as casting or traction, one can decrease the effects of immobility by isometric exercise of the muscles of the immobilized part. Isometric exercise involves active muscular contraction performed against stable resistance, such as tightening the muscles of the thigh and/or tightening the muscles of the buttocks. Active exercise of uninjured parts of the body helps prevent muscle atrophy.

continued

LIFE SPAN CONSIDERATIONS
A special feature that presents interesting facts about the human body as it relates to the child and the older adult.

TERMINOLOGY WITH SURGICAL PROCEDURES AND PATHOLOGY
This built-in dictionary includes pronunciations and identifies and defines word parts.

VOCABULARY WORDS
Lists common words or specialized terms to help you better understand the subject matter. Organized alphabetically, each term includes a definition and pronunciation guide.

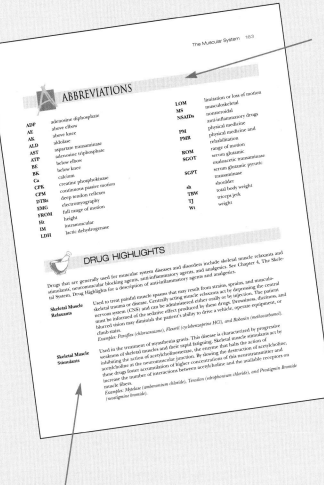

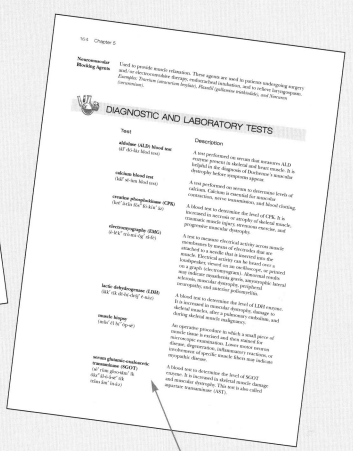

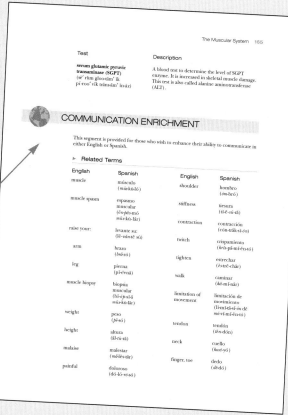

ABBREVIATIONS
Selected abbreviations are included in each chapter where appropriate.

DRUG HIGHLIGHTS
Presents essential and relevant drug information.

COMMUNICATION ENRICHMENT
Offers you an optional opportunity to learn English and/or Spanish for selected general terms and certain medical conditions.

DIAGOSTIC AND LABORATORY TESTS
Provides current tests and procedures used in the physical assessment and diagnosis of certain conditions and diseases.

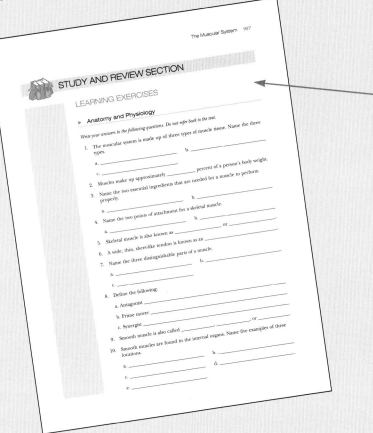

STUDY AND REVIEW SECTION

Provides an excellent opportunity to reinforce material. Includes learning exercises, spelling exercises, word parts study sheets, and review questions.

CRITICAL THINKING ACTIVITIES

Focused learning format highlights a disease, disorder, and/or condition. Questions are included that refer to the case study, and provide an opportunity to think critically.

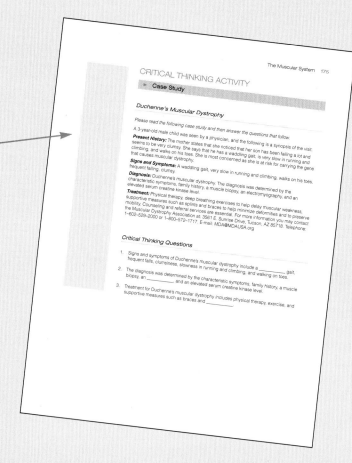

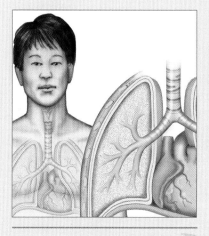

1

FUNDAMENTAL WORD STRUCTURE

OBJECTIVES

On completion of this chapter, you should be able to:

- Describe the fundamental elements that are used to build medical words.

- Use the learning aids to gain an understanding of medical terminology.

- List three guidelines that will assist you with the identification and spelling of medical words.

- Analyze, build, spell, and pronounce medical words that relate to surgical procedures and pathology.

- Identify and give the meaning of selected vocabulary words.

- Describe selected medical and surgical specialties, giving the scope of practice and the physician's title.

- Identify and define selected abbreviations.

- Successfully complete the study and review section.

► UNDERSTANDING FUNDAMENTAL WORD STRUCTURE

Medical terminology is the study of terms that are used in the art and science of medicine. It is a specialized language with its origin arising from the Greek influence on medicine. Hippocrates was a Greek physician who lived from 460 to 377 BC and whose vital role in medicine is still recognized today. He is called "The Father of Medicine" and is credited with establishing early ethical standards for physicians. Because of advances in scientific computerized technology, many new terms are coined daily; however, most of these terms are composed of word parts that have their origins in ancient Greek or Latin. Because of this foreign origin, it is necessary to learn the English translation of terms when learning the fundamentals of word structure.

► FUNDAMENTALS OF WORD STRUCTURE

The fundamental elements in medical terminology are the component parts used to build medical words. The terms for component parts used in this text are *P = prefix, R = root, CF = combining form,* and *S = suffix.* Each of these component parts is described in detail below.

PREFIX

The term *prefix* means to fix before or to fix to the beginning of a word. A prefix may be a syllable or a group of syllables united with or placed at the beginning of a word to alter or modify the meaning of the word or to create a new word.

For example: the word *abnormal* means pertaining to away from the normal. Note its component parts below:

ab	P or prefix meaning	away from
norm	R or root meaning	rule
al	S or suffix meaning	pertaining to

WORD ROOT

A *root* is a word or word element from which other words are formed. It is the foundation of the word. The root conveys the central meaning of the word and forms the base to which prefixes and suffixes are attached for word modification.

For example: the word *autonomy* means condition of being self-governed. Note its component parts below:

auto	P or prefix meaning	self
nom	R or root meaning	law
y	S or suffix meaning	condition

COMBINING FORM

A *combining form* is a word root to which a vowel has been added to join the root to a second root or to a suffix. The vowel "o" is used more often than any other to make combining forms. Combining forms may be found at the beginning of a word or within the word.

For example: the word *chemotherapy* means treatment of disease by using chemical agents. Note the relation of its component parts:

| chemo | CF or combining form meaning | chemical |
| therapy | S or suffix meaning | treatment |

SUFFIX

The term *suffix* means to fasten on beneath or under. A suffix or pseudo suffix may be a syllable or group of syllables united with or placed at the end of a word to alter or modify the meaning of the word or to create a new word.

For example: the word *centigrade* means having 100 steps or degrees and the word *centimeter* means one-hundredth of a meter:

centi	P or prefix meaning	a hundred
grade	S or suffix meaning	a step
centi	P or prefix meaning	a hundred
meter	S or suffix meaning	measure

In many medical terminology textbooks, all the prefixes, suffixes, and pseudo suffixes used throughout the text are grouped into one or two beginning chapters. Under this arrangement, you are forced to refer repeatedly back to these chapters to identify or define these word elements. In this book, however, prefixes, suffixes, and pseudo suffixes, along with their definitions, are integrated into each chapter throughout the text and provide a ready reference. Naturally, many of these same prefixes, suffixes, and pseudo suffixes will be used in each chapter. This repetition serves to reinforce the learning of the terms and their definitions and makes this text an improved learning tool.

Word roots and combining forms, together with their definitions, are included in each chapter according to the cell, tissue, organ, system, or element they describe. This arrangement makes it possible for you to form associations between medical terms and the various body systems. To reinforce this relation, this text provides you with a general anatomy and physiology overview for each of the body systems that it includes.

▶ PRINCIPLES OF COMPONENT PARTS

As you learn definitions for prefixes, roots, combining forms, and suffixes, you will discover that some component parts have the same meanings as others. This occurs most often with words that relate to the organs of the body and the diseases that affect them. The existence of more than one component part for a particular meaning can be traced to differences in the Greek or Latin words from which they originated. Most of the terms for the body's organs originated from Latin words, whereas terms describing diseases that affect these organs have their origins in Greek.

For example:

- **Uterus**—a Latin word for one of the organs of the female reproductive system
- **Hyster**—a Greek R (root) for womb
- **Hysterectomy**—surgical excision of the womb from hyster R (root) meaning womb + ectomy S (suffix) meaning surgical excision
- **Metri**—a Greek CF (combining form) for uterus
- **Myometrium**—muscular tissue of the uterus from myo CF meaning muscle + metri CF meaning uterus + um S meaning tissue

Many prefixes and suffixes have more than a single definition. When learning medical terminology, you must learn to use the definition that best describes the term. The following are commonly used prefixes that have more than a single definition:

Prefix	Meanings	Prefix	Meanings
a-, an-	no, not, without, lack of, apart	extra-	outside, beyond
ad-	toward, near, to	hyper-	above, beyond, excessive
bi-	two, double	hypo-	below, under, deficient
de-	down, away from		
di-	two, double	in-	in, into, not
dia-	through, between	mega-	large, great
dif-, dis-	apart, free from, separate	meta-	beyond, over, between, change
dys-	bad, difficult, painful	para-	beside, alongside, abnormal
ec-, ecto-	out, outside, outer	poly-	many, much, excessive
		post-	after, behind
end-, endo-	within, inner	pre-	before, in front of
ep-, epi-	upon, over, above	pro-	before, in front of
eu-	good, normal	super-	above, beyond
ex-, exo-	out, away from	supra-	above, beyond

The following prefixes and their meanings have been selected to aid you in building a medical vocabulary:

PREFIXES THAT PERTAIN TO POSITION OR PLACEMENT

Prefix	Meanings	Prefix	Meanings
ab-	away from	hyper-	above, excessive
ad-	toward	hypo-	below, deficient
ana-	up	infra-	below
ante-	before	inter-	between
cata-	down	intra-	within
circum-, peri-	around	meso-	middle
endo-	within	para-	beside
epi-	upon, above	retro-	backward
ex-	out, away from	sub-	below, under
extra-	outside, beyond	supra-	above, beyond

PREFIXES THAT PERTAIN TO NUMBERS AND AMOUNTS

Prefix	Meanings	Prefix	Meanings
ambi-	both	poly-	many
bi-	two, double	primi-	first
centi-	a hundred	quadri-	four
deca-	ten	quint-	five
dipl-	double	semi-, hemi-	half
di(s)-	two	tetra-	four
milli-	one-thousandth	tri-	three
multi-	many, much	uni-	one
nulli-	none		

PREFIXES THAT ARE DESCRIPTIVE AND ARE USED IN GENERAL

Prefix	Meanings	Prefix	Meanings
a, an-	without, lack of	hetero-	different
anti-, contra-	against	homeo-	similar, same
auto-	self	hydro-	water
brachy-	short	mega-	large, great
brady-	slow	micro-	small
cac-, mal-	bad	oligo-	scanty, little
dia-	through	pan-	all
dys-	bad, difficult	pseudo-	false
eu-	good, normal	sym-, syn-	together

The following are commonly used suffixes that have more than a single definition:

Suffix	Meanings	Suffix	Meanings
-ate	use, action	-plasm	a thing formed, plasma
-blast	immature cell, germ cell		
-ectasis	dilatation, dilation, distention	-plegia	stroke, paralysis
-gen	formation, produce	-ptosis	prolapse, drooping
-genesis	formation, produce	-rrhea	flow, discharge
-genic	formation, produce	-scopy	to view, examine
-gram	weight, mark, record	-spasm	tension, spasm
-ic	pertaining to, chemical	-stasis	control, stopping
-ive	nature of, quality of	-staxia	dripping, trickling
-lymph	serum, clear fluid	-trophy	nourishment, development
-lysis	destruction, to separate		
-megaly	enlargement, large	-y	process, condition, pertaining to
-penia	lack of, deficiency		

The following suffixes and their meanings have been selected to aid you in building a medical vocabulary:

SUFFIXES THAT PERTAIN TO PATHOLOGIC CONDITIONS

Suffix	Meanings	Suffix	Meanings
-algia, -dynia	pain	-pathy	disease
-cele	hernia, tumor, swelling	-penia	deficiency
-emesis	vomiting	-phobia	fear
-itis	inflammation	-plegia	paralysis, stroke
-lith	stone	-ptosis	drooping
-lysis	destruction, separation	-ptysis	spitting
-malacia	softening	-rrhage	bursting forth
-megaly	enlargement, large	-rrhagia	bursting forth
-oid	resemble	-rrhea	flow, discharge
-oma	tumor	-rrhexis	rupture
-osis	condition of		

SUFFIXES USED IN DIAGNOSTIC AND SURGICAL PROCEDURES

Suffix	Meanings	Suffix	Meanings
-centesis	surgical puncture	-pexy	surgical fixation
-desis	binding	-plasty	surgical repair
-ectomy	excision	-rrhaphy	suture
-gram	a weight, mark, record	-scope	instrument
-graph	to write, record	-scopy	to view
-graphy	recording	-stasis	control, stopping
-meter	instrument to measure, measure	-stomy	new opening
		-tome	instrument to cut
-opsy	to view	-tomy	incision

SUFFIXES THAT ARE USED IN GENERAL

Suffix	Meanings	Suffix	Meanings
-blast	immature cell, germ cell	-phraxis	to obstruct
-cyte	cell	-physis	growth
-ist	one who specializes, agent	-pnea	breathing
-logy	study of	-poiesis	formation
-phagia	to eat	-therapy	treatment
-plasia	formation, produce	-trophy	nourishment, development
-phasia	to speak		
-philia	attraction	-uria	urine

▶ IDENTIFYING MEDICAL TERMS

When identifying medical terms you will learn to distinguish between and select the appropriate component parts for the meaning of the term. It is most important that you learn the terms as they are listed, for the slightest change in the arrangement of a medical word's component parts can change its meaning.

For example: the word *microscope* means an instrument used to view small objects. Compare the following:

micro + scope	Proper placement of component parts (P + S) although the definitions translate micro = small and scope = instrument.
scope + micro	Improper placement of component parts (S + P). Although incorrect, this arrangement of word parts seems to correspond to the term's definition.

▶ SPELLING

Medical terms of Greek origin are often difficult to spell because many of them begin with a silent letter or have a silent letter within the word. The following are examples of words that begin with silent letters:

Silent Beginning	Pronounced	Medical Term	Pronunciation Guide
cn	n	**c**nemial	(nē′ mǐ-al)
gn	n	**g**nathic	(năth′ ǐk)
kn	n	**k**nuckle	(nŭk′ ě l)
mn	n	**m**nemic	(nē′ mǐk)
pn	n	**p**neumonia	(nū′-mō′ nǐ-ă)
ps	s	**p**sychiatrist	(sī-kī′ ă-trǐst)
pt	t	**p**tosis	(tō′ sǐs)

The following are examples of medical terms that contain silent letters within the word:

Silent Letter	Medical Term	Pronunciation Guide
g	phle**g**m	(flĕm)
p	ble**p**haroptosis	(blĕf″ ă-rō-tō′ sis)

Correct spelling is extremely important in medical terminology as the addition or omission of a single letter may change the meaning of a term to something entirely different. The following examples illustrate this point:

Term/Letter Change	Meaning of Term	Term/Letter Change	Meaning of Term
a**b**duct	To lead **away** from the middle	ar**te**ritis	Inflammation of an **artery**
a**d**duct	To lead **toward** the middle	ar**th**ritis	Inflammation of a **joint**

Listed below are some of the component parts that often contribute to spelling errors:

Prefix	Meaning	Suffix	Meaning
ante-	before	-poiesis	formation
anti-	against	-ptosis	prolapse, drooping
		-ptysis	spitting
ecto-	outside		
endo-	within	-rrhagia	bursting forth
		-rrhage	bursting forth
hyper-	above, beyond, excessive		
hypo-	below, under, deficient	-rrhaphy	suture
		-rrhea	flow
		-rrhexis	rupture

continued

Prefix	Meaning		Suffix	Meaning
inter-	between		-scope	instrument
intra-	within		-scopy	to view
para-	beside		-tome	instrument to cut
peri-	around		-tomy	incision
per-	through		-tripsy	crushing
pre-	before		-trophy	nourishment
pro-	before			
super-	above, beyond			
supra-	above, beyond			

The following guidelines are provided to help with the identification and spelling of medical terms:

1. If the suffix begins with a vowel, drop the combining vowel from the combining form and add the suffix.

   For example: hemat*o* + *o*ma becomes hematoma when we drop the "o" from hemat*o*.

2. If the suffix begins with a consonant, keep the combining vowel and add the suffix to the combining form.

   For example, kil*o* + gram becomes kilogram and we keep the "o" on the combining form kil*o*.

3. Keep the combining vowel between two or more roots in a term.

   For example: electr*o* + cardi*o* + gram becomes electr*o*cardi*o*gram and we keep the combining vowels.

► FORMING PLURAL ENDINGS

To change the following singular endings to plural endings, substitute the plural endings as illustrated:

Singular Ending	Plural Ending	Singular Ending	Plural Ending
a as in burs**a**	to **ae** as in burs**ae**	**ix** as in append**ix**	to **ices** as in append**ices**
ax as in thor**ax**	to **aces** as in thor**aces** or **es** as in thorax**es**	**nx** as in phala**nx**	to **ges** as in phalan**ges**
		on as in spermatoz**on**	to **a** as in spermatoz**a**
en as in foram**en**	to **ina** as in foram**ina**	**um** as in ov**um**	to **a** as in ov**a**
		us as in nucle**us**	to **i** as in nucle**i**
is as in cris**is**	to **es** as in cris**es**	**y** as in arter**y**	to **i** and add **es** as in arter**ies**
is as in ir**is**	to **ides** as in ir**ides**		
is as in femor**is**	to **a** as in femor**a**		

▶ PRONUNCIATION

Pronunciation of medical words may seem difficult; however, it is very important to pronounce medical words with the same or very similar sounds to convey their correct meanings. As in spelling, one mispronounced syllable can change the meaning of a medical word. This text uses a phonetically spelled pronunciation guide adapted from *Taber's Cyclopedic Medical Dictionary,* and you should practice speaking each term aloud when working with the various lists of medical terms or vocabulary words. Accent marks are used to indicate stress on certain syllables. A single accent mark (′) is called a primary accent and is used with the syllable that has the strongest stress. A double accent (″) is called a secondary accent and is given to syllables that are stressed less than primary syllables.

Diacritics are marks placed over or under vowels to indicate the long or short sound of the vowel. In this text, the macron (¯) shows the long sound of the vowel, the breve (˘) shows the short sound of the vowel, and the schwa (ə) indicates the uncolored, central vowel sound of most unstressed syllables [for example: antiseptic (an″ ti-sep′ tik) or diathermy (di′ ə-thĕr″ mē)].

▶ LEARNING AIDS

There are various methods that can be used to learn medical terminology. Some of these methods are:

- Use the **flash cards** in the back of the book or make additional flash cards for any word parts not included by using small cards or cutting paper into small pieces. Write the word part on one side and its meaning on the other side. You can arrange the cards in alphabetical order or, if preferred, according to the chapter being studied. These cards can be kept in a box or an envelope, or placed in a pocket in the back of your text. Flash cards are an excellent method for learning word parts.
- **Learning Exercises** included at the end of each chapter provide you with the opportunity to write in correct answers that relate to important topics of the chapter. The Word Parts section is arranged in alphabetical order and includes all of the word parts presented in the chapter.
- **Word Parts Study Sheets** are provided in each chapter. Selected word parts are listed and a place is provided for you to give the meaning. By using these study sheets you will learn the component parts that are used to build medical words.
- **Review Questions** included in each chapter are based on the vocabulary words, abbreviations, and diagnostic and laboratory tests.

Note: Using the word parts study sheets, making flash cards, and completing the learning exercises and review questions will help you develop a medical vocabulary.

TERMINOLOGY
WITH SURGICAL PROCEDURES & PATHOLOGY

TERM	WORD PARTS			DEFINITION
abnormal (ăb-nōr′ măl)	ab norm al	P R S	away from rule pertaining to	Pertaining to away from the normal
adhesion (ăd′ hē-zhŭn)	adhes ion	R S	stuck to process	The process of being stuck together
antipyretic (ăn″ tĭ-pī-rĕt′ ĭk)	anti pyret ic	P R S	against fever pertaining to	Pertaining to an agent that works against fever
antiseptic (ăn″ tĭ-sĕp′ tĭk)	anti sept ic	P R S	against putrefaction pertaining to	Pertaining to an agent that works against sepsis; *putrefaction*
antitussive (ăn″ tĭ-tŭs′ ĭv)	anti tuss ive	P R S	against cough nature of, quality of	Pertaining to an agent that works against coughing
asepsis (ā-sĕp′ sĭs)	a sepsis	P S	without decay	Without decay; *sterile,* free from all living microorganisms
autoclave (ŏ′ tō-klāv)	auto clave	P S	self a key	An apparatus used to sterilize articles by steam under pressure
autonomy (ăw-tŏ′ nōm-ē) (ŏ-tŏ′ nōmē)	auto nom y	P R S	self law condition	The condition of being self-governed; to function independently
axillary (ăks′ ĭ-lār-ē)	axill ary	R S	armpit pertaining to	Pertaining to the armpit
cachexia (kă-kĕks′ ĭ-ă)	cac hexia	P S	bad condition	A condition of ill health, malnutrition, and wasting
centigrade (sĕn′ tĭ-grād)	centi grade	P S	a hundred a step	Having 100 steps or degrees, like the Celsius temperature scale; boiling point = 100°C and freezing point = 0°C
centimeter (sĕn′ tĭ-mē-tĕr)	centi meter	P S	a hundred measure	Unit of measurement in the metric system; one hundredth of a meter

Terminology - continued

TERM	WORD PARTS			DEFINITION
centrifuge (sĕn' trĭ-fū j)	centri fuge	CF S	center to flee	A device used in a laboratory to separate solids from liquids
chemotherapy (kē" mō-thĕr' ă-pē)	chemo therapy	CF S	chemical treatment	Treatment using chemical agents
diagnosis (di" ăg-nō' sĭs)	dia gnosis	P S	through knowledge	Determination of the cause and nature of a disease
diaphoresis (di" ă-fō-rē' sĭs)	dia phoresis	P S	through to carry	To carry through sweat glands; *profuse sweating*
diathermy (dī' ă-thĕr" mē)	dia thermy	P S	through heat	Treatment using high-frequency current to produce heat within a part of the body
heterogeneous (hĕt" ĕr-ō-jē' nĭ-ŭs)	hetero gene ous	P R S	different formation, produce pertaining to	Pertaining to a different formation
kilogram (kĭl' ō-grăm)	kilo gram	CF S	a thousand a weight	Unit of weight in the metric system; *1000 g*
macroscopic (măk" rō-skŏp' ĭk)	macro scop ic	CF R S	large to examine pertaining to	Pertaining to objects large enough to be examined by the naked eye
malformation (măl" fōr-mā' shŭn)	mal format ion	P R S	bad a shaping process	The process of being badly shaped, deformed
microgram (mī' krō-grăm)	micro gram	P S	small a weight	A unit of weight in the metric system; *0.001 mg*
microorganism (mī" krō-ōr'găn-ĭzm)	micro organ ism	P R S	small organ condition	Small living organisms that are not visible to the naked eye
microscope (mī' krō-skōp)	micro scope	P S	small instrument	An instrument used to view small objects
milligram (mĭl' ĭ-grăm)	milli gram	P S	one-thousandth a weight	A unit of weight in the metric system; *0.001 g*
milliliter (mĭl' ĭ-lē" tĕr)	milli liter	P S	one-thousandth liter	A unit of volume in the metric system; *0.001 L*
multiform (mŭl' tĭ-form)	multi form	P S	many, much shape	Occurring in or having many shapes

continued

Terminology - continued

TERM	WORD PARTS			DEFINITION
necrosis (nĕ-krō′ sis)	necr osis	R S	death condition of	A condition of death of tissue
neopathy (nē-ŏp′ ă-thē)	neo pathy	P S	new disease	A new disease
oncology (ŏng-kŏl′ ō-jē)	onco logy	CF S	tumor study of	The study of tumors
paracentesis (păr″ ă-sĕn-tē′ sĭs)	para centesis	P S	beside surgical puncture	Surgical puncture of a body cavity for fluid removal
prognosis (prŏg-nō′ sĭs)	pro gnosis	P S	before knowledge	A condition of foreknowledge; the prediction of the course of a disease and the recovery rate
pyrogenic (pī″ rō-jĕn′ ĭk)	pyro genic	CF S	heat, fire formation, produce	Pertaining to the production of heat; *a fever*
radiology (rā″ dē-ŏl′ ō-jē)	radio logy	CF S	ray study of	The study of radioactive substances
syndrome (sĭn′ drōm)	syn drome	P S	together, with a course	A combination of signs and symptoms occurring together that characterize a specific disease
thermometer (thĕr-mŏm′ ĕ-tĕr)	thermo meter	CF S	hot, heat instrument to measure	An instrument used to measure degree of heat
topography (tō-pŏg′ răh-fē)	topo graphy	CF S	place recording	A recording of a special place of the body
triage (trē-ahzh′)	tri age	P S	three related to	The sorting and classifying of injuries to determine priority of need and treatment

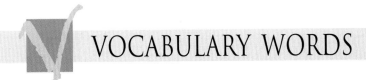

VOCABULARY WORDS

Vocabulary words are terms that have not been divided into component parts. They are common words or specialized terms associated with the subject of this chapter. These words are provided to enhance your medical vocabulary.

WORD	DEFINITION
abate (ă-bāt′)	To lessen, decrease, or cease
abscess (ăb′ sĕs)	A localized collection of pus, which may occur in any part of the body
acute (ă-cūt′)	Sudden, sharp, severe; a disease that has a sudden onset, severe symptoms, and a short course
afferent (ăf′ ĕr ĕnt)	Carrying impulses toward a center
ambulatory (ăm′ bŭ-lăh-tŏr″ē)	The condition of being able to walk, not confined to bed
antidote (ăn′ tĭ-dōt)	A substance given to counteract poisons and their effects
apathy (ăp′ ă-thē)	A condition in which one lacks feelings and emotions and is indifferent
biopsy (bī′ŏp-sē)	Surgical removal of a small piece of tissue for microscopic examination; used to determine a diagnosis of cancer or other disease processes in the body
chronic (krŏn′ ik)	Pertaining to time; a disease that continues over a long time, showing little change in symptoms or course
disease (dĭ-zēz′)	Lack of ease; an abnormal condition of the body that presents a series of symptoms that sets it apart from normal or other abnormal body states
disinfectant (dĭs″ ĭn-fĕk′ tănt)	A chemical substance that destroys bacteria
efferent (ĕf′ ĕr ĕnt)	Carrying impulses away from a center
empathy (ĕm′ pă-thē)	A state of projecting one's own personality into the personality of another to understand the feelings, emotions, and behavior of the person

Vocabulary - continued

WORD	DEFINITION
epidemic (ĕp″ i-dĕm′ ik)	Pertaining to among the people; the rapid, widespread occurrence of an infectious disease
etiology (ē″ tē-ŏl′ ō-jē)	The study of the cause(s) of disease
excision (ĕk-si′ zhŭn)	The process of cutting out, surgical removal
febrile (fē brĭl)	Pertaining to fever
gram (grăm)	A unit of weight in the metric system; a cubic centimeter or a milliliter of water is equal to the weight of a gram
illness (ĭl′ nĭs)	A state of being sick
incision (ĭn-sĭzh′ ŭn)	The process of cutting into
liter (lē′ tĕr)	A unit of volume in the metric system; equal to 33.8 fl oz or 1.0567 qt
malaise (mă-lāz′)	A bad feeling; a condition of discomfort, uneasiness; often felt by a patient with a chronic disease
malignant (mă-lĭg′ nănt)	A bad wandering; pertaining to the spreading process of cancer from one area of the body to another area
maximal (măks′ ĭ-măl)	Pertaining to the greatest possible quantity, number, or degree
minimal (mĭn′ ĭ-măl)	Pertaining to the least possible quantity, number, or degree
pallor (păl′ or)	Paleness, a lack of color
palmar (păl′ mar)	Pertaining to the palm of the hand
prognostication (prŏg-nŏs′ tĭ-cā-shŭn)	The study of the likely course of a disease and the signs of a patient's failure to thrive
prophylactic (prō-fi-lăk′ tĭk)	Pertaining to preventing or protecting against disease
rapport (ră-pōr′)	A relationship of understanding between two individuals, especially between the patient and the physician

▶ MEDICAL AND SURGICAL SPECIALTIES

The practice of medicine has evolved from the customs of ancient times.

- Circa 8000 BC prehistoric people practiced the first-known surgical treatment.
- Circa 2500 BC Egyptian physicians developed a system for treating diseases.
- Circa 400 BC, a Greek physician, Hippocrates, who is known as the "Father of Medicine," showed that diseases have natural, rather than supernatural causes. He established the foundation for the scientific basis of medical practice. He is also responsible for the Hippocratic Oath, a standard of medical ethics for physicians.

Today, the practice of medicine involves many areas of specialization. The American Board of Medical Specialists (ABMS) was founded in 1933. This board established standards for and monitoring of specialty practice areas. A physician who has met standards beyond those of admission to licensure and has passed an examination in a specialty area becomes board certified. There are various medical professional organizations that establish their own standards and administer their own board certification examinations. Individuals successfully completing all requirements are called Fellows, such as Fellow of the American College of Surgeons (FACS) or Fellow of the American College of Physicians (FACP). Board certification may be required by a hospital for admission to the medical staff or for determination of a staff member's rank. See Table 1–1 for selected medical and surgical specialties and Table 1–2 for types of surgical specialties with description of practice.

TABLE 1–1   Selected Medical and Surgical Specialties

Specialty and Scope of Practice/Physician/Word Parts

Allergy and Immunology: The branch of medicine concerned with diseases of an allergic nature. The physician is an **allergist** or **immunologist** (immuno—immune; log—study of; -ist—one who specializes).

Anesthesiology: The branch of medicine concerned with appropriate anesthesia for partial or complete loss of sensation. The physician is an **anesthesiologist** (an—without; esthesio—feeling; log—study of; -ist—one who specializes).

Cardiology: The branch of medicine concerned with diseases of the heart, arteries, veins, and capillaries. The physician is a **cardiologist** (cardio—heart; log—study of; -ist—one who specializes).

Dermatology: The branch of medicine concerned with diseases of the skin. The physician is a **dermatologist** (dermato—skin; log—study of; -ist—one who specializes).

Endocrinology: The branch of medicine concerned with diseases of the endocrine system. The physician is an **endocrinologist** (endo—within; crino—to secrete; log—study of; -ist—one who specializes).

Epidemiology: The branch of medicine concerned with epidemic diseases. The physician is an **epidemiologist** (epi—upon; demio—people; log—study of; -ist—one who specializes).

Family Practice: The branch of medicine concerned with the care of members of the family regardless of age and/or sex. The physician is a **Family Practitioner.**

Gastroenterology: The branch of medicine concerned with diseases of the stomach and intestines. The physician is a **gastroenterologist** (gastro—stomach; entero—intestine; log—study of; -ist—one who specializes).

Geriatrics: The branch of medicine concerned with aspects of aging. The physician is a **gerontologist** (geronto—old age; log—study of; -ist—one who specializes).

continued

TABLE 1–1   continued

***

Gynecology: The branch of medicine that studies diseases of the female reproductive system. The physician is a **gynecologist** *(gyneco—female; log—study of; -ist—one who specializes).*

Hematology: The branch of medicine that studies diseases of the blood and blood-forming tissues. The physician is a **hematologist** *(hemato—blood; log—study of; -ist—one who specializes).*

Infectious Disease: The branch of medicine concerned with diseases caused by the growth of pathogenic microorganisms within the body.

Internal Medicine: The branch of medicine concerned with diseases of internal origin, those not usually treated surgically. The physician is an **internist** *(intern—within; -ist—one who specializes).*

Nephrology: The branch of medicine concerned with diseases of the kidney and urinary system. The physician is a **nephrologist** *(nephro—kidney; log—study of; -ist—one who specializes).*

Neurology: The branch of medicine concerned with diseases of the nervous system. The physician is a **neurologist** *(neuro—nerve; log—study of; -ist—one who specializes).*

Obstetrics: The branch of medicine concerned with treating the female during pregnancy, childbirth, and the postpartum. The physician is an **obstetrician.** The Latin word element *obstetrix* means midwife.

Oncology: The branch of medicine that studies tumors. The physician is an **oncologist** *(onco—tumor; log—study of; -ist—one who specializes).*

Ophthalmology: The branch of medicine concerned with diseases of the eye. The physician is an **ophthalmologist** *(ophthalmo—eye; log—study of; -ist—one who specializes).*

Orthopedic Surgery *(Orthopaedic)***:** The branch of medicine concerned with diseases and disorders involving locomotor structures of the body. The physician is an **orthopedist** *(orthopaedist) (ortho—straight; ped—child; -ist—one who specializes).*

Otorhinolaryngology: The branch of medicine concerned with diseases of the ear, nose, and larynx. The physician is an **otorhinolaryngologist** *(oto—ear; rhino—nose; laryngo—larynx; log—study of; -ist—one who specializes).*

Pathology: The branch of medicine that studies structural and functional changes in tissues and organs caused by disease. The physician is a **pathologist** *(patho—disease; log—study of; -ist—one who specializes).*

Pediatrics: The branch of medicine concerned with diseases of children. The physician is a **pediatrician** *(ped—child; iatr—treatment; -ician—physician).*

Physical Medicine and Rehabilitation: The branch of medicine concerned with the treatment of disease by physical agents. The physician is a **physiatrist** *(phys—nature; iatr—treatment; -ist—one who specializes).*

Psychiatry: The branch of medicine concerned with diseases of the mind. The physician is a **psychiatrist** *(psycho—mind; iatr—treatment; -ist—one who specializes).*

Pulmonary Disease: The branch of medicine concerned with diseases of the lungs. The physician is a **pulmonologist** *(pulmono—lung; log—study of; -ist—one who specializes).*

Radiology: The branch of medicine that studies radioactive substances and their relationship to prevention, diagnosis, and treatment of disease. The physician is a **radiologist** *(radio—ray; log—study of; -ist—one who specializes).*

Rheumatology: The branch of medicine concerned with rheumatic diseases. The physician is a **rheumatologist** *(rheumato—rheumatism; log—study of; -ist—one who specializes).*

Urology: The branch of medicine concerned with diseases of the urinary system. The physician is a **urologist** *(uro—urine; log—study of; -ist—one who specializes).*

TABLE 1–2 Types of Surgical Specialties With Description of Practice

Surgical Specialty	Description of Practice
Surgery is defined as the branch of medicine dealing with manual and operative procedures for correction of deformities and defects, repair of injuries, and diagnosis and cure of certain diseases.	
Cardiovascular	Surgical repair and correction of cardiovascular dysfunctions
Colon and Rectum	Surgical repair and correction of colon and rectal dysfunctions
Cosmetic, Reconstructive, Plastic	Surgical repair, reconstruction, revision, or change the texture, configuration, or relationship of contiguous structures of any part of the human body
General	Surgical repair and correction of various body parts and/or organs
Maxillofacial	Surgical treatment of diseases, injuries, and defects of the human mouth and dental structures
Neurologic	Surgical repair and correction of neurologic dysfunctions
Orthopedic *(Orthopaedic)*	Surgical prevention and repair of musculoskeletal dysfunctions
Thoracic	Surgical repair and correction of organs within the rib cage
Trauma	Surgical repair and correction of traumatic injuries
Vascular	Surgical repair and correction of vascular (vessels) dysfunctions

ABBREVIATIONS

AB	abnormal	**FACS**	Fellow of the American College of Surgeons
ABMS	American Board of Medical Specialists		
ac	acute	**FP**	family practice
ax	axillary	**g, gm**	gram
Bx	biopsy	**Gyn**	gynecology
C	centigrade, Celsius	**kg**	kilogram
cm	centimeter	**L**	liter
CT	computerized tomography	**mcg**	microgram
CVD	cardiovascular disease	**mg**	milligram
D/C	discontinue	**mL, ml**	milliliter
derm	dermatology	**Ob**	obstetrics
Dx	diagnosis	**Peds**	pediatrics
DRGs	diagnosis-related groups	**Psy**	psychiatry, psychology
ENT	otorhinolaryngology		
FACP	Fellow of the American College of Physicians		

COMMUNICATION ENRICHMENT

This segment is provided for those who wish to enhance their ability to communicate in either English or Spanish.

▶ **Communication Enrichment Pronunciation Guide**

Short Vowel Sounds	*Long Vowel Sounds*	*In Spanish, It Is Important to Remember . . .*
ă—ăpple	ā—cāke	*G is like H before E or I*
ĕ—ĕgg	ē—lēaf	*J is like H*
ĭ—ĭgloo	ī—nīne	*H is always silent*
ŏ—ŏctopus	ō—cōat	*A at the end of a word is the*
ŭ—ŭp	ū—sūit	*feminine ending*

▶ **Weights and Measures   Peso y Medidas**
(pĕ-sō ĭ mĕ-dĭ-dăs)

English	Spanish
length	longitud (lōn-hĭ-*tūd*)
width	anchura (ăn-*chū*-ră)
height	altura (ăl-*tū*-ră)
volume	volumen; tomo (vō-*lū*-mĕn; *tō*-mō)
weight	peso (*pĕ*-sō)
microgram	microgramo (mĭ-krō-*gră*-mō)
milligram	miligramo (mĭ-lĭ-*gră*-mō)
gram	gramo (*gră*-mō)
kilogram	kilogramo (kĭ-lō-*gră*-mō)

English	Spanish
liter	litro (*lĭ*-trō)
millimeter	milímetro (mĭ-*lĭ*-mĕ-trō)
centimeter	centímetro (sĕn-*tĭ*-mĕ-trō)
cubic centimeter	centímetro cubico (sĕn-*tĭ*-mĕ-trō *kŭ*-bĭ-kō)
square	cuadrado (kū-ă-*dră*-dō)

▶ **Descriptive Words**

English	Spanish	English	Spanish
large	grande (*grăn*-dĕ)	weak	débil (*dĕ*-bĭl)
small	pequeño (pĕ-*kĕ*-ñyō)	strong	fuerte (*fŭ*-ĕr-tĕ)
tall	alto (*ăl*-tō)	better	mejor (mĕ-*hōr*)
short	bajo (*bă*-hō)	worse	peor (pĕ-*ōr*)
fat	gordo (*gōr*-dō)	alive	vivo (*vĭ*-vō)
thin	flaco (*flă*-kō)	dead	muerto (*mŭ*-ĕr-tō)
dark	obscuro (ŏs-*kŭ*-rō)	healthy	sano (*să*-nō)
light	claro (*clă*-rō)	sick	enfermo (ĕn-*fĕr*-mō)
soft	blando (*blăn*-dō)	sweet	dulce (*dūl*-sĕ)
hard	duro (*dŭ*-rō)	sour	agrio (*ăg*-rĭ-ō)

English	Spanish	English	Spanish
hot	caliente (kă-*lĭ-ĕn*-tĕ)	bitter	amargo (ă-*măr*-gō)
wet	mojado (mō-*hă*-dō)	good	bueno (*bway*-no)
dry	seco (*sĕ*-kō)	bad	malo (*mă*-lō)
open	abierto (ă-*bĭ-ĕr*-tō)	pain	dolor (dō-*lŏr*)
closed	cerrado (sĕ-*ră*-dō)	loud	fuerte (*fŭ-ĕr*-tĕ)

▶ Essential Phrases

English	Spanish
Good day	Buenos días (*bway*-nōs *dee*-ahs)
What is your name?	¿Cómo se llama usted? (*cō*-mō sĕ *yă*-mă ūs-*tĕd*)
How old are you?	¿Cuántos años tiene? (*kwan*-tos ă-ñōs *tĭ-ĕ*-nĕ)
Do you understand me?	¿Me entiende? (me en-tē-*en*-dā)
Yes	Sí (sĭ)
No	No (nō)

▶ Cardinal Numbers

English	Spanish	English	Spanish
1	uno (*oo*-nō)	4	cuatro (*kwa*-trō)
2	dos (dōs)	5	cinco (*sĭn*-kō)
3	tres (trĕs)	6	seis (sē-ĭs)

English	Spanish	English	Spanish
7	siete (*sĭ-ĕ*-tĕ)	20	veinte (*vĕn*-tĕ)
8	ocho (*ŏ*-chō)	30	treinta (*trĕn*-tă)
9	nueve (*nŭ-ĕ*-vĕ)	40	cuarenta (kŭ-ă-*rĕn*-tā)
10	diez (d'*yehs*)	50	cincuenta (sĭn-*kwen*-tă)
11	once (*ōn*-sĕ)	60	sesenta (sĕ-*sĕn*-tă)
12	doce (*dō*-sĕ)	70	setenta (sĕ-*tĕn*-tă)
13	trece (*trĕ*-sĕ)	80	ochenta (ō-*chĕn*-tă)
14	catorce (kă-*tŏr*-sĕ)	90	noventa (nō-*vĕn*-tă)
15	quince (*kĭn*-sĕ)	100	cien (sĭ-*ĕn*)

▶ Ordinal Numbers

English	Spanish	English	Spanish
first	primero (prĭ-*mĕ*-rō)	seventh	séptimo (*sĕp*-tĭ-mō)
second	segundo (sĕ-*gŭn*-dō)	eighth	octavo (ōk-*tă*-vō)
third	tercero (tĕr-*sĕ*-rō)	ninth	noveno (nō-*vĕn*-nō)
fourth	cuarto (*kwar*-tō)	tenth	décimo (*dĕ*-sĭ-mō)
fifth	quinto (*kĭn*-tō)	eleventh	décimo primero (*dĕ*-sĭ-mō prĭ-*mĕ*-rō)
sixth	sexto (*sĕk*-tō)	twelfth	décimo segundo (*dĕ*-sĭ-mō sĕ-*gŭn*-dō)

▶ Time

English	Spanish
hour	hora (ō-ră)
minute	minuto (mĭ-*n*ŭ-tō)
second	segundo (sĕ-*g*ŭn-dō)
at noon	al medio dia (ăl *m*ĕ-dĭ-ō *di*-ă)
at midnight	a la media noche (ă lă *m*ĕ-dĭ-ă *n*ō-chĕ)

▶ Months of the Year

English	Spanish	English	Spanish
January	enero (ĕ-*n*ĕ-rō)	July	julio (*h*ŭ-lĭ-ō)
February	febrero (fĕ-*br*ĕ-rō)	August	agosto (a-*g*ōs-tō)
March	marzo (*m*ăr-zō)	September	septiembre (sĕp-*t*ĭ-*ĕm*-brĕ)
April	abril (ă-*br*ĭl)	October	octubre (ōk-*t*ŭ-brĕ)
May	mayo (*m*ă-yō)	November	noviembre (no-*v*ĭ-*ĕm*-brĕ)
June	junio (*h*ŭ-nĭ-ō)	December	diciembre (dĭ-*c*ĭ-*ĕm*-brĕ)

▶ Holidays   (Dias de Fiesta)

English	Spanish
Christmas	Navidad (Nă-vĭ-*dă*d)
New Year	Año Nuevo (*A*-nyō *N*ŭ-ĕ-vō)
Easter	Pascuas (*Pă*s-qŭ-ăs)

English	Spanish
Holy Week	Semana Santa (Sĕ-*mă*-nă *săn*-tă)
Valentine's Day	Dia de los enamorados (*Dĭ*-ă dĕ lōs ĕ-nă-mō-*ră*-dōs)
July 4	Cuatro de julio (*Qŭ*-*ă*-trō dĕ *hŭ*-lĭ-ō)
Halloween	Dia de Todos los Santos (*Dĭ*-ă dĕ *tō*-dōs loš *Săn*-tōs)
birthday	cumpleaños (qŭm-plĕ-*ă*-nyōs)
anniversary	aniversario (ă-nĭ-vĕr-*să*-rĭ-ō)

► **Days of the Week**

English	Spanish	English	Spanish
Monday	lunes (*lŭ*-nĕs)	Friday	viernes (*vĭĕr*-ñes)
Tuesday	martes (*măr*-tĕs)	Saturday	sábado (*să*-bă-dō)
Wednesday	miércoles (*mĭĕr*-qō-lĕs)	Sunday	domingo (dō-*mĭn*-gō)
Thursday	jueves (hŭ-*ĕ*-vĕs)		

STUDY AND REVIEW SECTION

LEARNING EXERCISES

▶ Word Parts

1. In the spaces provided, write the definition of these prefixes, roots, combining forms, and suffixes. Do not refer to the listings of terminology words. Leave blank those terms you cannot define.

2. After completing as many as you can, refer back to the terminology word listings to check your work. For each word missed or left blank, write the term and its definition several times on the margins of these pages or on a separate sheet of paper.

3. To maximize the learning process, it is to your advantage to do the following exercises as directed. To refer to the terminology listings before completing these exercises invalidates the learning process.

Prefixes

Give the definitions of the following prefixes:

1. a- _____   2. ab- _____

3. anti- _____   4. auto- _____

5. cac- _____   6. centi- _____

7. dia- _____   8. hetero- _____

9. mal- _____   10. micro- _____

11. milli- _____   12. multi- _____

13. neo- _____   14. para- _____

15. pro- _____   16. syn- _____

17. tri- _____

Roots and Combining Forms

Give the definitions of the following roots and combining forms:

1. adhes _____   2. axill _____

3. centri _____   4. chemo _____

5. format _____   6. gene _____

7. kilo _____   8. macro _____

9. necr _____   10. nom _____

11. norm _____   12. onco _____

13. organ _____   14. pyret _____

15. pyro _____   16. radio _____

17. scop _____   18. sept _____

19. thermo _____   20. topo _____

21. tuss _____

Suffixes

Give the definitions of the following suffixes:

1. -age _____   2. -al _____

3. -ary _____   4. -centesis _____

5. -clave _____   6. -drome _____

7. -form _____   8. -fuge _____

9. -genic _____   10. -gnosis _____

11. -grade _____   12. -gram _____

13. -graphy _____   14. -hexia _____

15. -ic _____   16. -ion _____

17. -ism _____   18. -ive _____

19. -liter _____   20. -logy _____

21. -meter _____   22. -osis _____

23. -ous _____   24. -pathy _____

25. -phoresis _____   26. -scope _____

27. -sepsis _____   28. -therapy _____

29. -thermy _____   30. -y _____

▶ Identifying Medical Terms

In the spaces provided, write the medical terms for the following meanings:

1. _____   Process of being stuck together

2. _____ Without decay

3. _____ Pertaining to the armpit

4. _____ Treatment using chemical agents

5. _____ Pertaining to a different formation

6. _____ Process of being badly shaped, deformed

7. _____ An instrument used to view small objects

8. _____ Occurring in or having many shapes

9. _____ A new disease

10. _____ The study of tumors

▶ Spelling

In the spaces provided, write the correct spelling of these misspelled terms:

1. antseptic _____ 2. autnomy _____

3. centmeter _____ 4. diphoresis _____

5. miligram _____ 6. necosis _____

7. parcentesis _____ 8. radilogy _____

WORD PARTS STUDY SHEET

<u>Word Parts</u>	<u>Give the Meaning</u>

Prefixes: Pertaining to Position or Placement

ab- _____

ad- _____

ana- _____

ante- _____

cata- _____

circum-, peri- _____

endo- _____

epi- _____

ex- _____

extra- _____

hyper- _____

hypo- _____

infra- _____

inter- _____

intra- _____

meso- _____

para- _____

retro- _____

sub- _____

supra- _____

Prefixes: Pertaining to Numbers and Amounts

ambi- _____

bi- _____

centi- _____

deca- _____

dipl- _____

di(s)- _____

milli- _____

multi- _____

nulli- _____

poly- _____

primi- _____

quadri- _____

quint- _____

semi-, hemi- _____

tetra- _____

tri- _____

uni- _____

Suffixes

-algia and -dynia

_____

-blast

_____

-cele

_____

-centesis

_____

-cyte

_____

-ectomy

_____

-emesis

_____

-gram

_____

-graph

_____

-graphy

_____

-ist

_____

-itis

_____

-logy

_____

-lysis

_____

-malacia

_____

-megaly

_____

-meter

_____

-oid

_____

-oma

_____

-osis

_____

-opsy

_____

-pathy

_____

-penia

_____

-pexy

_____

-phagia

_____

-phobia

_____

-plegia   _____

-plasty   _____

-pnea   _____

-ptosis   _____

-rrhage   _____

-rrhea   _____

-rrhexis   _____

-scope   _____

-stomy   _____

-tome   _____

-tomy   _____

-trophy   _____

-uria   _____

REVIEW QUESTIONS

▶ **Matching**

Select the appropriate lettered meaning for each numbered line.

_____ 1. abate

_____ 2. antipyretic

_____ 3. cachexia

_____ 4. diagnosis

_____ 5. disease

_____ 6. etiology

_____ 7. illness

_____ 8. prognosis

_____ 9. prognostication

_____ 10. triage

a. Lack of ease
b. A state of being sick
c. The study of the likely course of a disease and the signs of a patient's failure to thrive
d. Pertaining to an agent that works against fever
e. The sorting and classifying of injuries to determine priority of need and treatment
f. To lessen, decrease, or cease
g. Determination of the cause and nature of a disease
h. A new disease
i. The prediction of the course of a disease and the recovery rate
j. A condition of ill health, malnutrition, and wasting
k. The study of the cause(s) of disease

▶ **Abbreviations**

Place the correct word, phrase, or abbreviation in the space provided.

1. AB _____

2. ax _____

3. biopsy _____

4. CVD _____

5. DRGs _____

6. otorhinolaryngology _____

7. family practice _____

8. gram _____

9. Gyn _____

10. Peds _____

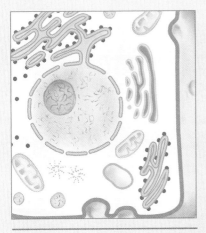

2

THE ORGANIZATION OF THE BODY

OBJECTIVES

On completion of this chapter, you should be able to:

- Define terms that describe the body and its structural units.

- List the systems of the body and give the organs in each system.

- Define terms that are used to describe direction, planes, and cavities of the body.

- Analyze, build, spell, and pronounce medical words that relate to surgical procedures and pathology.

- Identify and give the meaning of selected vocabulary words.

- Identify and define selected abbreviations.

- Review Drug Highlights presented in this chapter.

- Understand word analysis as it relates to Head-to-Toe Assessment.

- Successfully complete the study and review section.

▶ ANATOMY AND PHYSIOLOGY OVERVIEW

This chapter introduces you to terms describing the body and its structural units. To aid you, these terms have been grouped into two major sections: the first offering an overview of the units that make up the human body, and the second covering terms used to describe anatomical positions and locations. The human body is made up of atoms, molecules, organelles, cells, tissues, organs, and systems. See Figure 2–1. All of these parts normally function together in a unified and complex process. During *homeostasis* these processes allow the body to perform at its maximum potential.

▶ THE HUMAN BODY: LEVELS OF ORGANIZATION

ATOMS

An *atom* is the smallest chemical unit of matter. It consists of a nucleus that contains protons and neutrons and is surrounded by electrons. The *nucleus* is at the center of the atom and a *proton* is a positively charged particle, while a *neutron* is without an electrical charge. The *electron* is a negatively charged particle that revolves about the nucleus of an atom.

Chemical elements are made up of atoms. In chemistry, an *element* is a substance that cannot be separated into substances different from itself by ordinary chemical means. It is the basic component of which all matter is composed. There are at least 105 different chemical elements that have been identified.

Elements found in the human body include aluminum, carbon, calcium, chlorine, cobalt, copper, fluorine, hydrogen, iodine, iron, maganese, magnesium, nitrogen, oxygen, phosphorus, potassium, sodium, sulfur, and zinc.

ELEMENTS FOUND IN THE HUMAN BODY

Symbol	Element	Atomic Weight
Al	aluminum	13
C	carbon	6
Ca	calcium	20
Cl	chlorine	17
Co	cobalt	27
Cu	copper	29
F	fluorine	9
H	hydrogen	1
I	iodine	53
Fe	iron	26
Mn	manganese	25
Mg	magnesium	12
N	nitrogen	7
O	oxygen	8
P	phosphorus	15
K	potassium	19
Na	sodium	11
S	sulfur	16
Zn	zinc	30

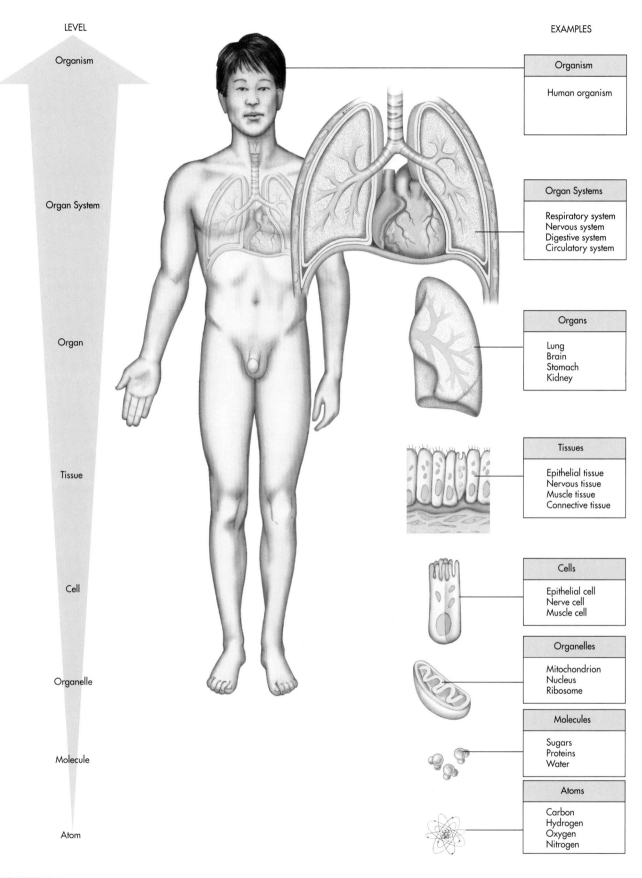

FIGURE 2–1

The human body: levels of organization.

MOLECULES

A *molecule* is a chemical combination of two or more atoms that form a specific chemical compound. In a water molecule (H_2O), oxygen forms polar covalent bonds with two hydrogen atoms. *Water* is a tasteless, clear, odorless liquid that makes up 65% of a male's body weight and 55% of a female's body weight. Water is the most important constituent of all body fluids, secretions, and excretions. It is an ideal transportation medium for inorganic and organic compounds.

CELLS

The body consists of millions of cells working individually and with each other to sustain life. For the purposes of this book, *cells* are considered the basic building blocks for the various structures that together make up the human being. There are several types of cells, each specialized to perform specific functions. The size and shape of a cell are generally related directly to its function. See Figure 2–2. For example, cells forming the skin overlap each other to form a protective barrier, whereas nerve cells are usually elongated with branches connecting to other cells for the transmission of sensory impulses. Despite these differences, however, cells can generally be said to have a number of common components. The common parts of the cell are the *cell membrane* and the *protoplasm*.

The Cell Membrane

The outer covering of the cell is called the *cell membrane*. Cell membranes have the capability of allowing some substances to pass into and out of the cell while denying passage to other substances. This selectivity allows cells to receive nutrition and dispose of waste just as the human being eats food and disposes of waste.

Protoplasm

The substance within the cell membrane is called *protoplasm*. Protoplasm is composed of cytoplasm and karyoplasm. These substances and their functions are described below.

Karyoplasm.   Enclosed by its own membrane, *karyoplasm* is the substance of the cell's nucleus and contains the genetic matter necessary for cell reproduction as well as control over activity within the cell's cytoplasm.

Cytoplasm.   All protoplasm outside the nucleus is called *cytoplasm*. The cytoplasm provides storage and work areas for the cell. The work and storage elements of the cell, called organelles, are the endoplasmic reticulum, ribosomes, Golgi apparatus, mitochondria, lysosomes, and centrioles. See Figure 2–3 and Table 2–1.

TISSUES

A *tissue* is a grouping of similar cells that together perform specialized functions. There are four basic types of tissue in the body: *epithelial, connective, muscle,* and *nerve.* Each of the four basic tissues has several subtypes named for their shape, appearance, arrangement, or function. The four basic types of tissue are described for you.

Epithelial Tissue

Epithelial tissue appears as sheet-like arrangements of cells, sometimes several layers thick, that form the outer layer of the skin, cover the surfaces of organs, line the walls of cavities, and form tubes, ducts, and portions of certain glands. The functions of epithelial tissues are protection, absorption, secretion, and excretion.

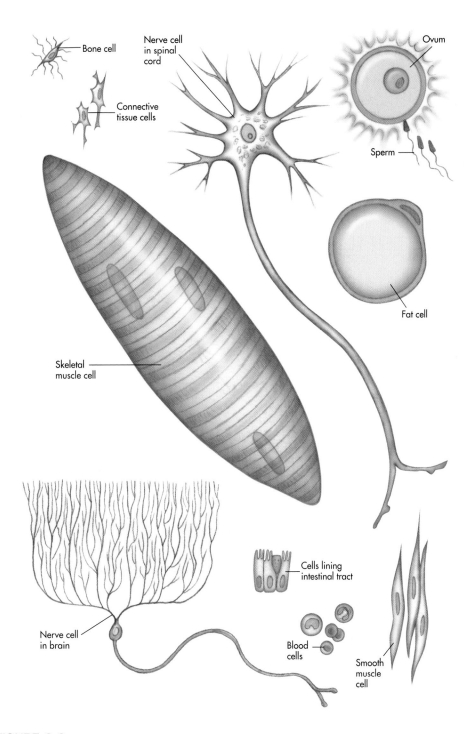

FIGURE 2-2

Cells may be described as the basic building blocks of the human body. They have many different shapes and vary in size and function. These examples show the range of forms and sizes with the dimensions they would have if magnified approximately 500 times.

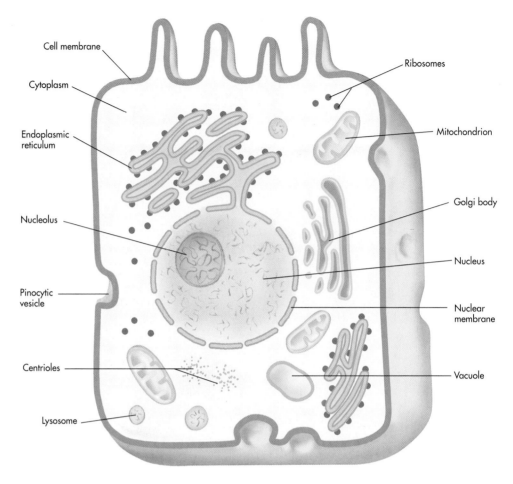

FIGURE 2–3

The major parts of a cell.

Connective Tissue

The most widespread and abundant of the body tissues, *connective tissue* forms the supporting network for the organs of the body, sheaths the muscles, and connects muscles to bones and bones to joints. Bone is a dense form of connective tissue.

Muscle Tissue

There are three types of *muscle tissue:* voluntary or striated, cardiac, and involuntary or smooth. Striated and smooth muscles are so described because of their appearance. Cardiac muscle is a specialized form of striated tissue under the control of the autonomic nervous system. Involuntary or smooth muscles are also controlled by this system. The striated or voluntary muscles are controlled by the person's will.

Nerve Tissue

Nerve tissue consists of nerve cells (neurons) and interstitial tissue. It has the properties of excitability and conductivity, and functions to control and coordinate the activities of the body.

TABLE 2–1   Major Cell Structures and Primary Functions

Cell Structures	Primary Functions
Cell membrane	Protects the cell; provides for communication via receptor proteins; surface proteins serve as positive identification tags; allow some substances to pass into and out of the cell while denying passage to other substances; this selectivity allows cells to receive nutrition and dispose of waste
Protoplasm	Composed of cytoplasm and karyoplasm
Karyoplasm	Substance of the cell's nucleus; contains the genetic matter necessary for cell reproduction as well as control over activity within the cell's cytoplasm
Cytoplasm	All protoplasm outside the nucleus. The cytoplasm provides storage and work areas for the cell:
Ribosomes	Make enzymes and other proteins; nicknamed "protein factories"
Endoplasmic reticulum (ER)	Carries proteins and other substances through the cytoplasm
Golgi apparatus	Chemically processes the molecules from the endoplasmic reticulum, then packages them into vesicles; nicknamed "chemical processing and packaging center"
Mitochondria	Complex, energy-releasing chemical reactions occur continuously; nicknamed "power plants"
Lysosomes	Contain enzymes that can digest food compounds; nicknamed "digestive bags"
Centrioles	Play an important role in cell reproduction
Cilia	Hair-like processes that project from epithelial cells; help propel mucus, dust particles, and other foreign substances from the respiratory tract
Flagellum	"Tail" of the sperm that makes it possible for the sperm to "swim" or move toward the ovum
Nucleus	Controls every organelle (little organ) in the cytoplasm; contains the genetic matter necessary for cell reproduction as well as control over activity within the cell's cytoplasm

ORGANS

Tissues serving a common purpose or function make up structures called *organs*. Organs are specialized components of the body such as the brain, skin, or heart.

SYSTEMS

A group of organs functioning together for a common purpose is called a *system*. The various body systems function in support of the body as a whole. Listed in Figure 2–4 are the organ systems of the body.

▶ ANATOMICAL LOCATIONS AND POSITIONS

Four primary reference systems have been adopted to provide uniformity to the anatomical description of the body. These reference systems are *direction, planes, cavities,* and *structural unit.* The standard anatomical position for the body is erect, head facing forward, arms by the sides with palms to the front. Left and right are from the subject's point of view, not the examiner's.

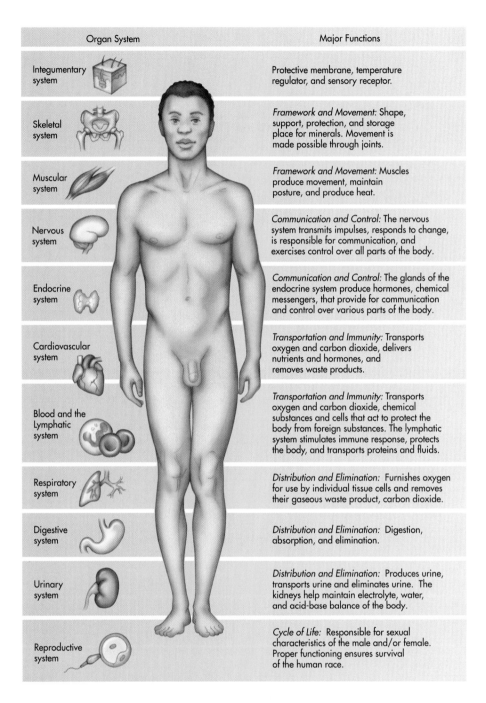

Organ System	Major Functions
Integumentary system	Protective membrane, temperature regulator, and sensory receptor.
Skeletal system	*Framework and Movement:* Shape, support, protection, and storage place for minerals. Movement is made possible through joints.
Muscular system	*Framework and Movement:* Muscles produce movement, maintain posture, and produce heat.
Nervous system	*Communication and Control:* The nervous system transmits impulses, responds to change, is responsible for communication, and exercises control over all parts of the body.
Endocrine system	*Communication and Control:* The glands of the endocrine system produce hormones, chemical messengers, that provide for communication and control over various parts of the body.
Cardiovascular system	*Transportation and Immunity:* Transports oxygen and carbon dioxide, delivers nutrients and hormones, and removes waste products.
Blood and the Lymphatic system	*Transportation and Immunity:* Transports oxygen and carbon dioxide, chemical substances and cells that act to protect the body from foreign substances. The lymphatic system stimulates immune response, protects the body, and transports proteins and fluids.
Respiratory system	*Distribution and Elimination:* Furnishes oxygen for use by individual tissue cells and removes their gaseous waste product, carbon dioxide.
Digestive system	*Distribution and Elimination:* Digestion, absorption, and elimination.
Urinary system	*Distribution and Elimination:* Produces urine, transports urine and eliminates urine. The kidneys help maintain electrolyte, water, and acid-base balance of the body.
Reproductive system	*Cycle of Life:* Responsible for sexual characteristics of the male and/or female. Proper functioning ensures survival of the human race.

FIGURE 2–4

Organ systems of the body with major functions.

DIRECTION

The following terms are used to describe direction:

- **Superior.** Above, in an upward direction
- **Anterior.** In front of or before
- **Posterior.** Toward the back
- **Cephalad.** Toward the head
- **Medial.** Nearest the midline
- **Lateral.** To the side
- **Proximal.** Nearest the point of attachment
- **Distal.** Away from the point of attachment
- **Ventral.** The same as anterior, the front side
- **Dorsal.** The same as posterior, the back side

PLANES

The terms defined below are used to describe the imaginary planes that are depicted in Figure 2–5 as passing through the body and dividing it into various sections.

Midsagittal Plane

The *midsagittal plane* vertically divides the body as it passes through the midline to form a *right* and *left half.*

Transverse or Horizontal Plane

A *transverse* or *horizontal plane* is any plane that divides the body into *superior* and *inferior* portions.

Coronal or Frontal Plane

A *coronal* or *frontal plane* is any plane that divides the body at right angles to the midsagittal plane. The coronal plane divides the body into *anterior* (ventral) and *posterior* (dorsal) portions.

CAVITIES

A *cavity* is a hollow space containing body organs. Body cavities are classified into two groups according to their location. On the front are the *ventral* or *anterior cavities* and on the back are the *dorsal* or *posterior cavities.* The various cavities found in the human body are depicted in Figure 2–6.

The Ventral Cavity

The *ventral cavity* is the hollow portion of the human torso extending from the neck to the pelvis and containing the heart and the organs of respiration, digestion, reproduction, and elimination. The ventral cavity can be subdivided into three distinct areas: thoracic, abdominal, and pelvic.

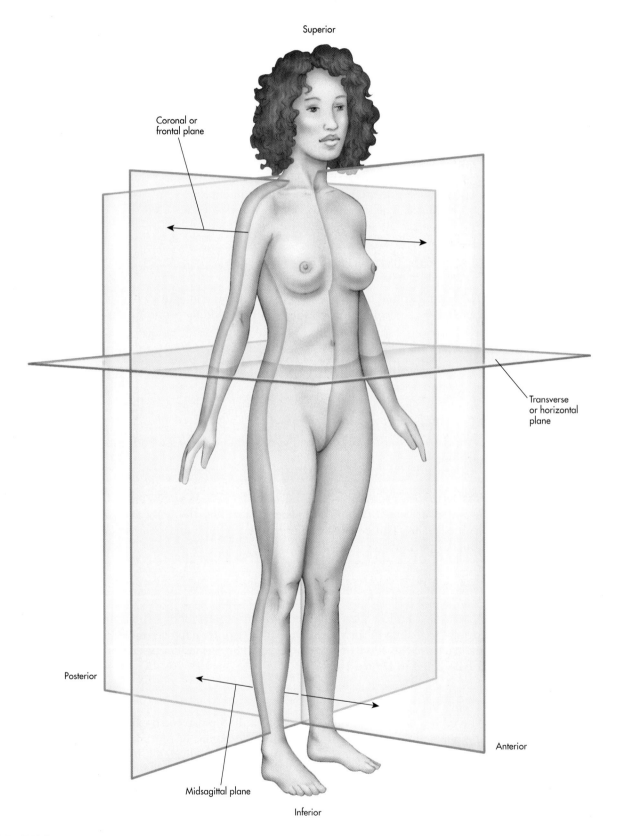

FIGURE 2–5

Planes of the body: coronal or frontal, transverse, and midsagittal.

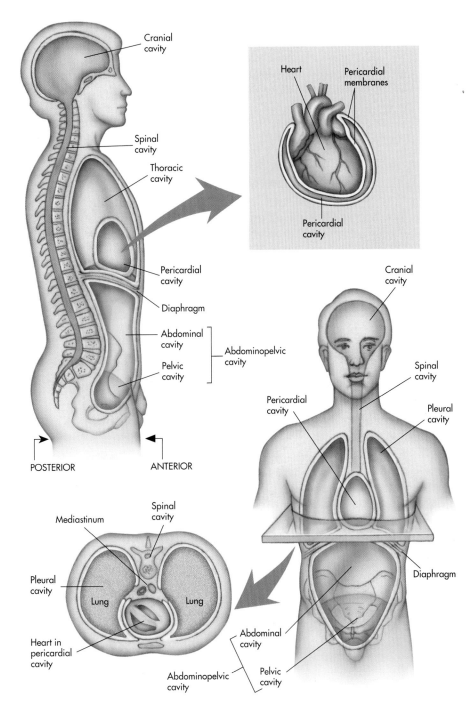

FIGURE 2-6

Body cavities.

The Thoracic Cavity.   The *thoracic cavity* is the area of the chest containing the heart and the lungs. Within this cavity, the space containing the *heart* is called the *pericardial* cavity and the spaces surrounding each *lung* are known as the *pleural* cavities. Other organs located in the thoracic cavity are the esophagus, trachea, thymus, and certain large blood and lymph vessels.

The Abdominal Cavity.   The *abdominal cavity* is the space below the diaphragm, commonly referred to as the belly. It contains the kidneys, stomach, intestines, and other organs of digestion.

The Pelvic Cavity.   The *pelvic cavity* is the space formed by the bones of the pelvic area and contains the organs of reproduction and elimination.

The Dorsal Cavity

Containing the structures of the nervous system, the *dorsal cavity* is subdivided into the cranial cavity and the spinal cavity.

The Cranial Cavity.   The *cranial cavity* is the space in the skull containing the brain.

The Spinal Cavity.   The *spinal cavity* is the space within the bony spinal column that contains the spinal cord and spinal fluid.

The Abdominopelvic Cavity

The *abdominopelvic cavity* is the combination of the abdominal and pelvic cavities. It is divided into nine regions.

NINE REGIONS OF THE ABDOMINOPELVIC CAVITY

As a ready reference for locating visceral organs, anatomists divided the abdominopelvic cavity into nine regions. A tic-tac-toe pattern drawn across the abdominopelvic cavity (Fig. 2–7A) delineates these regions:

- **Right hypochondriac**—upper right region at the level of the ninth rib cartilage
- **Left hypochondriac**—upper left region at the level of the ninth rib cartilage
- **Epigastric**—region over the stomach
- **Right lumbar**—right middle lateral region
- **Left lumbar**—left middle lateral region
- **Umbilical**—in the center, between the right and left lumbar region; at the navel
- **Right iliac (inguinal)**—right lower lateral region
- **Left iliac (inguinal)**—left lower lateral region
- **Hypogastric**—lower middle region below the navel

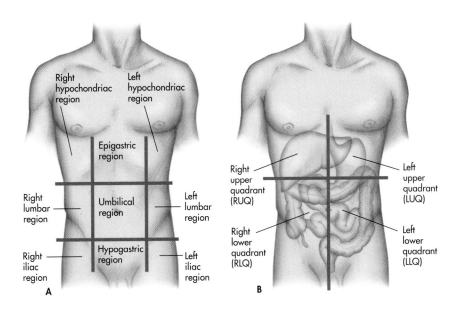

FIGURE 2-7

(A) The nine regions of the abdominopelvic cavity. **(B)** The four regions of the abdomen that are referred to as quadrants.

ABDOMEN DIVIDED INTO QUADRANTS

The *abdomen* is divided into four corresponding regions that are used for descriptive and diagnostic purposes. By using these regions one may describe the exact location of pain, a skin lesion, surgical incision, and/or abdominal tumor. The four *quadrants* are (Fig. 2–7B):

- Right upper (RUQ)
- Left upper (LUQ)
- Right lower (RLQ)
- Left lower (LLQ)

TERMINOLOGY
WITH SURGICAL PROCEDURES & PATHOLOGY

TERM	WORD PARTS			DEFINITION
adipose (ăd″ ĭ-pōs)	adip ose	R S	fat like	Fatty tissue throughout the body
ambilateral (ăm″ bĭ-lăt′ ĕr-ăl)	ambi later al	P R S	both side pertaining to	Pertaining to both sides
anatomy (ăn-ăt′ ō-mē)	ana tomy	P S	up incision	Literally means to cut up; the study of the structure of an organism such as humans
android (ăn′ droyd)	andr oid	R S	man resemble	To resemble man
bilateral (bī-lăt′ ĕr-ăl)	bi later al	P R S	two side pertaining to	Pertaining to two sides
biology (bi-ŏl′ ō-jē)	bio logy	CF S	life study of	The study of life
caudal (kŏd′ ăl)	caud al	R S	tail pertaining to	Pertaining to the tail
chromosome (krō-mō-sōm)	chromo some	P S	color body	Microscopic bodies that carry the genes that determine hereditary characteristics
cytology (sī-tŏl′ ō-jē)	cyto logy	CF S	cell study of	The study of cells
dehydrate (dē-hī′ drāt)	de hydr ate	P R S	down, away from water use, action	To remove water away from the body
diffusion (di-fū′ zhŭn)	dif fus ion	P R S	apart to pour process	A process in which parts of a substance move from areas of high concentration to areas of lower concentration
ectogenous (ĕk-tŏj′ ĕ-nŭs)	ecto gen ous	P R S	outside formation, produce pertaining to	Pertaining to formation outside the organism or body

Terminology - continued

TERM	WORD PARTS			DEFINITION
ectomorph (ĕk′ tō-morf)	ecto morph	P S	outside form, shape	A slender physical body form
endomorph (ĕn″ dō-morf)	endo morph	P S	within form, shape	A round physical body form
histology (hĭs-tŏl′ ō-jē)	histo logy	CF S	tissue study of	The study of tissue
homeostasis (hō″ mē-ō-stā′ sĭs)	homeo stasis	P S	similar, same control, stopping	The state of equilibrium maintained in the body's internal environment

TERMINOLOGY SPOTLIGHT

To maintain **homeostasis** it is essential that the body be supplied with adequate fluids. Water is the most important constituent of the human body and is essential to every body process. Bones depend on water intake to provide adequate blood for delivery and removal of calcium. The intestines and kidneys use water to remove waste. Muscles need water to remove acids that would otherwise build up, causing cramps and diminishing muscle action. Nerve function depends on the presence of certain minerals, which are kept in balance by water levels in the body. The immune system depends on sufficient water to ensure blood flow for delivery of immune cells and removal of diseased cells. Water in saliva and the stomach aids digestion and absorption of nutrients.

It is recommended that the average healthy adult drink eight 8-ounce glasses of water per day. One may need more than eight glasses of water per day before, during, and after exercise, in warm weather, during and after drinking alcohol or caffeine, when breast-feeding, during illness, with certain medications, after surgery, and/or with severe burns or bleeding.

karyogenesis (kăr″ i-ō-jĕn′ ĕ-sĭs)	karyo genesis	CF S	cell's nucleus formation, produce	Formation of a cell's nucleus
mesomorph (mĕs′ ō-morf)	meso morph	P S	middle form, shape	A well-proportioned body form
pathology (pă-thŏl′ ō-jē)	patho logy	CF S	disease study of	The study of disease
perfusion (pur-fū′ zhŭn)	per fus ion	P R S	through to pour process	The process of pouring through
physiology (fiz″ i-ŏl′ ō-jē)	physio logy	CF S	nature study of	The study of the nature of living organisms

continued

Terminology - continued

TERM	WORD PARTS			DEFINITION
pinocytosis (pī″ nō-si-tō′ sis)	pino cyt osis	CF R S	to drink cell condition of	The condition whereby a cell absorbs or ingests nutrients and fluids
protoplasm (prō-tō-plăzm)	proto plasm	P S	first a thing formed, plasma	The essential matter of a living cell
somatotrophic (sō″ mă-tō-trŏf′ ĭk)	somato troph ic	CF R S	body a turning pertaining to	Pertaining to stimulation of body growth
topical (tŏp′ ĭ-kăl)	topic al	R S	place pertaining to	Pertaining to a place, definite locale
unilateral (ū″ nĭ-lăt′ ĕr-ăl)	uni later al	P R S	one side pertaining to	Pertaining to one side
visceral (vĭs′ ĕr-ăl)	viscer al	R S	body organs pertaining to	Pertaining to body organs enclosed within a cavity, especially abdominal organs

 # VOCABULARY WORDS

Vocabulary words are terms that have not been divided into component parts. They are common words or specialized terms associated with the subject of this chapter. These words are provided to enhance your medical vocabulary.

WORD	DEFINITION
anterior (an-tĕr′ ē-ōr)	In front of, before
anthropometry (ăn-thrō-pŏm′ ĕt-rē)	The measurement of the human body; includes measurement of the skull, bones, height, weight, and skin fold evaluation for subcutaneous fat estimation
apex (ā′ pĕks)	The pointed end of a cone-shaped structure

Vocabulary - continued

WORD	DEFINITION
base (bās)	The lower part or foundation of a structure
center (sĕn′ tĕr)	The midpoint of a body or activity
cephalad (sĕf′ ă-lăd)	Toward the head
cilia (sĭl′ ē-ă)	Hair-like processes that project from epithelial cells; they help propel mucus, dust particles, and other foreign substances from the respiratory tract
deep (dēp)	Far down from the surface
distal (dĭs′ tăl)	Farthest from the center or point of origin
dorsal (dōr′ săl)	Pertaining to the back side of the body
filtration (fĭl-trā′ shŭn)	The process of filtering or straining particles from a solution
gene (jēn)	The hereditary unit that transmits and determines one's characteristics or hereditary traits
horizontal (hŏr′ă-zŏn′ tăl)	Pertaining to the horizon, of or near the horizon, lying flat, even, level
human genome (hū′ măn jē′ nōm)	The complete set of genes and chromosomes tucked inside each of the body's trillions of cells
inferior (ĭn-fē′ rē-or)	Located below or in a downward direction
inguinal (ĭng′ gwĭ-năl)	Pertaining to the groin, of or near the groin
internal (ĭn-tĕr′ nal)	Pertaining to within or the inside
lateral (lăt′ ĕr-ăl)	Pertaining to the side

continued

Vocabulary - continued

WORD	DEFINITION
medial (mē′ dē al)	Pertaining to the middle or midline
organic (or-găn′ĭk)	Pertaining to an organ
phenotype (fē′ nō-tīp)	The physical appearance or type of makeup of an individual
posterior (pŏs-tē′ rĭ-ōr)	Toward the back
prions (prē′ ons)	An entirely new genre of disease-causing agents that are made of proteins and do not contain any genes or genetic material. This detail distinguishes them from all other kinds of infectious agents such as viruses, bacteria, fungi, and parasites. In 1997, Doctor Stanley B. Prusiner, an American scientist, was awarded the Nobel Prize in Medicine for his discovery of prions. His work has proved invaluable in the study of mad cow disease and the human brain disease "new variant" Creutzfeldt-Jakob disease, believed to be caused by eating beef from affected cattle. Prusiner's discovery may lead to a better understanding of Alzheimer's disease and other neurodegenerative syndromes.
proximal (prŏk′ sĭm-ăl)	Nearest the center or point of origin; nearest the point of attachment
superficial (sū″ pĕr-fĭsh′ ăl)	Pertaining to the surface, on or near the surface
superior (sū-pēr′ rĭ-ōr)	Located above or in an upward direction
systemic (sis-tĕm′ ĭk)	Pertaining to the body as a whole
ventral (vĕn′ trăl)	Pertaining to the front side of the body, abdomen, belly surface
vertex (vĕr′ tĕks)	The top or highest point; the top or crown of the head

ABBREVIATIONS

abd	abdomen, abdominal	**lat**	lateral
A&P	anatomy and physiology	**LLQ**	left lower quadrant
AP	anterior–posterior	**LUQ**	left upper quadrant
CNS	central nervous system	**PA**	posterior–anterior
CV	cardiovascular	**resp**	respiratory
ER	endoplasmic reticulum	**RLQ**	right lower quadrant
GI	gastrointestinal	**RUQ**	right upper quadrant

DRUG HIGHLIGHTS

A drug is a medicinal substance that may alter or modify the functions of a living organism. There are thousands of drugs that are available as over-the-counter (OTC) medicines and do not need a prescription. A prescription is a written legal document that gives directions for compounding, dispensing, and administering a medication to a patient.

In general, there are five medical uses for drugs and these are: therapeutic, diagnostic, curative, replacement, and preventive or prophylactic.

- **Therapeutic Use.** Used in the treatment of a disease or condition, such as an allergy, to relieve the symptoms or to sustain the patient until other measures are instituted.
- **Diagnostic Use.** Certain drugs are used in conjunction with radiology to allow the physician to pinpoint the location of a disease process.
- **Curative Use.** Certain drugs, such as antibiotics, kill or remove the causative agent of a disease.
- **Replacement Use.** Certain drugs, such as hormones and vitamins, are used to replace substances normally found in the body.
- **Preventive or Prophylactic Use.** Certain drugs, such as immunizing agents, are used to ward off or lessen the severity of a disease.

Drug Names

Most drugs may be cited by their chemical, generic, and trade or brand (proprietary) name. The chemical name is usually the formula that denotes the composition of the drug. It is made up of letters and numbers that represent the drug's molecular structure. The generic name is the drug's official name and is descriptive of its chemical structure. The generic name is written in lowercase letters. A generic drug can be manufactured by more than one pharmaceutical company. When this is the case, each company markets the drug under its own unique trade or brand name. A trade or brand name is registered by the US Patent Office as well as approved by the US Food and Drug Administration (FDA). A trade or brand name is written with a capital.

Undesirable Actions of Drugs

Most drugs have the potential for causing an action other than their intended action. For example, antibiotics that are administered orally may disrupt the normal bacterial flora of the gastrointestinal tract and cause gastric discomfort. This type of reaction is known as a side effect. An adverse reaction is an unfavorable or harmful unintended action of a drug. For example, the adverse reaction of Demerol may be lightheadedness, dizziness, sedation, nausea, and sweating. A drug interaction may occur when one drug potentiates or diminishes the action of another drug. These actions may be desirable or undesirable. Drugs may also interact with foods, alcohol, tobacco, and other substances.

Medication Order and Dosage   The medication order is given for a specific patient and denotes the name of the drug, the dosage, the form of the drug, the time for or frequency of administration, and the route by which the drug is to be given.

The dosage is the amount of medicine that is prescribed for administration. The form of the drug may be liquid, solid, semisolid, tablet, capsule, transdermal therapeutic patch, etc. The route of administration may be by mouth, by injection, into the eye(s), ear(s), nostril(s), rectum, vagina, etc.

It is important for the patient to know when and how to take a medication. The following are some hows, whens, and directions for taking medications. To assist you in communicating this information to a patient, both English and Spanish are provided for you to use.

English	Spanish	English	Spanish
When	*Cuándo*	*When*	*Cuándo*
every hour	cada hora (că-dă ŏ-ră)	after meals	después de comer (děs-pū-ĕs dĕ cō-mĕr)
every two hours	cada dos horas (că-dă dōs ō-răs)	before breakfast	antes de desayunar (ăn-tĕs dĕ dĕ-să-jū-năr)
every three hours	cada tres horas (că-dă trĕs ō-răs)	after breakfast	después de desayunar (děs-pū-ĕs dĕ dĕ-să-jū-năr)
every four hours	cada cuatro horas (că-dă kū-ă-trō ō-răs)	before lunch	antes de merendar (ăn-tĕs dĕ mĕ-rĕn-dăr)
every six hours	cada seis horas (că-dă sĕ-ĭs ō-răs)	after dinner	después de cenar (děs-pū-ĕs dĕ sĕ-năr)
every eight hours	cada ocho horas (că-dă ō-chō ō-răs)	at night	por la noche (pōr lă nō-chĕ)
every twelve hours	cada doce horas (că-dă dō-sĕ ō-răs)	in the morning	por la mañana (pōr lă mă-nyă-nă)
before meals	antes de comer (ăn-tĕs dĕ cō-mĕr)	at bedtime	al acostarse (ăl ă-cōs-tăr-sĕ)
How	*Cómo*	*How*	*Cómo*
with meals	con la comida (kōn lă kō-mĭ-dă)	in the right eye	en el ojo derecho (ĕn ĕl ō-hō dĕ-rĕ-chō)
with milk	con leche (kōn lĕ-chĕ)	in the left eye	en el ojo izquierdo (ĕn ĕl ō-hō ĭs-kĭ-ĕr-dō)
with food	con alimento (kōn ă-lĭ-mĕn-tō)	in both eyes	en los dos ojos (ĕn lōs dōs ō-hōs)
with antacid	con anti-acido (kōn ăn-tĭ ă-cĭ-dō)	in the right ear	en el oido derecho (ĕn ĕl ō-ĭ-dō dĕ-rĕ-chō)

How	*Cómo*	*How*	*Cómo*
in the left ear	en el oido izquierdo (ĕn ĕl ō-ĭ-dō ĭs-kĭ-*ĕr*-dō)	into the rectum	en el recto (ĕn ĕl *rĕc*-tō)
in both ears	en los dos oidos (ĕn lōs dōs ō-ĭ-dōs)	into the vagina	en la vagina (ĕn lă vă-*hĭ*-nă)
into the nostrils	en la nariz (ĕn lă nă-*rĭz*)		

Directions	*Dirección*	*Directions*	*Dirección*
chew	mascar (măs-*kăr*)	shake well	agitar bien (ă-hĭ-tăr bĭ-ĕn)
do not chew	no mascar (nō măs-*kăr*)	for external use	para uso externo (pă-ră ū-sō ĕx-*tĕr*-nō)
avoid sunlight	evitar sol (ĕ-vĭ-tăr sōl)	keep refrigerated	mantener en el refrigerador (măn-tĕ-*nĕr* ĕn ĕl rĕ-frĭ-hĕ-ră-*dōr*)
avoid alcohol	evitar alcohol (ĕ-vĭ-tăr ăl-kō ōhl)		

COMMUNICATION ENRICHMENT

This segment is provided for those who wish to enhance their ability to communicate in either English or Spanish.

▶ Head-to-Toe Assessment

Body Area	Spanish	Component Part/Terminology
abdomen (belly)	vientre (vĭ-*ĕn*-trĕ)	abdomino (ăb-*dō*-mĭ-nō)
ankle	tobillo (*tō*-bĭ-yō)	ankylo (ăn-*kĭ*-lō)
arm	brazo (*bră*-zō)	brachi (*bră*-chĭ)
back	espalda (ĕs-*păl*-dă)	posterior (pōs-tĕ-rĭ-ōr)
bones	huesos (*wĕ*-sos)	osteo (ōs-tĕ-ō)

Body Area	Spanish	Component Part/Terminology
breast	ceno (sĕ-nō)	mast/mammo/mammary (măst; măm-ō; măm-ă-rē)
cheek	mejilla (mĕ-jĭ-yă)	bucco/buccal (bŭk-kō; bŭk-ăl)
chest	pecho (pĕ-chō)	thoraco (thō-ră-kō)
ear	oido (ō-ē-dō)	oto (ō-tō)
elbow	codo (kō-dō)	cubital (cū-bĭ-tăl)
eye	ojo (ō-hō)	ophthalmo; oculo; opto (ōp-thăl-mō; ō-kū-lō; ōp-tō)
finger	dedo (dĕ-dow)	dactylo/digit/phalanx (dăk-tĭ-lō; dĭj-ĭt; făl-ănks)
foot	pie (pĭĕ)	illus (il-lus-)
gums	encías (ĕn-sĭ-ăs)	gingiv (gĭn-gĭv-)
hand	mano (mă-nō)	manus (mă-nūs)
head	cabeza (că-bē-ză)	cephalo (sĕ-fă-lō)
heart	corazón (kō-ră-zōn)	cardio (kăr-dĭ-ō)
hip	cadera (kă-dĕ-ră)	coxa (kŏk-să)
leg	pierna (pī-ĕr-nă)	crural; femoral (crū-răl; fĕ-mō-răl)
liver	higado (hĭ-gă-dō)	hepato (hĕ-pă-tō)
lungs	pulmones (pūl-mō-nĕs)	pulmo (pūl-mō)
mouth	boca (bō-kă)	oro (ō-rō)

Body Area	Spanish	Component Part/Terminology
muscles	músculos (*mūs*-kū-lōs)	musculo (mūs-cū-lō)
navel	ombligo (*om*-blĭ-gō)	umbilic/umbilicus (ŭm-bĭ-*lĭ*-k; ŭm-bĭ-*lĭ*-kŭs)
neck	cuello (*kŭe*-jō)	cervico *sĕr*-vĭ-cō)
nerves	nervios (*ner*-vĭ-ōs)	neuro (*nū*-rō)
nose	nariz (*nă*-rĭz)	rhino; naso (*rĭ*-nō; *nă*-sō)
ribs	costillas (cōs-*tĭ*-yăs)	costo (*cō*s-tō)
side	costado (cōs-*tă*-dō)	lateral (lă-tĕ-*răl*)
skin	piel (pē-ĕl)	derma (*dĕr*-mă)
skull	cráneo (*krā*-nĕ-ō)	cranio; cranial (*kră*-nĭ-ō; *kră*-nē-ăl)
stomach	estómago (ĕs-tō-*mă*-gō)	gastro (*gă*s-trō)
teeth	dientes (*dĭĕn*-tĕs)	denti (*dĕn*-tĭ)
temples	templo (*ti*-ĕm-plō)	tempora (tĕm-*pō*-ră)
thigh	muslo (*mŭs*-lō)	femoral; crural (fĕ-mō-răl; crŭ-răl)
throat	garganta (găr-*găn*-tă)	pharyngo (fă-*rĭn*-hō)
thumb	dedo pulgar (*dĕ*-dow *pŭl*-găr)	pollex (*pōl*-lĕx)
tongue	lengua (*lĕn*-gŭ-ă)	linguo; glosso (lĭn-gū-ō; glōs-sō)
wrist	muñeca (*mŭ*-ñĕ-kă)	carpo (*căr*-pō)

▶ PATIENT INFORMATION FORM (INFORMACIÓN DE PACIENTE)

The patient information form is an essential part of the patient's record. This form is filled out by the patient on the first visit to the physician's office and then updated as necessary. It provides data that relate directly to the patient including last name, first name, sex, date of birth, marital status, street address, city, state, zip code, telephone number, social security number, employment status, address of employer, telephone number at employment agency, and vital information concerning who should be contacted in case of an emergency. Also included is information about who is responsible for the patient's bill.

The following is an example of a patient information form. *Note that it is in **Spanish** with English subtitles.*

INFORMACIÓN DE PACIENTE
(Patient Information)

Apellido _____ **Nombre** _____ **Sexo** _____
(Last Name)   (First Name)   (Sex)

Fecha de Nacamiento _____ **Estado Civil: C_____   S_____   V _____   D_____**
(Date of Birth)   (Marital Status: M, S, W, D)

Dirección _____ **Ciudad** _____ **Estado** _____
(Street Address)   (City)   (State)

Código Postal _____ **Teléfono** (____) _____ **# Seg. Social** _____
(Zip Code)   (Telephone)   (Social Security #)

Empleo _____ **Dirección de Empleo** _____
(Employment)   (Address of Employment)

Teléfono de Empleo (____) _____
(Work Telephone)

Contacto Emergencia (Alguien Qué No Vive En Su Casa)
(Who to Contact in Case of an Emergency)

Nombre _____ **Relación** _____
(Name)   (Relationship)

Dirección _____ **Ciudad** _____ **Estado** _____
(Street Address)   (City)   (State)

Código Postal _____ **Teléfono** (____) _____
(Zip Code)   (Telephone)

Quién Es Resposable de la Cuenta de Paciente
(Who is responsible for the patient's bill?)

Apellido _____ **Nombre** _____ **Sexo** _____
(Last Name)   (First Name)   (Sex)

Fecha de Nacamiento _____ **Teléfono** (____) _____ **# Seg. Social** _____
(Date of Birth)   (Telephone)   (Social Security #)

Dirección _____ **Ciudad** _____ **Estado** _____
(Street Address)   (City)   (State)

STUDY AND REVIEW SECTION

LEARNING EXERCISES

▶ **Anatomy and Physiology**

Write your answers to the following questions. Do not refer back to the text.

1. The _____ consist of millions of _____ working individually and with each other to _____ life.

2. The outer covering of the cell is known as the _____ which has the capability of allowing some substances to pass into and out of the cell.

3. The substance within the cell is known as _____ and is composed of _____ and _____.

4. The cell's nucleus is composed of _____, which contains its genetic material.

5. The two primary functions of the cell's nucleus are _____ and _____.

6. List the four functions of epithelial tissue.

   a. _____   b. _____

   c. _____   d. _____

7. _____ tissue is the most widespread and abundant of the four body tissues.

8. Name the three types of muscle tissue.

   a. _____   b. _____   c. _____

9. Two properties of nerve tissue are _____ and _____.

10. Define organ. _____.

11. Define body system. _____.

12. Name the organ systems listed in this text.

   a. _____   b. _____

   c. _____   d. _____

   e. _____   f. _____

   g. _____   h. _____

   i. _____   j. _____

   k. _____

13. Define the following directional terms:

    a. Superior _____   b. Anterior _____

    c. Posterior _____   d. Cephalad _____

    e. Medial _____   f. Lateral _____

    g. Proximal _____   h. Distal _____

    i. Ventral _____   j. Dorsal _____

14. The _____ _____ vertically divides the body. It passes through the midline to form a right and left half.

15. The _____ plane is any plane that divides the body into superior and inferior portions.

16. The _____ plane is any plane that divides the body at right angles to the plane described in question 14.

17. List the three distinct cavities that are located in the ventral cavity.

    a. _____   b. _____   c. _____

18. Name the two distinct cavities located in the dorsal cavity.

    a. _____   b. _____

▶ Word Parts

1. In the spaces provided, write the definition of these prefixes, roots, combining forms, and suffixes. Do not refer to the listings of terminology words. Leave blank those terms you cannot define.

2. After completing as many as you can, refer back to the terminology word listings to check your work. For each word missed or left blank, write the term and its definition several times on the margins of these pages or on a separate sheet of paper.

3. To maximize the learning process, it is to your advantage to do the following exercises as directed. To refer to the terminology listings before completing these exercises invalidates the learning process.

Prefixes

Give the definitions of the following prefixes:

1. ambi- _____   2. ana- _____

3. bi- _____   4. chromo- _____

5. de- _____   6. dif- _____

7.   ecto- _____

8.   endo- _____

9.   homeo- _____

10.   meso-_____

11.   per- _____

12.   proto- _____

13.   uni- _____

Roots and Combining Forms

Give the definitions of the following roots and combining forms:

1.   adip _____

2.   andr _____

3.   bio _____

4.   caud _____

5.   cyt _____

6.   cyto _____

7.   fus _____

8.   gen _____

9.   histo _____

10.   hydr _____

11.   karyo _____

12.   later _____

13.   patho _____

14.   physio _____

15.   pino _____

16.   somato _____

17.   topic _____

18.   troph _____

19.   viscer _____

Suffixes

Give the definitions for the following suffixes:

1.   -al _____

2.   -ate _____

3.   -genesis _____

4.   -ic _____

5.   -ion _____

6.   -logy _____

7.   -morph _____

8.   -oid _____

9.   -ose _____

10.   -osis _____

11.   -ous _____

12.   -plasm _____

13.   -some _____

14.   -stasis _____

15.   -tomy _____

Identifying Medical Terms

In the spaces provided, write the medical terms for the following meanings:

1. _____ To resemble man

2. _____ Pertaining to two sides

3. _____ The study of cells

4. _____ A slender physical body form

5. _____ Formation of a cell's nucleus

6. _____ Pertaining to the stimulation of body growth

7. _____ Pertaining to one side

Spelling

In the spaces provided, write the correct spelling of these misspelled terms:

1. adpose _____   2. caual _____

3. cytlogy _____   4. difusion _____

5. histlogy _____   6. mesmorph _____

7. prefusion _____   8. pincytosis _____

9. somattrophic _____ 10. unlateral _____

WORD PARTS STUDY SHEET

Word Parts	Give the Meaning
Head-to-Toe-Assessment	
abdomino-	_____
ankylo-	_____
brachi-	_____
posterior-	_____
osteo-	_____
bucco-	_____
mast-, mammo-	_____
thoraco-	_____

oto- _____

cubital- _____

ophthalmo-, oculo-, opto- _____

dactylo- _____

illus- _____

gingiv- _____

manus- _____

cephalo- _____

cardio- _____

coxa- _____

crural-, femoral- _____

hepato- _____

pulmo- _____

oro- _____

musculo- _____

umbilic- _____

cervico- _____

neuro- _____

rhino-, naso- _____

costo- _____

lateral- _____

derma- _____

cranio- _____

gastro- _____

denti- _____

tempora- _____

pharyngo- _____

linguo-, glosso- _____

carpo- _____

REVIEW QUESTIONS

▶ Matching

Select the appropriate lettered meaning for each numbered line.

_____	1.	ambilateral
_____	2.	anatomy
_____	3.	anthropometry
_____	4.	chromosome
_____	5.	cilia
_____	6.	homeostasis
_____	7.	human genome
_____	8.	phenotype
_____	9.	physiology
_____	10.	vertex

a. Hair-like processes that project from epithelial cells
b. The top or highest point
c. Pertaining to both sides
d. The study of the structure of an organism such as humans
e. The measurement of the human body
f. Microscopic bodies that carry the genes that determine hereditary characteristics
g. The complete set of genes and chromosomes
h. The physical appearance or type of makeup of an individual
i. The state of equilibrium maintained in the body's internal environment
j. The study of the nature of living organism
k. The study of disease

▶ Abbreviations

Place the correct word, phrase, or abbreviation in the space provided.

1. abdomen _____

2. A&P _____

3. CNS _____

4. cardiovascular _____

5. gastrointestinal _____

6. lat _____

7. resp _____

8. ER _____

9. AP _____

10. PA _____

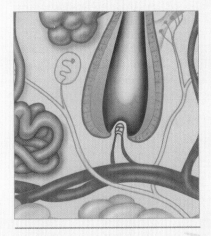

3

THE INTEGUMENTARY SYSTEM

OBJECTIVES

On completion of this chapter, you should be able to:

- Describe the integumentary system and its accessory structures.

- List the functions of the skin.

- Describe various types of skin signs.

- Describe skin differences of the child and the older adult.

- Analyze, build, spell, and pronounce medical words that relate to surgical procedures and pathology.

- Identify and give the meaning of selected vocabulary words.

- Identify and define selected abbreviations.

- Review Drug Highlights presented in this chapter.

- Provide the description of diagnostic and laboratory tests related to the integumentary system.

- Successfully complete the study and review section.

▶ ANATOMY AND PHYSIOLOGY OVERVIEW

The integumentary system is composed of the *skin* and its accessory structures: *hair, nails, sebaceous glands,* and *sweat glands.* This overview of the anatomy and physiology of the skin offers a general description of the integumentary system as an aid to those learning the terminology associated with its functions.

▶ FUNCTIONS OF THE SKIN

The *skin* is the external covering of the body. In an average adult it covers more than 3000 square inches of surface area, weighs more than 6 pounds, and is the largest organ in the body. The skin is well supplied with blood vessels and nerves and has four main functions: *protection, regulation, sensation,* and *secretion.*

PROTECTION

The skin serves as a *protective membrane* against invasion by bacteria and other potentially harmful agents that might try to penetrate to deeper tissues. It also protects against mechanical injury of delicate cells located beneath its epidermis or outer covering. The skin also serves to inhibit excessive loss of water and electrolytes and provides a reservoir for food and water storage. The skin guards the body against excessive exposure to the sun's ultraviolet rays by producing a protective pigmentation, and it helps to produce the body's supply of vitamin D.

REGULATION

The skin serves to raise or lower body temperature as necessary. When the body needs to lose heat, the blood vessels in the skin dilate, bringing more blood to the surface for

THE INTEGUMENTARY SYSTEM

ORGAN/STRUCTURE	PRIMARY FUNCTIONS
Skin	Protection, regulation, sensation, and secretion
The Epidermis	The outer layer of the skin. It is divided into four strata:
Stratum corneum	Forms protective covering for the body
Stratum lucidum	Translucent layer that is frequently absent and not seen in thinner skin
Stratum granulosum	Active in the keratinization process, its cells become hard or horny
Stratum germinativum	Responsible for the regeneration of the epidermis
The Dermis	Nourishes the epidermis, provides strength, and supports blood vessels
Papillae	Produce ridges that are one's fingerprints
Subcutaneous Tissue	Supports, nourishes, insulates, and cushions the skin
Hair	Provides sensation and some protection for the head. Hair around the eyes, in the nose, and in the ears serves to filter out foreign particles.
Nails	Protects ends of fingers and toes
Sebaceous Glands	Lubricates the hair and skin
Sweat (Sudoriferous) Glands	Secretes sweat or perspiration, which helps to cool the body by evaporation. Sweat also rids the body of waste.

cooling by *radiation*. At the same time, the sweat glands are secreting more sweat for cooling by means of *evaporation*. Conversely, when the body needs to conserve heat, the reflex actions of the nervous system cause constriction of the skin's blood vessels, thereby allowing more heat-carrying blood to circulate to the muscles and vital organs.

SENSATION

The skin contains millions of microscopic nerve endings that act as *sensory receptors* for pain, touch, heat, cold, and pressure. When stimulation occurs, nerve impulses are sent to the cerebral cortex of the brain. The nerve endings in the skin are specialized according to the type of sensory information transmitted and, once this information reaches the brain, any necessary response is triggered. For example, touching a hot surface with the hand causes the brain to recognize the senses of *touch, heat,* and *pain* and results in the immediate removal of the hand from the hot surface.

SECRETION

The skin contains millions of sweat glands, which secrete *perspiration* or *sweat,* and sebaceous glands, which secrete *oil* for lubrication. Perspiration is largely water with a small amount of salt and other chemical compounds. This secretion, when left to accumulate, causes body odor, especially where it is trapped among hairs in the axillary region. Sebaceous glands produce *sebum,* which acts to protect the body from dehydration and possible absorption of harmful substances.

▶ LAYERS OF THE SKIN

The skin is essentially composed of two layers, the *epidermis* and the *dermis.*

THE EPIDERMIS

The *epidermis* can be divided into four strata: the stratum corneum, the stratum lucidum, the stratum granulosum, and the stratum germinativum. See Figure 3–1 for the locations of these strata within the epidermis.

The Stratum Corneum

The *stratum corneum* is the outermost, horny layer, consisting of dead cells filled with a protein substance called *keratin*. It forms the protective covering for the body, and its thickness varies with the use made of the particular body part. Because of the pressure on their surfaces during use, the soles of the feet and palms of the hands have thicker layers of stratum corneum than do the eyelids or the forehead.

The Stratum Lucidum

The *stratum lucidum* is a translucent layer lying directly beneath the stratum corneum. It is frequently absent and is not seen in thinner skin. Cells in this layer are also dead or dying.

The Stratum Granulosum

The *stratum granulosum* consists of several layers of living cells that are in the process of becoming a part of the previously mentioned strata. Its cells are active in the *keratinization* process, during which they lose their nuclei and become hard or horny.

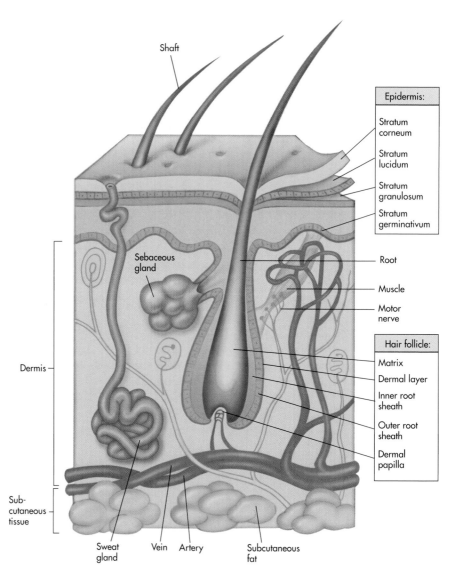

FIGURE 3–1

The integument: the epidermis, dermis, subcutaneous tissue, and its appendages.

The Stratum Germinativum

The *stratum germinativum* is composed of several layers of living cells capable of *mitosis* or cell division. Sometimes called the *mucosum* or *Malpighii,* the stratum germinativum is the innermost layer and is responsible for the regeneration of the epidermis. Damage to this layer, as in severe burns, necessitates the use of skin grafts. *Melanin,* the pigment that gives color to the skin, is formed in this layer. The more abundant the melanin, the darker the color of the skin.

THE DERMIS

Sometimes called the *corium* or *true skin,* the *dermis* is composed of connective tissue containing lymphatics, nerves and nerve endings, blood vessels, sebaceous and sweat glands, elastic fibers, and hair follicles. It is divided into two layers: the *upper* or *papillary layer* and the *lower* or *reticular layer.* The papillary layer is arranged into parallel rows of microscopic structures called *papillae*. The papillae produce the ridges of the skin that are one's fingerprints or footprints. The reticular layer is composed of white fibrous tissue that supports the blood vessels. The dermis is attached to underlying structures by the *subcutaneous tissue*. This tissue supports, nourishes, insulates, and cushions the skin.

▶ ACCESSORY STRUCTURES OF THE SKIN

The hair, nails, sebaceous glands, and sweat glands are the accessory structures of the skin.

HAIR

A *hair* is a thin, thread-like structure formed by a group of cells that develop within a hair *follicle* or *socket*. Each hair is composed of a *shaft,* which is the visible portion, and a *root,* which is embedded within the follicle. At the base of each follicle is a loop of capillaries enclosed within connective tissue called the *hair papilla. The pilomotor muscle* attaches to the side of each follicle. When the skin is cooled or the individual has an emotional reaction, the skin often forms *"goose pimples"* as a result of contraction by these muscles. Hair is distributed over the whole body with the exception of the palms of the hands and soles of the feet. It is thicker on the scalp and thinner on the other parts of the body. Hair around the eyes, in the nose, and in the ears serves to filter out foreign particles. The color of one's hair is a product of genetic background and is determined by the amount of pigmentation within the hair shaft. Hair grows at approximately 0.5 inch a month, and its growth is not affected by cutting.

NAILS

Finger- and *toenails* are horny cell structures of the epidermis and are composed of hard keratin. A nail consists of a *body*, a *root*, and a *matrix* or *nailbed* (Fig. 3–2). The crescent-shaped white area of the nail is the *lunula*. Nail growth may vary with age, disease, and hormone deficiency. Average growth is 1 mm per week, and a lost fingernail

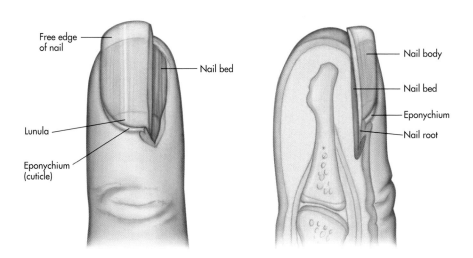

FIGURE 3–2

The fingernail, an appendage of the integument.

usually regenerates in 3½ to 5½ months. A lost toenail may require 6 to 8 months for regeneration.

SEBACEOUS GLANDS

The oil-secreting glands of the skin are called *sebaceous glands*. They have tiny ducts that open into the hair follicles, and their secretion, *sebum,* lubricates the hair as well as the skin. The amount of secretion is controlled by the endocrine system and varies with age, puberty, pregnancy, and senility.

SWEAT (SUDORIFEROUS) GLANDS

There are approximately 2 million *sweat glands.* These coiled, tubular glands are distributed over the entire surface of the body with the exception of the margin of the lips, glans penis, and the inner surface of the prepuce. They are more numerous on the palms of the hands, soles of the feet, forehead, and axillae. Sweat glands secrete *sweat* or *perspiration,* which helps to cool the body by evaporation. Sweat also rids the body of waste through the pores of the skin. Left to accumulate, sweat becomes odorous by the action of bacteria. The body loses about 0.5 L of fluid per day through sweat.

► SKIN SIGNS

Skin signs are objective evidence of an illness or disorder. They can be seen, measured, or felt. They may be described as lesions that are circumscribed areas of pathologically altered tissue. Types of skin signs are shown and described in Figure 3–3.

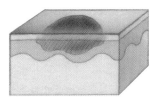

A macule is a discolored spot on the skin; freckle

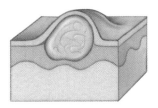

A pustule is a small, elevated, circumscribed lesion of the skin that is filled with pus; varicella (chickenpox)

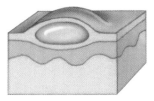

A wheal is a localized, evanescent elevation of the skin that is often accompanied by itching; urticaria

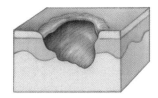

An erosion or ulcer is an eating or gnawing away of tissue; decubitus ulcer

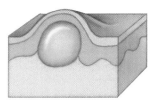

A papule is a solid, circumscribed, elevated area on the skin; pimple

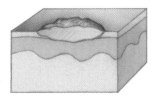

A crust is a dry, serous or seropurulent, brown, yellow, red, or green exudation that is seen in secondary lesions; eczema

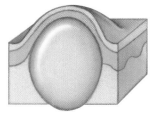

A nodule is a larger papule; acne vulgaris

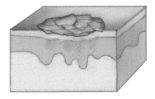

A scale is a thin, dry flake of cornified epithelial cells; psoriasis

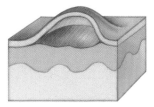

A vesicle is a small fluid filled sac; blister. A bulla is a large vesicle.

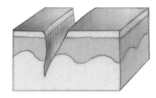

A fissure is a crack-like sore or slit that extends through the epidermis into the dermis; athlete's foot

FIGURE 3–3

Skin signs are objective evidence of an illness or disorder. They can be seen, measured, or felt.

▶ THE CHILD

Vernix caseosa, a cheese-like substance, covers the fetus until birth. At first the fetal skin is transparent and blood vessels are clearly visible. In about 13 to 16 weeks downy lanugo hair begins to develop, especially on the head. At 21 to 24 weeks, the skin is reddish and wrinkled and has little subcutaneous fat. At birth, the subcutaneous glands are developed and the skin is smooth and pink. Preterm and term newborns have less subcutaneous fat than adults; therefore, they are more sensitive to heat and cold. Babies can blister easily.

Skin conditions may be acute or chronic, local or systemic, and some are congenital, such as strawberry nevi and Mongolian spots. Certain children's skin conditions may be associated with age, such as milia in babies and acne in adolescents. **Milia** are white pinhead-size papules occurring on the face, and sometimes the trunk, of a newborn. They usually disappear in several weeks. **Acne** is an inflammatory condition of the sebaceous glands and the hair follicles (**pimples**). See Figure 3–4.

Skin infections in children generally produce systemic symptoms, such as fever and malaise. Sebaceous glands do not produce sebum until about 8 to 10 years of age; therefore, a child's skin is more dry and chaps easily.

The hair of the child will vary according to race, texture, quality, and distribution. A newborn may have no hair on its head or a head covered with hair. Hair can become dry and brittle, due to improper nutrition. During a severe illness hair loss and color change may occur.

▶ THE OLDER ADULT

With increasing years beyond reproductive maturity, the body begins the process of aging. By the year 2030 one in five people in the United States will be at least 65 years old. The process of aging varies with each individual. Aging is not a disease but rather a sequence of events regulated by complex processes.

The Integumentary System

As one ages, the skin becomes looser as the dermal papilla grows less dense. Collagen and elastic fibers of the upper dermis decrease and skin loses its elastic tone and wrinkles more easily. Skin conditions are common in the older adult. Dryness (**xerosis**) and itching (**pruritus**) are common. Premalignant and malignant skin lesions increase with aging. Carcinomas appear frequently on the nose, eyelid, or cheek. **Basal cell carcinomas** account for 80% of the skin cancers seen in the older adult. See Figure 3–5.

By age 50 approximately half of all people have some gray hair. Scalp hair thins in women and men. The hair becomes dry and often brittle. Older women may have an increase in facial hair. Men may have an increase in hair of the nares, eyebrows, or helix of the ear. In addition to the changes in the skin and hair, nails flatten and become discolored, dry, and brittle.

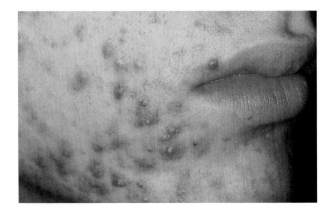

FIGURE 3–4

Acne. *(Courtesy of Jason L. Smith, MD.)*

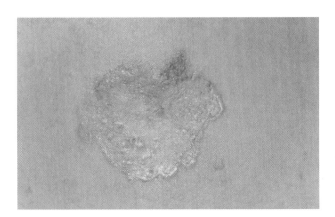

FIGURE 3–5

Basal cell carcinoma. *(Courtesy of Jason L. Smith, MD.)*

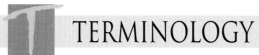

TERMINOLOGY

WITH SURGICAL PROCEDURES & PATHOLOGY

TERM	WORD PARTS			DEFINITION
acanthosis (ăk″ăn-thō′ sis)	acanth osis	R S	a thorn condition of	A condition of thickening of the prickle-cell layer of the skin
actinic dermatitis (ăk-tĭn′ ĭk dĕr″ mă-tī′ tĭs)	actin ic dermat itis	R S R S	ray pertaining to skin inflammation	Inflammation of the skin caused by exposure to radiant energy, such as x-rays, ultraviolet light, and sunlight. See Figure 3–6.
albinism (ăl′ bĭn-ĭsm)	albin ism	R S	white condition of	Absence of pigment in the skin, hair, and eyes
anhidrosis (ăn″ hī-drō′ sĭs)	an hidr osis	P R S	without, lack of sweat condition of	A condition in which there is a lack or complete absence of sweating
autograft (ŏ-tō-grăft)	auto graft	P S	self pencil	A graft taken from one part of the patient's body and transferred to another part
causalgia (kŏ-săl′ jĭ-ă)	caus algia	R S	heat pain	Intense burning pain associated with trophic skin changes in the hand or foot after trauma to the part
cutaneous (kū-tā′ nē-ŭs)	cutane ous	R S	skin pertaining to	Pertaining to the skin
dermatitis (dĕr″ mă-ti′ tĭs)	dermat itis	R S	skin inflammation	Inflammation of the skin. See Figures 3–7, 3–8, and 3–9.
dermatologist (dĕr″ mah-tol′ŏ-jĭst)	dermato log ist	CF R S	skin study of one who specializes	One who specializes in the study of the skin
dermatology (dĕr″ mă-tol′ŏ-jē)	dermato logy	CF S	skin study of	The study of the skin
dermatome (dĕr″ mah-tōm)	derma tome	CF S	skin instrument to cut	An instrument used to cut the skin for grafting
dermatopathy (dĕr″ mă-top′ ă-thē)	dermato pathy	CF S	skin disease	Skin disease

continued

Terminology - continued

TERM	WORD PARTS			DEFINITION
dermatoplasty (der′ mă-to-plas″ tē)	dermato plasty	CF S	skin surgical repair	Surgical repair of the skin
dermomycosis (dĕr′ mō-mī-kō′ sĭs)	dermo myc osis	CF R S	skin fungus condition of	A skin condition caused by a fungus
ecchymosis (ĕk-ĭ-mō′ sĭs)	ec chym osis	P R S	out juice condition of	A condition in which the blood seeps into the skin causing discolorations ranging from blue-black to greenish-yellow
eponychium (ĕp″ ō-nĭk′ ĭ-ŭm)	ep onychi um	P CF S	upon nail tissue	The horny embryonic tissue from which the nail develops
erysipelas (ĕr″ ĭ-sĭp′ ĕ-lăs)	erysi pelas	R S	red skin	Redness of the skin with inflammation caused by invasion by group A hemolytic streptococci. See Figure 3–10.
erythroderma (ĕ-rĭth″ rō-dĕr′-mă)	erythro derma	CF S	red skin	Abnormal redness of the skin occurring over widespread areas of the body. See Figure 3–11.
excoriation (ĕks-kō″ rē-ā′ shŭn)	ex coriat ion	P R S	out corium process	Abrasion of the epidermis by scratching, trauma, chemicals, burns, etc.
hidradenitis (hī-drăd-ĕ-nī′ tĭs)	hidr aden itis	R R S	sweat gland inflammation	Inflammation of the sweat glands
hyperhidrosis (hī″ pĕr-hī-drō′ sĭs)	hyper hidr osis	P R S	excessive sweat condition of	A condition of excessive sweating. See Figure 3–12.
hypertrichosis (hī″ pĕr-trĭ-kō′ sĭs)	hyper trich osis	P R S	excessive hair condition of	A condition of excessive hair growth
hypodermic (hī″ pō-dĕr′ mĭk)	hypo derm ic	P R S	under skin pertaining to	Pertaining to under the skin
hypodermoclysis (hī″ pō-dĕr-mŏk′ lĭ-sĭs)	hypo dermo clysis	P CF S	under skin injection	Injection of fluids under the skin to supply the body with a rapid replacement of fluids

Terminology - continued

TERM	WORD PARTS			DEFINITION
icteric (ik-tĕr′ ik)	icter ic	R S	jaundice pertaining to	Pertaining to jaundice
intradermal (in″ trăh-dĕr′ măl)	intra derm al	P R S	within skin pertaining to	Pertaining to within the skin
keloid (kē′ lŏyd)	kel oid	R S	tumor resemble	Overgrowth of scar tissue caused by excessive collagen formation. See Figure 3–13.
leukoderma (lū″ kō-dĕr′ mă)	leuko derma	CF S	white skin	Localized loss of pigmentation of the skin
melanoblast (mĕl′ ăn-ō-blăst″)	melano blast	CF S	black immature cell, germ cell	A germ cell found in the basal layers of the epidermis that is capable of forming melanin
melanocarcinoma (mĕl″ ă-nō-kar″ sĭn-ō′ mă)	melano carcin oma	CF R S	black cancer tumor	A cancerous tumor that has black pigmentation
melanoma (mĕl″ ă-nō′ mă)	melan oma	R S	black tumor	A malignant black mole or tumor. See Figures 3–14 and 3–15.

TERMINOLOGY SPOTLIGHT

Cancer that develops in the pigment cells is called **melanoma**. See Figures 3-14 and 3-15. Often the first sign of melanoma is change in the size, shape, or color of a mole. The **ABCD**s of melanoma describe the changes that can occur in a mole using the letters:

A—asymmetry—the shape of one half does not match the other.
B—border—the edges are ragged, notched, or blurred.
C—color—is uneven. Shades of black, brown, or tan are present. Areas of white, red, or blue may be seen.
D—diameter—there is a change in size.

TERM	WORD PARTS			DEFINITION
melanonychia (mĕl″ ă-nō-nĭk′ i-ă)	melan onych ia	R R S	black nail condition	A condition in which the nails are blackened by melanin pigmentation
onychectomy (ŏn″ ĭ-kĕk′ tō-mē)	onych ectomy	R S	nail excision	Surgical excision of a nail
onychitis (ŏn″ ĭ-kī′ tĭs)	onych itis	R S	nail inflammation	Inflammation of the nail
onychomalacia (ŏn″ ĭ-kō-mă-lā′ sĭ-ă)	onycho malacia	CF S	nail softening	Softening of the nail

continued

Terminology - continued

TERM	WORD PARTS			DEFINITION
onychomycosis (ŏn″ ĭ-kō-mī-kō′sĭs)	onycho myc osis	CF R S	nail fungus condition of	A condition of the nail caused by a fungus. See Figure 3–16.
onychophagia (ŏn″ ĭ-kŏf′ ă-jĭ-ă)	onycho phagia	CF S	nail to eat	Nail biting
pachyderma (păk-ē-der′ mă)	pachy derma	R S	thick skin	Thick skin
pachyonychia (păk″ ē-ō-nĭk′ ĭ-ă)	pachy onych ia	R R S	thick nail condition	A condition of thick nail or nails
paronychia (păr″ ō-nĭk′ ĭ-ă)	par onych ia	P R S	around nail condition	An infectious condition of the marginal structures around the nail
pediculosis (pĕ-dĭk″ ū-lō′ sĭs)	pedicul osis	R S	a louse condition of	A condition of infestation with lice. See Figure 3–17.
rhytidectomy (rĭt″ ĭ-dĕk′ tō-mē)	rhytid ectomy	R S	wrinkle excision	Surgical excision of wrinkles
rhytidoplasty (rĭt′ ĭ-dō-plăs″ tē)	rhytido plasty	CF S	wrinkle surgical repair	Plastic surgery for the removal of wrinkles
scleroderma (skli rō-děr′ mă)	sclero derma	CF S	hard skin	A chronic condition with hardening of the skin and other connective tissues of the body
seborrhea (sĕb″ or-ē′ ă)	sebo rrhea	CF S	oil flow	Excessive flow of oil from the sebaceous glands
senile keratosis (sĕn′ īl kĕr″ă-tō′sĭs)	senile kerat osis	R R S	old horn condition of	A condition occurring in older people wherein there is dry skin and localized scaling caused by excessive exposure to the sun. See Figure 3–18.
subcutaneous (sŭb″ kū-tā′ nē-ŭs)	sub cutane ous	P R S	below skin pertaining to	Pertaining to below the skin
subungual (sŭb-ŭng′ gwăl)	sub ungu al	P R S	below nail pertaining to	Pertaining to below the nail
thermanesthesia (thĕrm″ăn-ĕs-thē′ zē-ă)	therm an esthesia	R P S	hot, heat without, lack of sensation	Inability to distinguish between the sensations of heat and cold

Terminology - continued

TERM	WORD PARTS			DEFINITION
trichomycosis (trĭk″ ō-mi-kō′ sĭs)	tricho myc osis	CF R S	hair fungus condition of	A fungus condition of the hair
xanthoderma (zăn″ thō-dĕr′ mă)	xantho derma	CF S	yellow skin	Yellow skin
xanthoma (zăn-thō′mă)	xanth oma	R S	yellow tumor	Yellow tumor. See Figure 3–19.
xeroderma (zē″ rō-dĕr′ mă)	xero derma	CF S	dry skin	Dry skin
xerosis (zē- rō′sĭs)	xer osis	R S	dry condition of	Abnormal dryness of skin, mucous membranes, or the conjunctiva. See Figure 3–20.

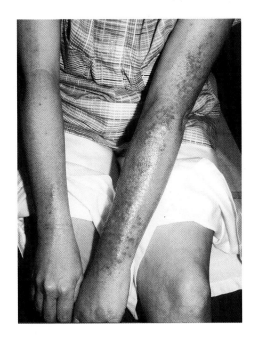

FIGURE 3–6

Photodermatitis. *(Courtesy of Jason L. Smith, MD.)*

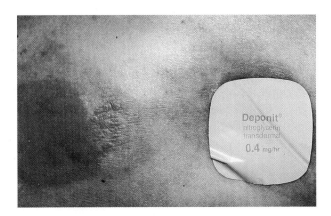

FIGURE 3–7

Contact dermatitis; adhesive reaction. *(Courtesy of Jason L. Smith, MD.)*

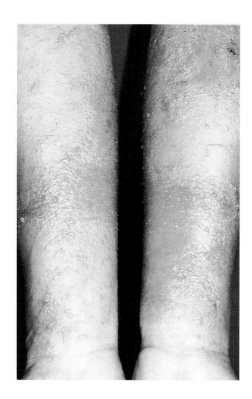

FIGURE 3–8

Dermatitis; poison ivy. *(Courtesy of Jason L. Smith, MD.)*

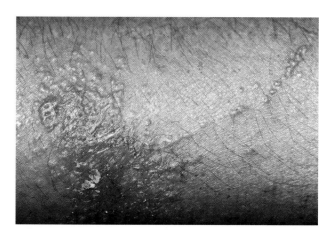

FIGURE 3–9

Dermatitis; poison ivy. *(Courtesy of Jason L. Smith, MD.)*

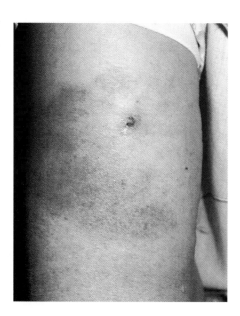

FIGURE 3–10

Erysipelas. *(Courtesy of Jason L. Smith, MD.)*

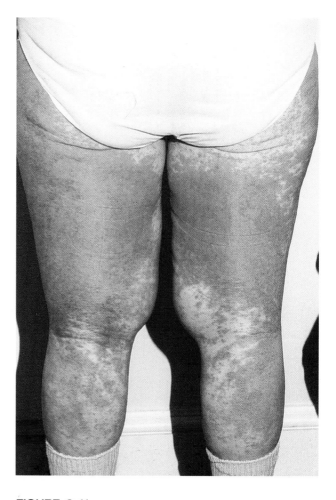

FIGURE 3–11

Erythroderma. *(Courtesy of Jason L. Smith, MD.)*

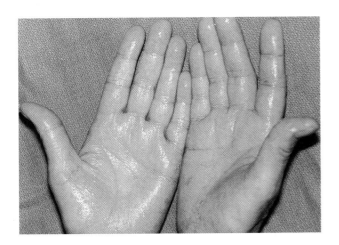

FIGURE 3–12

Hyperhidrosis. *(Courtesy of Jason L. Smith, MD.)*

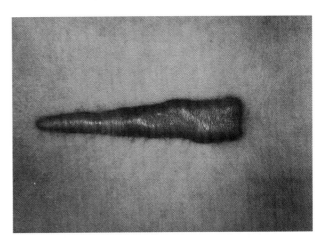

FIGURE 3–13

Keloid. *(Courtesy of Jason L. Smith, MD.)*

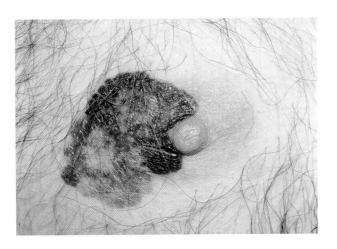

FIGURE 3–14

Melanoma. *(Courtesy of Jason L. Smith, MD.)*

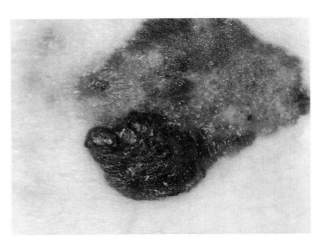

FIGURE 3–15

Melanoma, forearm. *(Courtesy of Jason L. Smith, MD.)*

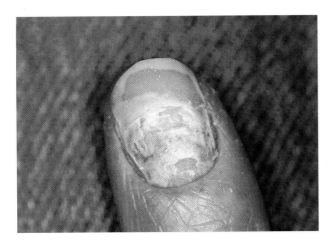

FIGURE 3–16

Onychomycosis. *(Courtesy of Jason L. Smith, MD.)*

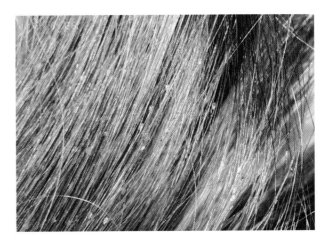

FIGURE 3–17

Pediculosis capitis. *(Courtesy of Jason L. Smith, MD.)*

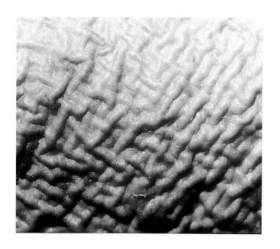

FIGURE 3–18

Photoaging solar elastosis; senile keratosis. *(Courtesy of Jason L. Smith, MD.)*

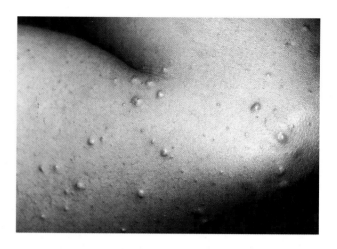

FIGURE 3–19

Eruptive xanthoma. *(Courtesy of Jason L. Smith, MD.)*

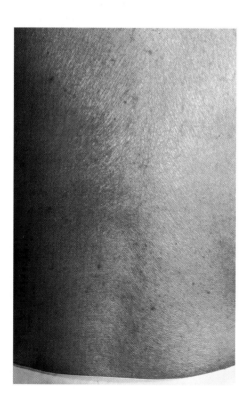

FIGURE 3–20

Xerosis. *(Courtesy of Jason L. Smith, MD.)*

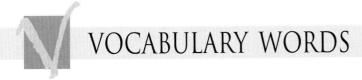

VOCABULARY WORDS

Vocabulary words are terms that have not been divided into component parts. They are common words or specialized terms associated with the subject of this chapter. These words are provided to enhance your medical vocabulary.

WORD	DEFINITION
acne (ăk′ nē)	An inflammatory condition of the sebaceous glands and the hair follicles; *pimples.* See Figure 3–4.
acrochordon (ăk″ rō-kor′ dŏn)	A small outgrowth of epidermal and dermal tissue; *skin tags.* See Figure 3–21.
alopecia (al″ ō-pē′ shĭ-ă)	Loss of hair, *baldness; alopecia areata* is loss of hair in defined patches usually involving the scalp. See Figure 3–22. Male pattern alopecia begins in the frontal area and proceeds until only a horseshoe area of the hair remains in the back and temples. See Figure 3–23.
avulsion (ă-vŭl′ shŭn)	The process of forcibly tearing off a part or structure of the body, such as a finger or toe
basal cell carcinoma bā′săl sel kăr″ sĭ-nō′mă	An epithelial malignant tumor of the skin that rarely metastasizes. It usually begins as a small, shiny papule and enlarges to form a whitish border around a central depression. See Figure 3–5.
bite (bīt)	An injury in which a part of the body surface is torn by an insect, animal, or human, resulting in an abrasion, puncture, or laceration. See Figures 3–24, 3–25, 3–26, and 3–27.
boil (boil)	An acute, painful nodule formed in the subcutaneous layers of the skin, gland, or hair follicle; most often caused by the invasion of staphylococci; *furuncle.* See Figure 3–28.
bulla (bŭl′ lă)	A larger blister; *a bleb.* See Figure 3–29.
burn (burn) (bərn)	An injury to tissue caused by heat, fire, chemical agents, electricity, lightning, or radiation; burns are classified according to degree or depth of skin damage. See Figure 3–30.
callus (kăl′ ŭs)	Hardened skin
candidiasis (kăn″ dĭ-dī′ă-sĭs)	An infection of the skin or mucous membranes with any species of *Candida,* but chiefly *Candida albicans. Candida* is a genus of yeasts and was formerly called *Monilia.* See Figure 3–31.

continued

Vocabulary - continued

WORD	DEFINITION
carbuncle (kăr′ bŭng″ kl)	An infection of the subcutaneous tissue, usually composed of a cluster of boils. See Figure 3–32.
cellulitis (sĕl-ū-lī′ tĭs)	Inflammation of cellular or connective tissue. See Figure 3–33.
cicatrix (sĭk′ ă-trĭks)	The scar left after the healing of a wound
comedo (kŏm′ ē-dō)	Blackhead
corn (korn) (ko(ə)rn)	A horny induration and thickening of the skin on the toes caused by ill-fitting shoes.
cyst (sĭst)	A bladder or sac; a closed sac that contains fluid, semifluid, or solid material
decubitus (dē-kū′ bĭ-tŭs)	Literally means a lying down; *a bedsore*
dehiscence (dē- hĭs′ ĕns)	The separation or bursting open of a surgical wound. See Figure 3–34.
eczema (ĕk′ zĕ-mă)	An inflammatory skin disease of the epidermis
erythema (ĕr″ ĭ-thē′ mă)	A redness of the skin; may be caused by capillary congestion, inflammation, heat, sunlight, or cold temperature. *Erythema infectiosum* is known as Fifth disease, a mild, moderately contagious disease caused by the human parvovirus B-19. It is most commonly seen in school-age children and is thought to be spread via respiratory secretions from infected persons. See Figure 3–35.
eschar (ĕs′ kăr)	A slough, scab
exudate (ĕks′ ū-dāt)	The production of pus or serum
folliculitis (fō-lĭk″ ū-lī′ tĭs)	Inflammation of a follicle or follicles. See Figure 3–36.
herpes simplex (hĕr′ pēz sĭm′ plĕks)	An inflammatory skin disease caused by a herpes virus (Type I); *cold sore* or *fever blister*. See Figures 3–37 and 3–38.
hives (hīvz)	Eruption of itching and burning swellings on the skin; *urticaria*. See Figure 3–39.

Vocabulary - continued

WORD	DEFINITION
impetigo (ĭm″ pĕ-tī′ gō)	A skin infection marked by vesicles or bullae; usually caused by streptococci or staphylococci. See Figure 3–40.
integumentary (ĭn-tĕg″ ū-mĕn′ tă-rē)	A covering; the skin, consisting of the dermis and the epidermis
intertrigo (ĭn″ tĕr-trī′ gō)	A superficial dermatitis that occurs in the folds of the skin
jaundice (jawn′ dĭs)	Yellow; a symptom of a disease in which there is excessive bile in the blood; the skin, whites of the eyes, and mucous membranes are yellow; *icterus*
lentigo (lĕn-tī′ gō)	A flat, brownish spot on the skin sometimes caused by exposure to the sun and weather; *freckle.* See Figure 3–41.
leukoplakia (loo″ kō-plā′ kē-ă)	White spots or patches formed on the mucous membrane of the tongue or cheek; the spots are smooth, hard, and irregular in shape and may become malignant
lupus (lū′ pŭs)	Originally used to describe a destructive type of skin lesion; current usage of the word is usually in combination with the words *vulgaris* or *erythematosus: lupus vulgaris* or *lupus erythematosus*
miliaria (mĭl-ē-ā′ rē-ă)	Is called *prickly heat* and is commonly seen in newborns and/or infants. It is caused by excessive body warmth. There is retention of sweat in the sweat glands, which have become blocked or inflamed, and then rupture or leak into the skin. *Miliaria* appears as a rash with tiny pinhead-sized papules, vesicles, and/or pustules. See Figure 3–42.
mole (mōl)	A pigmented, elevated spot above the surface of the skin; a *nevus.* See Figure 3–43.
petechiae (pē- tē′ kĭ-ē)	Small, pinpoint, purplish hemorrhagic spots on the skin
pityriasis (pĭt″ ĭ-rī′ ă-sĭs)	A skin disease characterized by branny (like bran) scales. See Figure 3–44.
pruritus (proo-rī′ tŭs)	A severe itching
psoriasis (sō-rī′ ă-sĭs)	A chronic skin disease characterized by pink or dull-red lesions surmounted by silvery scaling. See Figures 3–45, 3–46, and 3–47.
purpura (pur′ pū-ră)	A purplish discoloration of the skin caused by extravasation of blood into the tissues. See Figures 3–48 and 3–49.
roseola (rō-zē′ ō-lă)	Any rose-colored rash marked by *maculae* or red spots on the skin. See Figure 3–50.

continued

Vocabulary - continued

WORD	DEFINITION
rubella (roo-běl′ lă)	A systemic disease caused by a virus and characterized by a rash and fever; also called *German measles* and *three-day measles*
rubeola (roo-bē′ ō-lă)	A contagious disease characterized by fever, inflammation of the mucous membranes, and rose-colored spots on the skin; also called *measles*
scabies (skā′ bēz) or (skā′ bǐ-ēz)	A contagious skin disease characterized by papules, vesicles, pustules, burrows, and intense itching; it is caused by the itch mite and is also called *"the itch"* or the *"seven-year itch."* See Figure 3–51.
scar (skahr)	The mark left by the healing process of a wound, sore, or injury
sebum (sē′ bŭm)	The fatty or oil secretion of sebaceous glands of the skin
striae (plural) (strī′ ē)	Streaks or lines on the breasts, thighs, abdomen, or buttocks caused by weakening of elastic tissue. See Figure 3–52.
taut (tot)	Tight, firm; to pull or draw tight a surface, such as the skin
telangiectasia (těl-ăn″ jē-ěk-tā′ zē-ă)	Dilatation of small blood vessels that may appear as a *"birthmark"*
tinea (tǐn′ ē-ă)	Contagious skin diseases affecting both man and domestic animals, caused by certain fungi, and marked by the localized appearance of discolored, scaly patches on the skin; also called *ringworm*. See Figures 3–53, 3–54, 3–55, and 3–56.
ulcer (ŭl′ sěr)	An open lesion or sore of the epidermis or mucous membrane. See Figures 3–57 and 3–58.
varicella (văr″ i-sěl′ ă)	A contagious viral disease characterized by fever, headache, and a crop of red spots that become macules, papules, vesicles, and crusts; also called *chickenpox*. See Figure 3–59.
vitiligo (vǐt″ ǐl-ǐ′ gō)	A skin condition characterized by milk-white patches surrounded by areas of normal pigmentation. See Figures 3–60 and 3–61.
wart (wōrt)	An elevation of viral origin on the epidermis; *verruca*. See Figures 3–62, 3–63, and 3–64. A plantar wart is known as *verruca plantaris*. It occurs on a pressure-bearing area, especially the sole of the foot. See Figure 3–65.
wen (wěn)	A sebaceous cyst; *steatoma*
wound (woond)	An injury to soft tissue caused by trauma; generally classified as open or closed

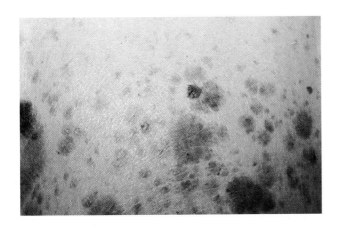

FIGURE 3–21

Acrochordon (skin tags). *(Courtesy of Jason L. Smith, MD.)*

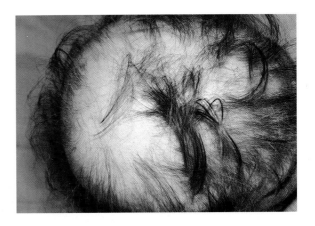

FIGURE 3–22

Alopecia areata. *(Courtesy of Jason L. Smith, MD.)*

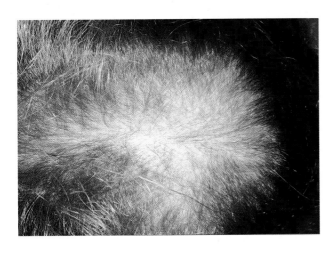

FIGURE 3–23

Male pattern alopecia. *(Courtesy of Jason L. Smith, MD.)*

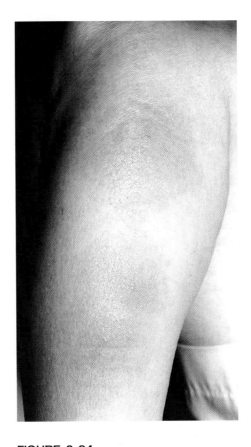

FIGURE 3–24

Fire ant bites. *(Courtesy of Jason L. Smith, MD.)*

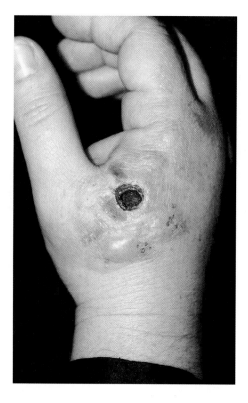

FIGURE 3–25

Brown recluse spider bite. *(Courtesy of Jason L. Smith, MD.)*

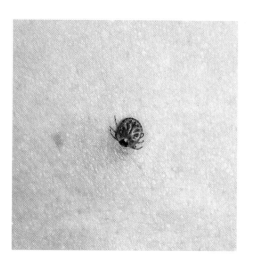

FIGURE 3–26

Tick bite. *(Courtesy of Jason L. Smith, MD.)*

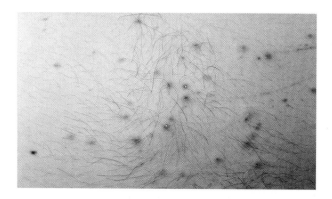

FIGURE 3–27

Flea bites. *(Courtesy of Jason L. Smith, MD.)*

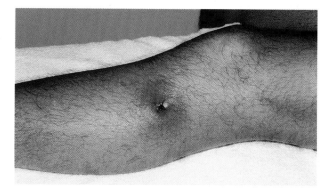

FIGURE 3–28

Furuncle. *(Courtesy of Jason L. Smith, MD.)*

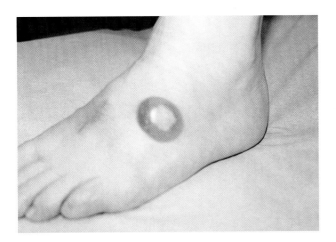

FIGURE 3–29

Bulla. *(Courtesy of Jason L. Smith, MD.)*

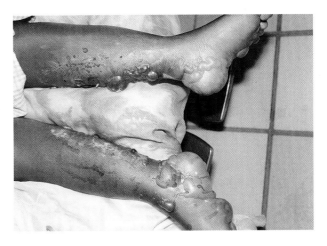

FIGURE 3–30

Burn, second degree. *(Courtesy of Jason L. Smith, MD.)*

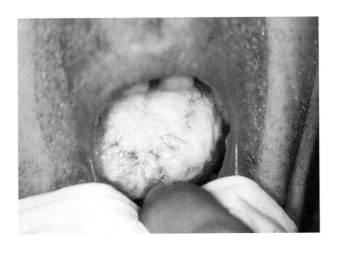

FIGURE 3–31

Candidiasis. *(Courtesy of Jason L. Smith, MD.)*

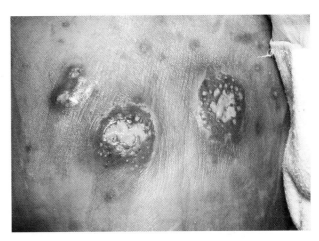

FIGURE 3–32

Carbuncles. *(Courtesy of Jason L. Smith, MD.)*

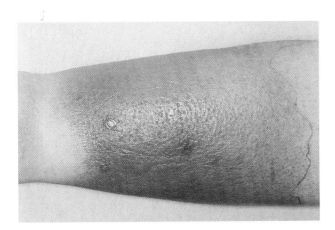

FIGURE 3–33

Cellulitis. *(Courtesy of Jason L. Smith, MD.)*

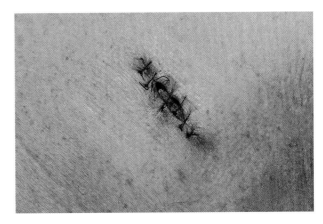

FIGURE 3–34

Wound dehiscence, back. *(Courtesy of Jason L. Smith, MD.)*

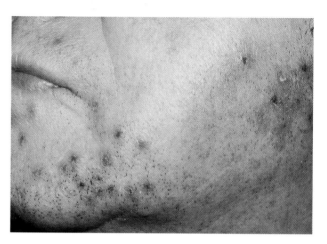

FIGURE 3–35

Erythema infectiosum (Fifth disease). *(Courtesy of Jason L. Smith, MD.)*

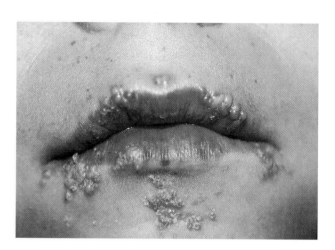

FIGURE 3–36

Staphylococcal folliculitis. *(Courtesy of Jason L. Smith, MD.)*

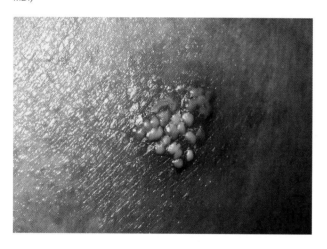

FIGURE 3–37

Herpes simplex. *(Courtesy of Jason L. Smith, MD.)*

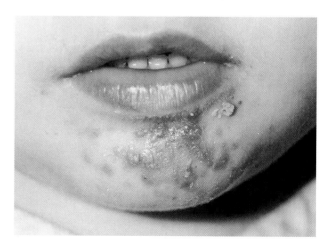

FIGURE 3–38

Herpes labialis. *(Courtesy of Jason L. Smith, MD.)*

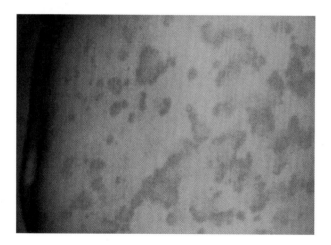

FIGURE 3–39

Urticaria (hives). *(Courtesy of Jason L. Smith, MD.)*

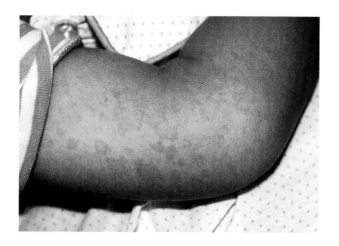

FIGURE 3–40

Impetigo. *(Courtesy of Jason L. Smith, MD.)*

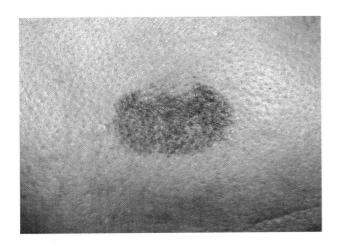

FIGURE 3-41

Lentigo. *(Courtesy of Jason L. Smith, MD.)*

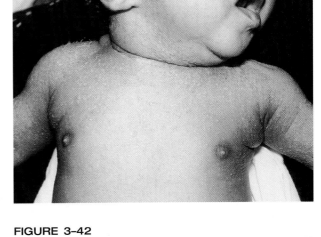

FIGURE 3-42

Miliaria. *(Courtesy of Jason L. Smith, MD.)*

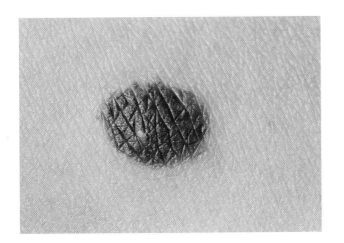

FIGURE 3-43

Nevus (mole). *(Courtesy of Jason L. Smith, MD.)*

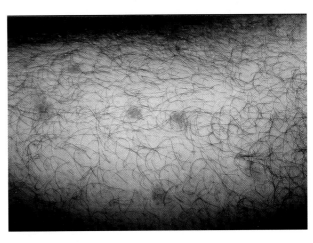

FIGURE 3-44

Pityriasis rosea. *(Courtesy of Jason L. Smith, MD.)*

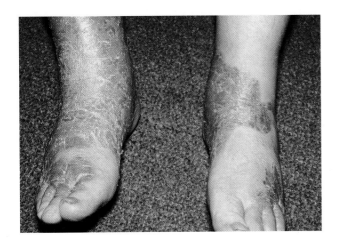

FIGURE 3-45

Psoriasis lower extremities. *(Courtesy of Jason L. Smith, MD.)*

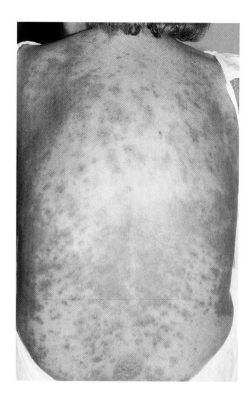

FIGURE 3–46

Psoriasis, back. *(Courtesy of Jason L. Smith, MD.)*

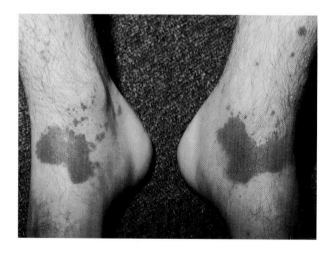

FIGURE 3–48

Purpura. *(Courtesy of Jason L. Smith, MD.)*

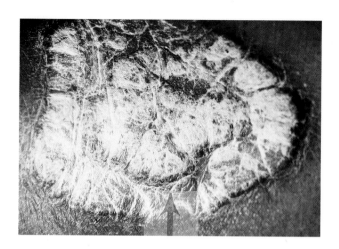

FIGURE 3–47

Psoriasis. *(Courtesy of Jason L. Smith, MD.)*

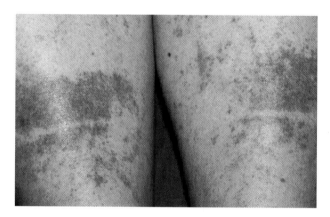

FIGURE 3–49

Benign pigmented purpura. *(Courtesy of Jason L. Smith, MD.)*

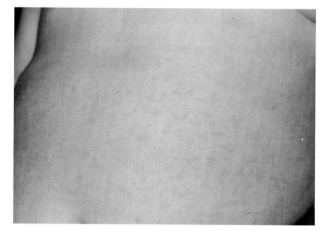

FIGURE 3–50

Roseola. *(Courtesy of Jason L. Smith, MD.)*

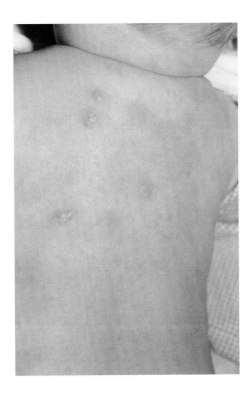

FIGURE 3-51

Scabies. *(Courtesy of Jason L. Smith, MD.)*

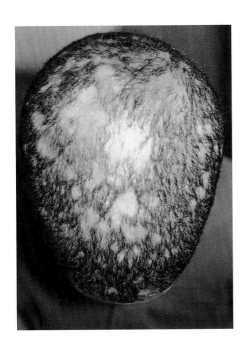

FIGURE 3-53

Tinea capitis. *(Courtesy of Jason L. Smith, MD.)*

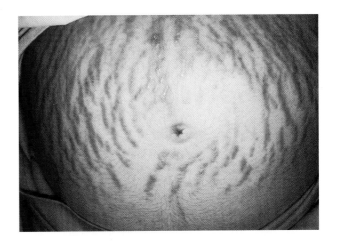

FIGURE 3-52

Striae. *(Courtesy of Jason L. Smith, MD.)*

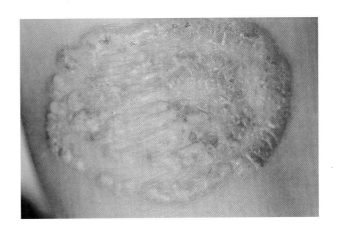

FIGURE 3-54

Tinea corporis. *(Courtesy of Jason L. Smith, MD.)*

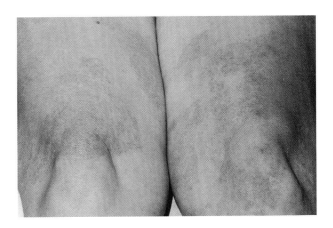

FIGURE 3-55

Tinea corporis. *(Courtesy of Jason L. Smith, MD.)*

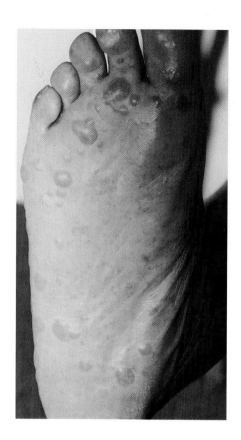

FIGURE 3–56

Tinea pedis. *(Courtesy of Jason L. Smith, MD.)*

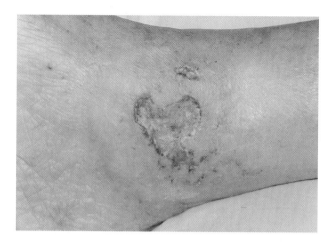

FIGURE 3–57

Ulcer (vasculitis). *(Courtesy of Jason L. Smith, MD.)*

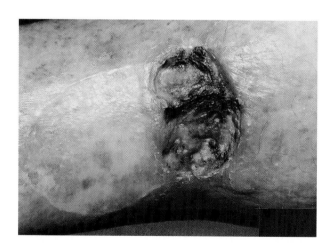

FIGURE 3–58

Leg ulcer radiation site. *(Courtesy of Jason L. Smith, MD.)*

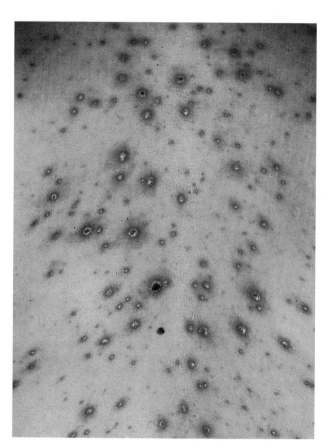

FIGURE 3–59

Varicella (chickenpox). *(Courtesy of Jason L. Smith, MD.)*

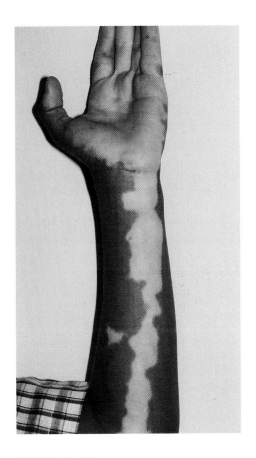

FIGURE 3–60

Vitiligo. *(Courtesy of Jason L. Smith, MD.)*

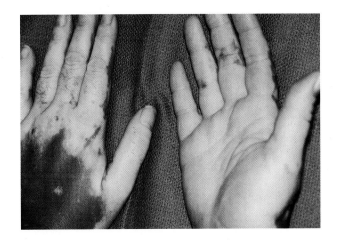

FIGURE 3–61

Vitiligo. *(Courtesy of Jason L. Smith, MD.)*

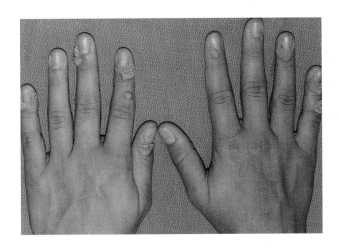

FIGURE 3–62

Verrucae (warts). *(Courtesy of Jason L. Smith, MD.)*

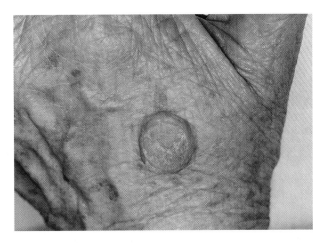

FIGURE 3–63

Verruca vulgaris. *(Courtesy of Jason L. Smith, MD.)*

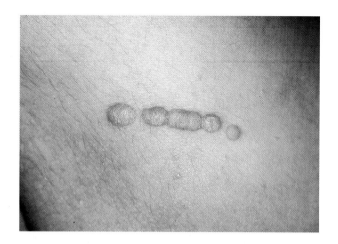

FIGURE 3-64

Verruca vulgaris. *(Courtesy of Jason L. Smith, MD.)*

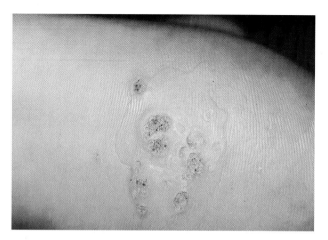

FIGURE 3-65

Plantar wart. *(Courtesy of Jason L. Smith, MD.)*

ABBREVIATIONS

decub	decubitus	**SG**	skin graft
derm	dermatology	**SLE**	systemic lupus erythematosus
FB	foreign body	**STD**	skin test done
FUO	fever of unknown origin	**STSG**	split thickness skin graft
H	hypodermic	**subcu**	subcutaneous
Hx	history	**subq**	subcutaneous
ID	intradermal	**T**	temperature
I&D	incision and drainage	**TTS**	transdermal therapeutic system
PUVA	psoralen-ultraviolet light	**ung**	ointment
		UV	ultraviolet

DRUG HIGHLIGHTS

Drugs that are used for dermatologic diseases or disorders include emollient, keratolytic, local anesthetic, antipruritic, antibiotic, antifungal, antiviral, anti-inflammatory, and antiseptic agents. Other drugs include Retin-A and Rogaine.

Emollients   Substances that are generally oily in nature. These substances are used for dry skin caused by aging, excessive bathing, and psoriasis.
Examples: Dermassage, Neutrogena, and Desitin.

Keratolytics   Agents that cause or promote loosening of horny (keratin) layers of the skin. These agents may be used for acne, warts, psoriasis, corns, calluses, and fungal infections.
Examples: Duofilm, Keralyt, and Compound W.

Local Anesthetic Agents	Agents that inhibit the conduction of nerve impulses from sensory nerves and thereby reduce pain and discomfort. These agents may be used topically to reduce discomfort associated with insect bites, burns, and poison ivy. *Examples: Solarcaine, Xylocaine, and Dyclone.*
Antipruritic Agents	Agents that prevent or relieve itching. *Examples: Topical—PBZ (tripelennamine HCl); Oral—Benadryl (diphenhydramine HCl) and Atarax (hydroxyzine HCl).*
Antibiotic Agents	Agents that destroy or stop the growth of microorganisms. These agents are used to prevent infection associated with minor skin abrasions and to treat superficial skin infections and acne. Several antibiotic agents are combined in a single product to take advantage of the different antimicrobial spectrum of each drug. *Examples: Neosporin, Polysporin, and Mycitracin.*
Antifungal Agents	Agents that destroy or inhibit the growth of fungi and yeast. These agents are used to treat fungus and/or yeast infection of the skin, nails, and scalp. *Examples: Fungizone (amphotericin B), Micatin (miconazole nitrate), and Desenex.*
Antiviral Agents	Agents that combat specific viral diseases. *Zovirax (acyclovir)* is used in the treatment of herpes simplex virus types 1 and 2, varicella-zoster, Epstein-Barr, and cytomegalovirus.
Anti-inflammatory Agents	Agents used to relieve the swelling, tenderness, redness, and pain of inflammation. Topically applied corticosteroids are used in the treatment of dermatitis and psoriasis. *Examples: Hydrocortisone, Decadron (dexamethasone), and Temovate (clobetasol propionate).* Oral corticosteroids are used in the treatment of contact dermatitis, such as in poison ivy, when the symptoms are severe. *Example: Sterapred (prednisone) 12-day unipak.*
Antiseptic Agents	Agents that prevent or inhibit the growth of pathogens. Antiseptics are generally applied to the surface of living tissue. *Examples: Isopropyl alcohol and Zephrian (benzalkonium chloride)*
Other Drugs	*Retin-A (tretinoin)* is available as a cream, gel, or liquid. It is used in the treatment of acne vulgaris. *Rogaine (minoxidil)* is available as a topical solution to stimulate hair growth. It was first approved as a treatment of male pattern baldness.

DIAGNOSTIC AND LABORATORY TESTS

Test	Description
tuberculosis skin tests (tū-bĕr″ kū-lō′ sĭs)	Tests performed to identify the presence of the *Tubercle bacilli*. The tine, Heaf, or Mantoux test may be used. The tine test and Heaf test are intradermal tests performed using a sterile, disposable, multiple-puncture lancet. The tuberculin is on metal tines that are pressed into the skin. A hardened raised area at the test site 48 to 72 hours later indicates the presence of the pathogens in the blood.

Test	Description
	In the **Mantoux** test 0.1 mL of purified protein derivative (PPD) tuberculin is intradermally injected. Test results are read 48 to 72 hours after administration.
sweat test (chloride) (swĕt)	A test performed on **sweat** to determine the level of chloride concentration on the skin. In **cystic fibrosis,** there is an increase in skin chloride.
Tzanck test (tsănk)	A microscopic examination of a small piece of tissue that has been surgically scraped from a pustule. The specimen is placed on a slide and stained, and the type of viral infection can be identified.
wound culture (woond)	A test done on wound exudate to determine the presence of microorganisms. An effective antibiotic can be prescribed for identified microbes.
biopsy (skin) (bī′ ŏp-sē)	Any skin lesion that exhibits signs or characteristics of malignancy may be excised and examined microscopically to establish a diagnosis. Usually only a small piece of living tissue is needed for examination.

COMMUNICATION ENRICHMENT

This segment is provided for those who wish to enhance their ability to communicate in either English or Spanish.

▶ **Related Terms**

English	Spanish	English	Spanish
skin	piel (pĭ-*ĕl*)	hair	pelo (*pĕ*-lō)
glands	glándulas (*glăn*-dŭ-lăs)	perspiration	perspiracion (pers-pir-a-*sion*)
bald	calvo (*căl*-vō)	rash	erupción (ĕ-*rŭp*-sĭ-ō n)
chickenpox	varicela (*vă*-rĭ-cĕ-lă)	redness	enrojecimiento (ĕn-rō-*hĕ*-sĭ-mĭ-ĕn-tō)
heat, warmth	calor (*că*-lō r)	sores	úlceros (ŭl-*sĕ*-răs)

English	Spanish	English	Spanish
itching	picazón (pĭ-*că*-zōn)	sweating	sudar (*sŭ*-dăr)
jaundice	ictericia (ĭk-tĕ-rĭ-sĭ-ă)	wound	herida (ĕ-*rĭ*-dă)
measles	sarampión (*să*-răm-pĭ-ōn)		

▶ **Colors**

English	Spanish (Colores)	Combining Form
red	rojo (*rō*-hō)	erythro; rubeo; rhodo (ĕ-*rĭ*-thrō; rū-bĕ-ō; *rō*-dō)
white	blanco (*blăn*-cō)	leuko; albin (lĕ-ō-kō; *ăl*-bĭn)
green	verde (*vĕr*-dĕ)	chloro (*klō*-rō)
blue	azul (*ă*-zŭl)	cyano (sĭ-*ă*-nō)
black	negro (*nĕ*-grō)	melano (*mĕ*-lă-nō)
gray	gris (grĭs)	polio (*pō*-lĭ-ō)
yellow	amarillo (*ă*-mă-ri-yō)	xantho (*zăn*-thō)
purple	morado (mō-*ră*-dō)	purpura (pūr-*pū*-rā)
pink	rosado (rō-*să*-dō)	
rose	rosa (*rō*-să)	
orange-yellow	cirrho (*sĭr*-ō)	

STUDY AND REVIEW SECTION

LEARNING EXERCISES

▶ Anatomy and Physiology

Write your answers to the following questions. Do not refer back to the text.

1.   Name the primary organ of the integumentary system. _____

2.   Name the four accessory structures of the integumentary system.

  a. _____   b. _____

  c. _____   d. _____

3.   State the four main functions of the skin.

  a. _____   b. _____

  c. _____   d. _____

4.   The skin is essentially composed of two layers, the _____ and

  the _____.

5.   Name the four strata of the epidermis.

  a. _____   b. _____

  c. _____   d. _____

6.   _____ is a protein substance found in the dead cells of the epidermis.

7.   _____ is a pigment that gives color to the skin.

8.   The _____ is known as the corium or true skin.

9.   Name the two layers of the part of the skin described in question 8.

  a. _____   b. _____

10.   The crescent-shaped white area of the nail is the _____.

▶ Word Parts

1.   In the spaces provided, write the definition of these prefixes, roots, combining
   forms, and suffixes. Do not refer to the listings of terminology words. Leave blank
   those terms you cannot define.

2. After completing as many as you can, refer back to the terminology word listings to check your work. For each word missed or left blank, write the term and its definition several times on the margins of these pages or on a separate sheet of paper.

3. To maximize the learning process, it is to your advantage to do the following exercises as directed. To refer to the terminology listings before completing these exercises invalidates the learning process.

Prefixes

Give the definitions of the following prefixes:

1. an- _____

2. auto- _____

3. ec- _____

4. ep- _____

5. ex- _____

6. hyper- _____

7. hypo- _____

8. intra- _____

9. par- _____

10. sub- _____

Roots and Combining Forms

Give the definitions of the following roots and combining forms:

1. acanth _____

2. actin _____

3. aden _____

4. albin _____

5. carcin _____

6. caus _____

7. chym _____

8. coriat _____

9. cutane _____

10. derm _____

11. derma _____

12. dermat _____

13. dermato _____

14. dermo _____

15. erysi _____

16. erythro _____

17. hidr _____

18. icter _____

19. kel _____

20. kerat _____

21. leuko _____

22. log _____

23. melan _____

24. melano _____

25. myc _____

26. onych _____

27. onychi _____

28. onycho _____

29. pachy _____   30. pedicul _____

31. rhytid _____   32. rhytido _____

33. sclero _____   34. sebo _____

35. senile _____   36. therm _____

37. trich _____   38. tricho _____

39. ungu _____   40. xantho _____

41. xero _____

Suffixes

Give the definitions of the following suffixes:

1. -al _____   2. -algia _____

3. -blast _____   4. -clysis _____

5. -derma _____   6. -ectomy _____

7. -esthesia _____   8. -graft _____

9. -ia _____   10. -ic _____

11. -ion _____   12. -ism _____

13. -ist _____   14. -itis _____

15. -logy _____   16. -malacia _____

17. -oid _____   18. -oma _____

19. -osis _____   20. -ous _____

21. -pathy _____   22. -pelas _____

23. -phagia _____   24. -plasty _____

25. -rrhea _____   26. -tome _____

27. -um _____

▶ Identifying Medical Terms

In the spaces provided, write the medical terms for the following meanings:

1. _____   Inflammation of the skin caused by exposure to actinic rays

2. _____   Pertaining to the skin

3. _____   Inflammation of the skin

4. _____   The study of the skin

5. _____   Skin disease

6. _____   Condition of excessive sweating

7. _____   Pertaining to under the skin

8. _____   Pertaining to jaundice

9. _____   Surgical excision of a nail

10. _____   Thick skin

11. _____   Inability to distinguish between the sensations of heat and cold

12. _____   Yellow skin

▶ Spelling

In the spaces provided, write the correct spelling of these misspelled terms.

1. caualgia _____   2. dermomcosis _____

3. echymosis _____   4. ersipelas _____

5. hypdermoclysis _____   6. melnoma _____

7. onchophagia _____   8. rhytiectomy _____

9. sleroderma _____   10. sebrrhea _____

WORD PARTS STUDY SHEET

Word Parts	Give the Meaning
ec-	_____
ep-	_____
hyper-	_____
hypo-	_____
par-	_____
sub-	_____
cutane-	_____
derm-, dermat-	_____

dermo-, dermato- _____

erythro- _____

hidr- _____

icter- _____

kel- _____

leuko- _____

melan-, melano- _____

myc- _____

onych-, onychi-, onycho- _____

pachy- _____

pedicul- _____

rhytid-, rhytido- _____

sebo- _____

tricho- _____

ungu- _____

xantho- _____

xero- _____

-al _____

-clysis _____

-derma _____

-ia, -osis _____

-ist _____

-itis _____

-logy _____

-oid _____

-oma _____

-phagia _____

-plasty _____

-rrhea _____

-tome   _____

-um   _____

REVIEW QUESTIONS

▶ ## Matching

Select the appropriate lettered meaning for each numbered line.

_____	1. acne	a. Small, pinpoint, purplish hemorrhagic spots on the skin
_____	2. alopecia	b. The production of pus or serum
_____	3. cicatrix	c. A severe itching
_____	4. comedo	d. An inflammatory condition of the sebaceous gland and the hair follicles
_____	5. decubitus	e. The scar left after the healing of a wound
_____	6. dehiscence	f. Loss of hair, baldness
_____	7. exudate	g. White spots or patches formed on the mucous membrane of the tongue or cheek
_____	8. leukoplakia	h. Blackhead
_____	9. petechiae	i. The separation or bursting open of a surgical wound
_____	10. pruritus	j. A bedsore
		k. A slough, scab

▶ ## Abbreviations

Place the correct word, phrase, or abbreviation in the space provided.

1. fever of unknown origin _____

2. transdermal therapeutic system _____

3. H _____

4. incision and drainage _____

5. skin graft _____

6. ID _____

7. temperature _____

8. ultraviolet _____

9. FB _____

10. PUVA _____

▶ Diagnostic and Laboratory Tests

Select the best answer to each multiple choice question. Circle the letter of your choice.

1. The _____ _____ is an intradermal test performed using a sterile, disposable, multiple puncture lancet.
   a. sweat test
   b. Mantoux test
   c. tine test
   d. Tzanck test

2. A test done on wound exudate to determine the presence of microorganisms is:
   a. sweat test
   b. biopsy
   c. Tzanck test
   d. wound culture

3. A microscopic examination of a small piece of tissue that has been surgically scraped from a pustule is:
   a. Tzanck test
   b. sweat test
   c. biopsy
   d. wound culture

4. Tests performed to identify the presence of the *Tubercle bacilli* include the:
   a. tine, Heaf, and sweat
   b. tine, Heaf, and Mantoux
   c. tine, Tzanck, and Mantoux
   d. tine, Mantoux, and sweat

5. The _____ test may be used to determine the level of chloride concentration on the skin.
   a. sweat
   b. Tzanck
   c. tine
   d. Mantoux

CRITICAL THINKING ACTIVITY

► Case Study

Contact Dermatitis, Poison Ivy

Please read the following case study and then answer the questions that follow.

A 42-year-old male was seen by a dermatologist, and the following is a synopsis of his visit.

Present History: The patient states that he apparently came into contact with poison oak or poison ivy while working in the yard.

Signs and Symptoms: Chief Complaint: moderate itching at first and then severe (pruritus); small blisters (vesicles) on right and left forearms; redness of skin (erythroderma) with moderate to severe swelling (edema) of surrounding tissue.

Diagnosis: Contact Dermatitis Poison Ivy. See Figure 3–8.

Treatment: Antipruritic agent—hydroxyzine HCl 25 mg Tab; corticosteroid therapy—Temovate 0.05% cream—apply twice a day to affected area; and Sterapred 12 day unipak—take as directed.

Prevention: Stay away from poison oak and/or poison ivy. When working outside in the yard, wear clothing that covers arms and legs. After working in the yard, immediately take a bath or shower to remove any possible contamination of skin with poison oak or poison ivy.

Critical Thinking Questions

1. What is the medical term that means severe itching? _____

2. What is the medical term that means a papule with a fluid core; blister? _____

3. A person who is sensitive to poison oak or poison ivy may develop _____.

4. An antipruritic agent is used to help relieve _____.

5. Temovate 0.05% cream is a form of _____ therapy.

6. Prevention is a key concept in today's health care delivery system. List three preventive measures that the patient with contact dermatitis may use to help and/or prevent his condition.

   a. _____

   b. _____

   c. _____

7. The medical term for redness of the skin is _____.

8. The medical term for swelling is _____.

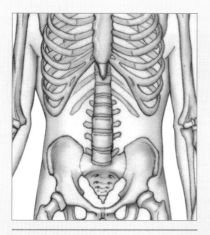

THE SKELETAL SYSTEM

OBJECTIVES

On completion of this chapter, you should be able to:

- Describe the skeletal system.
- Describe various types of body movement.
- Describe the vertebral column.
- Identify abnormal curvatures of the spine.
- Describe the male and female pelvis.
- Describe various types of fractures.
- Describe skeletal differences of the child and the older adult.
- Analyze, build, spell, and pronounce medical words that relate to surgical procedures and pathology.
- Identify and give the meaning of selected vocabulary words.
- Identify and define selected abbreviations.
- Review Drug Highlights presented in this chapter.
- Provide the description of diagnostic and laboratory tests related to the skeletal system.
- Successfully complete the study and review section.

▶ ANATOMY AND PHYSIOLOGY OVERVIEW

The skeletal system is composed of 206 *bones* that, together with *cartilage* and *ligaments,* make up the *framework* or skeleton of the body. The skeleton can be divided into two main groups of bones: the *axial skeleton* consisting of 80 bones and the *appendicular skeleton* with the remaining 126 bones (see Fig. 4–1). The principal bones of the axial skeleton are the skull, spine, ribs, and sternum. The shoulder girdle, arms, and hands and the pelvic girdle, legs, and feet are the primary bones of the appendicular skeleton (Fig. 4–2).

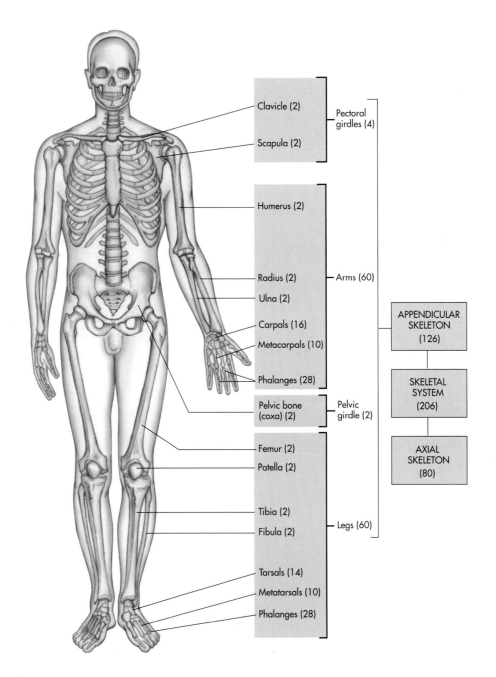

FIGURE 4–1

The principal bones of the appendicular skeleton.

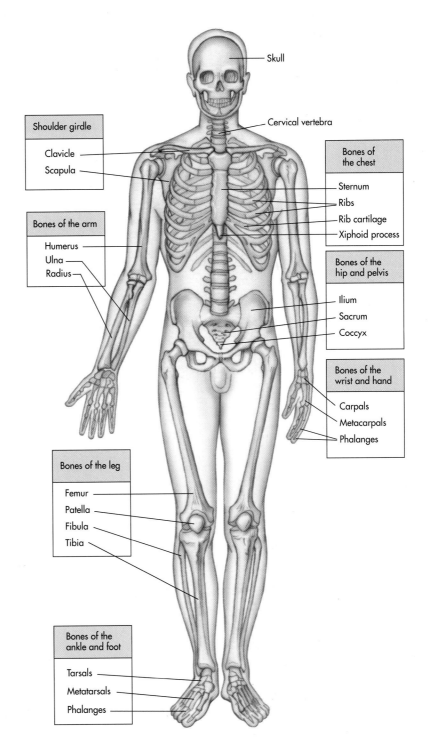

Skull

Cervical vertebra

Shoulder girdle

Clavicle

Scapula

Bones of the arm

Humerus

Ulna

Radius

Bones of the chest

Sternum

Ribs

Rib cartilage

Xiphoid process

Bones of the hip and pelvis

Ilium

Sacrum

Coccyx

Bones of the wrist and hand

Carpals

Metacarpals

Phalanges

Bones of the leg

Femur

Patella

Fibula

Tibia

Bones of the ankle and foot

Tarsals

Metatarsals

Phalanges

FIGURE 4–2

The skull, cervical vertebra, and principal bones of the axial and appendicular skeleton.

THE SKELETAL SYSTEM

ORGAN/STRUCTURE	PRIMARY FUNCTIONS
Bones	Provide shape, support, protection, and the framework of the body
	Serve as a storage place for mineral salts, calcium, and phosphorus
	Play an important role in the formation of blood cells
	Provide areas for the attachment of skeletal muscles
	Help make movement possible
Cartilages	Form the major portion of the embryonic skeleton and part of the skeleton in adults
Ligaments	Connect the articular ends of bones, binding them together and facilitating or limiting motion
	Connect cartilage and other structures
	Serve to support or attach fascia or muscles

► BONES

The *bones* are the primary organs of the skeletal system and are composed of about 50% water and 50% solid matter. The solid matter in bone is a calcified, rigid substance known as *osseous tissue.*

CLASSIFICATION OF BONES

Bones are classified according to their shapes. The following table classifies the bones and gives an example of each type:

SHAPE	EXAMPLE OF THIS CLASSIFICATION
Flat	Ribs, scapula, parts of the pelvic girdle, bones of the skull
Long	Tibia, femur, humerus, radius
Short	Carpal, tarsal
Irregular	Vertebrae, ossicles of the ear
Sesamoid	Patella

FUNCTIONS OF BONES

The following are the main functions of bones:

1. Provide shape and support and form the framework of the body
2. Provide protection for internal organs
3. Serve as a storage place for mineral salts, calcium, and phosphorus
4. Play an important role in the formation of blood cells as *hemopoiesis* takes place in the bone marrow
5. Provide areas for the attachment of skeletal muscles
6. Help to make movement possible through *articulation*

THE STRUCTURE OF A LONG BONE

Long bones, such as the tibia, femur, humerus, or radius, have most of the features found in all bones. These features are shown in Figure 4–3.

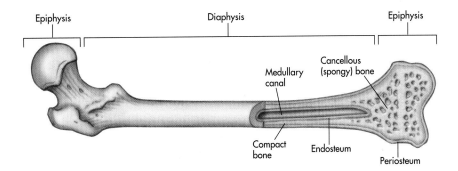

FIGURE 4-3

The features found in a long bone.

Epiphysis. The ends of a developing bone

Diaphysis. The shaft of a long bone

Periosteum. The membrane that forms the covering of bones except at their articular surfaces

Compact bone. The dense, hard layer of bone tissue

Medullary canal. A narrow space or cavity throughout the length of the diaphysis

Endosteum. A tough, connective tissue membrane lining the medullary canal and containing the bone marrow

Cancellous or spongy bone. The reticular tissue that makes up most of the volume of bone

BONE MARKINGS

There are certain commonly used terms that describe the *markings of bones*. These markings are listed for your better understanding of their role in joining bones together, providing areas for muscle attachments, and serving as a passageway for blood vessels, ligaments, and nerves.

MARKING	DESCRIPTION OF THE BONE STRUCTURE
Condyle	A rounded process that enters into the formation of a joint, articulation
Crest	A ridge on a bone
Fissure	A slit-like opening between two bones
Foramen	An opening in the bone for blood vessels, ligaments, and nerves
Fossa	A shallow depression in or on a bone
Head	The rounded end of a bone
Meatus	A tube-like passage or canal
Process	An enlargement or protrusion of a bone
Sinus	An air cavity within certain bones
Spine	A pointed, sharp, slender process
Sulcus	A groove, furrow, depression, or fissure
Trochanter	A very large process of the femur
Tubercle	A small, rounded process
Tuberosity	A large, rounded process

▶ JOINTS AND MOVEMENT

A *joint* is an articulation, a place where two or more bones connect. The manner in which bones connect determines the type of movement allowed at the joint. Joints are classified as:

Synarthrosis. Does not permit movement. The bones are in close contact with each other and there is no joint cavity. An example is the *cranial sutures.*

Amphiarthrosis. Permits very slight movement. An example of this type of joint is the *vertebrae.*

Diarthrosis. Allows free movement in a variety of directions. Examples of this type of joint are the *knee, hip, elbow, wrist,* and *foot.*

The following terms describe types of body movement that occur at the *diarthrotic joints* (Fig. 4–4):

Abduction. The process of moving a body part away from the middle

Adduction. The process of moving a body part toward the middle

Circumduction. The process of moving a body part in a circular motion

Dorsiflexion. The process of bending a body part backward

Eversion. The process of turning outward

Extension. The process of straightening a flexed limb

Flexion. The process of bending a limb

Inversion. The process of turning inward

Pronation. The process of lying prone or face downward; also the process of turning the hand so the palm faces downward

Protraction. The process of moving a body part forward

Retraction. The process of moving a body part backward

Rotation. The process of moving a body part around a central axis

Supination. The process of lying supine or face upward; also the process of turning the palm or foot upward

▶ THE VERTEBRAL COLUMN

The *vertebral column* is composed of a series of separate bones *(vertebrae)* connected in such a way as to form four spinal curves. These curves have been identified as the cervical, thoracic, lumbar, and sacral. The *cervical curve* consists of the first 7 vertebrae, the *thoracic curve* consists of the next 12 vertebrae, the *lumbar curve* consists of the next 5 vertebrae, and the *sacral curve* consists of the sacrum and coccyx (tailbone) (Fig. 4–5).

It is known that a curved structure has more strength than a straight structure. The spinal curves of the human body are most important, as they help support the weight of the body and provide the balance that is necessary to walk on two feet.

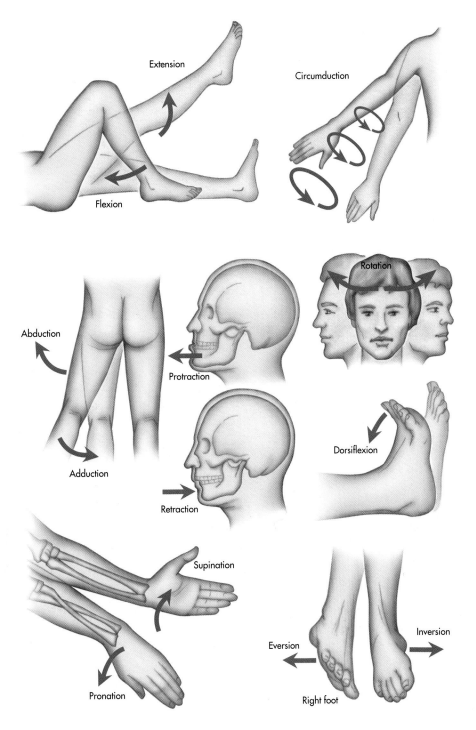

FIGURE 4–4

Types of body movements.

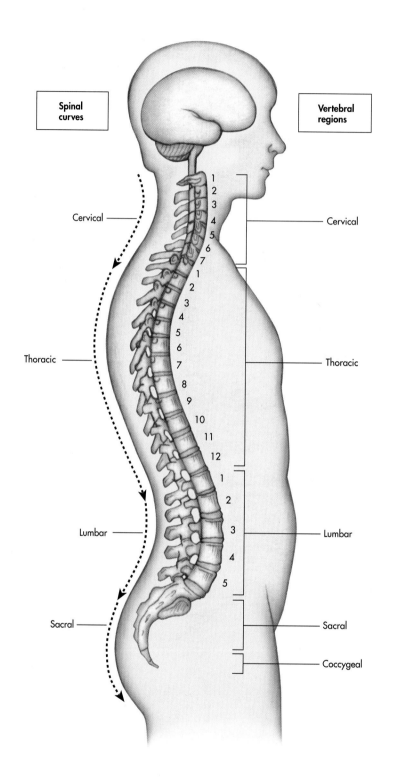

FIGURE 4–5

Vertebral regions, showing the four spinal curves.

► ABNORMAL CURVATURES OF THE SPINE

SCOLIOSIS, LORDOSIS, AND KYPHOSIS

In *scoliosis*, there is an abnormal lateral curvature of the spine. This condition usually appears in adolescence, during periods of rapid growth. Treatment modalities may include the application of a cast, brace, traction, electrical stimulation, and/or surgery. See Figure 4–6A.

In *lordosis*, there is an abnormal anterior curvature of the spine. This condition may be referred to as *"swayback"* as the abdomen and buttocks protrude due to an exaggerated lumbar curvature. See Figure 4–6B.

In *kyphosis*, the normal thoracic curvature becomes exaggerated, producing a *"humpback"* appearance. This condition may be caused by a congenital defect, a disease process such as tuberculosis and/or syphilis, a malignancy, compression fracture, faulty posture, osteoarthritis, rheumatoid arthritis, rickets, osteoporosis, or other conditions. See Figure 4–6C.

► THE MALE AND FEMALE PELVIS

The *pelvis* is the lower portion of the trunk of the body. It forms a basin bound anteriorly and laterally by the hip bones and posteriorly by the sacrum and coccyx.

The bony pelvis is formed by the sacrum, the coccyx, and the bones that form the hip and pubic arch, the ilium, pubis, and ischium. These bones are separate in the child, but become fused in adulthood.

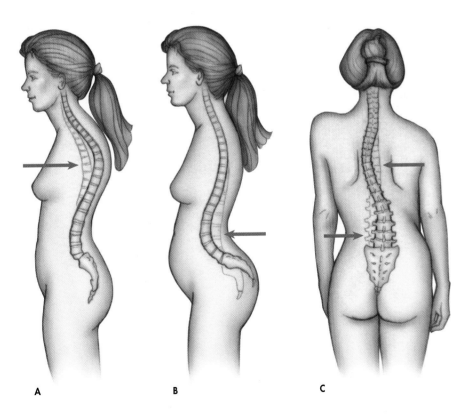

A   B   C

FIGURE 4–6

Abnormal curvatures of the spine: **(A)** kyphosis, **(B)** lordosis, **(C)** scoliosis.

THE MALE PELVIS

The *male pelvis* is shaped like a *funnel*, forming a narrower outlet than the female. It is heavier and stronger than the female pelvis; therefore, it is more suited for lifting and running. See Figure 4–7A.

THE FEMALE PELVIS

The *female pelvis* is shaped like a *basin*. It may be oval to round, and it is wider than the male pelvis. The female pelvis is constructed to accommodate the fetus during pregnancy and to facilitate its downward passage through the pelvic cavity in childbirth. In general the female pelvis is broader and lighter than the male pelvis. See Figure 4–7B.

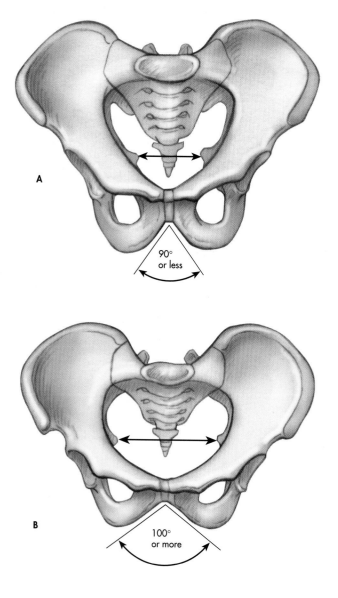

FIGURE 4–7

(A) The male pelvis is shaped like a funnel, forming a narrower outlet than the female. **(B)** The female pelvis is shaped like a basin.

▶ FRACTURES

Fractures are classified according to their external appearance, the site of the fracture, and the nature of the crack or break in the bone. Important fracture types are indicated in Figure 4–8 and several have been paired with representative x-rays. Many fractures fall in more than one category. For example, Colles' fracture is a transverse fracture, but depending on the injury it may also be a comminuted fracture that can be either open or closed.

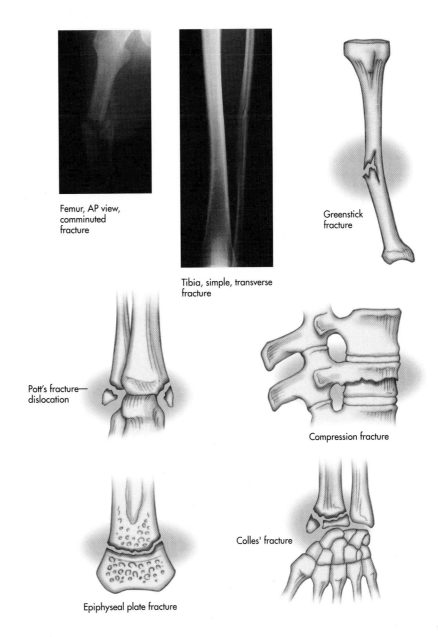

Femur, AP view, comminuted fracture

Tibia, simple, transverse fracture

Greenstick fracture

Pott's fracture— dislocation

Compression fracture

Epiphyseal plate fracture

Colles' fracture

FIGURE 4–8

Various types of fractures.

TYPES OF FRACTURES (SEE FIGURE 4–8)

- **Closed,** or **simple,** fractures do not involve a break in the skin; they are completely internal.
- **Open,** or **compound,** fractures are more dangerous because the fracture projects through the skin and there is a possibility of infection or hemorrhage.
- **Comminuted** fractures shatter the affected part into a multitude of bony fragments.
- **Transverse** fractures break the shaft of a bone across its longitudinal axis.
- **Greenstick** fractures usually occur in children whose long bones have not fully ossified; only one side of the shaft is broken, and the other is bent (like a green stick).
- **Spiral** fractures are spread along the length of a bone and are produced by twisting stresses.
- **Colles'** fracture is often the result of reaching out to cushion a fall; there is a break in the distal portion of the radius.
- **Pott's** fracture occurs at the ankle and affects both bones of the lower leg (fibula and tibia).
- **Compression** fractures occur in vertebrae subjected to extreme stresses, as when one falls and lands on his/her bottom.
- **Epiphyseal** fractures usually occur where the matrix is undergoing calcification and chondrocytes (cartilage cells) are dying; this type of fracture is seen in children.

LIFE SPAN CONSIDERATIONS

▶ THE CHILD

Bone begins to develop during the second month of fetal life as cartilage cells enlarge, break down, disappear, and are replaced by bone-forming cells called **osteoblasts.** Most bones of the body are formed by this process, known as **endochondral ossification.** In this process, the bone cells deposit organic substances in the spaces vacated by cartilage to form bone matrix. As this process proceeds, blood vessels form within the bone and deposit salts such as calcium and phosphorus that serve to harden the developing bone.

The **epiphyseal plate** is the center for longitudinal bone growth in children. See Figure 4–9. It is possible to determine the biological age of a child from the development of epiphyseal ossification centers as shown radiographically.

About 3 years from the onset of puberty the ends of the long bones **(epiphyses)** knit securely to their shafts **(diaphysis),** and further growth can no longer take place.

The bones of children are more resilient, tend to bend, and before breaking may become deformed. Fracture healing occurs more quickly in children because there is a rich blood supply to bones and

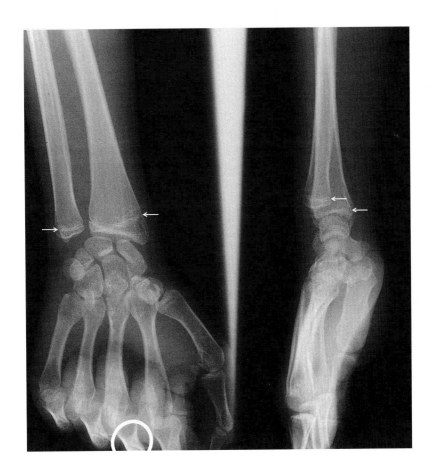

FIGURE 4–9

Epiphyseal plate (arrows). *(Courtesy of Teresa Resch.)*

their periosteum is thick and osteogenic activity is high.

Calcium is critical to the strength of bones. The daily recommendations of calcium by age group are:

- 1 to 3 years   500 mg
- 4 to 8 years   800 mg
- 9 to 13 years   1300 mg
- 14 to 18 years   1300 mg

▶ THE OLDER ADULT

Women build bone until about age 35, then begin to lose about 1% of bone mass annually. Men usually start losing bone mass 10 to 20 years later. Most of the skeletal system changes that take place during the aging process involve changes in connective tissue. There is a loss of bone mass and bone strength due to the loss of bone mineral content during later life. Calcium salts may be deposited in the matrix and cartilage becomes hard and brittle.

Age-related **osteoporosis,** loss of bone mass, is often seen in older women and men. Other changes that may occur involve the joints as there is diminished viscosity of the synovial fluid, degeneration of collagen and elastin cells, outgrowth of cartilaginous clusters in response to continuous wear and tear, and formation of scar tissues and calcification in the joint capsules.

Low levels of calcium can make people more susceptible to osteoporosis and stress fractures, especially those that are commonly seen in the older adult. Bone healing in the older adult is slower and impaired due to osteoblasts being less able to use calcium to restructure bone tissue. The National Academy of Sciences suggests that people 51 and older consume 1200 mg of calcium per day to help strengthen their bones. See Table 4–1 for good sources of calcium.

TABLE 4–1   Good Sources of Calcium

1 cup skim milk	300 mg
1 cup yogurt	450 mg
1 cup calcium-fortified orange juice	300 mg
1 ounce cheddar cheese	205 mg
1 ounce Swiss cheese	270 mg
1 cup tofu (processed with calcium sulfate)	520 mg
1 cup turnip greens, cooked	200 mg
3 ounces canned salmon (with bones)	205 mg
7-inch homemade waffle	179 mg
1 cup broccoli, cooked	90 mg

Dairy foods supply 75% of all the calcium in the U.S. food supply. People who get 2 to 3 servings of dairy products a day are most likely meeting the recommended requirements. For those who do not like milk or dairy products, there are other ways of getting enough calcium per day.

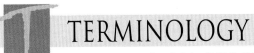

TERMINOLOGY
WITH SURGICAL PROCEDURES & PATHOLOGY

TERM	WORD PARTS			DEFINITION
acetabular (ăs″ ĕ-tăb′ ū-lăr)	acetabul ar	R S	vinegar cup pertaining to	The cup-shaped socket of the hipbone into which the thighbone fits
achillobursitis (ă-kil″ ō-bŭr-sī′ tĭs)	achillo burs itis	CF R S	achilles, heel a pouch inflammation	Inflammation of the bursa lying over the Achilles' tendon
achondroplasia (ă-kŏn″ drō-plā′ sĭ-ă)	a chondro plasia	P CF S	without cartilage formation	A defect in the formation of cartilage at the epiphyses of long bones
acroarthritis (ăk″ rō-ăr-thrī′ tĭs	acro arthr itis	CF R S	extremity joint inflammation	Inflammation of the joints of the hands or feet
acromion (ă-krō′ mĭ-ŏn)	acr omion	R S	extremity, point shoulder	The projection of the spine of the scapula that forms the point of the shoulder and articulates with the clavicle
ankylosis (ăng″ kĭ-lō′ sĭs)	ankyl osis	R S	stiffening, crooked condition of	A condition of stiffening of a joint
arthralgia (ăr-thrăl′ jĭ-ă)	arthr algia	R S	joint pain	Pain in a joint
arthrectomy (ăr-thrĕk′ tō-mē)	arthr ectomy	R S	joint excision	Surgical excision of a joint
arthredema (ăr″ thrĕ-dē′ mă)	arthr edema	R S	joint swelling	Swelling of a joint
arthritis (ăr-thrī′ tĭs)	arthr itis	R S	joint inflammation	Inflammation of a joint
arthrocentesis (ăr″ thrō-sĕn-tē′ sĭs)	arthro centesis	CF S	joint surgical puncture	Surgical puncture of a joint for removal of fluid
arthrodesis (ăr″ thrō-dē′ sĭs)	arthro desis	CF S	joint binding	The surgical binding of a joint for immobilization
arthropathy (ăr-thrŏp′ ă-thē)	arthro pathy	CF S	joint disease	Any joint disease

continued

Terminology - continued

TERM	WORD PARTS			DEFINITION
arthroplasty (ăr″ thrō-plăs′ tē)	arthro plasty	CF S	joint surgical repair	Surgical repair of a joint
arthropyosis (ăr″ thrō-pī-ō′ sĭs)	arthro py osis	CF R S	joint pus condition of	A condition of pus at a joint
bursectomy (bŭr-sĕk′ tō-mē)	burs ectomy	R S	a pouch excision	Surgical excision of a bursa
bursitis (bŭr-sī′ tĭs)	burs itis	R S	a pouch inflammation	Inflammation of a bursa
calcaneal (kăl-kā′ nē-ăl)	calcane al	R S	heel bone pertaining to	Pertaining to the heel bone
calcaneodynia (kăl-kā″ nē-ō-dĭn′ ĭ-ă)	calcaneo dynia	CF S	heel bone pain	Pain in the heel bone
carpal (kär′ pəl)	carp al	R S	wrist pertaining to	Pertaining to the wristbone
carpopedal (kär″ pō-pēd′ ăl)	carpo ped al	CF R S	wrist foot pertaining to	Pertaining to the wrist and the foot
carpoptosis (kär″ pŏp-tō′ sĭs)	carpo ptosis	CF S	wrist drooping	Wrist drop
chondral (kŏn′ drăl)	chondr al	R S	cartilage pertaining to	Pertaining to cartilage
chondralgia (kŏn-drăl′ jĭ-ă)	chondr algia	R S	cartilage pain	Pain in or around cartilage
chondrectomy (kŏn-drĕk′ tō-mē)	chondr ectomy	R S	cartilage excision	Surgical excision of a cartilage
chondroblast (kŏn′ drō-blăst)	chondro blast	CF S	cartilage immature cell, germ cell	A cell that forms cartilage
chondrocostal (kŏn″ drō-kŏs′ tăl)	chondro cost al	CF R S	cartilage rib pertaining to	Pertaining to the rib cartilage
chondropathology (kŏn″ drō-pă-thŏl′ ō-jē)	chondro patho logy	CF CF S	cartilage disease study of	The study of the diseases of cartilage

Terminology - continued

TERM	WORD PARTS			DEFINITION
clavicular (klă-vĭk′ ū-lăr)	clavicul ar	R S	little key pertaining to	Pertaining to the clavicle
cleidorrhexis (klī″ dō-rĕks′ sĭs)	cleido rrhexis	CF S	clavicle rupture	Rupture of the clavicle of the fetus to facilitate delivery
coccygeal (kŏk-sĭj′ ĭ-ăl)	coccyge al	CF S	tailbone pertaining to	Pertaining to the coccyx
coccygodynia (kŏk-sĭ-gō-dĭn′ ĭ-ă)	coccygo dynia	CF S	tailbone pain	Pain in the coccyx
collagen (kŏl′ ă-jĕn)	colla gen	CF S	glue formation, produce	A fibrous insoluble protein found in the connective tissue, skin, ligaments, and cartilage
connective (kə′ nĕk′ tĭv)	connect ive	R S	to bind together nature of	That which connects or binds together
costal (käst′ əl)	cost al	R S	rib pertaining to	Pertaining to the rib
costosternal (kŏs″ tō-stĕr′ năl)	costo stern al	CF R S	rib sternum pertaining to	Pertaining to a rib and the sternum
coxalgia (kŏk-săl′ jĭ-ă)	cox algia	R S	hip pain	Pain in the hip
coxofemoral (kŏk″ sō-fĕm′ ŏ-răl)	coxo femor al	CF R S	hip femur pertaining to	Pertaining to the hip and femur
craniectomy (krā″ nĭ-ĕk′ tŏ-mē)	crani ectomy	R S	skull excision	Surgical excision of a portion of the skull
cranioplasty (krā′ nĭ-ō-plăs″ tē)	cranio plasty	CF S	skull surgical repair	Surgical repair of the skull
craniotomy (krā″ nĭ-ŏt′ ō-mē)	cranio tomy	CF S	skull incision	Incision into the skull
dactylic (dăk′ tĭl′ ĭk)	dactyl ic	R S	finger or toe pertaining to	Pertaining to the finger or toe
dactylogram (dăk-til′ə grăm	dactylo gram	CF S	finger or toe mark, record	A fingerprint

continued

Terminology - continued

TERM	WORD PARTS			DEFINITION
dactylogryposis (dăk″ tĭ-lō-grĭ-pō′ sĭs)	dactylo gryp osis	CF R S	finger or toe curve condition of	Permanent contraction of the fingers
dactylomegaly (dăk″ tĭ-lō-měg′ ă-lē)	dactylo megaly	CF S	finger or toe enlargement, large	Enlargement of the fingers and toes
epicondyle (ĕp-ĭ-kŏn′ dīl)	epi condyle	P R	upon, above knuckle	A projection from a long bone near the articular extremity above or upon the condyle
femoral (fĕm′ ŏr-ăl)	femor al	R S	femur pertaining to	Pertaining to the femur; the thighbone
fibular (fĭb′ ū-lăr)	fibul ar	R S	fibula pertaining to	Pertaining to the fibula
humeral (hū′ měr-ăl)	humer al	R S	humerus pertaining to	Pertaining to the humerus
hydrarthrosis (hi″ drăr-thrō′ sĭs)	hydr arthr osis	P R S	water joint condition of	Condition of fluid in a joint
iliac (ĭl′ ē-ăk)	ili ac	R S	ilium pertaining to	Pertaining to the ilium
iliosacral (ĭl″ ĭ-ō-sā′ krăl)	ilio sacr al	CF R S	ilium sacrum pertaining to	Pertaining to the ilium and the sacrum
iliotibial (ĭl″ ĭ-ō-tĭb′ ĭ-ăl)	ilio tibi al	CF R S	ilium tibia pertaining to	Pertaining to the ilium and tibia
intercostal (ĭn″ tēr-kŏs′ tăl)	inter cost al	R R S	between rib pertaining to	Pertaining to between the ribs
ischial (ĭs′ kĭ-al)	ischi al	R S	ischium, hip pertaining to	Pertaining to the ischium, hip
ischialgia (ĭs″ kĭ-ăl′ jĭ-ă)	ischi algia	R S	ischium, hip pain	Pain in the ischium, hip
kyphosis (kī-fō′ sĭs)	kyph osis	R S	a hump condition of	Humpback
laminectomy (lăm″ ĭ-něk′ tō-mē)	lamin ectomy	R S	lamina (thin plate) excision	Surgical excision of a vertebral posterior arch

Terminology - continued

TERM	WORD PARTS			DEFINITION
lordosis (lŏr-dō′ sĭs)	lord osis	R S	bending condition of	Abnormal anterior curvature of the spine
lumbar (lŭm′ băr)	lumb ar	R S	loin pertaining to	Pertaining to the loins
lumbodynia (lŭm″ bō-dĭn′ ĭ-ă)	lumbo dynia	CF S	loin pain	Pain in the loins
mandibular (măn-dĭb′ ū-lăr)	mandibul ar	R S	lower jawbone pertaining to	Pertaining to the lower jawbone
maxillary (măk′ sĭ-lĕr″ ē)	maxill ary	R S	jawbone pertaining to	Pertaining to the upper jawbone
metacarpal (mĕt″ ă-kär′ pəl)	meta carp al	P R S	beyond wrist pertaining to	Pertaining to the bones of the hand
metacarpectomy (mĕt″ ă-kăr-pĕk′ tō-mē)	meta carp ectomy	P R S	beyond wrist excision	Surgical excision of one or more bones of the hand
myelitis (mī-ĕ-lī′ tĭs)	myel itis	R S	marrow inflammation	Inflammation of the bone marrow
myeloma (mī-ĕ-lō′ mă)	myel oma	R S	marrow tumor	A tumor of the bone marrow
myelopoiesis (mī′ ĕl-ō-poy-ē′ sĭs)	myelo poiesis	CF S	marrow formation	The formation of bone marrow
olecranal (ō-lĕk′ răn-ăl)	olecran al	R S	elbow pertaining to	Pertaining to the elbow
osteoarthritis (ŏs″ tē-ō-ăr-thrī′ tĭs)	osteo arthr itis	CF R S	bone joint inflammation	Inflammation of the bone and joint
osteoarthropathy (ŏs″ tē-ō-ăr-thrŏp′ ă-thē)	osteo arthro pathy	CF CF S	bone joint disease	Any disease of the bones and joints
osteoblast (ŏs′ tē-ō-blăst″)	osteo blast	CF S	bone immature cell, germ cell	A bone-forming cell
osteocarcinoma (ŏs″ tē-ō-kăr″ sĭn-ō mă)	osteo carcin oma	CF R S	bone cancer tumor	A cancerous tumor of a bone; new growth of epithelial tissue

continued

Terminology - continued

TERM	WORD PARTS			DEFINITION
osteochondritis (ŏs″ tē-ō-kŏn-drī′ tĭs)	osteo	CF	bone	Inflammation of the bone and cartilage
	chondr	R	cartilage	
	itis	S	inflammation	
osteoclasia (ŏs″ tē-ō-klā′ zĭ-ă)	osteo	CF	bone	Surgical fracture of a bone to correct a deformity
	clasia	S	a breaking	
osteodynia (ŏs″ tē-ō-dĭn′ ĭ-ă)	osteo	CF	bone	Pain in a bone
	dynia	S	pain	
osteofibroma (ŏs″ tē-ō-fī-brō′ mă)	osteo	CF	bone	A tumor of bone and fibrous tissues
	fibr	R	fibrous	
	oma	S	tumor	
osteogenesis (ŏs″ tē-ō-jĕn′ ĕ-sĭs)	osteo	CF	bone	The formation of bone
	genesis	S	formation, produce	
osteomalacia (ŏs″ tē- ō-măl-ā′ shĭ-ă)	osteo	CF	bone	Softening of the bones
	malacia	S	softening	
osteomyelitis (ŏs″ tē-ō-mī″ ĕl-ī′ tĭs)	osteo	CF	bone	Inflammation of the bone marrow
	myel	R	marrow	
	itis	S	inflammation	
osteonecrosis (ŏs″ tē-ō-nē-krō′ sĭs)	osteo	CF	bone	A condition in which there is death of bone tissue
	necr	R	death	
	osis	S	condition of	
osteopenia (ŏs″ tē-ō-pē′ nĭ-ă)	osteo	CF	bone	A lack of bone tissue
	penia	S	lack of	
osteoporosis (ŏs″ tē-ō-por-ō′ sĭs)	osteo	CF	bone	A condition that results in reduction of bone mass
	por	R	a passage	
	osis	S	condition of	

TERMINOLOGY SPOTLIGHT

Osteoporosis affects more than 25 million Americans, most of them women 50 to 70 years of age. Each year, the disease leads to 1.4 million bone fractures, including more than 500,000 vertebral fractures, 300,000 hip fractures, and 200,000 wrist fractures. Osteoporosis frequently occurs when there is not enough calcium in the diet. The body then uses calcium stored in bones, weakening them and making them vulnerable to breaking. See Table 4–1 for good sources of calcium.

There are some risk factors involved in developing osteoporosis and these are:

- Family history of osteoporosis
- Lack of exercise
- Thin, petite build
- Never been pregnant
- Early menopause (before 45 years)

- Prone to fractures, and loss of height in the past few years
- Avoided dairy products as a child
- Smoking, drinking alcoholic beverages
- Diet high in salt, caffeine, or fat

Terminology - continued

TERM	WORD PARTS			DEFINITION
osteorrhagia (ŏs″ tē-ō-ră′ jĭ-ă)	osteo rrhagia	CF S	bone to burst forth	Hemorrhage from a bone
osteorrhaphy (ŏs-tē-or′ ă-fē)	osteo rrhaphy	CF S	bone suture	Suture of a bone
osteosarcoma (ŏs″ tē-ō-săr-kō′ mă)	osteo sarc oma	CF R S	bone flesh tumor	A malignant tumor of the bone; cancer arising from connective tissue
osteosclerosis (ŏs″ tē-ō-sklĕ-rō′ sĭs)	osteo scler osis	CF R S	bone hardening condition of	A condition of hardening of the bone
osteotome (ŏs′ tē-ō-tōm″)	osteo tome	CF S	bone instrument to cut	An instrument used for cutting bone
patellapexy (pă-tĕl′ ă-pĕk″ sē)	patella pexy	R S	kneecap fixation	Surgical fixation of the patella
patellar (pă-tĕl′ ăr)	patell ar	R S	kneecap pertaining to	Pertaining to the patella
pedal (pĕd ′l)	ped al	R S	foot pertaining to	Pertaining to the foot
perichondral (pĕr″ i-kŏn′ drăl)	peri chondr al	P R S	around cartilage pertaining to	Pertaining to the membrane that covers cartilage
periosteoedema (pĕr″ ĭ-ŏs″ tē-ō- ĕ-dē′ mă)	peri osteo edema	P CF S	around bone swelling	Swelling around a bone
phalangeal (fā-lăn′ jē-ăl)	phalange al	CF S	closely knit row pertaining to	Pertaining to the bones of the fingers and the toes
polyarthritis (pŏl″ ē-ăr-thrī′ tĭs)	poly arthr itis	P R S	many, much joint inflammation	Inflammation of more than one joint
rachialgia (rā″ kĭ-ăl′ jĭ-ă)	rachi algia	CF S	spine pain	Pain in the spine
rachigraph (rā′ kĭ-grăf)	rachi graph	CF S	spine to write	An instrument used to measure the curvature of the spine
rachiotomy (rā″ kĭ-ŏt′ ō-mē)	rachio tomy	CF S	spine incision	Surgical incision of the spine

continued

Terminology - continued

TERM	WORD PARTS			DEFINITION
radial (rā′ dĭ-ăl)	radi al	CF S	radius pertaining to	Pertaining to the radius
scapular (skăp′ ū-lăr)	scapul ar	R S	shoulder blade pertaining to	Pertaining to the shoulder blade
scoliosis (skō″ lĭ-ō′ sĭs)	scoli osis	R S	curvature condition of	A condition of lateral curvature of the spine
scoliotone (skō′ lĭ-ō-tōn)	scolio tone	CF S	curvature tension	A device for correcting the curve in scoliosis by stretching the spine
spinal (spī′ năl)	spin al	R S	spine pertaining to	Pertaining to the spine
spondylitis (spŏn-dĭl-ī′ tĭs)	spondyl itis	R S	vertebra inflammation	Inflammation of one or more vertebrae
sternal (stēr′ năl)	stern al	R S	sternum pertaining to	Pertaining to the sternum
sternalgia (stēr-năl′ jĭ-ă)	stern algia	R S	sternum pain	Pain in the sternum
sternotomy (stēr-nŏt′ ō-mē)	sterno tomy	CF S	sternum incision	Surgical incision of the sternum
subclavicular (sŭb″ klă-vĭk′ ū-lăr)	sub clavicul ar	P R S	under, beneath a little key pertaining to	Pertaining to beneath the clavicle
subcostal (sŭb-kŏs′ tăl)	sub cost al	P R S	under, beneath rib pertaining to	Pertaining to beneath the ribs
submaxilla (sŭb″ măk-sĭl′ ă)	sub maxilla	P R	under, beneath jaw	The lower jaw or mandible
symphysis (sĭm′ fĭ-sĭs)	sym physis	P S	together growth	A growing together
syndesis (sĭn′ dē-sĭs)	syn desis	P S	together binding	Binding together; surgical fixation or ankylosis of a joint
tendoplasty (tĕn′ dō-plăs″ tē)	tendo plasty	CF S	tendon surgical repair	Surgical repair of a tendon
tenonitis (tĕn″ ō-nī′ tĭs)	tenon itis	R S	tendon inflammation	Inflammation of a tendon

Terminology - continued

TERM	WORD	PARTS		DEFINITION
tibial (tĭb′ ĭ-ăl)	tibi al	R S	tibia pertaining to	Pertaining to the tibia
ulnar (ŭl′ năr)	uln ar	R S	elbow pertaining to	Pertaining to the elbow
ulnocarpal (ŭl″ nō-kăr′ păl)	ulno carp al	CF R S	elbow wrist pertaining to	Pertaining to the ulna side of the wrist
ulnoradial (ŭl″ nō-rā′ dĭ-ăl)	ulno radi al	CF CF S	elbow radius pertaining to	Pertaining to the ulna and radius
vertebral (vĕr′ tĕ-brăl)	vertebr al	R S	vertebra pertaining to	Pertaining to a vertebra
vertebrectomy (vĕr″ tĕ-brĕk′ tō-mē)	vertebr ectomy	R S	vertebra excision	Surgical excision of a vertebra
vertebrosternal (vĕr″ tĕ-brō-ster′ năl)	vertebro stern al	CF R S	vertebra sternum pertaining to	Pertaining to a vertebra and the sternum
xiphoid (zĭf′ oyd)	xiph oid	R S	sword resemble	Resembling a sword

VOCABULARY WORDS

Vocabulary words are terms that have not been divided into component parts. They are common words or specialized terms associated with the subject of this chapter. These words are provided to enhance your medical vocabulary.

WORD	DEFINITION
arthroscope (ăr-thrŏs′ kōp)	An instrument used to examine the interior of a joint
bone marrow transplant (bōn măr′ ō trăns′ plănt)	The surgical process of transferring bone marrow from a donor to a patient

continued

Vocabulary - continued

WORD	DEFINITION
breakbone fever (brāk′ bōn fē′ vėr)	An acute febrile disease characterized by intense, arthritis-like pain; also known as *dengue fever*
bursa (bŭr′ sah)	A small space between muscles, tendons, and bones that is lined with synovial membrane and contains a fluid, *synovia*
calcium (kăl′ sĭ-ŭm)	A mineral that is essential for bone growth, teeth development, blood coagulation, and many other functions
carpal tunnel syndrome (kär′ pĕl tŭn′ ĕl sĭn′ drōm)	A condition caused by compression of the median nerve by the carpal ligament; symptoms: soreness, tenderness, weakness, pain, tingling, and numbness at the wrist
cartilage (kär′ tĭ-lĭj)	A specialized type of fibrous connective tissue present in adults, which forms the major portion of the embryonic skeleton
cast (kåst)	A type of material, made of plaster of paris, sodium silicate, starch, or dextrin used to immobilize a fractured bone, a dislocation, or a sprain
clawfoot (klō fút)	A deformity of the foot characterized by an abnormally high arch; *also known as pes cavus*
dislocation (dĭs″ lō-kā′ shŭn)	The displacement of a bone from a joint
fixation (fĭks-ā′ shŭn)	The process of holding or fastening in a fixed position; making rigid, immobilizing
flatfoot (flăt fút)	An abnormal flatness of the sole and arch of the foot; *also known as pes planus*
genu valgum (jē′ nū văl′ gŭm)	Knock-knee
genu varum (jē′ nū vā′ rŭm)	Bowleg
gout (gowt)	A hereditary metabolic disease that is a form of acute arthritis; usually begins in the knee or foot but can affect any joint
hallux (hăl″ ŭks)	The big or great toe
hammertoe (hăm′ er-tō)	An acquired flexion deformity of the interphalangeal joint

Vocabulary - continued

WORD	DEFINITION
ligament (lĭg′ ă-mĕnt)	A band of fibrous connective tissue that connects bones, cartilages, and other structures; also serves as a place for the attachment of fascia or muscle
meniscus (mĕn-ĭs′kŭs)	Crescent-shaped interarticular fibrocartilage found in certain joints, especially the lateral and medial *menisci* (semilunar cartilages) of the knee joint
phosphorus (fŏs′ fō-rŭs)	A mineral that is essential in bone formation, muscle contraction, and many other functions
radiograph (rā′ dĭ-ō-grăf)	An x-ray photograph of a body part
reduction (rē-dŭk′ shŭn)	The manipulative or surgical procedure used to correct a fracture or hernia
rheumatoid arthritis (roo′ mă-toyd ăr-thrī′ tĭs)	A chronic systemic disease characterized by inflammation of the joints, stiffness, pain, and swelling that results in crippling deformities. See Figure 4–10.
rickets (rĭk′ ĕts)	A deficiency condition in children primarily caused by a lack of vitamin D; may also result from inadequate intake or excessive loss of calcium
sequestrum (sē-kwĕs′ trŭm)	A fragment of a dead bone that has become separated from its parent bone
splint (splĭnt)	An appliance used for fixation, support, and rest of an injured body part
sprain (sprān)	Twisting of a joint that causes pain and disability
spur (spər)	A sharp or pointed projection, as on a bone
tennis elbow (tĕn′ ĭs ĕl′ bō)	A chronic condition characterized by pain caused by excessive pronation and supination activities of the forearm; usually caused by strain, as in playing tennis
traction (trăk′ shŭn)	The process of drawing or pulling on bones or muscles to relieve displacement and facilitate healing

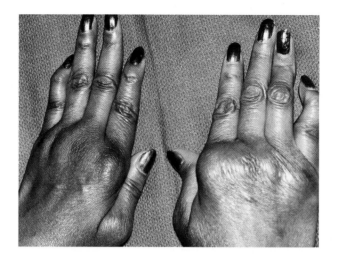

FIGURE 4–10

Rheumatoid arthritis. *(Courtesy of Jason L. Smith, MD.)*

 ## ABBREVIATIONS

AP	anteroposterior		**C-1**	cervical vertebra, first
CDH	congenital dislocation of hip		**C-2**	cervical vertebra, second
C-3	cervical vertebra, third		**ortho**	orthopedics, orthopaedics
Ca	calcium		**OA**	osteoarthritis
DJD	degenerative joint disease		**PEMFs**	pulsing electromagnetic fields
Fx	fracture		**PWB**	partial weight bearing
JRA	juvenile rheumatoid arthritis		**RA**	rheumatoid arthritis
jt	joint		**SAC**	short arm cast
KJ	knee jerk		**SLC**	short leg cast
L-1	lumbar vertebra, first		**SPECT**	single-photon emission
L-2	lumbar vertebra, second			computed tomography
L-3	lumbar vertebra, third		**T-1**	thoracic vertebra, first
LAC	long arm cast		**T-2**	thoracic vertebra, second
lig	ligament		**T-3**	thoracic vertebra, third
LLC	long leg cast		**TMJ**	temporomandibular joint
LLCC	long leg cylinder cast		**Tx**	traction

DRUG HIGHLIGHTS

Drugs that are generally used for skeletal system diseases and disorders include anti-inflammatory drugs, antirheumatic drugs, and analgesics. Fractures, arthritis, rheumatoid arthritis, bursitis, carpal tunnel syndrome, dislocation, and pain are some of the conditions involving the skeletal system and the need for pharmacologic therapy.

Anti-inflammatory Agents
Relieve the swelling, tenderness, redness, and pain of inflammation. These agents may be classified as steroidal (corticosteroids) and nonsteroidal.

Corticosteroids
Steroid substance with potent anti-inflammatory effects.
Examples: Depo-Medrol (methylprednisolone acetate), Aristocort (triamcinolone), Celestone (betamethasone), and Decadron (dexamethasone).

Nonsteroidal (NSAIDs)
Agents that are used in the treatment of arthritis and related disorders.
Examples: Bayer Aspirin (acetylsalicylic acid), Motrin (ibuprofen), Feldene (piroxicam), and Orudis (ketoprofen).

Antirheumatic Drugs
Prevent or relieve rheumatism. Rheumatism is defined as an acute or chronic condition characterized by inflammation, soreness and stiffness of muscles, and pain in joints and associated structures. *Gold therapy* and *Rheumatrex (methotrexate)* are used in the treatment of rheumatoid arthritis.

Gold therapy (chrysotherapy)
Used in the long-term treatment of rheumatoid arthritis. Gold preparations have been shown to be effective in reducing the progression of the disease, as well as relieving inflammation, but its use is limited by the toxicity of the gold compound.
Examples: Ridaura (auranofin), Myochrysine (gold sodium thiomalate), and Solganal (aurothioglucose).

Rheumatrex
A low-dose form of *methotrexate* approved for adult rheumatoid arthritis. It is recommended for selected adults with severe, active, classical, or definite rheumatoid arthritis who have had insufficient response to other forms of treatment. The patient may see improvement within 3 to 6 weeks.

Analgesics
Agents that relieve pain without causing loss of consciousness. They are classified as narcotic or non-narcotic.

Narcotic
Examples: Demerol (meperidine HCl) and morphine sulfate.

Non-narcotic
Examples: Tylenol (acetaminophen), aspirin, ibuprofen (Advil, Motrin, Nuprin), and Naprosyn (naproxen).

DIAGNOSTIC AND LABORATORY TESTS

Test	Description
arthrography (ăr-thrŏg′ ră-fē)	A diagnostic examination of a joint (usually the knee) in which air and, then, a radiopaque contrast medium are injected into the joint space, x-rays are taken, and internal injuries of the meniscus, cartilage, and ligaments may be seen, if present.
arthroscopy (ăr-thrŏs′ kō-pē)	The process of examining internal structures of a joint via an arthroscope; usually done after an arthrography and before joint surgery.
goniometry (gŏ″ nē-ŏm′ ĕt-rē)	The measurement of joint movements and angles via a goniometer.
photon absorptiometry (fō′ tŏn ăb-sorp′ shē-ŏm′ ĕt-rē)	A bone scan that uses a low beam of radiation to measure bone-mineral density and bone loss in the lumbar vertebrae; useful in monitoring osteoporosis.
thermography (thĕr-mŏg′ ră-fē)	The process of recording heat patterns of the body's surface; can be used to investigate the pathophysiology of rheumatoid arthritis.
x-ray (ĕks′ rā)	The examination of bones by use of an electromagnetic wave of high energy produced by the collision of a beam of electrons with a target in a vacuum tube; used to identify fractures and pathologic conditions of the bones and joints such as rheumatoid arthritis, spondylitis, and tumors.
alkaline phosphatase blood test (ăl′ kă-lĭn fŏs′ fă-tās)	A blood test to determine the level of alkaline phosphatase; increased in osteoblastic bone tumors, rickets, osteomalacia, and during fracture healing.
antinuclear antibodies (ANA) (ăn″ tĭ-nū′ klē-ăr ăn′ tĭ-bŏd″ ēs)	Present in a variety of immunologic diseases; positive result may indicate rheumatoid arthritis.
calcium (Ca) blood test (kăl′ sē- ŭm)	The calcium level of the blood may be increased in metastatic bone cancer, acute osteoporosis, prolonged immobilization, and during fracture healing; may be decreased in osteomalacia and rickets.
C-Reactive protein blood test (sē-rē-ăk″ tĭv prō′ tē-in)	Positive result may indicate rheumatoid arthritis, acute inflammatory change, and widespread metastasis.
phosphorus (P) blood test (fŏs′ fō-rŭs)	Phosphorus level of the blood may be increased in osteoporosis and fracture healing.

Test	Description
serum rheumatoid factor (RF) (sē′ rŭm roo′ mă-toyd făk′ tōr)	An immunoglobulin present in the serum of 50 to 95% of adults with rheumatoid arthritis.
uric acid blood test (ū′ rĭk ăs′ ĭd)	Uric acid is increased in gout, arthritis, multiple myeloma, and rheumatism.

COMMUNICATION ENRICHMENT

This segment is provided for those who wish to enhance their ability to communicate in either English or Spanish.

▶ Related Terms

English	Spanish	English	Spanish
fracture	fractura (frăc-*tŭ*-ră)	plaster	yeso (*jĕ*-sō)
sprain	torcer (*tōr*-sĕr)	ray	rayo (*ră*-jō)
bones	huesos (*wĕ*-sŏs)	crutches	muletas (mŭ-*lĕ*-tăs)
shoulder	hombros (*ōm*-brōs)	foot	pie (*pĭ*-ĕ)
elbow	codo (*kō*-dō)	hands	manos (*mă*-nōs)
wrist	muñeca (mŭ-*ñĕ*-kă)	joint	cojuntura (kō-jŭn-*tŭ*-ră)
fingers, toes	dedos (*dĕ*-dōs)	leg	pierna (pĭ′-*ĕr*-nă)
hip	cadera (kă-*dĕ*-ră)	neck	cuello (*kū*-ĕ-jŏ)
knee	rodilla (rō-*dĭ*-jă)	chest x-ray	radiografia del tórax (*ră*-dĭ-ō-gră-fĭ-ă dĕl *tō*-răx)
ankle	tobillo (tō-*bĭ*-jō)	rib	costilla (kōs-*tĭ*-jă)

English	Spanish	English	Spanish
cartilage	cartilago (*kăr*-tĭ-lă-gō)	water	agua (*ă*-gŭ-ă)
ligament	ligamento (*lĭ*-gă-mĭĕn-tō)	thigh	muslo (*mŭs*-lō)
skeleton	esqueleto (*ĕs*-kĕ-lĕ-tō)	pelvis	pelvis (*pĕl*-vĭs)
skull	craneo (*kră*-nĕ-ō)	shape	forma (*fōr*-mă)
spine	espinazo (ĕs-pĭ-*nă*-zō)	support	sustento (*sūs*-tĕn-tō)
calcium	calcio (*kăl*-sĭ-ō)	protection	protección (*prō*-tĕk-sĭ-ōn)
phosphorus	fósforo (*fōs*-fō-rō)	reduction	reducción (*rĕ*-dŭk-sĭ-ōn)

STUDY AND REVIEW SECTION

LEARNING EXERCISES

▶ Anatomy and Physiology

Write your answers to the following questions. Do not refer back to the text.

1. The skeletal system is composed of _____ bones.

2. Name the two main divisions of the skeletal system.

   a. _____   b. _____

3. Name the five classifications of bone and give an example of each.

   a. _____   Example _____

   b. _____   Example _____

   c. _____   Example _____

   d. _____   Example _____

   e. _____   Example _____

4. State the six main functions of the skeletal system.

    a. _____   b. _____

    c. _____   d. _____

    e. _____   f. _____

5. Define the following features of a long bone:

    a. Epiphysis _____

    b. Diaphysis _____

    c. Periosteum _____

    d. Compact bone _____

    e. Medullary canal _____

    f. Endosteum _____

    g. Cancellous or spongy bone _____

6. Match the term in column one with its definition from column two. Place the correct number from column two in the space provided in column one.

    _____ a. Meatus
    _____ b. Head
    _____ c. Tuberosity
    _____ d. Process
    _____ e. Condyle
    _____ f. Tubercle
    _____ g. Crest
    _____ h. Trochanter
    _____ i. Sinus
    _____ j. Fissure
    _____ k. Fossa
    _____ l. Spine
    _____ m. Foramen
    _____ n. Sulcus

    1. An air cavity within certain bones
    2. A shallow depression in or on a bone
    3. A pointed, sharp, slender process
    4. A large, rounded process
    5. A groove, furrow, depression, or fissure
    6. A tube-like passage or canal
    7. An opening in the bone for blood vessels, ligaments, and nerves
    8. A rounded process that enters into the formation of a joint, articulation
    9. A ridge on a bone
    10. A small, rounded process
    11. The rounded end of a bone
    12. A slit-like opening between two bones
    13. An enlargement or protrusion of a bone
    14. A very large process of the femur

7. Name the three classifications of joints.

    a. _____   b. _____

    c. _____

8. _____ is the process of moving a body part away from the middle.

9. Adduction is _____.

10. _____ is the process of moving a body part in a circular motion.

11. Dorsiflexion is _____.

12. _____ is the process of turning outward.

13. Extension is _____.

14. _____ is the process of bending a limb.

15. Inversion is _____.

16. _____ is the process of lying face downward.

17. Protraction is _____.

18. _____ is the process of moving a body part backward.

19. Rotation is _____.

20. _____ is the process of lying face upward.

▶ Word Parts

1. In the spaces provided, write the definition of these prefixes, roots, combining forms, and suffixes. Do not refer to the listings of terminology words. Leave blank those terms you cannot define.

2. After completing as many as you can, refer back to the terminology word listings to check your work. For each word missed or left blank, write the term and its definition several times on the margins of these pages or on a separate sheet of paper.

3. To maximize the learning process, it is to your advantage to do the following exercises as directed. To refer to the terminology listings before completing these exercises invalidates the learning process.

Prefixes

Give the definitions of the following prefixes:

1. a- _____   2. epi- _____

3. hydr- _____   4. inter- _____

5. meta- _____   6. peri- _____

7. poly- _____   8. sub- _____

9. sym- _____   10. syn- _____

Roots and Combining Forms

Give the definitions of the following roots and combining forms:

1. acetabul _____
2. achillo _____
3. acr _____
4. acro _____
5. ankyl _____
6. arthr _____
7. arthro _____
8. burs _____
9. calcane _____
10. calcaneo _____
11. carcin _____
12. carp _____
13. carpo _____
14. chondr _____
15. chondro _____
16. clavicul _____
17. cleido _____
18. coccyge _____
19. coccygo _____
20. colla _____
21. condyle _____
22. connect _____
23. cost _____
24. costo _____
25. cox _____
26. coxo _____
27. crani _____
28. cranio _____
29. dactyl _____
30. dactylo _____
31. femor _____
32. fibr _____
33. fibul _____
34. gryp _____
35. humer _____
36. ili _____
37. ilio _____
38. ischi _____
39. kyph _____
40. lamin _____
41. lord _____
42. lumb _____
43. lumbo _____
44. mandibul _____
45. maxill _____
46. maxilla _____
47. myel _____
48. myelo _____
49. necr _____
50. olecran _____
51. osteo _____
52. patell _____
53. patella _____
54. patho _____
55. ped _____
56. phalange _____

57. por _____   58. py _____

59. rachi _____   60. rachio _____

61. radi _____   62. sacr _____

63. sarc _____   64. scapul _____

65. scler _____   66. scoli _____

67. scolio _____   68. spin _____

69. spondyl _____   70. stern _____

71. sterno _____   72. tendo _____

73. tenon _____   74. tibi _____

75. uln _____   76. ulno _____

77. vertebr _____   78. vertebro _____

79. xiph _____

Suffixes

Give the definitions of the following suffixes:

1. -ac _____   2. -al _____

3. -algia _____   4. -ar _____

5. -ary _____   6. -blast _____

7. -centesis _____   8. -clasia _____

9. -desis _____   10. -dynia _____

11. -ectomy _____   12. -edema _____

13. -gen _____   14. -genesis _____

15. -gram _____   16. -graph _____

17. -ic _____   18. -itis _____

19. -ive _____   20. -logy _____

21. -malacia _____   22. -megaly _____

23. -oid _____   24. -oma _____

25. -omion _____   26. -osis _____

27. -pathy _____   28. -penia _____

29. -pexy _____   30. -physis _____

31. -plasia _____   32. -plasty _____

33. -poiesis _____   34. -ptosis _____

35. -rrhagia _____   36. -rrhaphy _____

37. -rrhexis _____   38. -tome _____

39. -tomy _____   40. -tone _____

▶ **Identifying Medical Terms**

In the spaces provided, write the medical term for the following meanings:

1. _____   Inflammation of the joints of the hands or feet

2. _____   The condition of stiffening of a joint

3. _____   Surgical excision of a joint

4. _____   Inflammation of a joint

5. _____   Any joint disease

6. _____   Pertaining to the heel bone

7. _____   Wrist drop

8. _____   Pertaining to cartilage

9. _____   Study of the diseases of cartilage

10. _____   Pain in the coccyx

11. _____   Pertaining to the rib

12. _____   Surgical excision of a portion of the skull

13. _____   Pertaining to the finger or toe

14. _____   Condition of fluid in a joint

15. _____   Pertaining to between the ribs

16. _____   Pain in the hip

17. _____   Pertaining to the loins

18. _____   A tumor of the bone marrow

19. _____   Inflammation of the joint and bone

20. _____   Pain in a bone

21. _____   Inflammation of the bone marrow

22. _____   A lack of bone tissue

23. _____   Pertaining to the foot

24. _____   Pain in the sternum

25. _____   Resembling a sword

▶ Spelling

In the spaces provided, write the correct spelling of these misspelled terms:

1. acrmoin _____   2. arthedema _____

3. buritis _____   4. chondblast _____

5. conective _____   6. cranplasty _____

7. dactlomegaly _____   8. ischal _____

9. melyitis _____   10. ostchonditis _____

11. ostnecrosis _____   12. patelar _____

13. phalangal _____   14. rachgraph _____

15. scolosis _____   16. spondlitis _____

17. symphsis _____   18. tennitis _____

19. ulncarpal _____   20. vertbral _____

WORD PARTS STUDY SHEET

Word Parts	Give the Meaning
epi-	_____
hydr-	_____
inter-	_____
meta-	_____
peri-	_____
poly-	_____
sym-, syn-	_____
acr-, acro-	_____
arthr-, arthro-	_____

burs- _____

chondr-, chondro- _____

dactyl-, dactylo- _____

fibr- _____

ischi- _____

kyph- _____

lord- _____

myel-, myelo- _____

osteo- _____

ped- _____

por- _____

scoli- _____

-algia _____

-al, -ic _____

-blast _____

-centesis _____

-clasia _____

-desis _____

-dynia _____

-ectomy _____

-itis _____

-ive _____

-logy _____

-malacia _____

-omnion _____

-osis _____

-pathy _____

-plasty _____

-tomy _____

REVIEW QUESTIONS

▶ Matching

Select the appropriate lettered meaning for each numbered line.

_____ 1. arthroscope

_____ 2. carpal tunnel syndrome

_____ 3. clawfoot

_____ 4. gout

_____ 5. hammertoe

_____ 6. kyphosis

_____ 7. metacarpal

_____ 8. rickets

_____ 9. tennis elbow

_____ 10. ulnar

a. A deficiency condition in children primarily caused by a lack of vitamin D
b. An acquired flexion deformity of the interphalangeal joint
c. A hereditary metabolic disease that is a form of acute arthritis
d. A chronic condition characterized by pain that is caused by excessive pronation and supination activities of the forearm
e. A deformity of the foot characterized by an abnormally high arch
f. Pertaining to the elbow
g. Pertaining to the bones of the hand
h. Humpback
i. An instrument used to examine the interior of a joint
j. A condition caused by compression of the median nerve by the carpal ligament
k. Pertaining to the knee

▶ Abbreviations

Place the correct word, phrase, or abbreviation in the space provided.

1. congenital dislocation of hip _____

2. degenerative joint disease _____

3. LLC _____

4. OA _____

5. pulsing electromagnetic fields _____

6. RA _____

7. single-photon emission computed tomography _____

8. T-1 _____

9. TMJ _____

10. traction _____

▶ Diagnostic and Laboratory Test

Select the best answer to each multiple choice question. Circle the letter of your choice.

1. _____ is a diagnostic examination of a joint in which air and, then, a radiopaque contrast medium are injected into the joint space, x-rays are taken, and internal injuries of the meniscus, cartilage, and ligaments may be seen, if present.
   a. Arthroscopy
   b. Goniometry
   c. Arthrography
   d. Thermography

2. The process of recording heat patterns of the body's surface is:
   a. arthrography
   b. arthroscopy
   c. goniometry
   d. thermography

3. _____ is increased in gout, arthritis, multiple myeloma, and rheumatism.
   a. Calcium
   b. Phosphorus
   c. Uric acid
   d. Alkaline phosphatase

4. _____ level of the blood may be increased in osteoporosis and fracture healing.
   a. Antinuclear antibodies
   b. Phosphorus
   c. Uric acid
   d. Alkaline phosphatase

5. _____ is/are present in a variety of immunologic diseases.
   a. Alkaline phosphatase
   b. Antinuclear antibodies
   c. C-Reactive protein
   d. Uric acid

CRITICAL THINKING ACTIVITY

▶ **Case Study**

Osteoporosis

Please read the following case study and then answer the questions that follow.

A 62-year-old female was seen by a physician, and the following is a synopsis of her visit.

Present History: The patient states that she seems to be shorter, her back "hurts" all the time, and she has developed a humpback.

Signs and Symptoms: Loss of height, kyphosis, and pain in the back.

Diagnosis: Osteoporosis (postmenopausal)

Treatment: Estrogen replacement therapy (ESTRADERM—Estradiol Transdermal System), begin a regular exercise program, a diet rich in calcium, phosphorus, magnesium, and vitamins A, C, D, the B-complex vitamins, and analgesics for pain.

Prevention: Know the risk factors involved in developing osteoporosis, follow a regular exercise program, and include a diet rich in calcium, phosphorus, magnesium, and vitamins A, C, D, and the B-complex vitamins. For more information on osteoporosis you can call the National Osteoporosis Foundation at 1–800–464–6700.

Good sources of **vitamin A** are dairy products, fish, liver oils, animal liver, green and yellow vegetables. Good sources of **vitamin D** are ultraviolet rays, dairy products, and commercial foods that contain supplemental vitamin D (milk and cereals). Good sources of **vitamin C** are citrus fruits, tomatoes, melons, fresh berries, raw vegetables, and sweet potatoes. Good sources of the **B-complex vitamins** are organ meats, dried beans, poultry, eggs, yeast, fish, whole grains, and dark-green vegetables. Good sources of **calcium** are dairy products, beans, cauliflower, egg yolk, molasses, leafy green vegetables, tofu, sardines, clams, and oysters. Good sources of **phosphorus** are dairy products, eggs, fish, poultry, meats, dried peas and beans, whole grain cereals, and nuts. Good sources of **magnesium** are whole grain cereals, fruits, milk, nuts, vegetables, seafood, and meats.

Critical Thinking Questions

1. Signs and symptoms of osteoporosis include loss of height, _____, and pain in the back.

2. _____ is an Estradiol Transdermal System.

3. Good sources of vitamin A are dairy products, fish, liver oils, _____ _____, green and yellow vegetables.

4. Good sources of magnesium are whole grain cereals, fruits, milk, _____, vegetables, seafood, and meats.

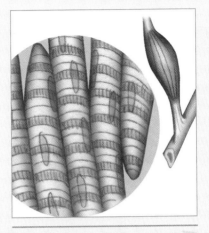

5

THE MUSCULAR SYSTEM

OBJECTIVES

On completion of this chapter, you should be able to:

- Describe the muscular system.
- Describe types of muscle tissue.
- Provide the functions of muscles.
- Describe muscular differences of the child and the older adult.
- Analyze, build, spell, and pronounce medical words that relate to surgical procedures and pathology.
- Identify and give the meaning of selected vocabulary words.
- Identify and define selected abbreviations.
- Review Drug Highlights presented in this chapter.
- Provide the description of diagnostic and laboratory tests related to the muscular system.
- Successfully complete the study and review section.

▶ ANATOMY AND PHYSIOLOGY OVERVIEW

The muscular system is composed of all the *muscles* in the body. This overview will describe the three basic types of muscles and some of their functions. The muscles are the primary tissues of the system. They make up approximately 42% of a person's body weight and are composed of long, slender cells known as *fibers*. Muscle fibers are of different lengths and shapes and vary in color from white to deep red. Each muscle consists of a group of fibers held together by connective tissue and enclosed in a fibrous sheath or *fascia*. See Figure 5–1. Each fiber within a muscle receives its own nerve impulses and has its own stored supply of glycogen, which it uses as fuel for energy. Muscle has to be supplied with proper nutrition and oxygen to perform properly; therefore, blood and lymphatic vessels permeate its tissues.

▶ TYPES OF MUSCLE TISSUE

Skeletal muscle, smooth muscle, and *cardiac muscle* are the three basic types of muscle tissue classed according to their functions and appearance (Fig. 5–2).

SKELETAL MUSCLE

Also known as *voluntary* or *striated* muscles, *skeletal muscles* are controlled by the conscious part of the brain and attach to the bones. There are 600 skeletal muscles that, through contractility, extensibility, and elasticity, are responsible for the movement of the body. These muscles have a cross-striped appearance and thus are known as striated muscles. They vary in size, shape, arrangement of fibers, and means of attachment to bones. Selected skeletal muscles are listed with their functions in Tables 5–1 and 5–2 and shown in Figures 5–3 and 5–4.

Skeletal muscles have two or more attachments. The more fixed attachment is known as the *origin*, and the point of attachment of a muscle to the part that it moves is the *insertion*. The means of attachment is called a *tendon*, which can vary in length from less than 1 inch to more than 1 foot. A wide, thin, sheet-like tendon is known as an *aponeurosis*.

A muscle has three distinguishable parts: the *body* or main portion, an *origin*, and an *insertion*. The skeletal muscles move body parts by pulling from one bone across its joint

THE MUSCULAR SYSTEM

ORGAN/STRUCTURE	PRIMARY FUNCTIONS
Muscles	Responsible for movement, help to maintain posture, and produce heat
Skeletal	Through contractility, extensibility, and elasticity, are responsible for the movement of the body
Smooth	Produce relatively slow contraction with greater degree of extensibility in the internal organs, especially organs of the digestive, respiratory, and urinary tract, plus certain muscles of the eye and skin, and walls of blood vessels
Cardiac	Muscle of the heart, controlled by the autonomic nervous system and specialized neuromuscular tissue located within the right atrium that is capable of causing cardiac muscle to contract rhythmically. The neuromuscular tissue of the heart comprises the sinoatrial node, the atrioventricular node, and the atrioventricular bundle
Tendons	A band of connective tissue serving for the attachment of muscles to bones

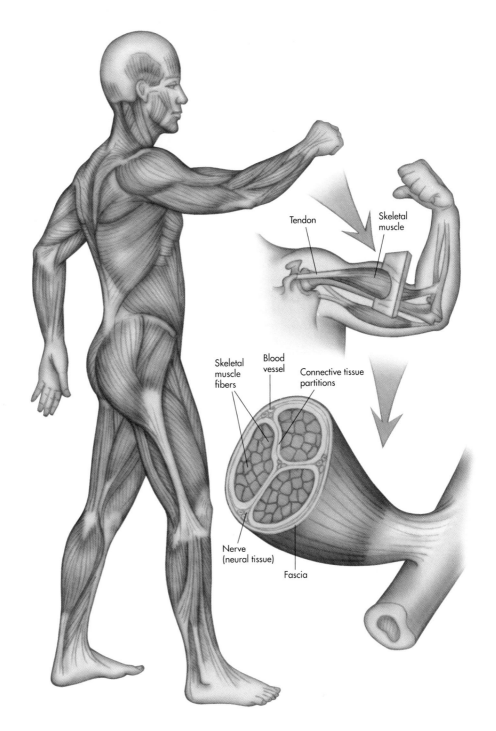

FIGURE 5–1

A skeletal muscle consists of a group of fibers held together by connective tissue. It is enclosed in a fibrous sheath (fascia).

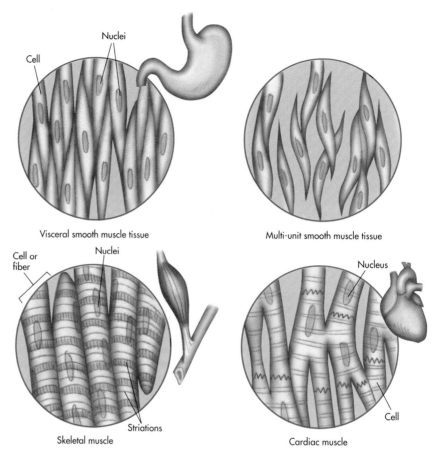

FIGURE 5–2

Types of muscle tissue.

TABLE 5–1   Selected Skeletal Muscles (Anterior View)

Muscle	Action
Sternocleidomastoid	Rotates and laterally flexes neck
Trapezius	Draws head back and to the side, rotates scapula
Deltoid	Raises and rotates arm
Rectus femoris	Extends leg and assists flexion of thigh
Sartorius	Flexes and rotates the thigh and leg
Tibialis anterior	Dorsiflexes foot and increases the arch in the beginning process of walking
Pectoralis major	Flexes, adducts, and rotates arm
Biceps brachii	Flexes arm and forearm and supinates forearm
Rectus abdominis	Compresses or flattens abdomen
Gastrocnemius	Plantar flexes foot and flexes knee
Soleus	Plantar flexes foot

TABLE 5-2   Selected Skeletal Muscles (Posterior View)

Muscle	Action
Trapezius	Draws head back and to the side, rotates scapula
Deltoid	Raises and rotates arm
Triceps	Extends forearm
Latissimus dorsi	Adducts, extends, and rotates arm. Used during swimming
Gluteus maximus	Extends and rotates thigh
Biceps femoris	Flexes knee and rotates it outward
Gastrocnemius	Plantar flexes foot and flexes knee
Semitendinosus	Flexes and rotates leg, extends thigh

to another bone with movement occurring at the diarthrotic joint. The types of body movement occurring at the diarthrotic joints are described in the chapter entitled The Skeletal System.

Muscles and nerves function together as a motor unit. For skeletal muscles to contract, it is necessary to have stimulation by impulses from motor nerves. Muscles perform in groups and are classified as:

- **Antagonist.** A muscle that counteracts the action of another muscle
- **Prime mover.** A muscle that is primary in a given movement. Its contraction produces the movement.
- **Synergist.** A muscle that acts with another muscle to produce movement

SMOOTH MUSCLE

Also called *involuntary, visceral,* or *unstriated, smooth muscles* are not controlled by the conscious part of the brain. They are under the control of the autonomic nervous system and, in most cases, produce relatively slow contraction with greater degree of extensibility. These muscles lack the cross-striped appearance of skeletal muscle and are smooth. Included in this type are the muscles of internal organs of the digestive, respiratory, and urinary tract, plus certain muscles of the eye and skin.

CARDIAC MUSCLE

The muscle of the heart *(myocardium)* is *involuntary* but *striated* in appearance. It is controlled by the autonomic nervous system and specialized neuromuscular tissue located within the right atrium.

▶ FUNCTIONS OF MUSCLES

The following is a list of the primary functions of muscles:

1. Muscles are responsible for movement. The types of movement are locomotion, propulsion of substances through tubes as in circulation and digestion, and changes in the size of openings as in the contraction and relaxation of the iris of the eye.
2. Muscles help to maintain posture through a continual partial contraction of skeletal muscles. This process is known as *tonicity.*
3. Muscles help to produce heat through the chemical changes involved in muscular action.

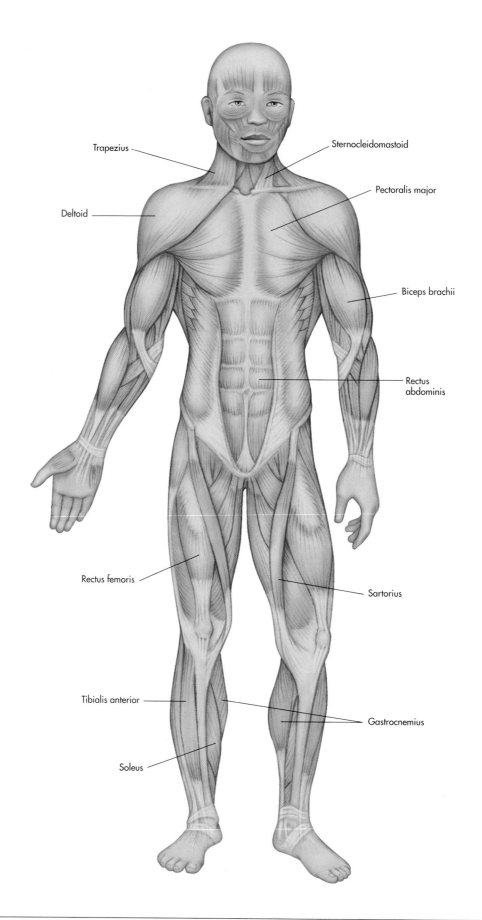

FIGURE 5–3

Selected skeletal muscles (anterior view).

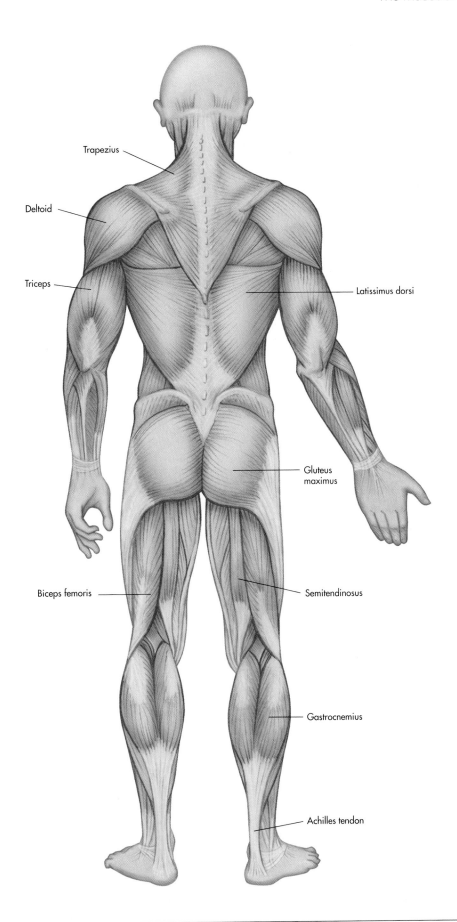

Trapezius

Deltoid

Triceps

Latissimus dorsi

Gluteus
maximus

Biceps femoris

Semitendinosus

Gastrocnemius

Achilles tendon

FIGURE 5–4

Selected skeletal muscles and the Achilles tendon (posterior view).

LIFE SPAN CONSIDERATIONS

▶ THE CHILD

At about 6 weeks the size of the embryo is 12 mm (0.5 inch). The limb buds are extending and the skeletal and muscular systems are developing. At about 7 weeks the **diaphragm,** a partition of muscles and membranes that separates the chest cavity and the abdominal cavity, is completely developed. At the end of 8 weeks, the embryo is now known as the **fetus.** Fetal growth proceeds from head to tail **(cephalo** to **caudal),** with the head being larger in comparison to the rest of the body.

During fetal development the bones and muscles continue growing and developing. At about 32 weeks the developed skeletal system is soft and flexible. Muscle and fat accumulate and the fetus weighs approximately 2000 g (4 lb, 7 oz). At about 40 weeks the fetus is ready for birth and extrauterine life.

The movements of the newborn are uncoordinated and random. Muscular development proceeds from head to foot and from the center of the body to the periphery. Head and neck muscles are the first ones that can be controlled by the baby. A baby can hold his head up before he can sit erect. The baby needs freedom of movement. The bath is an excellent time for the newborn to exercise.

▶ THE OLDER ADULT

With aging changes related to mobility are most significant. There is a decrease in muscle strength, endurance, range of motion, coordination and elasticity, and flexibility of connective tissue. There is an actual loss in the number of muscle fibers due to **myofibril atrophy** with fibrous tissue replacement, which begins in the fourth decade of life.

To prevent loss of strength, muscles need to be exercised. Regular exercise strengthens muscles and keeps joints, tendons, and ligaments more flexible, allowing active people to move freely and carry out routine activities easily. Exercises such as aerobic dance, brisk walking, and bicycling improve muscle tone and heart and lung function. To maintain aerobic fitness one needs to participate in such activities for 20 minutes or more at least three times a week and work at one's target heart rate. The target range declines with age and the following table shows the correct range during exercise for women between 45 and 65 years old.

AGE	TARGET HEART RATE (BEATS PER MINUTE)
45 years old	108 to 135
50 years old	102 to 127
55 years old	99 to 123
60 years old	96 to 120
65 years old	93 to 116

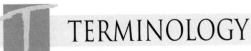

TERMINOLOGY
WITH SURGICAL PROCEDURES & PATHOLOGY

TERM	WORD PARTS			DEFINITION
abductor (ăb-dŭk′ tōr)	ab duct or	P R S	away from to lead a doer	A muscle that, on contraction, draws away from the middle
adductor (ă-dŭk′ tōr)	ad duct or	P R S	toward to lead a doer	A muscle that draws a part toward the middle
antagonist (ăn-tăg′ ō-nĭst)	ant agon ist	P R S	against agony, a contest agent	A muscle that counteracts the action of another muscle
aponeurorrhaphy (ăp″ ō-nū-ror′ ă-fē)	apo neuro rrhaphy	P CF S	separation nerve suture	Suture of an aponeurosis
aponeurosis (ăp″ ō-nū-rō′ sĭs)	apo neur osis	P R S	separation nerve condition of	A fibrous sheet of connective tissue that serves to attach muscle to bone or to other tissues
ataxia (ă-tăks′ ĭ-ă)	a taxia	P S	lack of order	A lack of muscular coordination
atonic (ă-tŏn′ ĭk)	a ton ic	P R S	lack of tone, tension pertaining to	Pertaining to a lack of normal tone or tension
atrophy (ăt′ rō-fē)	a trophy	P S	lack of nourishment, development	A lack of nourishment; a wasting of muscular tissue that may be caused by lack of use

TERMINOLOGY SPOTLIGHT

Atrophy occurs with the disuse of muscles over a long period of time. Bedrest and immobility can cause loss of muscle mass and strength. When immobility is due to a treatment mode, such as casting or traction, one can decrease the effects of immobility by isometric exercise of the muscles of the immobilized part. Isometric exercise involves active muscular contraction performed against stable resistance, such as tightening the muscles of the thigh and/or tightening the muscles of the buttocks. Active exercise of uninjured parts of the body helps prevent muscle atrophy.

continued

TERM	WORD PARTS			DEFINITION

Other benefits of exercise:

- It may slow down the progression of osteoporosis.
- It reduces the levels of triglycerides and raises the "good" cholesterol (high-density lipoproteins).
- It can lower systolic and diastolic blood pressure.
- It may improve blood glucose levels in the diabetic person.
- Combined with a low-fat, low-calorie diet, it is effective in preventing obesity and helping individuals maintain a proper body weight.
- It can elevate one's mood and reduce anxiety and tension.

Lipoatrophy is atrophy of fat tissue. This condition may occur at the site of an insulin and/or corticosteroid injection. It is also known as lipodystrophy. See Figure 5–5.

TERM	WORD PARTS			DEFINITION
biceps (bī′ sĕps)	bi ceps	P S	two head	A muscle with two heads or points of origin
brachialgia (brā″ kǐ-ăl′ jǐ-ă)	brachi algia	CF S	arm pain	Pain in the arm
bradykinesia (brăd″ ǐ-kǐ-nē′ sǐ-ă)	brady kinesia	P S	slow motion	Slowness of motion or movement
clonic (klŏn′ ǐk)	clon ic	R S	turmoil pertaining to	Pertaining to alternate contraction and relaxation of muscles
contraction (kŏn-trăk′ shŭn)	con tract ion	P R S	with, together to draw process	The process of drawing up and thickening of a muscle fiber
dactylospasm (dăk′ tǐ-lō-spăzm)	dactylo spasm	CF S	finger or toe tension, spasm	Cramp of a finger or toe
diaphragm (dī′ ă-frăm)	dia phragm	P S	through a fence, partition	The partition, of muscles and membranes, that separates the chest cavity and the abdominal cavity
dystonia (dǐs′ tō′ nǐ-ă)	dys ton ia	P R S	difficult tone, tension condition	A condition of impaired muscle tone
dystrophy (dǐs′ trō-fē)	dys trophy	P S	difficult nourishment, development	Faulty muscular development caused by lack of nourishment

Terminology - continued

TERM	WORD PARTS			DEFINITION
fascia (făsh′ ĭ-ă)	fasc ia	R S	a band condition	A thin layer of connective tissue covering, supporting, or connecting the muscles or inner organs of the body
fasciectomy (făsh″ ĭ-ĕk′ tō-mē)	fasci ectomy	CF S	a band excision	Surgical excision of fascia
fasciodesis (făsh ĭ-ŏd′ ĕ-sĭs)	fascio desis	CF S	a band binding	Surgical binding of a fascia to a tendon or another fascia
fascioplasty (făsh′ ĭ-ō-plăs″ tē)	fascio plasty	CF S	a band surgical repair	Surgical repair of a fascia
fascitis (fă-sī′ tĭs)	fasc itis	R S	a band inflammation	Inflammation of a fascia
fibromyitis (fī″ brō-mī-ī′ tĭs)	fibro my itis	CF R S	fiber muscle inflammation	Inflammation of muscle and fibrous tissue
insertion (ĭn″ sûr′ shŭn)	in sert ion	P R S	into to gain process	The point of attachment of a muscle to the part that it moves
intramuscular (ĭn″ tră-mŭs′kū-lər)	intra muscul ar	P R S	within muscle pertaining to	Pertaining to within a muscle
isometric (ī″ sō-mĕt′ rĭk)	iso metr ic	CF R S	equal to measure pertaining to	Pertaining to having equal measure
isotonic (ī″ sō-tŏn′ ĭk)	iso ton ic	CF R S	equal tone, tension pertaining to	Pertaining to having the same tone or tension
levator (lē-vā′ tər	levat or	R S	lifter a doer	A muscle that raises or elevates a part
lordosis (lŏr-dō′ sĭs)	lord osis	R S	bending condition of	Abnormal anterior curve of the spine
myalgia (mī-ăl′ jĭ-ă)	my algia	R S	muscle pain	Pain in the muscle
myasthenia (mī-ăs-thē′ nĭ-ă)	my asthenia	R S	muscle weakness	Muscle weakness

continued

Terminology - continued

TERM	WORD PARTS			DEFINITION
myitis (mī-ī′ tĭs)	my itis	R S	muscle inflammation	Inflammation of a muscle
myoblast (mī′ ō blăst)	myo blast	CF S	muscle immature cell, germ cell	An embryonic cell that develops into a cell of muscle fiber
myofibroma (mī″ ō fī-brō′ mă)	myo fibr oma	CF R S	muscle fiber tumor	A tumor that contains muscle and fiber
myogenesis (mī″ō-jĕn′ ĕ-sĭs)	myo genesis	CF F	muscle formation, produce	Formation of muscle tissue
myograph (mī′ ō-grăf)	myo graph	CF S	muscle to write, record	An instrument used to record muscular contractions
myoid (mī′ oid)	my oid	R S	muscle resemble	Resembling muscle
myokinesis (mī″ ō-kĭn-ē′ sĭs)	myo kinesis	CF S	muscle motion	Muscular motion or activity
myology (mĭ-ōl ō-jē)	myo logy	CF S	muscle study of	The study of muscles
myolysis (mī-ŏl′ ĭ-sĭs)	myo lysis	CF S	muscle destruction	Destruction of muscle tissue
myoma (mī-ō′ mă)	my oma	R S	muscle tumor	A tumor containing muscle tissue
myomalacia (mī″ ō-mă-lā′ sĭ-ă)	myo malacia	CF S	muscle softening	Softening of muscle tissue
myomelanosis (mī″ ō-mĕl-ă-nō′ sĭs)	myo melan osis	CF R S	muscle black condition of	A condition of abnormal darkening of muscle tissue
myoparesis (mī″ ō-păr′ ĕ-sĭs)	myo paresis	CF S	muscle weakness	Weakness or slight paralysis of a muscle
myopathy (mī-ŏp′ ă-thē)	myo pathy	CF S	muscle disease	Muscle disease
myoplasty (mī′-ŏ-plăs″tē)	myo plasty	CF S	muscle surgical repair	Surgical repair of a muscle

Terminology - continued

TERM	WORD PARTS			DEFINITION
myorrhaphy (mī-ŏr′ ă-fē)	myo rrhaphy	CF S	muscle suture	Suture of a muscle wound
myorrhexis (mī-ŏr-ĕk′ sĭs)	myo rrhexis	CF S	muscle rupture	Rupture of a muscle
myosarcoma (mī″ ō-sar-kō′ mă)	myo sarc oma	CF R S	muscle flesh tumor	A malignant tumor derived from muscle tissue
myosclerosis (mī″ ō-sklĕr-ō′ sĭs)	myo scler osis	CF R S	muscle hardening condition of	A condition of hardening of muscle
myospasm (mī″ ō-spăzm)	myo spasm	CF S	muscle tension, spasm	Spasmodic contraction of a muscle
myotenositis (mī″ ō-tĕn″ ō-sī′ tĭs)	myo tenos itis	CF R S	muscle tendon inflammation	Inflammation of a muscle and its tendon
myotome (mī′ ō-tōm)	myo tome	CF S	muscle instrument to cut	An instrument used to cut muscle
myotomy (mī″ŏt′ ō-mē)	myo tomy	CF S	muscle incision	Incision into a muscle
myotrophy (mī″ŏt′ rō-fē)	myo trophy	CF S	muscle nourishment, development	Nourishment of muscle tissue
neuromuscular (nū″ rō-mŭs′ kū-lăr)	neuro muscul ar	CF R S	nerve muscle pertaining to	Pertaining to both nerves and muscles
neuromyopathic (nū″ rō-mī″ ō-păth′ ĭk)	neuro myo path ic	CF CF R S	nerve muscle disease pertaining to	Pertaining to disease of both nerves and muscles
neuromyositis (nū″ rō-mī″ ō-sī′ tĭs)	neuro myos itis	CF R S	nerve muscle inflammation	Inflammation of nerves and muscles
polymyoclonus (pŏl″ ē-mī ŏk′ lō-nŭs)	poly myo clon us	P CF R S	many muscle turmoil pertaining to	Pertaining to a shock-like muscular contraction occurring in various muscles at the same time

continued

Terminology - continued

TERM	WORD PARTS			DEFINITION
polyplegia (pŏl″ē-plē′jĭ-ă)	poly plegia	P S	many stroke, paralysis	Paralysis affecting many muscles
quadriceps (kwŏd′rĭ-sĕps)	quadri ceps	P S	four head	A muscle that has four heads or points of origin
relaxation (rē-lăk-sā′shŭn)	relaxat ion	R S	to loosen process	The process in which a muscle loosens and returns to a resting stage
rhabdomyoma (răb″dō-mī-ō′mă)	rhabdo my oma	CF R S	rod muscle tumor	A tumor of striated muscle tissue
rotation (rō-tā′shŭn)	rotat ion	R S	to turn process	The process of moving a body part around a central axis
sarcitis (sar-sī′tĭs)	sarc itis	R S	flesh inflammation	Inflammation of muscle tissue
sarcolemma (sar″kō-lĕm′ă)	sarco lemma	CF R	flesh a rind	A plasma membrane surrounding each striated muscle fiber
spasticity (spăs-tĭs′ĭ-tē)	spastic ity	R S	convulsive condition	A condition of increased muscular tone causing stiff and awkward movements
sternocleidomas-toid (stur″nō-klī″ dō-măs′toyd)	sterno cleido mast oid	CF CF R S	sternum clavicle breast resemble	Muscle arising from the sternum and clavicle with its insertion in the mastoid process
synergetic (sin″ĕr-jĕt′ĭk)	syn erget ic	P R S	with, together work pertaining to	Pertaining to certain muscles that work together
tenodesis (tĕn-ōd′ĕ-sĭs)	teno desis	CF S	tendon binding	Surgical binding of a tendon
tenodynia (tĕn″ō-dĭn-ĭ-ă)	teno dynia	CF S	tendon pain	Pain in a tendon
tenorrhaphy (tĕn-ōr′ă-fē)	teno rrhaphy	CF S	tendon suture	Suture of a tendon
tenotomy (tĕn-ŏt′ō-mē)	teno tomy	CF S	tendon incision	Surgical incision of a tendon

Terminology - continued

TERM	WORD PARTS			DEFINITION
tonic (tŏn′ ĭk)	ton ic	R S	tone, tension pertaining to	Pertaining to tone, especially muscular tension
torticollis (tŏr″ tĭ-kŏl′ ĭs)	torti collis	CF R	twisted neck	Stiff neck caused by spasmodic contraction of the muscles of the neck; wry neck
triceps (trī′ sĕps)	tri ceps	P S	three head	A muscle having three heads with a single insertion
voluntary (vŏl′ ŭn-tĕr″ ē)	volunt ary	R S	will pertaining to	Pertaining to under the control of one's will

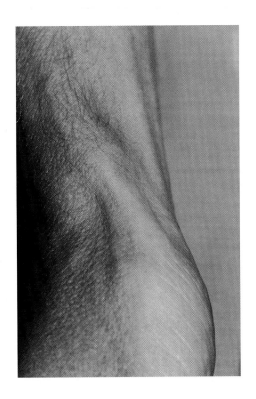

FIGURE 5–5

Lipoatrophy, wrist. *(Courtesy of Jason L. Smith, MD.)*

VOCABULARY WORDS

Vocabulary words are terms that have not been divided into component parts. They are common words or specialized terms associated with the subject of this chapter. These words are provided to enhance your medical vocabulary.

WORD	DEFINITION
amputation (ăm″ pū-tā′ shŭn)	Surgical excision of a limb, part, or other appendage
contracture (kōn-trăk′ chūr)	A condition in which a muscle shortens and renders the muscle resistant to the normal stretching process
degeneration (dē-gĕn″ ĕ-rā′ shŭn)	The process of deteriorating; to change from a higher to a lower form
dermatomyositis (dĕr″ mă-tō-mī″ ō-sī′ tĭs)	Inflammation of the muscles and the skin; a connective tissue disease characterized by edema, dermatitis, and inflammation of the muscles. See Figure 5–6.
diathermy (dī′ ă-thĕr″ mē)	Treatment using high-frequency current to produce heat within a part of the body; used to increase blood flow and should not be used in acute stage of recovery from trauma. Types: **Microwave.** Electromagnetic radiation is directed to specified tissues **Short-wave.** High-frequency electric current (wavelength of 3–30 m) is directed to specified tissues **Ultrasound.** High-frequency sound waves (20,000–10 billion cycles/sec) are directed to specified tissues
Dupuytren's contracture (dū-pwē- tranz′ kŏn-trăk′ chŭr)	A slow, progressive contracture of the palmar fascia causing the ring and little fingers to bend into the palm so that they cannot be extended. See Figure 5–7.
dystrophin (dĭs-trōf′ ĭn)	A protein found in muscle cells; when the gene that is responsible for this protein is defective and sufficient dystrophin is not produced, muscle wasting occurs
exercise (ĕk′ sĕr-sīz)	Performed activity of the muscles for improvement of health or correction of deformity. Types: **Active.** The patient contracts and relaxes his or her muscles **Assistive.** The patient contracts and relaxes his or her muscles with the assistance of a therapist **Isometric.** Active muscular contraction performed against stable resistance, thereby not shortening the muscle length **Passive.** Exercise is performed by another individual without the assistance of the patient

Vocabulary - continued

WORD	DEFINITION
	Range of Motion. Movement of each joint through its full range of motion. Used to prevent loss of motility or to regain usage after an injury or fracture **Relief of Tension.** Technique used to promote relaxation of the muscles and provide relief from tension
extrinsic (ĕks-trĭn′ sĭk)	Pertaining to external origin; a muscle or muscles partly attached to the trunk and partly to a limb
fatigue (fă-tēg′)	A state of tiredness or weariness occurring in a muscle as a result of repeated contractions
fibromyalgia (fī″ brō-mī-ăl′ jē-ă)	A condition with widespread muscular pain and debilitating fatigue; believed to have an organic or biochemical cause. Diagnosis may be made by testing for unusual tenderness at specific body points.
First Aid Treatment—RICE **Rest** **Ice** **Compression** **Elevation**	**Cryotherapy** (use of cold) is the treatment of choice for soft tissue injuries and muscle injuries. It causes vasoconstriction of blood vessels and is effective in diminishing bleeding and edema. Ice should not be placed directly onto the skin. **Compression** by an elastic bandage is generally determined by the type of injury and the preference of the physician. Some experts disagree on the use of elastic bandages. When used, the bandage should be 3 to 4 inches wide and applied firmly, and toes or fingers should be periodically checked for blue or white discoloration, indicating that the bandage is too tight. **Elevation** is used to reduce swelling. The injured part should be elevated on two or three pillows.
flaccid (flăk′ sĭd)	Lacking muscle tone; *weak, soft,* and *flabby*
heat (hēt)	**Thermotherapy.** The treatment using scientific application of heat may be used 48 to 72 hours after the injury. Types: heating pad, hot water bottle, hot packs, infrared light, and immersion of body part in warm water. Extreme care should be followed when using or applying heat.
hydrotherapy (hī-drō-thĕr′ă-pē)	Treatment using scientific application of water; types: hot tub, cold bath, whirlpool, and vapor bath
intrinsic (ĭn-trĭn′ sĭk)	Pertaining to internal origin; a muscle or muscles that have their origin and insertion within a structure
involuntary (ĭn-vŏl′ ŭn-tăr″ ē)	Pertaining to action independent of the will

continued

Vocabulary - continued

WORD	DEFINITION
manipulation (măh-nĭp″ ŭ-lā′ shŭn)	The process of using the hands to handle or manipulate as in massage of the body
massage (măh-săhzh)	To knead, apply pressure and friction to external body tissues
muscular dystrophy (mŭs′ kū-lār dĭs′ trō-fē)	A chronic, progressive wasting and weakening of muscles. It is a familial disease and onset is usually at an early age
myositis (mī-ō-sī′ tĭs)	Inflammation of muscle tissue
origin (ŏr′ ĭ-jĭn)	The beginning of anything; the more fixed attachment of a skeletal muscle
position (pō-zĭsh′ ŭn)	Bodily posture or attitude; the manner in which a patient's body may be arranged for examination

Types of positions and their descriptions:

Anatomic. Body is erect, head facing forward, arms by the sides with palms to the front; used as the position of reference in designating the site or direction of a body structure

Dorsal Recumbent. Patient is on back with lower extremities flexed and rotated outward; used in application of obstetric forceps, vaginal and rectal examination, and bimanual palpation

Fowler's. The head of the bed or examining table is raised about 18 inches or 46 cm, and the patient sits up with knees also elevated

Knee–Chest. Patient on knees, thighs upright, head and upper part of chest resting on bed or examining table, arms crossed and above head; used in sigmoidoscopy, displacement of prolapsed uterus, rectal exams, and flushing of intestinal canal

Lithotomy. Patient is on back with lower extremities flexed and feet placed in stirrups; used in vaginal examination, Pap smear, vaginal operations, and diagnosis and treatment of diseases of the urethra and bladder

Orthopneic. Patient sits upright or erect; used for patients with dyspnea

Prone. Patient lying face downward; used in examination of the back, injections, and massage

Sims'. Patient is lying on left side, right knee and thigh flexed well up above left leg that is slightly flexed, left arm behind the body, and right arm forward, flexed at elbow; used in examination of rectum, sigmoidoscopy, enema, and intrauterine irrigation after labor

Supine. Patient lying flat on back with face upward and arms at the sides; used in examining the head, neck, chest, abdomen, and extremities and in assessing vital signs

Vocabulary - continued

WORD	DEFINITION
	Trendelenburg. Patient's body is supine on a bed or examining table that is tilted at about 45° angle with the head lower than the feet; used to displace abdominal organs during surgery and in treating cardiovascular shock; also called the "shock position"
prosthesis (prŏs′ thē-sĭs)	An artificial device, organ, or part such as a hand, arm, leg, or tooth
rheumatism (roo′ mă-tĭzm)	A general term used to describe conditions characterized by inflammation, soreness and stiffness of muscles, and pain in joints
rigor mortis (rĭg′ ur mȯr tĭs)	Stiffness of skeletal muscles seen in death
rotator cuff (rō-tā′ tor kŭf)	A term used to describe the muscles immediately surrounding the shoulder joint. They stabilize the shoulder joint while the entire arm is moved.
strain (strān)	Excessive, forcible stretching of a muscle or the musculotendinous unit
synovectomy (sĭn″ ō-vĕk′ tō-mē)	Surgical excision of a synovial membrane
tendon (tĕn′ dŭn)	A band of fibrous connective tissue serving for the attachment of muscles to bones; a giant cell tumor of a tendon sheath is a benign, small, yellow, tumor-like nodule. See Figure 5–8.
torsion (tȯr′ shŭn)	The process of being twisted

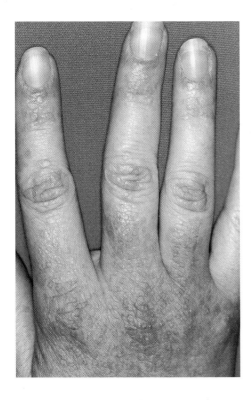

FIGURE 5–6

Dermatomyositis. *(Courtesy of Jason L. Smith, MD.)*

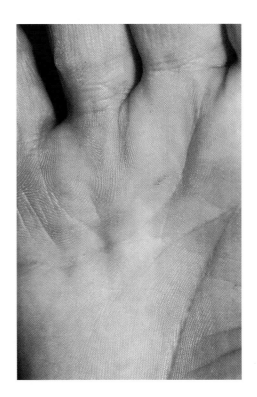

FIGURE 5–7

Dupuytren's contracture. *(Courtesy of Jason L. Smith, MD.)*

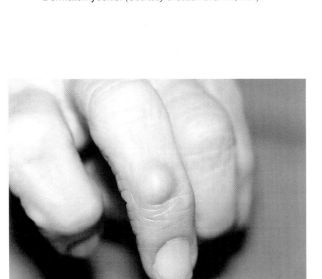

FIGURE 5–8

Giant cell tumor of tendon sheath. *(Courtesy of Jason L. Smith, MD.)*

The Muscular System **163**

ABBREVIATIONS

ADP	adenosine diphosphate		**LOM**	limitation or loss of motion
AE	above elbow		**MS**	musculoskeletal
AK	above knee		**NSAIDs**	nonsteroidal anti-inflammatory drugs
ALD	aldolase			
AST	aspartate transaminase		**PM**	physical medicine
ATP	adenosine triphosphate		**PMR**	physical medicine and rehabilitation
BE	below elbow			
BK	below knee		**ROM**	range of motion
Ca	calcium		**SGOT**	serum glutamic oxaloacetic transaminase
CPK	creatine phosphokinase			
CPM	continuous passive motion		**SGPT**	serum glutamic pyruvic transaminase
DTRs	deep tendon reflexes			
EMG	electromyography		**sh**	shoulder
FROM	full range of motion		**TBW**	total body weight
Ht	height		**TJ**	triceps jerk
IM	intramuscular		**Wt**	weight
LDH	lactic dehydrogenase			

DRUG HIGHLIGHTS

Drugs that are generally used for muscular system diseases and disorders include skeletal muscle relaxants and stimulants, neuromuscular blocking agents, anti-inflammatory agents, and analgesics. See Chapter 4, The Skeletal System, Drug Highlights for a description of anti-inflammatory agents and analgesics.

Skeletal Muscle Relaxants	Used to treat painful muscle spasms that may result from strains, sprains, and musculoskeletal trauma or disease. Centrally acting muscle relaxants act by depressing the central nervous system (CNS) and can be administered either orally or by injection. The patient must be informed of the sedative effect produced by these drugs. Drowsiness, dizziness, and blurred vision may diminish the patient's ability to drive a vehicle, operate equipment, or climb stairs. *Examples: Paraflex (chlorzoxazone), Flexeril (cyclobenzaprine HCl), and Robaxin (methocarbamol).*
Skeletal Muscle Stimulants	Used in the treatment of myasthenia gravis. This disease is characterized by progressive weakness of skeletal muscles and their rapid fatiguing. Skeletal muscle stimulants act by inhibiting the action of acetylcholinesterase, the enzyme that halts the action of acetylcholine at the neuromuscular junction. By slowing the destruction of acetylcholine, these drugs foster accumulation of higher concentrations of this neurotransmitter and increase the number of interactions between acetylcholine and the available receptors on muscle fibers. *Examples: Mytelase (ambenonium chloride), Tensilon (edrophonium chloride), and Prostigmin Bromide (neostigmine bromide).*

Neuromuscular Blocking Agents   Used to provide muscle relaxation. These agents are used in patients undergoing surgery and/or electroconvulsive therapy, endotracheal intubation, and to relieve laryngospasm. *Examples: Tracrium (atracurium besylate), Flaxedil (gallamine triethiodide), and Norcuron (vecuronium).*

DIAGNOSTIC AND LABORATORY TESTS

Test	Description
aldolase (ALD) blood test (ăl′ dŏ-lāz blod test)	A test performed on serum that measures ALD enzyme present in skeletal and heart muscle. It is helpful in the diagnosis of Duchenne's muscular dystrophy before symptoms appear.
calcium blood test (kăl′ sē-ŭm blod test)	A test performed on serum to determine levels of calcium. Calcium is essential for muscular contraction, nerve transmission, and blood clotting.
creatine phosphokinase (CPK) (krē′ ă-tĭn fŏs″ fō-kīn′ āz)	A blood test to determine the level of CPK. It is increased in necrosis or atrophy of skeletal muscle, traumatic muscle injury, strenuous exercise, and progressive muscular dystrophy.
electromyography (EMG) (ē-lĕk″ trō-mī-ŏg′ ră-fē)	A test to measure electrical activity across muscle membranes by means of electrodes that are attached to a needle that is inserted into the muscle. Electrical activity can be heard over a loudspeaker, viewed on an oscilloscope, or printed on a graph (electromyogram). Abnormal results may indicate myasthenia gravis, amyotrophic lateral sclerosis, muscular dystrophy, peripheral neuropathy, and anterior poliomyelitis.
lactic dehydrogenase (LDH) (lăk′ tĭk dē-hī-drŏj′ ĕ-nāz)	A blood test to determine the level of LDH enzyme. It is increased in muscular dystrophy, damage to skeletal muscles, after a pulmonary embolism, and during skeletal muscle malignancy.
muscle biopsy (mŭs′ ĕl bī′ ŏp-sē)	An operative procedure in which a small piece of muscle tissue is excised and then stained for microscopic examination. Lower motor neuron disease, degeneration, inflammatory reactions, or involvement of specific muscle fibers may indicate myopathic disease.
serum glutamic-oxaloacetic transaminase (SGOT) (sē′ rŭm gloo-tăm′ ĭk ŏks″ ăl-ō-ă-sē′ tĭk trăns ăm′ ĭn-āz)	A blood test to determine the level of SGOT enzyme. It is increased in skeletal muscle damage and muscular dystrophy. This test is also called aspartate transaminase (AST).

Test	Description
serum glutamic pyruvic transaminase (SGPT) (sē′ rŭm gloo-tăm′ ĭk pī-roo′ vĭk trăns-ăm′ ĭn-āz)	A blood test to determine the level of SGPT enzyme. It is increased in skeletal muscle damage. This test is also called alanine aminotransferase (ALT).

COMMUNICATION ENRICHMENT

This segment is provided for those who wish to enhance their ability to communicate in either English or Spanish.

▶ Related Terms

English	Spanish	English	Spanish
muscle	músculo (*mūs*-kū-lō)	shoulder	hombro (*ōm*-brō)
muscle spasm	espasmo muscular (ĕs-*păs*-mō *mŭs*-kū-lăr)	stiffness	tiesura (tĭ-ĕ-*sū*-ră)
		contraction	contracción (cōn-trăk-sĭ-*ōn*)
raise your:	levante su: (lĕ-*văn*-tĕ sū)	twitch	crispamiento (*krĭs*-pă-mĭ-ĕn-tō)
arm	brazo (*bră*-zō)	tighten	estrechar (ĕs-trĕ-*chăr*)
leg	pierna (pĭ-*ĕr*-nă)	walk	caminar (kă-mĭ-*năr*)
muscle biopsy	biopsia muscular (bĭ-*ōp*-sĭ-ă *mŭs*-kū-lăr)	limitation of movement	limitación de movimiento (lĭ-mĭ-tă-sĭ-*ōn* dĕ *mō*-vĭ-mĭ-ĕn-tō)
weight	peso (*pĕ*-sō)	tendon	tendón (*tĕn*-dōn)
height	altura (ăl-*tū*-ră)	neck	cuello (*kwā*-yō)
malaise	malestar (*mă*-lĕs-tăr)	finger, toe	dedo (*dĕ*-dō)
painful	doloroso (dō-lō-*rō*-sō)		

English	Spanish	English	Spanish
fiber	fibra (*fĭ*-bră)	amputate	amputar (ăm-pū-*tăr*)
bend	vuelta (*vū*-ĕl-tă)	sport	deporte (dĕ-*pōr*-tĕ)
motion	moción (*mō*-sĭ-ōn)	heat	calor (kă-*lōr*)
weakness	debilidad (dĕ-bĭ-lĭ-*dăd*)	massage	masaje (mă-*să*-hĕ)
fatigue	fatiga (*fă*-tĭ-gă)	harden	endurecer (ĕn-*dū*-rĕ-sĕr)
tone	tono (*tō*-nō)	tense	tenso (*tĕn*-sō)
flaccid	flacido (*flă*-sĭ-dō)	nourishment	nutrimento (nū-trĭ-mĭ-*ĕn*-tō)
position	posición (pō-sĭ-sĭ-*ōn*)	two	dos (dōs)
development	desarrollo (dĕ-să-*rō*-jō)	slow	lento (*lĕn*-tō)
exercise	ejercicio (ĕ-hĕr-*sĭ*-sĭ-ō)		

STUDY AND REVIEW SECTION

LEARNING EXERCISES

▶ **Anatomy and Physiology**

Write your answers to the following questions. Do not refer back to the text.

1. The muscular system is made up of three types of muscle tissue. Name the three types.

   a. _____   b. _____

   c. _____

2. Muscles make up approximately _____ percent of a person's body weight.

3. Name the two essential ingredients that are needed for a muscle to perform properly.

   a. _____   b. _____

4. Name the two points of attachment for a skeletal muscle.

   a. _____   b. _____

5. Skeletal muscle is also known as _____ or _____.

6. A wide, thin, sheet-like tendon is known as an _____.

7. Name the three distinguishable parts of a muscle.

   a. _____   b. _____

   c. _____

8. Define the following:

   a. Antagonist _____

   b. Prime mover _____

   c. Synergist _____

9. Smooth muscle is also called _____, _____, or _____.

10. Smooth muscles are found in the internal organs. Name five examples of these locations.

    a. _____   b. _____

    c. _____   d. _____

    e. _____

11. _____ is the muscle of the heart.

12. Name the three primary functions of the muscular system.

   a. _____   b. _____

   c. _____

▶ **Word Parts**

1. In the spaces provided, write the definition of these prefixes, roots, combining forms, and suffixes. Do not refer to the listings of terminology words. Leave blank those terms you cannot define.

2. After completing as many as you can, refer back to the terminology word listings to check your work. For each word missed or left blank, write the term and its definition several times on the margins of these pages or on a separate sheet of paper.

3. To maximize the learning process, it is to your advantage to do the following exercises as directed. To refer to the terminology listings before completing these exercises invalidates the learning process.

Prefixes

Give the definitions of the following prefixes:

1. a- _____   2. ab- _____

3. ad- _____   4. ant- _____

5. apo- _____   6. bi- _____

7. brady- _____   8. con- _____

9. dia- _____   10. dys- _____

11. in- _____   12. intra- _____

13. poly- _____   14. quadri- _____

15. syn- _____   16. tri- _____

Roots and Combining Forms

Give the definitions of the following roots and combining forms:

1. agon _____   2. brachi _____

3. cleido _____   4. clon _____

5. collis _____   6. dactylo _____

7. duct _____   8. erget _____

9. fasc _____
10. fasci _____
11. fascio _____
12. fibr _____
13. fibro _____
14. iso _____
15. lemma _____
16. levat _____
17. lord _____
18. mast _____
19. melan _____
20. metr _____
21. muscul _____
22. my _____
23. myo _____
24. myos _____
25. neur _____
26. neuro _____
27. path _____
28. relaxat _____
29. rhabdo _____
30. rotat _____
31. sarc _____
32. sarco _____
33. scler _____
34. sert _____
35. spastic _____
36. sterno _____
37. teno _____
38. tenos _____
39. ton _____
40. torti _____
41. tract _____
42. volunt _____

Suffixes

Give the definitions of the following suffixes:

1. -algia _____
2. -ar _____
3. -ary _____
4. -asthenia _____
5. -blast _____
6. -ceps _____
7. -desis _____
8. -dynia _____
9. -ectomy _____
10. -genesis _____
11. -graph _____
12. -ia _____
13. -ic _____
14. -ion _____
15. -ist _____
16. -itis _____
17. -ity _____
18. -kinesia _____
19. -kinesis _____
20. -logy _____

21. -lysis _____   22. -malacia _____

23. -oid _____   24. -oma _____

25. -or _____   26. -osis _____

27. -paresis _____   28. -pathy _____

29. -phragm _____   30. -plasty _____

31. -plegia _____   32. -rrhaphy _____

33. -rrhexis _____   34. -spasm _____

35. -taxia _____   36. -tome _____

37. -tomy _____   38. -trophy _____

39. -us _____

▶ Identifying Medical Terms

In the spaces provided, write the medical terms for the following meanings:

1. _____   Suture of an aponeurosis

2. _____   Pertaining to a lack of normal tone or tension

3. _____   Slowness of motion or movement

4. _____   Cramp of a finger or toe

5. _____   Faulty muscular development caused by lack of nourishment

6. _____   Surgical repair of a fascia

7. _____   Pertaining to within a muscle

8. _____   A muscle that raises or elevates a part

9. _____   Muscle weakness

10. _____   Formation of muscle tissue

11. _____   Study of muscles

12. _____   Weakness or slight paralysis of a muscle

13. _____   Surgical repair of a muscle

14. _____   A malignant tumor derived from muscle tissue

15. _____   Inflammation of a muscle and its tendon

16. _____   Incision into a muscle

17. _____   Inflammation of nerves and muscles

18. _____   Paralysis affecting many muscles

19. _____   Surgical binding of a tendon

20. _____   Pertaining to certain muscles that work together

21. _____   A muscle having three heads with a single insertion

▶ Spelling

In the spaces provided, write the correct spelling of these misspelled terms:

1. facia _____   2. mykinesis _____

3. polymyclonus _____   4. rhadomyoma _____

5. sarclemma _____   6. sterncleidomastoid _____

7. tentomy _____   8. torticolis _____

WORD PARTS STUDY SHEET

Word Parts	Give the Meaning
a-	_____
dys-	_____
intra-	_____
quadri-	_____
brachi-	_____
fasci-, fascio-	_____
fibr-, fibro-	_____
iso-	_____
lemma-	_____
levat-	_____
melan-	_____
metr-	_____
muscul-	_____

my-, myo-, myos-   _____

rhabdo-   _____

rotat-   _____

sarc-, sarco-   _____

sert-   _____

teno-, tenos-   _____

torti-   _____

-ar, -ic   _____

-algia, -dynia   _____

-asthenia   _____

-ceps   _____

-desis   _____

-ectomy   _____

-ist   _____

-itis   _____

-logy   _____

-lysis   _____

-malacia   _____

-oma   _____

-osis   _____

-plasty   _____

-rrhaphy   _____

-rrhexis   _____

-tomy   _____

-trophy   _____

REVIEW QUESTIONS

▶ Matching

Select the appropriate lettered meaning for each numbered line.

_____	1. dermatomyositis	a. A term used to describe the muscles immediately surrounding the shoulder joint
_____	2. fibromyalgia	b. The process of being twisted
_____	3. muscular dystrophy	c. Pain in a tendon
_____	4. myositis	d. Inflammation of the muscles and the skin
_____	5. prosthesis	e. Inflammation of muscle tissue
_____	6. rotator cuff	f. Pertaining to under the control of one's will
_____	7. strain	g. A chronic, progressive wasting and weakening of muscles
_____	8. tenodynia	h. Excessive, forcible stretching of a muscle or the musculotendinous unit
_____	9. torsion	i. A condition with widespread muscular pain and debilitating fatigue
_____	10. voluntary	j. An artificial device, organ, or part
		k. Pain in a joint

▶ Abbreviations

Place the correct word, phrase, or abbreviation in the space provided.

1. AE _____

2. AST _____

3. calcium _____

4. electromyography _____

5. FROM _____

6. MS _____

7. range of motion _____

8. shoulder _____

9. TBW _____

10. TJ _____

▶ Diagnostic and Laboratory Tests

Select the best answer to each multiple choice question. Circle the letter of your choice.

1. A diagnostic test to help diagnose Duchenne's muscular dystrophy before symptoms appear.
   a. creatine phosphokinase
   b. aldolase blood test
   c. calcium blood test
   d. muscle biopsy

2. A test to measure electrical activity across muscle membranes by means of electrodes that are attached to a needle that is inserted into the muscle.
   a. muscle biopsy
   b. lactic dehydrogenase
   c. creatine phosphokinase
   d. electromyography

3. This test is also called aspartate transaminase.
   a. lactic dehydrogenase
   b. serum glutamic oxaloacetic transaminase
   c. serum glutamic pyruvic transaminase
   d. creatine phosphokinase

4. This test is also called alanine aminotransferase.
   a. lactic dehydrogenase
   b. serum glutamic oxaloacetic transaminase
   c. serum glutamic pyruvic transaminase
   d. creatine phosphokinase

5. For a/an _____, a small piece of muscle tissue is excised and then stained for microscopic examination.
   a. muscle biopsy
   b. electromyography
   c. bone biopsy
   d. electrocardiography

CRITICAL THINKING ACTIVITY

▶ **Case Study**

Duchenne's Muscular Dystrophy

Please read the following case study and then answer the questions that follow.

A 3-year-old male child was seen by a physician, and the following is a synopsis of the visit.

Present History: The mother states that she noticed that her son has been falling a lot and seems to be very clumsy. She says that he has a waddling gait, is very slow in running and climbing, and walks on his toes. She is most concerned as she is at risk for carrying the gene that causes muscular dystrophy.

Signs and Symptoms: A waddling gait, very slow in running and climbing, walks on his toes, frequent falling, clumsy.

Diagnosis: Duchenne's muscular dystrophy. The diagnosis was determined by the characteristic symptoms, family history, a muscle biopsy, an electromyography, and an elevated serum creatine kinase level.

Treatment: Physical therapy, deep breathing exercises to help delay muscular weakness, supportive measures such as splints and braces to help minimize deformities and to preserve mobility. Counseling and referral services are essential. For more information you may contact the Muscular Dystrophy Association at: 3561 E. Sunrise Drive, Tucson, AZ 85718. Telephone: 1–602–529–2000 or 1–800–572–1717. E-mail: MDA@MDAUSA.org

Critical Thinking Questions

1. Signs and symptoms of Duchenne's muscular dystrophy include a _____ gait, frequent falls, clumsiness, slowness in running and climbing, and walking on toes.

2. The diagnosis was determined by the characteristic symptoms, family history, a muscle biopsy, an _____, and an elevated serum creatine kinase level.

3. Treatment for Duchenne's muscular dystrophy includes physical therapy, exercise, and supportive measures such as braces and _____.

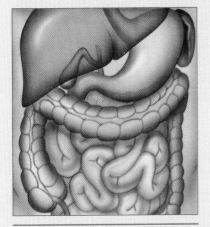

6

THE DIGESTIVE SYSTEM

OBJECTIVES

On completion of this chapter, you should be able to:

- Describe the digestive system.
- Describe the primary organs of the digestive system and state their functions.
- Describe the accessory organs of the digestive system and state their functions.
- Describe digestive differences of the child and the older adult.
- Analyze, build, spell, and pronounce medical words that relate to surgical procedures and pathology.
- Identify and give the meaning of selected vocabulary words.
- Identify and define selected abbreviations.
- Review Drug Highlights presented in this chapter.
- Provide the description of diagnostic and laboratory tests related to the digestive system.
- Successfully complete the study and review section.

► ANATOMY AND PHYSIOLOGY OVERVIEW

A general description of the digestive system is that of a continuous tube beginning with the mouth and ending at the anus. This tube is known as the *alimentary canal* and/or *gastrointestinal tract*. It measures about 30 feet in adults and contains both primary and accessory organs for the conversion of food and fluids into a semiliquid that can be absorbed for use by the body. The three main functions of the digestive system are *digestion, absorption,* and *elimination*. Each of the various organs commonly associated with digestion is described in this chapter. The organs of digestion are shown in Figure 6–1.

► THE MOUTH

The *mouth* is the cavity formed by the palate or roof, the lips and cheeks on the sides, and the tongue at its floor. Contained within are the teeth and salivary glands. The cheeks form the lateral walls and are continuous with the lips. The vestibule includes the space between the cheeks and the teeth. The *gingivae* (gums) surround the necks of the teeth. The hard and soft palates provide a roof for the oral cavity, with the tongue at its floor. The free portion of the tongue is connected to the underlying epithelium by a thin fold of mucous membrane, the *lingual frenulum*. The *tongue* is made of skeletal muscle and is covered with mucous membrane. The tongue can be divided into a blunt rear portion called the *root*, a *pointed tip*, and a *central body*. Located on the surface of the tongue are *papillae* (elevations) and *taste buds* (sweet, salt, sour, and bitter). Three pairs of salivary glands secrete fluids into the oral cavity. These glands are the *parotid, sublingual,* and *submandibular*. The posterior margin of the soft palate supports the dangling uvula and two pairs of muscular pharyngeal arches. On either side,

THE DIGESTIVE SYSTEM

ORGAN	FUNCTIONS
Mouth	Breaks food apart by the action of the teeth, moistens and lubricates food with saliva; food formed into a bolus
Pharynx	Common passageway for both respiration and digestion; muscular constrictions move the bolus into the esophagus
Esophagus	Peristalsis moves the food down the esophagus into the stomach
Stomach	Reduces food to a digestible state, converts the food to a semiliquid form
Small Intestine	Digestion and absorption take place. Nutrients are absorbed into tiny capillaries and lymph vessels in the walls of the small intestine and transmitted to body cells by the circulatory system
Large Intestine	Removes water from the fecal material, stores, and then eliminates waste from the body via the rectum and anus
Salivary Glands	Secrete saliva to moisten and lubricate food
Liver	Changes glucose to glycogen and stores it until needed; changes glycogen back to glucose; desaturates fats, assists in protein catabolism, manufactures bile, fibrinogen, prothrombin, heparin, and blood proteins, stores vitamins, produces heat, and detoxifies substances
Gallbladder	Stores and concentrates bile
Pancreas	Secretes pancreatic juice into the small intestine, contains cells that produce digestive enzymes, secretes insulin and glucagon

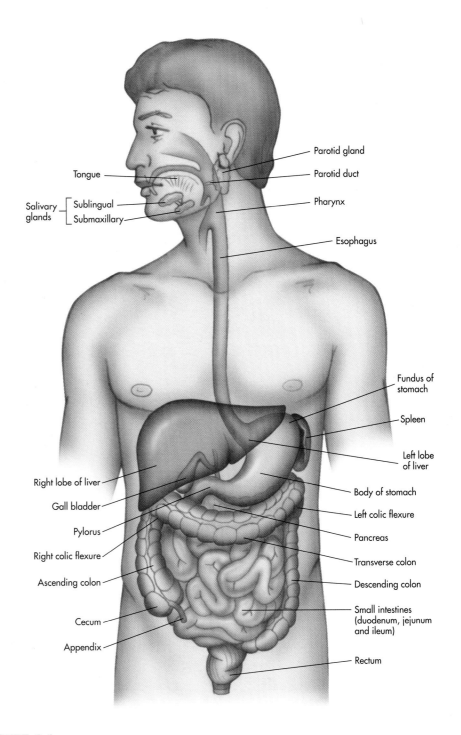

FIGURE 6–1

The digestive system.

a palatine tonsil lies between an anterior palatoglossal arch and a posterior palatopharyngeal arch. A curving line that connects the palatoglossal arches and uvula forms the boundaries of the fauces, the passageway between the oral cavity and the pharynx (Fig. 6–2). Digestion begins as food is broken apart by the action of the teeth, moistened and lubricated by saliva, and formed into a *bolus*. A bolus is a small mass of masticated food ready to be swallowed.

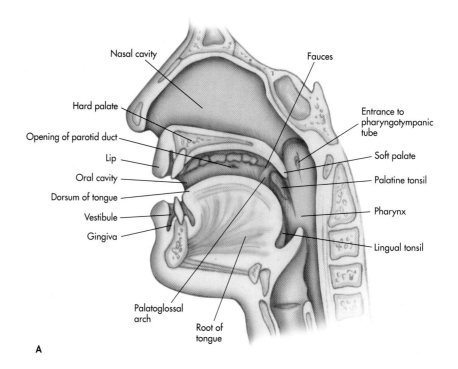

Nasal cavity

Fauces

Hard palate

Entrance to
pharyngotympanic
tube

Opening of parotid duct

Soft palate

Lip

Palatine tonsil

Oral cavity

Dorsum of tongue

Pharynx

Vestibule

Gingiva

Lingual tonsil

Palatoglossal
arch

Root of
tongue

A

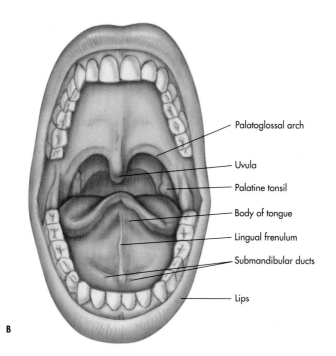

Palatoglossal arch

Uvula

Palatine tonsil

Body of tongue

Lingual frenulum

Submandibular ducts

Lips

B

FIGURE 6-2

The oral cavity: **(A)** sagittal section, **(B)** anterior view as seen through the open mouth.

▶ THE PHARYNX

Just beyond the mouth, at the beginning of the tube leading to the stomach, is the *pharynx*. Simply put, the pharynx is a common passageway for both respiration and digestion. Both the *larynx,* or voicebox, and the esophagus begin in the pharynx. Food that is swallowed passes through the pharynx into the esophagus reflexively. Muscular constrictions move the ball of food into the esophagus while, at the same time, blocking the opening to the larynx and preventing the food from entering the airway leading to the trachea or windpipe.

▶ THE ESOPHAGUS

The *esophagus* is a collapsible tube about 10 inches long that leads from the pharynx to the stomach. Food passes down the esophagus and into the stomach. Food is carried along the esophagus by a series of wave-like muscular contractions called *peristalsis.*

▶ THE STOMACH

The *stomach* is a large sac-like organ into which food passes from the esophagus for storage while undergoing the early processes of digestion. In the stomach, food is further reduced to a digestible state. Hydrochloric acid and gastric juices convert the food to a semiliquid state, which is passed, at intervals, into the small intestine.

▶ THE SMALL INTESTINE

The *small intestine* is about 21 feet long and 1 inch in diameter. It extends from the pyloric orifice at the base of the stomach to the entrance of the large intestine. The small intestine is considered to have three parts: the *duodenum,* the *jejunum,* and the *ileum.* The duodenum is the first 12 inches just beyond the stomach. The jejunum is the next 8 feet or so, and the ileum is the remaining 12 feet of the tube. Semiliquid food (called *chyme*) is received from the stomach through the pylorus and mixed with bile from the liver and gallbladder along with pancreatic juice from the pancreas. Digestion and absorption take place chiefly in the small intestine. Nutrients are absorbed into tiny capillaries and lymph vessels in the walls of the small intestine and transmitted to body cells by the circulatory system.

▶ THE LARGE INTESTINE

The *large intestine* is about 5 feet long and 2.5 inches in diameter. It extends from the ileocecal orifice at the small intestine to the anus. The large intestine may be divided into the *cecum,* the *colon,* the *rectum,* and the *anal canal.* The cecum is a pouch-like structure forming the beginning of the large intestine. It is about 3 inches long and has the appendix attached to it. The *colon* makes up the bulk of the large intestine and is divided into several parts—the ascending colon, the transverse colon, the descending colon, and, at its end, the sigmoid colon. Digestion and absorption continue in the large intestine on a reduced scale. The waste products of digestion are eliminated from the body via the rectum and the anus.

▶ ACCESSORY ORGANS

The *salivary glands,* the *liver,* the *gallbladder,* and the *pancreas* are not actually part of the digestive tube; however, they are closely related to it in their functions.

THE SALIVARY GLANDS

Located in or near the mouth, the *salivary glands* secrete *saliva* in response to the sight, smell, taste, or mental image of food. The various salivary glands are the *parotid,* located on either side of the face slightly below the ear; the *submandibular,* located in the floor of the mouth; and the *sublingual,* located below the tongue. All salivary glands secrete through openings into the mouth to moisten and lubricate food.

THE LIVER

The largest glandular organ in the body, the *liver* weighs about 3½ lb and is located in the upper right part of the abdomen. The liver plays an essential role in the normal metabolism of carbohydrates, fats, and proteins. In carbohydrate metabolism, it changes glucose to glycogen and stores it until needed by body cells. It also changes glycogen back to glucose. In fat metabolism, the liver serves as a storage place and acts to desaturate fats before releasing them into the bloodstream. In protein metabolism, the liver acts as a storage place and assists in protein catabolism.

The liver manufactures the following important substances:

- **Bile**—a digestive juice
- **Fibrinogen** and **prothrombin**—coagulants essential for blood clotting
- **Heparin**—an anticoagulant that helps to prevent the clotting of blood
- **Blood proteins**—albumin, gamma globulin

Additionally, the liver stores iron and vitamins B_{12}, A, D, E, and K. It also produces body heat and detoxifies many harmful substances such as drugs and alcohol.

THE GALLBLADDER

The *gallbladder* is a membranous sac attached to the liver in which excess bile is stored and concentrated. Bile leaving the gallbladder is 6 to 10 times as concentrated as that which comes to it from the liver. Concentration is accomplished by absorption of water from the bile into the mucosa of the gallbladder.

THE PANCREAS

The *pancreas* is a large, elongated gland situated behind the stomach and secreting pancreatic juice into the small intestine. The pancreas is 6 to 9 inches long and contains cells that produce digestive *enzymes*. Other cells in the pancreas secrete the hormones insulin and glucagon directly into the bloodstream.

LIFE SPAN CONSIDERATIONS

▶ THE CHILD

The primitive digestive tract is formed by the embryonic membrane (yolk sac) and is divided into three sections. The **foregut** evolves into the pharynx, lower respiratory tract, esophagus, stomach, duodenum, and beginning of the common bile duct. The **midgut** elongates in the 5th week to form the primary intestinal loop. The remainder of the large colon is derived from the primitive hindgut. The liver, pancreas, and biliary tract evolve from the **foregut.** At 8 weeks, the anal membrane ruptures, forming the anal canal and opening.

Normally the functioning of the gastrointestinal tract begins after birth. Food is prepared for absorption and absorbed, and waste products are eliminated. **Meconium,** the first stool, is a mixture of amniotic fluid and secretions of the intestinal glands. It is thick and sticky, and dark green in color. It is usually passed 8 to 24 hours following birth. The stools change during the first week and become loose and greenish-yellow. The stools of a breast-fed baby are bright yellow, soft, and pasty. The stools of a bottle-fed baby are more solid than those of the breast-fed baby and they vary from yellow to brown in color.

The infant's stomach is small and empties rapidly. Newborns produce very little saliva until they are 3 months of age. Swallowing is a reflex action for the first 3 months. The hepatic efficiency of the newborn is often immature; thereby, causing **jaundice.** Fat absorption is poor because of a decreased level of bile production.

▶ THE OLDER ADULT

With aging, the digestive system becomes less motile, as muscle contractions become weaker. Glandular secretions decrease, thus causing a drier mouth and a lower volume of gastric juices. Nutrient absorption is mildly reduced due to **atrophy** of the mucosal lining. The teeth are mechanically worn down with age and begin to recede away from the gums. There is a loss of tastebuds, and food preferences change. Gastric motor activity slows; as a result, gastric emptying is delayed and hunger contractions diminish. There are no significant changes in the small intestine, but in the large intestine, the muscle layer and mucosa atrophy. Smooth muscle tone and blood flow decrease, and connective tissue increases.

Constipation is a frequent problem among older adults. It is believed that constipation is not a normal age-related change, but is caused by low fluid intake, lack of dietary fiber, inactivity, medicines, depression, and other health-related conditions.

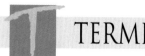

TERMINOLOGY

WITH SURGICAL PROCEDURES & PATHOLOGY

TERM	WORD PARTS			DEFINITION
amylase (ăm′ ĭ-lās)	amyl ase	R S	starch enzyme	An enzyme that breaks down starch
anabolism (ă-năb′ ō-lĭzm)	ana bol ism	P R S	up to cast, throw condition of	Literally "a throwing upward"; the building up of the body substance
anorexia (ăn″ ō-rĕks′ ĭ-ă)	an orexia	P S	lack of appetite	Lack of appetite
anoscope (ā′ nō-skōp)	ano scope	CF S	anus instrument	An instrument used to examine the anus
appendectomy (ăp″ ĕn-dĕk′ tō-mē)	append ectomy	R S	appendix excision	Surgical excision of the appendix
appendicitis (ă-pĕn″ dĭ-sī′ tĭs)	appendic itis	R S	appendix inflammation	Inflammation of the appendix
biliary (bĭl′ ĭ-ār″ ē)	bili ary	CF S	gall, bile pertaining to	Pertaining to or conveying bile
buccal (bək′ əl)	bucc al	R S	cheek pertaining to	Pertaining to the cheek
catabolism (kă-tăb′ ō-lĭzm)	cata bol ism	P R S	down to cast, throw condition of	Literally "a throwing down"; a breaking of complex substances into more basic elements
celiac (sē′ lĭ-ăk)	celi ac	R S	abdomen, belly pertaining to	Pertaining to the abdomen
cheilosis (kī-lō′ sĭs)	cheil osis	R S	lip condition of	An abnormal condition of the lip as seen in riboflavin and other B-complex deficiencies
cholecystectomy (kō″ lē-sĭs-tĕk′ tō-mē)	chole cyst ectomy	CF R S	gall, bile bladder excision	Surgical excision of the gallbladder
cholecystitis (kō″ lē- sĭs-tī′ tĭs)	chole cyst itis	CF R S	gall, bile bladder inflammation	Inflammation of the gallbladder

Terminology - continued

TERM	WORD PARTS			DEFINITION
choledochotomy (kō-lĕd″ ō-kŏt′ ō-mē)	choledocho tomy	CF S	common bile duct incision	Surgical incision of the common bile duct
colectomy (kō-lĕk′ tō-mē)	col ectomy	R S	colon excision	Surgical excision of part of the colon
colonic (kō-lŏn′ ĭk)	colon ic	R S	colon pertaining to	Pertaining to the colon
colonoscopy (kō-lŏn-ŏs′ kō-pē)	colono scopy	CF S	colon to view, examine	Examination of the upper portion of the colon
colorrhaphy (kŏ-lōr′ ăh-fē)	colo rrhaphy	CF S	colon suture	Suture of the colon
colostomy (kō-lŏs′ tō-mē)	colo stomy	CF S	colon new opening	The creation of a new opening into the colon
dentalgia (dĕn-tăl′ jĭ-ă)	dent algia	R S	tooth pain	Pain in a tooth; *toothache*
dentibuccal (dĕn″ tĭ-bŭk′ l)	denti bucc al	CF R S	tooth cheek pertaining to	Pertaining to the teeth and the cheek
dentist (dĕn′ təst)	dent ist	R S	tooth one who specializes	One who specializes in dentistry
diverticulitis (dī″ vĕr-tĭk″ ū-lī′ tĭs)	diverticul itis	R S	diverticula inflammation	Inflammation of the diverticula in the colon

 TERMINOLOGY SPOTLIGHT

Pain is a common symptom of **diverticulitis.** Diverticulitis occurs when a **diverticulum** (a pouch or sac in the walls of an organ or canal) become inflamed or infected. See Figure 6–3. The exact cause of this condition is unknown, but it generally begins when stool lodges in the diverticula. Infection can lead to complications such as swelling or rupturing of the diverticula. Symptoms include pain, fever, chills, cramping, bloating, constipation, or diarrhea. Treatment depends upon the severity of the condition. A liquid diet and oral antibiotics are used for mild conditions, generally followed by a high-fiber diet (see Table 6–1). If the condition is severe, hospitalization, bedrest, IV antibiotics and fluids, and/or surgery are recommended.

duodenal (dū″ ō-dē′ năl)	duoden al	R S	duodenum pertaining to	Pertaining to the duodenum; the first part of the small intestine

continued

Terminology - continued

TERM	WORD PARTS			DEFINITION
dyspepsia (dĭs-pĕp′ sĭ-ă)	dys pepsia	P S	difficult to digest	Difficulty in digestion; *indigestion*
dysphagia (dĭs-fā′ jĭ-ă)	dys phagia	P S	difficult to eat	Difficulty in swallowing
enteric (ĕn-tĕr′ ĭk)	enter ic	R S	intestine pertaining to	Pertaining to the intestine
enteritis (ĕn″ tĕr-ī′ tĭs)	enter itis	R S	intestine inflammation	Inflammation of the intestine
enteroclysis (ĕn″ tĕr-ŏk′ lĭ-sĭs)	entero clysis	CF S	intestine injection	Injection of a solution into the intestine
enterostomy (ĕn″ tĕr-ŏs′ tō-mē)	entero stomy	CF S	intestine new opening	The creation of a permanent opening into the intestine
epigastric (ĕp′ ĭ-găs′ trĭc)	epi gastr ic	P R S	above stomach pertaining to	Pertaining to the region above the stomach
esophageal (ē-sŏf″ ă-jē′ ăl)	esophage al	CF S	esophagus pertaining to	Pertaining to the esophagus
esophagoscope (ĕ-sŏf′ ă-gō-skōp″)	esophago scope	CF S	esophagus instrument	An instrument used to examine the esophagus
gastralgia (gās-trăl′ jĭ-ă)	gastr algia	R S	stomach pain	Pain in the stomach
gastrectomy (găs-trĕk′ tō-mē)	gastr ectomy	R S	stomach excision	Surgical excision of a part or the whole stomach
gastric (găs′ trĭk)	gastr ic	R S	stomach pertaining to	Pertaining to the stomach
gastrodynia (găs″ trō-dĭn′ ĭ-ă)	gastro dynia	CF S	stomach pain	Pain in the stomach
gastroenterology (găs″ trō-ĕn″ tĕr-ŏl′ ō-jē)	gastro entero logy	CF CF S	stomach intestine study of	Study of the stomach and the intestines
gastropexy (găs′ trō-pĕk″ sē)	gastro pexy	CF S	stomach fixation	Surgical fixation of the stomach to the abdominal wall
gastroscope (găs′ trō-skōp)	gastro scope	CF S	stomach instrument	An instrument used to view the interior of the stomach

Terminology - continued

TERM	WORD	PARTS		DEFINITION
gastrotomy (găs-trŏt′ ō-mē)	gastro tomy	CF S	stomach incision	Surgical incision into the stomach
gingivitis (jĭn″ jĭ-vī′ tĭs)	gingiv itis	R S	gums inflammation	Inflammation of the gums
glossotomy (glŏ-sŏt′ ō-mē)	glosso tomy	CF S	tongue incision	Surgical incision into the tongue
glycogenesis (glī″ kŏ-jĕn′ ĕ-sĭs)	glyco genesis	CF S	sweet, sugar formation, produce	The formation of glycogen from glucose
hematemesis (hĕm″ ăt-ēm′ ĕ-sĭs)	hemat emesis	R S	blood vomiting	Vomiting of blood
hepatitis (hĕp″ ă-tī′ tĭs)	hepat itis	R S	liver inflammation	Inflammation of the liver
hepatoma (hĕp″ ă-tŏ′ mă)	hepat oma	R S	liver tumor	A tumor of the liver
hepatomegaly (hĕp″ ă-tō-mĕg′ ă-lē)	hepato megaly	CF S	liver enlargement, large	Enlargement of the liver
hepatotoxin (hĕp″ ă-tō-tŏk′ sĭn)	hepato tox in	CF R S	liver poison pertaining to	Pertaining to a substance that is poisonous to the liver
herniotomy (hĕr″ nĭ-ŏt′ ō-mē)	hernio tomy	CF S	hernia incision	Surgical incision for the repair of a hernia
hyperemesis (hī″ pĕr-ĕm′ ĕ-sĭs)	hyper emesis	P S	excessive, above vomiting	Excessive vomiting
hypogastric (hī″ pō-găs′ trĭk)	hypo gastr ic	P R S	deficient, below stomach pertaining to	Pertaining to below the stomach
ileitis (ĭl″ ē-ī′ tis)	ile itis	R S	ileum inflammation	Inflammation of the ileum
ileostomy (ĭl″ ē-ŏs′ tō-mē)	ileo stomy	CF S	ileum new opening	The creation of a new opening through the abdominal wall into the ileum
labial (lā′ bĭ-ăl)	labi al	R S	lip pertaining to	Pertaining to the lip

continued

Terminology - continued

TERM	WORD PARTS			DEFINITION
laparotomy (lăp″ăr-ŏt′ ō-mē)	laparo tomy	CF S	flank, abdomen incision	Surgical incision into the abdomen
laxative (lăk′ să-tĭv)	laxat ive	R S	to loosen nature of, quality of	A substance that acts to loosen the bowels
lingual (lĭng′ gwal)	lingu al	R S	tongue pertaining to	Pertaining to the tongue

 TERMINOLOGY SPOTLIGHT

There are various conditions that can occur on the tongue. Two of these are **fibroma** and **black hairy tongue.** A fibroma is a fibrous, encapsulated connective tissue tumor. See Figures 6–4 and 6–5. Black hairy tongue is a tongue covered with hair-like papillae, entangled with threads produced by *Aspergillus niger* or *Candida albicans* fungi. This condition may be caused by poor oral hygiene and/or overgrowth of fungi due to antibiotic therapy. See Figure 6–6.

lipolysis (lĭp-ŏl′ ĭ-sĭs)	lipo lysis	CF S	fat destruction, to separate	The destruction of fat
malabsorption (măl″ăb-sōrp′ shŭn)	mal absorpt ion	P R S	bad to suck in process	The process of bad or inadequate absorption of nutrients from the intestinal tract
megacolon (měg′ ă-kō′ lŏn)	mega colon	P R	large, great colon	A condition in which the colon is extremely enlarged
mesentery (měs′ ĕn-tĕr″ ē)	mes enter y	R R S	middle intestine pertaining to	Pertaining to the peritoneal fold encircling the small intestines and connecting the intestines to the abdominal wall
pancreatectomy (păn″ krē-ăt-ĕk′ tō-mē)	pancreat ectomy	R S	pancreas excision	Surgical excision of the pancreas
pancreatitis (păn″ krē-ă-tī′ tĭs)	pancreat itis	R S	pancreas inflammation	Inflammation of the pancreas
peptic (pĕp′ tĭk)	pept ic	R S	to digest pertaining to	Pertaining to gastric digestion

Terminology - continued

TERM	WORD PARTS			DEFINITION
peristalsis (pĕr" ĭ-stăl' sĭs)	peri stalsis	P S	around contraction	A wave-like contraction that occurs involuntarily in hollow tubes of the body, especially the alimentary canal
pharyngeal (făr-ĭn' jē-ăl)	pharynge al	CF S	pharynx pertaining to	Pertaining to the pharynx
postprandial (pōst-prăn' dĭ-ăl)	post prandi al	P CF S	after meal pertaining to	Pertaining to after a meal
proctalgia (prŏk-tăl' jĭ-ă)	proct algia	R S	rectum, anus pain	Pain in the rectum and anus
proctologist (prŏk-tŏl' ō-jĭst)	procto log ist	CF R S	rectum, anus study of one who specializes	One who specializes in the study of the anus and the rectum
proctoscope (prŏk' tō-scōp)	procto scope	CF S	rectum, anus instrument	An instrument used to view the anus and rectum
pyloric (pī-lōr' ĭk)	pylor ic	R S	pylorus, gatekeeper pertaining to	Pertaining to the gatekeeper, the opening between the stomach and the duodenum
pyloroplasty (pī-lōr' ō-plăs" tē)	pyloro plasty	CF S	pylorus, gatekeeper surgical repair	Surgical repair of the pylorus
rectocele (rĕk' tō-sēl)	recto cele	CF S	rectum hernia	A hernia of part of the rectum into the vagina
retrolingual (rĕt" rō-lĭng' gwăl)	retro lingu al	P R S	backward tongue pertaining to	Pertaining to behind the tongue
sialadenitis (sī"ăl-ăd" ĕ-nī' tĭs)	sial aden itis	R R S	saliva gland inflammation	Inflammation of the salivary gland
sigmoidoscope (sĭg-moy' dō-skōp)	sigmoido scope	CF S	sigmoid instrument	An instrument used to view the sigmoid
splenomegaly (splē" nō-mĕg'ă-lē)	spleno megaly	CF S	spleen enlargement, large	Enlargement of the spleen

continued

Terminology - continued

TERM	WORD PARTS			DEFINITION
splenopathy (splē -nŏp′ ă-thē)	spleno pathy	CF S	spleen disease	Any disease of the spleen
stomatitis (stō″ mă-tī′ tĭs)	stomat itis	R S	mouth inflammation	Inflammation of the mouth
sublingual (sŭb-lĭng′ gwăl)	sub lingu al	P R S	below tongue pertaining to	Pertaining to below the tongue
vagotomy (vā-gŏt′ ō-mē)	vago tomy	CF S	vagus incision	Incision into the vagus nerve
vermiform (vēr′ mĭ-form)	vermi form	CF S	worm shape	Shaped like a worm

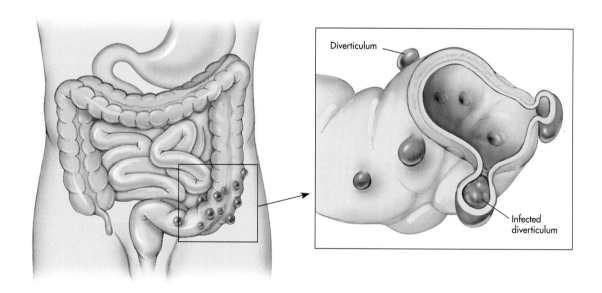

FIGURE 6–3

Diverticulitis.

TABLE 6–1   Good Choices of High-Fiber Foods

One needs 25 to 30 grams of fiber each day to keep the colon working at its best. The following are selected good choices of high-fiber foods.

Fruits

1 medium apple	4 grams
1 medium pear	4 grams
1 medium orange	3 grams
1 cup strawberries	3 grams
5 dried prunes (uncooked)	3 grams

Vegetables

1 baked potato (with skin)	5 grams
½ cup cooked frozen peas	4 grams
½ cup cooked fresh spinach	3 grams
½ cup cooked frozen corn	2 grams

Beans

½ cup cooked lentils	8 grams
½ cup cooked kidney beans	6 grams
½ cup cooked green beans	2 grams

Whole-Grain Cereals

⅓ cup all-bran cereal	10 grams
⅓ cup wheat flakes	3 grams
⅓ cup shredded wheat	3 grams

Whole-Bran Breads and Rice

2 slices whole-wheat bread	4 grams
2 slices rye bread	4 grams
½ cup cooked brown rice	2 grams

Pure Bran

3 T unprocessed wheat bran	6 grams
3 T unprocessed oat bran	3 grams

T = tablespoon

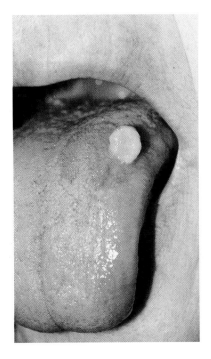

FIGURE 6–4

Fibroma. *(Courtesy of Jason L. Smith, MD.)*

FIGURE 6–5

Fibroma, mucosal. *(Courtesy of Jason L. Smith, MD.)*

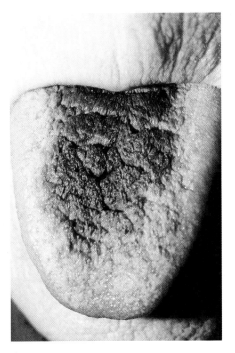

FIGURE 6–6

Black hairy tongue. *(Courtesy of Jason L. Smith, MD.)*

VOCABULARY WORDS

Vocabulary words are terms that have not been divided into component parts. They are common words or specialized terms associated with the subject of this chapter. These words are provided to enhance your medical vocabulary.

WORD	DEFINITION
absorption (ăb-sōrp′ shŭn)	The process whereby nutrient material is taken into the bloodstream or lymph
ascites (ă-sī′ tēz)	An accumulation of serous fluid in the peritoneal cavity
bilirubin (bĭl″ ĭ-roo′ bĭn)	The orange-colored bile pigment produced by the separation of hemoglobin into parts that are excreted by the liver cells
bowel (bou′ əl)	The intestine, gut, entrail
chyle (kīl)	The milky fluid of intestinal digestion, composed of lymph and emulsified fats
cirrhosis (sĭ-rō′ sĭs)	A chronic degenerative liver disease characterized by changes in the lobes; parenchymal cells and the lobules are infiltrated with fat
constipation (kon″ stĭ-pā′ shŭn)	Infrequent passage of unduly hard and dry feces; *difficult defecation*
defecation (dĕf-ĕ-kā′ shŭn)	The evacuation of the bowel
deglutition (dē″ gloo-tĭsh′ ŭn)	The act or process of swallowing
diarrhea (dī′ ă-rē′ ă)	Frequent passage of unformed watery stools
digestion (dī-jĕst′ chŭn)	The process by which food is changed in the mouth, stomach, and intestines by chemical, mechanical, and physical action so that it can be absorbed by the body
dysentery (dĭs′ ĕn-tĕr″ē)	An intestinal disease characterized by inflammation of the mucous membrane
emesis (ĕm′ ĕ-sĭs)	Vomiting
enzyme (ĕn′ zīm)	A protein substance capable of causing chemical changes in other substances without being changed itself

Vocabulary - continued

WORD	DEFINITION
epulis (ĕp-ū′lĭs)	Any tumor of the gingiva; a giant cell epulis is a pedunculated lesion of the gum caused by an inflammatory reaction to injury or hemorrhage. See Figure 6–7.
eructation (ē-rŭk-tā′ shŭn)	Belching
esophageal reflux (ē-sŏf″ă-jē-ăl rē′ flŭks)	A return or backward flow of gastric contents into the esophagus
feces (fē′ sēz)	Body waste expelled from the bowels; *stools, excreta*
fiberscope (fī′ bĕr-skōp)	A flexible scope that is equipped with fiberoptic lens; useful in endoscopic examination of the colon *(fibercolonoscope)* and the stomach *(fibergastroscope)*
flatus (flā′ tŭs)	Gas in the stomach or intestines
gavage (gă-văzh′)	To feed liquid or semiliquid food via a tube (stomach or nasogastric)
halitosis (hăl″ ĭ-tō′ sĭs)	Bad breath
hemorrhoid (hĕm′ ō-royd)	A mass of dilated, tortuous veins in the anorectum; may be internal or external
hernia (hĕr′ nē-ă)	The abnormal protrusion of an organ or a part of an organ through the wall of the body cavity that normally contains it. See Figure 6–8.
hyperalimentation (hī″ pĕr-ăl″ĭ mĕn-tā′ shŭn)	An intravenous infusion of a hypertonic solution to sustain life; used in patients whose gastrointestinal tracts are not functioning properly
lavage (lă-văzh′)	To wash out a cavity
liver transplant (lĭv′ ĕr trăns′ plănt)	The surgical process of transferring the liver from a donor to a patient
mastication (măs″ tĭ-kā′ shŭn)	Chewing
melena (mĕl′ ĕ-nă)	Black feces caused by the action of intestinal juices on blood

continued

Vocabulary - continued

WORD	DEFINITION
nausea (naw′ sē-ă)	The feeling of the inclination to vomit
pancreas transplant (păn′ krē-ăs trăns plănt)	The surgical process of transferring the pancreas from a donor to a patient
paralytic ileus (păr″ă-lĭt′ ĭk ĭl′ē-ŭs)	A paralysis of the intestines that causes distention and symptoms of acute obstruction and prostration
pilonidal cyst (pī″ lō-nī′ dăl sĭst)	A closed sac in the crease of the sacrococcygeal region caused by a developmental defect that permits epithelial tissue and hair to be trapped below the skin
ulcer (ŭl′sĕr)	An open lesion or sore of the epidermis or mucous membrane. A peptic ulcer forms in the mucosal wall of the stomach, the pylorus, the duodenum, or the esophagus. It is referred to as a *gastric, duodenal,* or *esophageal ulcer,* depending on the location. See Figure 6–9.
volvulus (vŏl′ vū-lŭs)	A twisting of the bowel on itself that causes an obstruction. See Figure 6–10.
vomit (vŏm′ ĭt)	To eject stomach contents through the mouth

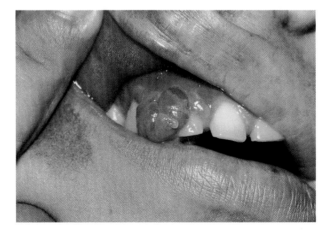

FIGURE 6–7

Giant cell epulis. *(Courtesy of Jason L. Smith, MD.)*

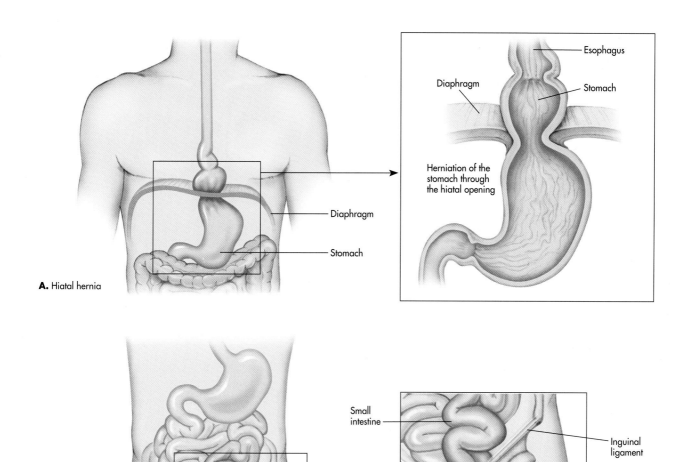

A. Hiatal hernia

Esophagus

Diaphragm

Stomach

Herniation of the
stomach through
the hiatal opening

Diaphragm

Stomach

B. Inguinal hernia

Small
intestine

Inguinal
ligament

Direct inguinal
hernia

FIGURE 6–8

Hernias.

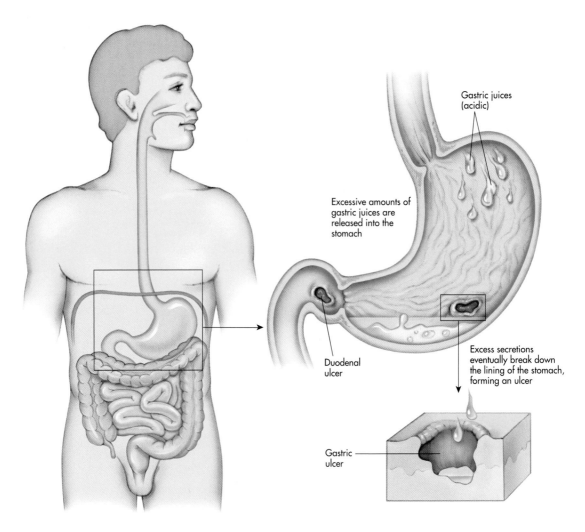

FIGURE 6–9

Peptic ulcer disease (PUD).

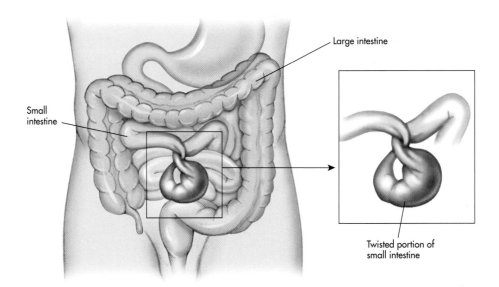

FIGURE 6–10

Volvulus.

ABBREVIATIONS

a.c.	before meals (ante cibum)	**HAV**	hepatitis A virus
A/G	albumin/globulin (ratio)	**HBIG**	hepatitis B immune globulin
ALP	alkaline phosphatase	**HBV**	hepatitis B virus
ATP	adenosine triphosphate	**HCl**	hydrochloric acid
Ba	barium	**IBS**	irritable bowel syndrome
BE	barium enema	**ICG**	indocyanine green
BAO	basal acid output	**IVC**	intravenous cholangiography
BM	bowel movement	**LDH**	lactic dehydrogenase
BRP	bathroom privileges	**NANBH**	non-A, non-B hepatitis virus
BS	bowel sounds	**NG**	nasogastric (tube)
BSP	bromsulphalein	**NH$_4$**	ammonia
CCK-PZ	cholecystokinin-pancreozymin	**n.p.o.**	nil per os (nothing by mouth)
CDCA	chenodeoxycholic acid	**OCG**	oral cholecystography
CHO	carbohydrate	**O&P**	ova and parasites
chol	cholesterol	**p.c.**	after meals (post cibum)
cib	food (cibus)	**PEG**	percutaneous endoscopic gastrostomy
CUC	chronic ulcerative colitis	**p.o.**	per os (by mouth)
E. coli	*Escherichia coli*	**PP**	postprandial (after meals)
ERCP	endoscopic retrograde cholangiopancreatography	**PTC**	percutaneous transhepatic cholangiography
GB	gallbladder	**PUD**	peptic ulcer disease
GERD	gastroesophageal reflux disease	**RDA**	recommended dietary or daily allowance
GGT	gamma-glutamyl transferase	**TPN**	total parenteral nutrition
GI	gastrointestinal	**UDCA**	ursodeoxycholic acid
GIP	gastric inhibitory peptide		
GTT	glucose tolerance test		
HAA	hepatitis-associated antigen		

DRUG HIGHLIGHTS

Drugs that are generally used for digestive system diseases and disorders include antacids, antacid mixtures, histamine H$_2$-receptor antagonists, other ulcer medicines, laxatives, antidiarrheal agents, and antiemetics.

Antacids	Neutralize hydrochloric acid in the stomach. Antacids are classified as nonsystemic and systemic.
Nonsystemic	*Examples: Amphojel (aluminum hydroxide), Tums (calcium carbonate), Riopan (magaldrate), and Milk of Magnesia (magnesium hydroxide).*
Systemic	*Example: sodium bicarbonate.*

Antacid Mixtures

Products that combine aluminum (may cause constipation) and/or calcium compounds with magnesium (may cause diarrhea) salts. By combining the antacid properties of two single-entity agents, these products provide the antacid action of both, yet tend to counter the adverse effects of each other.
Examples: Gaviscon, Gelusil, Maalox Plus, and Mylanta.

Histamine H$_2$-Receptor Antagonists

Inhibit both daytime and nocturnal basal gastric acid secretion and inhibit gastric acid stimulated by food, histamines, caffeine, insulin, and pentagastrin. These drugs are used in the treatment of active duodenal ulcer.
Examples: Tagamet (cimetidine), Pepcid (famotidine), Axid (nizatidine), and Zantac (ranitidine).

Other Ulcer Medications

Include *Carafate (sucralfate)* that is a cytoprotective agent that is used to prevent further damage by ulcers and to promote the healing process by coating the surface of the damaged mucosa. *Cytotec (misoprostol)* is an antiulcer agent that is used to prevent nonsteroidal anti-inflammatory drug (NSAID)–induced gastric ulcers.

In February 1994, it was announced that a bacterium called *Helicobacter pylori* plays a role in peptic ulcer disease. It is recommended that patients with peptic ulcer disease who test positive for *H. pylori* be treated with *bismuth* and a combination of antibiotic drugs, such as *tetracycline, metronidazole,* or *amoxicillin* for a period of 2 weeks.

Laxatives

Used to relieve constipation and to facilitate the passage of feces through the lower gastrointestinal tract.
Examples: Dulcolax (bisacodyl), Milk of Magnesia (magnesium hydroxide), Metamucil (psyllium hydrophilic muciloid), and Ex-Lax (phenolphthalein).

Antidiarrheal Agents

Used to treat diarrhea.
Examples: Pepto-Bismol (bismuth subsalicylate), Kaopectate (kaolin mixture with pectin), and Imodium (loperamide HCl).

Antiemetics

Prevent or arrest vomiting. These drugs are also used in the treatment of vertigo, motion sickness, and nausea.
Examples: Dramamine (dimenhydrinate), Phenergan (promethazine HCl), Tigan (trimethobenzamide HCl), and Transderm Scop (scopolamine).

DIAGNOSTIC AND LABORATORY TESTS

Test	Description
alcohol toxicology (ethanol and ethyl) (ăl′ kō-hōl tŏks″ ĭ-kŏl′ ō-jē)	A test performed on blood serum or plasma to determine levels of alcohol. Legally, 0.05% or 50 mg/dL is considered not under the influence. Increased values indicate alcohol consumption that may lead to cirrhosis of the liver, gastritis, malnutrition, vitamin deficiencies, and other gastrointestinal disorders.
ammonia (NH$_4$) (ă-mō′ nē-ă)	A test performed on blood plasma to determine the level of ammonia (end product of protein

Test	Description
	breakdown). Increased values may indicate hepatic failure, hepatic encephalopathy, portacaval anastomosis, high protein diet in hepatic failure, and Reye's syndrome.
barium enema (BE) (bă′ rē-ūm ĕn′ ĕ-mă)	A test performed by administering barium via the rectum to determine the condition of the colon. X-rays are taken to ascertain the structure and to check the filling of the colon. Abnormal results may indicate cancer of the colon, polyps, fistulas, ulcerative colitis, diverticulitis, hernias, and intussusception.
bilirubin blood test (total) (bĭl-ĭ-roo′ bĭn blod test)	A test done on blood serum to determine if bilirubin is conjugated and excreted in the bile. Abnormal results may indicate obstructive jaundice, hepatitis, and cirrhosis.
carcinoembryonic antigen (CEA) (kăr″ sĭn-ō-ĕm″ brē-ō n′ ĭk ăn′ tĭ-jĕn)	A test performed on whole blood or plasma to determine the presence of CEA (antigens originally isolated from colon tumors). Increased values may indicate stomach, intestinal, rectal, and various other cancers and conditions. This test is nonspecific and must be combined with other tests for a final diagnosis. It is being used to monitor the course of cancer therapy.
cholangiography (kō-lăn″ jē-ŏg′ ră-fē)	X-ray examination of the common bile duct, cystic duct, and hepatic ducts. A radiopaque dye is injected, and then films are taken. Abnormal results may indicate obstruction, stones, and tumors.
cholecystography (kō″ lē-sĭs-tŏg′ ră-fē)	X-ray examination of the gallbladder. A radiopaque dye is injected, and then films are taken. Abnormal results may indicate cholecystitis, cholelithiasis, and tumors.
colonofiberoscopy (kŏ′ lō-nŏ-fī″ bĕr-ŏs′ kō-pē)	Fiberoptic colonoscopy. The direct visual examination of the colon via a flexible colonoscope; used as a diagnostic aid, for removal of foreign bodies, polyps, and tissue.
endoscopic retrograde cholangiopancreatography (ERCP) (ĕn′ dō-skōp-ĭk rĕt′ rō-grād kō-lăn″ jē-ō-păn″ krē-ă-tŏg′ ră-fē)	X-ray examination of the biliary and pancreatic ducts. A contrast medium is injected, and then films are taken. Abnormal results may indicate fibrosis, biliary or pancreatic cysts, strictures, stones, and chronic pancreatitis.
esophagogastroduodenoscopy (ĕ-sŏf″ ă-gō′ găs″ trō-dū″ ō-dĕ-nŏs′ kō-pē)	An endoscopic examination of the esophagus, stomach, and small intestine. During the procedure, photographs, biopsy, or brushings may be done.

Test	Description
gamma-glutamyl tranferase (GGT) (găm′ ă glōō-tăm′ ĭl trăns′ fĕr-ās)	A test performed on blood serum to determine the level of GGT (enzyme found in the liver, kidney, prostate, heart, and spleen). Increased values may indicate cirrhosis, liver necrosis, hepatitis, alcoholism, neoplasms, acute pancreatitis, acute myocardial infarction, nephrosis, and acute cholecystitis.
gastric analysis (găs′ trĭk ă-năl′ ĭ sĭs)	A test performed to determine quality of secretion, amount of free and combined HCl, and absence or presence of blood, bacteria, bile, and fatty acids. Increased level of HCl may indicate peptic ulcer disease, Zollinger-Ellison syndrome, and hypergastremia. Decreased level of HCl may indicate stomach cancer, pernicious anemia, and atrophic gastritis.
gastrointestinal (GI) series (găs″ trō-ĭn-tes′ tĭn″ ăl sĕr′ ēz)	Fluoroscopic examination of the esophagus, stomach, and small intestine. Barium is given orally, and it is observed as it flows through the GI system. See Figure 6–11. Abnormal results may indicate esophageal varices, ulcers, gastric polyps, malabsorption syndrome, hiatal hernias, diverticuli, pyloric stenosis, and foreign bodies.
hepatic antigen (HAA) (hĕ-păt′ ĭk ăn′ tĭ-jĕn)	A test performed to determine the presence of the hepatitis B virus
liver biopsy (lĭv′ ĕr bī-ŏp-sē)	Microscopic examination of liver tissue. Abnormal results may indicate cirrhosis, hepatitis, and tumors
occult blood (ŭ-kŭlt blod)	A test performed on feces to determine gastrointestinal bleeding that is invisible (hidden). Positive results may indicate gastritis, stomach cancer, peptic ulcer, ulcerative colitis, bowel cancer, bleeding esophageal varices, portal hypertension, pancreatitis, and diverticulitis.
ova and parasites (O&P) (o′ vă păr′ ă-sīts)	A test performed on stool to identify ova and parasites. Positive results indicate protozoa infestation.
stool culture (stool kŭl′ tūr)	A test performed on stool to identify the presence of organisms.
ultrasonography, gallbladder (ŭl-tră-sŏn-ŏg′ ră-fē găl″ blăd′ dĕr)	A test to visualize the gallbladder by using high-frequency sound waves. The echoes are recorded on an oscilloscope and film. See Figure 6–12. Abnormal results may indicate biliary obstruction, cholelithiasis, and acute cholecystitis.
ultrasonography, liver (ŭl-tră-sōn-ŏg′ ră-fē lĭv′ ĕr)	A test to visualize the liver by using high-frequency sound waves. The echoes are recorded on an oscilloscope and film. See Figure 6–13. Abnormal

Test	Description
	results may indicate hepatic tumors, cysts, abscess, and cirrhosis.
upper gastrointestinal fiberoscopy (ŭp′ ir găs′ trō-ĭn-tĕs′ tĭn″ ăl fī′ bĕr-ŏs′ kō-pē)	The direct visual examination of the gastric mucosa via a flexible fiberscope. Colored photographs or motion pictures can be taken during the procedure; used when gastric neoplasm is suspected.

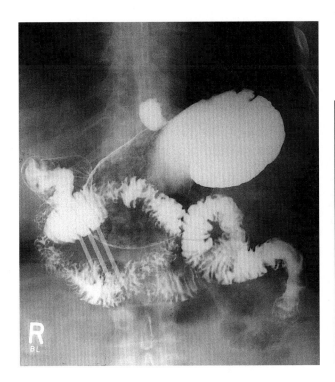

FIGURE 6–11

Upper GI series. *(Courtesy of Teresa Resch.)*

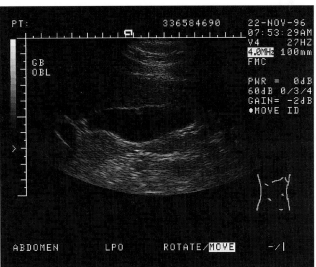

FIGURE 6–12

Gall bladder ultrasound. *(Courtesy of Teresa Resch.)*

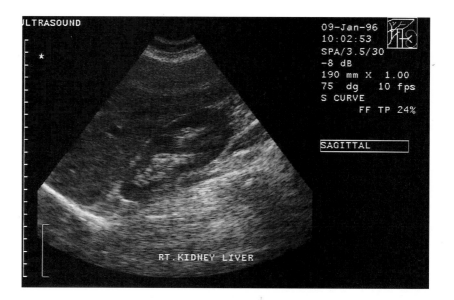

FIGURE 6–13

Ultrasound liver and right kidney. *(Courtesy of Teresa Resch.)*

COMMUNICATION ENRICHMENT

This segment is provided for those who wish to enhance their ability to communicate in either English or Spanish.

▶ **Related Terms**

English	Spanish	English	Spanish
swallowing	tragar (tră-*găr*)	beans	frijoles (frĭ-*hō*-lĕs)
nausea	nausea (*nă*-ū-sĕ-ă)	beer	cerveza (sĕr-*vĕ*-ză)
vomit	vomitos (*vō*-mĭ-tōs)	bread	pan (păn)
belch	eructos (ĕ-*rŭk*-tōs)	butter	mantequilla (măn-tĕ-*kĭ*-jă)
constipation	estreñimiento (ĕs-trĕ-ñĭ-mĭ-*ĕn*-tō)	cheese	queso (*kĕ*-sō)
diarrhea	diarrea (dĭ-ă-*rĕ*-ă)	coffee	café (că-*fĕ*)

English	Spanish	English	Spanish
gallbladder	vesicula biliar (vĕ-sĭ-kū-lă bĭ-lĭ-ăr)	cream	crema (crĕ-mă)
gallstones	cálculos biliares (kăl-kū-lōs bĭ-lĭ-ă-rĕs)	cup	taza (tă-să)
gingiva; gum	encias (ĕn-sĭ-ăs)	eggs	huevos (wĕ-vōs)
intestine	intestino (ĭn-tĕs-tĭ-nō)	diet	dieta (dī-ē-tă)
lips	labios (lă-bĭ-ōs)	fatty foods	comida grasosa (kō-mĭ-dă gră-sō-să)
liver	higado (ĭ-gă-dō)	fish	pescado (pĕs-kă-dō)
mouth	boca (bō-kă)	food	comida (kō-mĭ-dă)
rectum	recto (rĕk-tō)	fried	frito (frĭ-tō)
stomach	estomago (ĕs-tō-mă-gō)	fruit	fruta (frŭ-tă)
teeth	dientes (dĭ-ĕn-tĕs)	meat	carne (kăr-nĕ)
tongue	lengua (lĕn-gwā)	milk	leche (lĕ-chĕ)
chewing	masticar (măs-ti-kăr)	hunger	hambre (ăm-brĕ)
jaundice	ictericia (ĭk-tĕ-rĭ-sĭ-ă)	vegetable	vegetal (vĕ-hĕ-tăl)
laxative	purgante (pūr-găn-tĕ)	vitamins	vitaminas (vĭ-tă-mĭ-năs)
appetite	apetito (ă-pĕ-tĭ-tō)	bitter taste	sabor amargo (să-bōr ă-măr-gō)

STUDY AND REVIEW SECTION

LEARNING EXERCISES

▶ **Anatomy and Physiology**

Write your answers to the following questions. Do not refer back to the text.

1. Name the primary organs commonly associated with digestion.

   a. _____   b. _____

   c. _____   d. _____

   e. _____   f. _____

2. Name four accessory organs of digestion.

   a. _____   b. _____

   c. _____   d. _____

3. State the three main functions of the digestive system.

   a. _____

   b. _____

   c. _____

4. Define bolus. _____

   _____

5. Define peristalsis. _____

   _____

6. _____ _____ and _____ _____
   convert the food into a semiliquid state.

7. The _____ is the first portion of the small intestine.

8. Semiliquid food is called _____.

9. The _____ _____ transports nutrients to body cells.

10. The large intestine can be divided into four distinct sections called the

    _____, the _____,

    the _____, and the _____.

11. The _____ is the largest glandular organ in the body.

12. State the function of the gallbladder. _____

13. Name an important function of the pancreas. _____

14. State three functions of the liver.

    a. _____   b. _____

    c. _____

15. Where does digestion and absorption chiefly take place? _____

    _____

16. The salivary glands located in and about the mouth are called the _____,

    the _____, and the _____.

17. Name the two hormones secreted into the bloodstream by the pancreas.

    a. _____   b. _____

▶ Word Parts

1. In the spaces provided, write the definition of these prefixes, roots, combining forms, and suffixes. Do not refer to the listings of terminology words. Leave blank those terms you cannot define.

2. After completing as many as you can, refer back to the terminology word listings to check your work. For each word missed or left blank, write the term and its definition several times on the margins of these pages or on a separate sheet of paper.

3. To maximize the learning process, it is to your advantage to do the following exercises as directed. To refer to the terminology listings before completing these exercises invalidates the learning process.

Prefixes

Give the definitions of the following prefixes:

1. an- _____   2. ana- _____

3. cata- _____   4. dys- _____

5. epi- _____   6. hyper- _____

7. hypo- _____   8. mal- _____

9. mega- _____   10. peri- _____

11. post- _____   12. retro- _____

13. sub- _____

Roots and Combining Forms

Give the definitions of the following roots and combining forms:

1. absorpt _____
2. aden _____
3. amyl _____
4. ano _____
5. append _____
6. appendic _____
7. bili _____
8. bol _____
9. bucc _____
10. celi _____
11. cheil _____
12. chole _____
13. choledocho _____
14. col _____
15. colo _____
16. colon _____
17. colono _____
18. cyst _____
19. dent _____
20. denti _____
21. diverticul _____
22. duoden _____
23. enter _____
24. entero _____
25. esophage _____
26. esophago _____
27. gastr _____
28. gastro _____
29. gingiv _____
30. glosso _____
31. glyco _____
32. hemat _____
33. hepat _____
34. hepato _____
35. hernio _____
36. ile _____
37. ileo _____
38. labi _____
39. laparo _____
40. laxat _____
41. lingu _____
42. lipo _____
43. log _____
44. mes _____
45. pancreat _____
46. pept _____
47. pharynge _____
48. prandi _____
49. proct _____
50. procto _____
51. pylor _____
52. recto _____
53. sial _____
54. sigmoido _____
55. spleno _____
56. stomat _____

57. tox _____   58. vago _____

59. vermi _____

Suffixes

Give the definitions of the following suffixes:

1. -ac _____   2. -al _____

3. -algia _____   4. -ary _____

5. -ase _____   6. -cele _____

7. -clysis _____   8. -dynia _____

9. -ectomy _____   10. -emesis _____

11. -form _____   12. -genesis _____

13. -ic _____   14. -in _____

15. -ion _____   16. -ism _____

17. -ist _____   18. -itis _____

19. -ive _____   20. -logy _____

21. -lysis _____   22. -megaly _____

23. -oma _____   24. -orexia _____

25. -osis _____   26. -pathy _____

27. -pepsia _____   28. -pexy _____

29. -phagia _____   30. -plasty _____

31. -rrhaphy _____   32. -scope _____

33. -scopy _____   34. -stalsis _____

35. -stomy _____   36. -tomy _____

37. -y _____

▶ Identifying Medical Terms

In the spaces provided, write the medical terms for the following meanings:

1. _____   An enzyme that breaks down starch

2. _____   The building up of the body substances

3. _____   Lack of appetite

4. _____   Surgical excision of the appendix

5. _____   Inflammation of the appendix

6. _____   Pertaining to or conveying bile

7. _____   Pertaining to the abdomen

8. _____   Suture of the colon

9. _____   Difficulty in swallowing

10. _____   Inflammation of the liver

11. _____   Surgical incision for the repair of a hernia

12. _____   Pertaining to after meals

13. _____   Pain in the rectum and anus

14. _____   Enlargement of the spleen

15. _____   Instrument used to view the sigmoid

▶ Spelling

In the spaces provided, write the correct spelling of these misspelled terms:

1. bilery _____   2. colonscopy _____

3. enteroclsis _____   4. gastorentreology _____

5. heptotoxin _____   6. laxtive _____

7. persitalsis _____   8. salademitis _____

9. vaogtomy _____   10. verimform _____

WORD PARTS STUDY SHEET

Word Parts	Give the Meaning
dys-	_____
mega-	_____
peri-	_____
post-	_____
sub-	_____
appendic-	_____

bucc- _____

chole- _____

cirrh- _____

col-, colo-, colon-, colono- _____

cyst- _____

dent-, denti- _____

duoden- _____

enter-, entero- _____

esophage-, esophago- _____

gastr-, gastro- _____

gingiv- _____

glosso- _____

hepat-, hepato- _____

lingu- _____

pancreat- _____

prandi- _____

proct-, procto- _____

sigmoido- _____

-al, -ic _____

-algia, -dynia _____

-ase _____

-ectomy _____

-genesis _____

-ion _____

-ist _____

-itis _____

-megaly _____

-oma _____

-pathy _____

-pepsia _____

-plasty   _____

-rrhaphy   _____

-scopy   _____

-stalsis   _____

-stomy   _____

REVIEW QUESTIONS

▶ Matching

Select the appropriate lettered meaning for each numbered line.

_____   1. cirrhosis

_____   2. constipation

_____   3. diarrhea

_____   4. gavage

_____   5. hemorrhoid

_____   6. hernia

_____   7. hyperalimentation

_____   8. lavage

_____   9. pilonidal cyst

_____   10. volvulus

a. To wash out a cavity
b. To feed liquid or semiliquid food via a tube
c. A twisting of the bowel on itself
d. Frequent passage of unformed watery stools
e. A chronic degenerative liver disease
f. Infrequent passage of unduly hard and dry feces
g. A closed sac in the crease of the sacrococcygeal region
h. The abnormal protrusion of an organ or a part of an organ through the wall of the body cavity that normally contains it
i. A mass of dilated, tortuous veins in the anorectum
j. An intravenous infusion of a hypertonic solution to sustain life
k. The evacuation of the bowel

▶ Abbreviations

Place the correct word, phrase, or abbreviation in the space provided.

1. before meals _____

2. BM _____

3. BS _____

4. food _____

5. gallbladder _____

6. hepatitis A virus _____

7. NG _____

8. n.p.o. _____

9. after meals _____

10. total parenteral nutrition _____

▶ **Diagnostic and Laboratory Tests**

Select the best answer to each multiple choice question. Circle the letter of your choice.

1. X-ray examination of the common bile duct, cystic duct, and hepatic ducts.
   a. cholangiography
   b. cholecystography
   c. cholangiopancreatography
   d. ultrasonography

2. The direct visual examination of the colon via a flexible colonoscope.
   a. cholangiography
   b. ultrasonography
   c. colonofiberoscopy
   d. cholecystography

3. Fluoroscopic examination of the esophagus, stomach, and small intestine.
   a. barium enema
   b. ultrasonography
   c. cholangiography
   d. gastrointestinal series

4. An endoscopic examination of the esophagus, stomach, and small intestine.
   a. cholangiography
   b. gastroduodenoesophagoscopy
   c. esophagogastroduodenoscopy
   d. gastric analysis

5. A test performed to determine the presence of the hepatitis B virus.
   a. occult blood test
   b. stool culture
   c. hepatic antigen
   d. ova and parasites test

CRITICAL THINKING ACTIVITY

▶ Case Study

Peptic Ulcer Disease (PUD)

Please read the following case study and then answer the questions that follow.

A 35-year-old male was seen by a physician and the following is a synopsis of the visit.

Present History: The patient states that he has been under a lot of pressure at work lately and has noticed a dull, aching pain in his stomach and back. He states that he has heartburn and "belches" a lot.

Signs and Symptoms: Dull, gnawing pain and a burning sensation in the midepigastrium. Pyrosis (heartburn) and sour eructation (belching).

Diagnosis: Acute gastric ulcer; peptic ulcer disease. Diagnosis determined by a gastrointestinal (GI) series, gastric analysis, and histology with culture to determine presence of *Helicobacter pylori*. No *H. pylori* were found in the culture.

Treatment: Goal is to manage and reduce gastric acidity. This may be accomplished through various treatment regimens such as stress management, rest, diet, avoidance of tobacco, caffeine, and alcohol, and medication. The patient is placed on Mylanta 2 tablets every 2 to 4 hours between meals and at bedtime, and Zantac 300 mg at bedtime.

Prevention: Avoid substances that produce gastric acidity. Stress management, rest, diet, avoidance of tobacco, caffeine, and alcohol are recommended.

Critical Thinking Questions

1. Signs and symptoms of a gastric ulcer include a dull, gnawing pain and a burning sensation in the midepigastrium. Other indications are: _____, which is heartburn, and sour eructation.

2. The diagnosis of acute gastric ulcer was determined by a gastric analysis and a _____ series.

3. The goal of treatment for acute gastric ulcer is to manage and reduce gastric _____.

4. The medication regimen prescribed included _____ 2 tablets every 2 to 4 hours between meals and at bedtime and,

5. Zantac _____ mg at bedtime is also prescribed.

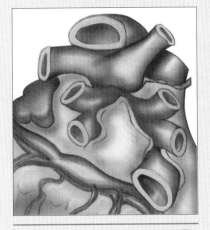

7

THE CARDIOVASCULAR SYSTEM

OBJECTIVES

On completion of this chapter, you should be able to:

- Describe the cardiovascular system.
- Describe and state the functions of arteries, veins, and capillaries.
- Describe cardiovascular differences of the child and the older adult.
- Identify the commonly used pulse checkpoints of the body.
- Describe blood pressure.
- Analyze, build, spell, and pronounce medical words that relate to surgical procedures and pathology.
- Identify and give the meaning of selected vocabulary words.
- Identify and define selected abbreviations.
- Review Drug Highlights presented in this chapter.
- Provide the description of diagnostic and laboratory tests related to the cardiovascular system.
- Successfully complete the study and review section.

▶ ANATOMY AND PHYSIOLOGY OVERVIEW

Through the cardiovascular system, blood is circulated to all parts of the body by the action of the heart. This process provides the body's cells with oxygen and nutritive elements and removes waste materials and carbon dioxide. The *heart,* a muscular pump, is the central organ of the system, which also includes *arteries, veins,* and *capillaries.* The various organs and components of the cardiovascular system are described in this chapter, along with some of their functions.

▶ THE HEART

The *heart* is a four-chambered, hollow muscular pump that circulates blood throughout the cardiovascular system. The heart is the center of the cardiovascular system from which the various blood vessels originate and later return. It is slightly larger than a man's fist and weighs approximately 300 g in the average adult male. It lies slightly to the left of the midline of the body and is shaped like an inverted cone with its apex downward. The heart has three layers or linings:

Endocardium. The inner lining of the heart
Myocardium. The muscular, middle layer of the heart
Pericardium. The outer, membranous sac surrounding the heart

CHAMBERS OF THE HEART

The human heart acts as a double pump and is divided into the right and left heart by a partition called the *septum.* Each side contains an upper and lower chamber. The *atria* or upper chambers are separated by the interatrial septum. The *ventricles* or lower chambers are separated by the interventricular septum. The atria receive blood from the various parts of the body, whereas the ventricles pump blood to body parts. A description of the heart's four chambers and some of their functions is given below.

The Right Atrium

The right upper portion of the heart is called the *right atrium.* It is a thin-walled space that receives blood from all body parts except the lungs. Two large veins bring the blood into the right atrium and are known as the superior and inferior vena cavae.

THE CARDIOVASCULAR SYSTEM

ORGAN/STRUCTURE	PRIMARY FUNCTIONS
Heart	Hollow muscular pump that circulates blood throughout the cardiovascular system
Arteries	Branching system of vessels that transports blood from the right and left ventricles of the heart to all body parts
Veins	Vessels that transport blood from peripheral tissues to the heart
Capillaries	Microscopic blood vessels that connect arterioles with venules; facilitate passage of life-sustaining fluids containing oxygen and nutrients to cell bodies and the removal of accumulated waste and carbon dioxide

The Right Ventricle

The right lower portion of the heart is called the *right ventricle*. It receives blood from the right atrium through the atrioventricular valve and pumps it through a semilunar valve to the lungs.

The Left Atrium

The left upper portion of the heart is called the *left atrium*. It receives blood rich in oxygen as it returns from the lungs via the left and right pulmonary veins.

The Left Ventricle

The left lower portion of the heart is called the *left ventricle*. It receives blood from the left atrium through an atrioventricular valve and pumps it through a semilunar valve to a large artery known as the aorta and from there to all parts of the body except the lungs.

HEART VALVES

The *valves* of the heart are located at the entrance and exit of each ventricle. The functions of each of the four heart valves are described below.

The Tricuspid Valve

The *right atrioventricular* or *tricuspid valve* guards the opening between the atrium and the right ventricle. The tricuspid valve allows the flow of blood into the ventricle and prevents its return to the right atrium.

The Pulmonary Semilunar Valve

The exit point for blood leaving the right ventricle is called the *pulmonary semilunar valve*. Located between the right ventricle and the pulmonary artery, it allows blood to flow from the right ventricle through the pulmonary artery to the lungs.

The Bicuspid or Mitral Valve

The left atrioventricular valve between the left atrium and ventricle is called the *bicuspid* or *mitral valve*. It allows blood to flow to the left ventricle and closes to prevent its return to the left atrium.

The Aortic Semilunar Valve

Blood exits from the left ventricle through the *aortic semilunar valve*. Located between the left ventricle and the aorta, it allows blood to flow into the aorta and prevents its return to the ventricle.

VASCULAR SYSTEM OF THE HEART

Due to the membranous lining of the heart *(endocardium)* and the thickness of the myocardium, it is essential that the heart have its own vascular system. The coronary arteries supply the heart with blood, and the cardiac veins, draining into the coronary sinus, collect the blood and return it to the right atrium (Fig. 7–1).

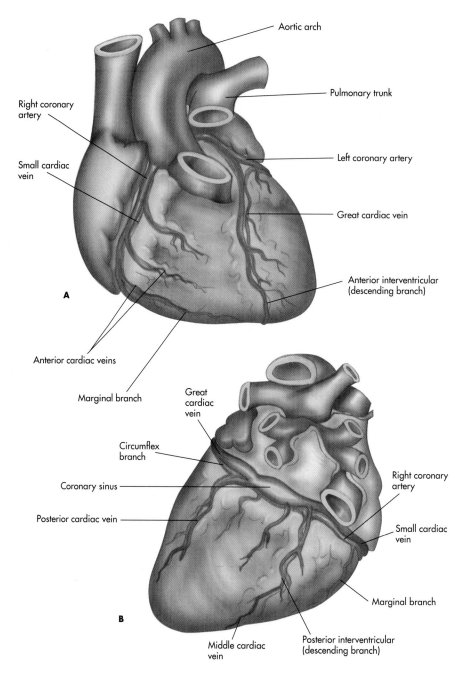

Aortic arch

Right coronary artery

Small cardiac vein

Pulmonary trunk

Left coronary artery

Great cardiac vein

Anterior interventricular (descending branch)

A

Anterior cardiac veins

Marginal branch

Great cardiac vein

Circumflex branch

Coronary sinus

Posterior cardiac vein

Right coronary artery

Small cardiac vein

Marginal branch

B

Middle cardiac vein

Posterior interventricular (descending branch)

FIGURE 7–1

Coronary circulation. **(A)** Coronary vessels portraying the complexity and extent of the coronary circulation. **(B)** Coronary vessels that supply the anterior surface of the heart.

▶ THE FLOW OF BLOOD

Blood flows through the heart, to the lungs, back to the heart, and on to the various body parts as indicated in Figure 7–2. Blood from the superior and inferior vena cavae enters the right atrium and subsequently passes through the tricuspid valve and into the right ventricle, which pumps it through the pulmonary semilunar valve into the left and right pulmonary arteries, which carry it to the lungs. In the lungs, the blood gives up wastes

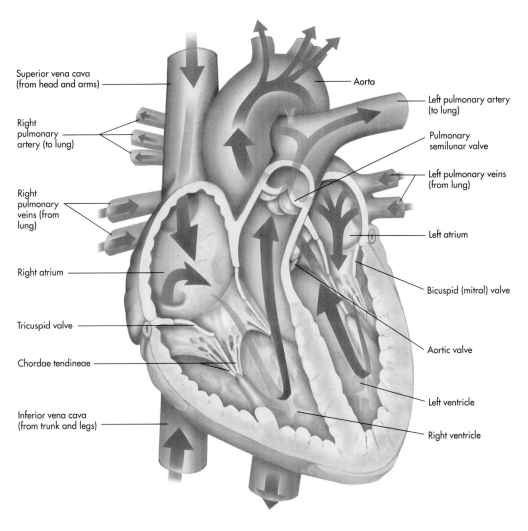

Superior vena cava (from head and arms)

Right pulmonary artery (to lung)

Right pulmonary veins (from lung)

Right atrium

Tricuspid valve

Chordae tendineae

Inferior vena cava (from trunk and legs)

Aorta

Left pulmonary artery (to lung)

Pulmonary semilunar valve

Left pulmonary veins (from lung)

Left atrium

Bicuspid (mitral) valve

Aortic valve

Left ventricle

Right ventricle

FIGURE 7-2

The flow of blood through the heart.

and takes on oxygen as it passes through capillaries into veins. Blood leaves the lungs through the left and right pulmonary veins, which carry it to the heart's left atrium. The oxygenated blood then passes through the bicuspid or mitral valve into the left ventricle, which pumps it out through the aortic valve and into the *aorta*. This large artery supplies a branching system of smaller arteries that connect to tiny capillaries throughout the body.

Capillaries are microscopic blood vessels with thin walls that allow the passage of oxygen and nutrients to the body and let the blood pick up waste and carbon dioxide. Veins lead away from the capillaries as tiny vessels and increase in size until they join the superior and inferior vena cavae as they return to the heart.

THE HEARTBEAT

The *heartbeat* is controlled by the autonomic nervous system. It is normally generated by specialized neuromuscular tissue of the heart that is capable of causing cardiac muscle to contract rhythmically. The neuromuscular tissue of the heart comprises the *sinoatrial node*, the *atrioventricular node*, and the *atrioventricular bundle* (Fig. 7–3).

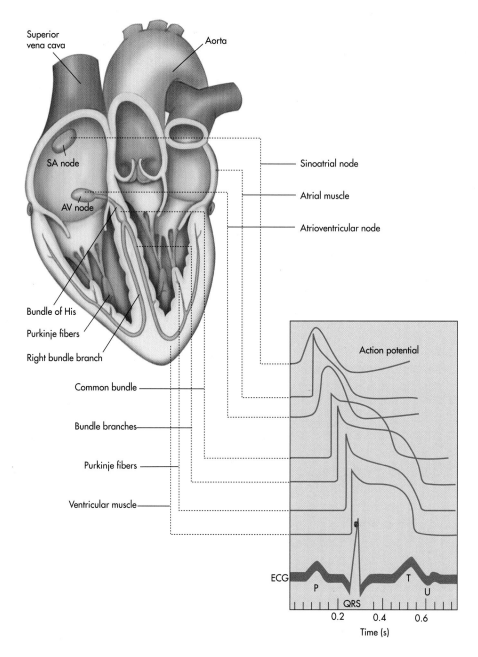

FIGURE 7-3

The conduction system of the heart. Action potentials for the SA and AV nodes, other parts of the conduction system, and the atrial and ventricular muscles are shown along with the correlation to recorded electrical activity (electrocardiogram ECG [EKG]).

Sinoatrial Node (SA Node)

Often called the *pacemaker of the heart,* the *SA node* is located in the upper wall of the right atrium, just below the opening of the superior vena cava. It consists of a dense network of *Purkinje fibers (atypical muscle fibers)* considered to be the source of impulses initiating the heartbeat. Electrical impulses discharged by the SA node are distributed to the right and left atria and cause them to contract.

Atrioventricular Node (AV Node)

Located beneath the endocardium of the right atrium, the *AV node* transmits electrical impulses to the *bundle of His (atrioventricular bundle).*

Atrioventricular Bundle (Bundle of His)

The *bundle of His* forms a part of the conducting system of the heart. It extends from the AV node into the intraventricular septum, where it divides into two branches within the two ventricles. The *Purkinje system* includes the bundle of His and the peripheral fibers. These fibers end in the ventricular muscles, where the excitation of muscle is initiated, causing contraction. The average heartbeat *(pulse)* is between 60 and 100 beats per minute for the average adult. The rate of heartbeat may be affected by emotions, smoking, disease, body size, age, stress, the environment, and many other factors.

ELECTROCARDIOGRAM

An *electrocardiogram* (ECG, EKG) records the electrical activity of the heart. A standard electrocardiogram consists of 12 different leads. With electrodes placed on the patient's arms, legs, and six positions on the chest, a 12-lead ECG can be recorded. The leads that are recorded on an electrocardiograph are I, II, III, aVR, aVL, aVF, and six chest leads V_1, V_2, V_3, V_4, V_5, and V_6. The standard limb leads, leads I, II, and III, each record the differences in potential between two limbs. Augmented limb leads, aVR, aVL, and aVF, record between one limb and the other two limbs. There are six unipolar chest leads that record electrical activity of different parts of the heart. An ECG provides valuable information in the diagnosing of cardiac abnormalities, such as myocardial damage and arrhythmias (Fig. 7–4).

▶ ARTERIES

The *arteries* constitute a branching system of vessels that transports blood from the right and left ventricles of the heart to all body parts (Table 7–1, and Fig. 7–5). In a normal state, arteries are elastic tubes that recoil and carry blood in pulsating waves. All arteries have a pulse, reflecting the rhythmical beating of the heart; however, certain points are commonly used to check the rate, rhythm, and condition of the arterial wall. These checkpoints are listed below and shown in Figure 7–6.

Radial. Located on the radial *(thumb side)* of the wrist. This is the most common site for taking a pulse

Brachial. Located in the antecubital space of the elbow. This is the most common site used to check blood pressure

Carotid. Located in the neck. In an emergency *(cardiac arrest),* this site is the most readily accessible

Temporal. Located at the temple

Femoral. Located in the groin

Popliteal. Located behind the knee

Dorsalis pedis. Located on the upper surface of the foot

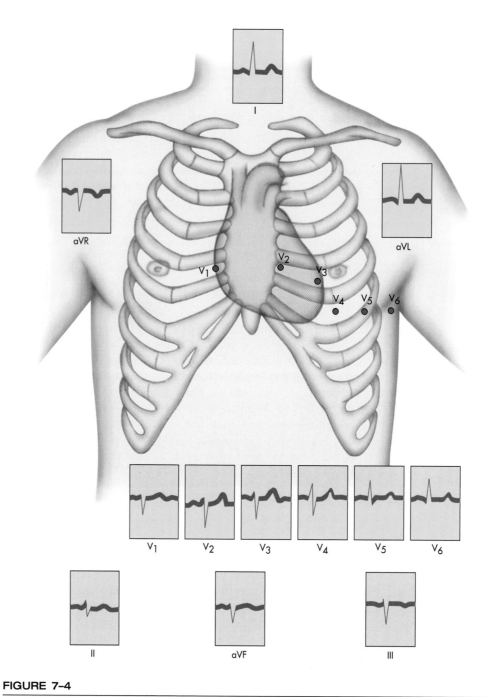

FIGURE 7–4

A normal electrocardiogram (ECG [EKG]).

▶ BLOOD PRESSURE

Blood pressure, generally speaking, is the pressure exerted by the blood on the walls of the vessels. The term most commonly refers to the pressure exerted in large arteries at the peak of the pulse wave. This pressure is measured with a *sphygmomanometer* used in concert with a *stethoscope*. Pressure is reported in millimeters of mercury as observed on a graduated column. With the use of a pressure cuff, circulation is interrupted in the brachial artery just above the elbow. Pressure from the cuff is shown on the graduated

TABLE 7–1   Selected Arteries

Artery	Tissue Supplied
Right common carotid	Right side of the head and neck
Left common carotid	Left side of the head and neck
Left subclavian	Left upper extremity
Brachiocephalic	Head and arm
Aortic arch	Branches to head, neck, and upper extremities
Celiac	Stomach, spleen, and liver
Renal	Kidneys
Superior mesenteric	Lower half of large intestine
Inferior mesenteric	Small intestines and first half of the large intestine
Axillary	Axilla
Brachial	Arm
Radial	Lateral side of the hand
Ulnar	Medial side of the hand
Internal iliac	Pelvic viscera and rectum
External iliac	Genitalia and lower trunk muscles
Deep femoral	Deep thigh muscles
Femoral	Thigh
Popliteal	Leg and foot
Anterior tibial	Leg
Dorsalis pedis	Foot

column of the sphygmomanometer, and as the pressure is released, blood again flows past the cuff. At this point, using a stethoscope, one hears a heartbeat and records the systolic pressure. Continued release of pressure results in a change in the heartbeat sound from loud to soft, at which point one records the diastolic pressure. This method results in a ratio of systolic over diastolic readings expressed in millimeters of mercury (mm Hg). In the average adult, the systolic pressure usually ranges from 100 to 140 mm Hg and the diastolic from 60 to 90 mm Hg. A typical blood pressure showing systolic over diastolic readings might be expressed as 120/80. Two types of sphygmomanometers are shown in Figure 7–7.

PULSE PRESSURE

The *pulse pressure* is the difference between the systolic and diastolic readings. This reading is an indication of the tone of the arterial walls. The normal pulse pressure is found when the systolic pressure is about 40 points higher than the diastolic reading. For example, if the blood pressure is 120/80, the pulse pressure would be 40.

▶ VEINS

The vessels that transport blood from peripheral tissues to the heart are the *veins* (see Table 7–2, and Fig. 7–8). In a normal state, veins have thin walls and valves that prevent the backflow of blood. Veins are the vessels used when blood is removed for analysis. The process of removing blood from a vein is called *venipuncture.*

▶ CAPILLARIES

The *capillaries* are microscopic blood vessels with single-celled walls that connect *arterioles* (small arteries) with *venules* (small veins). Blood, passing through capillaries, gives

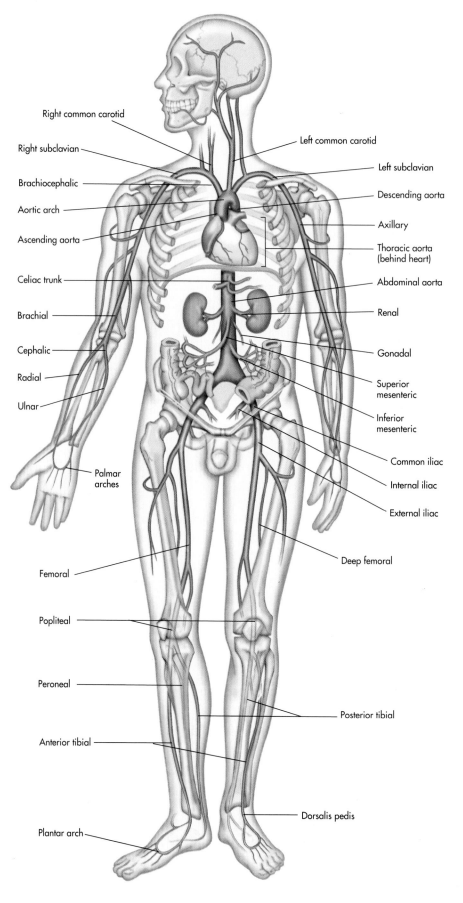

Right common carotid

Right subclavian

Brachiocephalic

Aortic arch

Ascending aorta

Celiac trunk

Brachial

Cephalic

Radial

Ulnar

Palmar arches

Femoral

Popliteal

Peroneal

Anterior tibial

Plantar arch

Left common carotid

Left subclavian

Descending aorta

Axillary

Thoracic aorta (behind heart)

Abdominal aorta

Renal

Gonadal

Superior mesenteric

Inferior mesenteric

Common iliac

Internal iliac

External iliac

Deep femoral

Posterior tibial

Dorsalis pedis

FIGURE 7–5

An overview of the arterial system.

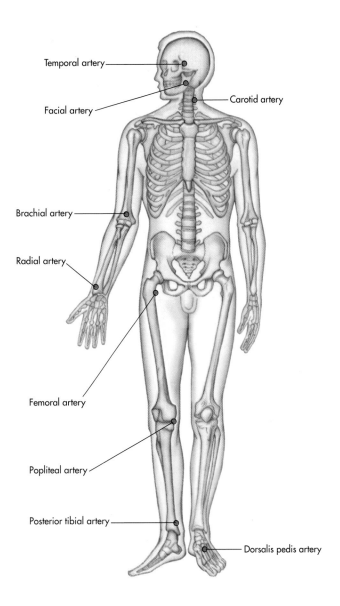

Temporal artery

Facial artery

Carotid artery

Brachial artery

Radial artery

Femoral artery

Popliteal artery

Posterior tibial artery

Dorsalis pedis artery

FIGURE 7-6

The primary pulse points of the body.

up the oxygen and nutrients carried to this point by the arteries and picks up waste and carbon dioxide as it enters veins. The extremely thin walls of capillaries facilitate passage of life-sustaining fluids containing oxygen and nutrients to cell bodies and the removal of accumulated waste and carbon dioxide.

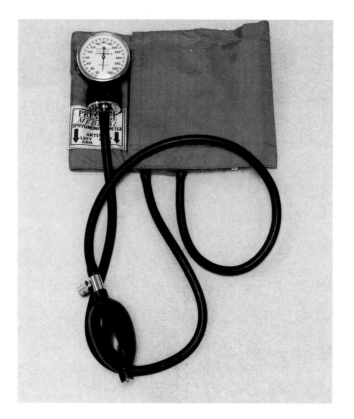
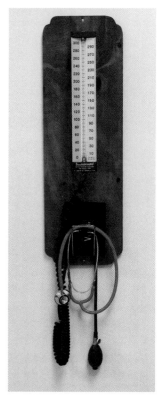

A   **B**

FIGURE 7–7

Sphygmomanometers: **(A)** aneroid type, **(B)** mercury type.

TABLE 7–2   Selected Veins

Vein	Tissue Drained
External jugular	Superficial tissues of the head and neck
Internal jugular	Sinuses of the brain
Subclavian	Upper extremities
Superior vena cava	Head, neck, and upper extremities
Inferior vena cava	Lower body
Hepatic	Liver
Hepatic portal	Liver and gallbladder
Superior mesenteric	Small intestine and most of the colon
Inferior mesenteric	Descending colon and rectum
Cephalic	Lateral arm
Axillary	Axilla and arm
Basilic	Medial arm
External iliac	Lower limb
Internal iliac	Pelvic viscera
Femoral	Thigh
Great saphenous	Leg
Popliteal	Lower leg
Peroneal	Foot
Anterior tibial	Deep anterior leg and dorsal foot

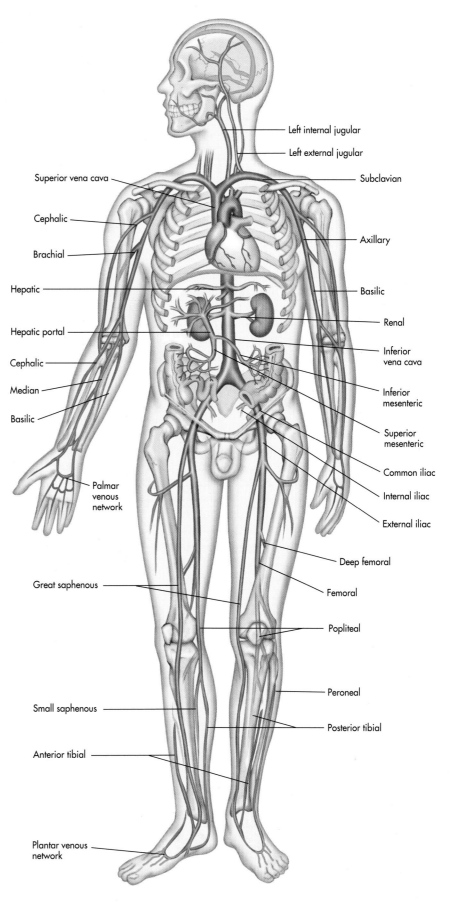

Left internal jugular

Left external jugular

Superior vena cava

Subclavian

Cephalic

Axillary

Brachial

Hepatic

Basilic

Hepatic portal

Renal

Cephalic

Inferior vena cava

Median

Inferior mesenteric

Basilic

Superior mesenteric

Palmar venous network

Common iliac

Internal iliac

External iliac

Deep femoral

Great saphenous

Femoral

Popliteal

Small saphenous

Peroneal

Posterior tibial

Anterior tibial

Plantar venous network

FIGURE 7–8

An overview of the venous system.

LIFE SPAN CONSIDERATIONS

▶ THE CHILD

The development of the fetal heart is usually completed during the first 2 months of intrauterine life. It is completely formed and functioning by 10 weeks. At 16 weeks fetal heart tones can be heard with a **fetoscope.** Oxygenated blood is transported by the umbilical vein from the placenta to the fetus. Fetal circulation is terminated at birth when the umbilical cord is clamped. The newborn's circulation begins to function shortly after birth and if proper adaptations do not take place, congenital heart disease may occur. Most congenital heart defects develop before the 10th week of pregnancy. Pediatric cardiologists have recognized more than 50 congenital heart defects. If the left side of the heart is not completely separated from the right side, various septal defects develop. If the four chambers of the heart do not occur normally, complex anomalies form, such as tetralogy of Fallot, a congenital heart defect involving pulmonary stenosis, ventricular septal defect, dextroposition of the aorta, and hypertrophy of the right ventricle.

The **pulse, blood pressure,** and **respirations** will vary according to the age of the child. A newborn's pulse rate is irregular and rapid, varying from 120 to 140 beats/minute. Blood pressure is low and may vary with the size of the cuff used. The average blood pressure at birth is 80/46. The respirations are approximately 35 to 50 per minute.

▶ THE OLDER ADULT

Current evidence indicates that cardiac changes that were once contributed to the aging process may be minimized by modifying lifestyle and personal habits, such as following a low-sodium, low-fat diet, not smoking, drinking in moderation, managing stress, and exercising regularly. Studies have shown that the normal aging heart is able to provide an adequate cardiac output. But in some older adults, the heart must work harder to pump blood because of hardening of the arteries **(arteriosclerosis)** and a buildup of fatty plaques in the arterial walls **(atherosclerosis).** Arteries may gradually become stiff and lose their elastic recoil. The aorta and arteries supplying the heart and brain are generally affected first. Reduced blood flow, elevated blood lipids, and defective endothelial repair that can be seen in aging accelerate the course of cardiovascular disease.

Some common symptoms seen in the older adult with cardiovascular disease are confusion, syncope, palpitations, shortness of breath, dry, hacking cough, fatigue, chest pain, weight gain, and fluid retention, especially in the legs.

TERMINOLOGY

WITH SURGICAL PROCEDURES & PATHOLOGY

TERM	WORD PARTS			DEFINITION
anginal (ăn′ jĭ-năl)	angin al	R S	to choke, quinsy pertaining to	Pertaining to attacks of choking or suffocation
angioblast (ăn′ jĭ-ō-blăst)	angio blast	CF S	vessel immature cell, germ cell	The germ cell from which blood vessels develop
angiocardiog- **raphy** (ăn″ jĭ-ō-kăr″ dĭ-ŏg′ ră-fē)	angio cardio graphy	CF CF S	vessel heart recording	The process of recording the heart and vessels after an intravenous injection of a radiopaque solution
angiocarditis (ăn″ jĭ-ō-kăr-dī′ tĭs)	angio card itis	CF R S	vessel heart inflammation	Inflammation of the heart and its great vessels
angioma (ăn″ jĭ-ō′ mă)	angi oma	CF S	vessel tumor	A tumor of a blood vessel. See Figure 7–9.
angionecrosis (ăn″ jĭ-ō-nĕc-rō′ sĭs)	angio necr osis	CF R S	vessel death condition of	A condition of the death of blood vessels
angiopathy (ăn″ jĭ-ŏp′ ă-thē)	angio pathy	CF S	vessel disease	Disease of blood vessels
angioplasty (ăn′ jĭ-ō-plăs″ tē)	angio plasty	CF S	vessel surgical repair	Surgical repair of a blood vessel or vessels
angiorrhaphy (ăn″ jĭ-or′ ă-fē)	angio rrhaphy	CF S	vessel suture	Suture of a blood vessel or vessels
angiospasm (ăn′ jĭ-ō-spăzm)	angio spasm	CF S	vessel contraction, spasm	Contraction or spasm of a blood vessel
angiostenosis (ăn″ jĭ-ō-stĕ-nō′ sĭs)	angio sten osis	CF R S	vessel narrowing condition of	A condition of narrowing of a blood vessel
aortitis (ā″ ōr-tī′ tĭs)	aort itis	R S	aorta inflammation	Inflammation of the aorta

continued

Terminology - continued

TERM	WORD PARTS			DEFINITION
aortomalacia (ā-ōr″ tō-mă-lā′ shĭ-ă)	aorto malacia	CF S	aorta softening	Softening of the walls of the aorta
arrhythmia (ă-rĭth′ mĭ-ă)	a rrhythm ia	P R S	lack of rhythm condition	A condition in which there is a lack of rhythm of the heartbeat
arterectomy (ăr″ tĕ-rĕk′ tō-mē)	arter ectomy	R S	artery excision	Surgical excision of an artery
arterial (ăr-tē′ rĭ-ăl)	arteri al	CF S	artery pertaining to	Pertaining to an artery
arteriolith (ăr-tē′ rĭ-ō-lĭth)	arterio lith	CF S	artery stone	An arterial stone
arteriosclerosis (ăr-tē″ rĭ-ō-sklĕ-rō′ sĭs)	arterio scler osis	CF R S	artery hardening condition of	A condition of hardening of an artery
arteriotome (ăr-tē′ rĭ-ō-tōm)	arterio tome	CF S	artery instrument to cut	An instrument used to cut an artery
arteriotomy (ăr″ tē-rĭ-ŏt′ ō-mē)	arterio tomy	CF S	artery incision	Incision into an artery
arteritis (ăr″ tĕ-rī′ tĭs)	arter itis	R S	artery inflammation	Inflammation of an artery. See Figure 7–10.
atheroma (ăth″ ĕr-ō′ mă)	ather oma	R S	fatty substance, porridge tumor	Tumor of an artery containing a fatty substance
atherosclerosis (ăth″ ĕr-ō-sklĕ-rō′ sĭs)	athero scler osis	CF R S	fatty substance, porridge hardening condition of	A condition of the arteries characterized by the buildup of fatty substances and hardening of the walls
atrioventricular (ăt″ rĭ-ō-vĕn-trĭk′ ū-lăr)	atrio ventricul ar	CF R S	atrium ventricle pertaining to	Pertaining to the atrium and the ventricle
bicuspid (bī-kŭs′ pĭd)	bi cuspid	P S	two point	Having two points or cusps; pertaining to the mitral valve

Terminology - continued

TERM	WORD PARTS			DEFINITION
bradycardia (brăd″ ĭ-kăr′ dĭ-ă)	brady card ia	P R S	slow heart condition	A condition of slow heartbeat
cardiac (kăr′ dĭ-ăk)	cardi ac	CF S	heart pertaining to	Pertaining to the heart
cardiocentesis (kăr″ dĭ-ō-sĕn-tē′ sĭs)	cardio centesis	CF S	heart surgical puncture	Surgical puncture of the heart
cardiodynia (kăr″ dĭ-ō-dĭn′ ĭ-ă)	cardio dynia	CF S	heart pain	Pain in the heart
cardiokinetic (kăr″ dĭ-ō-kĭ-nĕt′ ĭk)	cardio kinet ic	CF R S	heart motion pertaining to	Pertaining to heart motion
cardiologist (kăr-dē-ŏl′ ō-jĭst)	cardio log ist	CF R S	heart study of one who specializes	One who specializes in the study of the heart
cardiology (kăr″ dĭ-ŏl′ ō-jē)	cardio logy	CF S	heart study of	The study of the heart
cardiomegaly (kăr″ dĭ-ō-mĕg′ ă-lē)	cardio megaly	CF S	heart enlargement, large	Enlargement of the heart
cardiometer (kăr″ dĭ-ŏm′ ĕ-tĕr)	cardio meter	CF S	heart instrument to measure	An instrument used to measure the action of the heart
cardiopathy (kăr″ dĭ-ŏp′ ă-thē)	cardio pathy	CF S	heart disease	Heart disease
cardioplegia (kăr″ dĭ-ŏ-plē′ jĭ-ă)	cardio plegia	CF S	heart stroke, paralysis	Paralysis of the heart
cardioptosis (kăr″ dĭ-ō-tō′ sĭs)	cardio ptosis	CF S	heart prolapse, drooping	Prolapse of the heart; a downward displacement
cardiopulmonary (kăr″ dĭ-ō-pŭl′ mō-nĕr-ē)	cardio pulmonar y	CF R S	heart lung pertaining to	Pertaining to the heart and lungs

continued

Terminology - continued

TERM	WORD PARTS			DEFINITION
cardioscope (kăr′ dĭ-ō-skōp″)	cardio scope	CF S	heart instrument	An instrument used to examine the interior of the heart
cardiotonic (kăr″ dĭ-ō-tŏn′ ĭk)	cardio ton ic	CF R S	heart tone pertaining to	Pertaining to increasing the tone of the heart; a type of medication
cardiovascular (kăr″ dĭ-ō-văs′ kū-lar)	cardio vascul ar	CF R S	heart small vessel pertaining to	Pertaining to the heart and small blood vessels
carditis (kăr-dĭ′ tĭs)	card itis	R S	heart inflammation	Inflammation of the heart
constriction (kən-strĭk′ shən)	con strict ion	P R S	together, with to draw, to bind process	The process of drawing together as in the narrowing of a vessel
cyanosis (sī-ăn-ō′ sĭs	cyan osis	R S	dark blue condition of	A dark blue condition of the skin and mucus membranes caused by oxygen deficiency
dextrocardia (dĕks″ trō-kăr′ dĭ-ă)	dextro card ia	CF R S	to the right heart condition	The condition of the heart being on the right side of the body
electrocardio-graph (ē-lĕk″ trō-kăr′ dĭ-ō-grăf)	electro cardio graph	CF CF S	electricity heart to write, record	A device used for recording the electrical impulses of the heart muscle
electrocardio-phonograph (ē-lĕk″ trō-kăr″ dĭ-ō-fō′ nō-grăf)	electro cardio phono graph	CF CF CF S	electricity heart sound to write, record	A device used to record heart sounds
embolism (ĕm′ bō-lĭzm)	embol ism	R S	a throwing in condition of	A condition in which a blood clot obstructs a blood vessel; *a moving blood clot*
endarterectomy (ĕn″ dăr-tĕr-ĕk′ tō-mē)	end arter ectomy	P R S	within artery excision	Surgical excision of the inner portion of an artery
endocarditis (ĕn″ dō-kăr-dĭ′ tĭs)	endo card itis	P R S	within heart inflammation	Inflammation of the endocardium

Terminology - continued

TERM	WORD PARTS			DEFINITION
endocardium (ĕn″ dō-kăr′ dē-ŭm)	endo cardi um	P CF S	within heart tissue	The inner lining of the heart
extrasystole (ĕks″ tră-sĭs′ tō-lē)	extra systole	P S	outside contraction	A cardiac contraction caused by an impulse arising outside the sinoatrial node
hemangiectasis (hē″ măn-jĭ-ĕk′ tă-sĭs)	hem angi ectasis	R CF S	blood vessel dilatation	Dilatation of a blood vessel
hemangioma (hē-măn″ jĭ-ō′ mă)	hem angi oma	R CF S	blood vessel tumor	A benign tumor of a blood vessel. See Figures 7–11 and 7–12.
hypertension (hī″ pĕr-tĕn′ shŭn)	hyper tens ion	P R S	excessive, above pressure process	High blood pressure; a disease of the arteries caused by such pressure

TERMINOLOGY SPOTLIGHT

Hypertension is a medical term that is used to describe a blood pressure higher than normal: a systolic reading above 140 millimeter (mm) of mercury (Hg) and a diastolic reading above 90 mm Hg. With hypertension (HBP), the blood vessels can become tight and constricted. See Figure 7–13. These changes can cause the blood to press on the vessel walls with extra force. When this force exceeds a certain level and remains there, one has high blood pressure. Hypertension often has no symptoms and is frequently called "the silent killer," because if left untreated it can lead to kidney failure, stroke, heart attack, peripheral artery disease, and eye damage. See Figure 7–14. There are various factors that can contribute to developing hypertension (see Table 7–3).

Hypertension can be controlled by a variety of methods, such as taking blood pressure medicine as prescribed, seeing a physician on a regular basis, establishing healthy eating habits, exercising, avoiding stress, and making lifestyle changes.

TABLE 7–3   Contributing Factors to Hypertension

Those That One Can Control:

Smoking	Avoid the use of tobacco products
Overweight	Maintain a proper weight for age and body size
Lack of Exercise	Exercise regularly
Stress	Learn to manage stress
Alcohol	Limit intake of alcohol

Other Contributing Factors:

Heredity	Family history of high blood pressure, heart attack, stroke, or diabetes
Race	There is a greater incidence of hypertension among African-Americans
Sex	Males have a greater chance of developing hypertension
Age	The likelihood of hypertension increases with age

continued

Terminology - continued

TERM	WORD PARTS			DEFINITION
hypotension (hī″ pō-tĕn′ shŭn)	hypo	P	deficient, below	Low blood pressure
	tens	R	pressure	
	ion	S	process	
ischemia (ĭs-kē′ mĭ-ă)	isch	R	to hold back	A condition in which there is a lack of blood supply to a part caused by constriction or obstruction of a blood vessel
	emia	S	blood condition	
mitral stenosis (mī′ trăl stě-nō′ sĭs)	mitr	R	mitral valve	A condition of narrowing of the mitral valve
	al	S	pertaining to	
	sten	R	narrowing	
	osis	S	condition of	
myocardial (mī″ ō-kăr′ dĭ-ăl)	myo	CF	muscle	Pertaining to the heart muscle
	cardi	CF	heart	
	al	S	pertaining to	
myocarditis (mī″ ō-kăr-dī′ tĭs)	myo	CF	muscle	Inflammation of the heart muscle
	card	R	heart	
	itis	S	inflammation	
oxygen (ŏk′ sĭ-jĕn)	oxy	R	sour, sharp, acid	A colorless, odorless, tasteless gas essential in the respiration of animals
	gen	S	formation, produce	
pericardial (pĕr″ ĭ-kăr′ dĭ-ăl)	peri	P	around	Pertaining to the pericardium, the sac surrounding the heart
	cardi	CF	heart	
	al	S	pertaining to	
pericardio- rrhaphy (pĕr″ ĭ-kăr″ dĭ-ōr′ ă-fē)	peri	P	around	Suture of the pericardium
	cardio	CF	heart	
	rrhaphy	S	to suture	
pericarditis (pĕr″ ĭ-kăr-dī′ tĭs)	peri	P	around	Inflammation of the pericardium
	card	R	heart	
	itis	S	inflammation	
phlebitis (flĕ-bī′ tĭs)	phleb	R	vein	Inflammation of a vein
	itis	S	inflammation	
phlebolith (flĕb′ ō-lĭth)	phlebo	CF	vein	A stone within a vein
	lith	S	stone	
phlebotomy (flĕ-bŏt′ ō-mē)	phlebo	CF	vein	Incision into a vein
	tomy	S	incision	

Terminology - continued

TERM	WORD PARTS			DEFINITION
presystolic (prē″ sĭs-tōl′ ĭk)	pre systol ic	P R S	before contraction pertaining to	Pertaining to before the systole (regular contraction) of the heart
semilunar (sĕm″ ĭ-lū′ năr)	semi lun ar	P R S	half moon pertaining to	Valves of the aorta and pulmonary artery
sinoatrial (sīn″ ō-ā′ trĭ-ăl)	sino atri al	CF R S	a curve atrium pertaining to	Pertaining to the sinus venosus and the atrium
sphygmomano-meter (sfĭg″ mō-măn-ōm ĕt-ĕr)	sphygmo mano meter	CF CF S	pulse thin instrument to measure	An instrument used to measure the arterial blood pressure
stethoscope (stĕth′ ō-skōp)	stetho scope	CF S	chest instrument	An instrument used to listen to the sounds of the heart, lungs, and other internal organs
tachycardia (tăk″ ĭ-kăr′ dĭ-ă)	tachy card ia	P R S	fast heart condition	A fast heartbeat
thrombosis (thrŏm-bō′ sĭs) vascular	thromb osis	R S	clot of blood condition of	A condition in which there is a blood clot within the system; *a stationary blood clot*
tricuspid (trī-kŭs′ pĭd)	tri cuspid	P S	three a point	Having three points; pertaining to the tricuspid valve
triglyceride (trī-glĭs′ ĕr-īd)	tri glyc er ide	P R S S	three sweet, sugar relating to having a particular quality	Pertaining to a compound consisting of three molecules of fatty acids
vasoconstrictive (văs″ ō-kŏn-strĭk′ tĭv)	vaso con strict ive	CF P R S	vessel together to draw, to bind nature of, quality of	The drawing together, as in the narrowing of a blood vessel

continued

Terminology - continued

TERM	WORD PARTS			DEFINITION
vasodilator (văs″ ō-dī-lā′ tor)	vaso dilat or	CF R S	vessel to widen one who, a doer	A nerve or agent that causes dilation of blood vessels
vasospasm (văs′ ō-spăzm)	vaso spasm	CF S	vessel contraction, spasm	Contraction of a blood vessel
vasotonic (văs″ ō-tŏn′ ĭk)	vaso ton ic	CF R S	vessel tone pertaining to	Pertaining to the tone of a blood vessel
vasotripsy (văs′ ō-trĭp″ sē)	vaso tripsy	CF S	vessel crushing	The crushing of a blood vessel to arrest hemorrhaging
vectorcardiogram (vĕk″ tor-kăr′ dĭ-ō-grăm)	vector cardio gram	R CF S	a carrier heart a mark, record	A record of the direction and magnitude of the electromotive forces of the heart during one complete cycle
venipuncture (vĕn′ ĭ-pŭnk″ chūr)	veni puncture	CF S	vein to pierce	To pierce a vein
venoclysis (vē-nŏk′ lĭ-sĭs)	veno clysis	CF S	vein injection	The injection of medicine or nutritional fluid via a vein
venotomy (vē-nŏt′ ō-mē)	veno tomy	CF S	vein incision	Incision into a vein
ventricular (vĕn-trĭk′ ū-lăr)	ventricul ar	R S	ventricle pertaining to	Pertaining to a ventricle

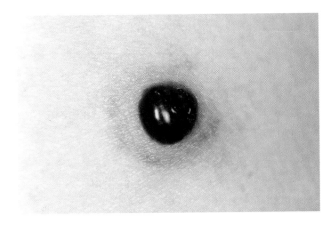

FIGURE 7–9

Infarction angioma. *(Courtesy of Jason L. Smith, MD.)*

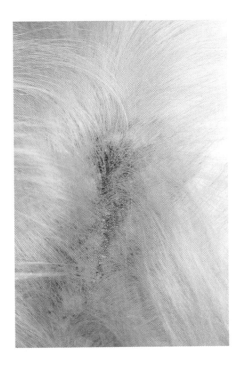

FIGURE 7–10

Temporal arteritis. *(Courtesy of Jason L. Smith, MD.)*

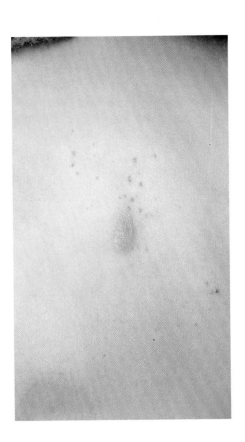

FIGURE 7–11

Hemangioma. *(Courtesy of Jason L. Smith, MD.)*

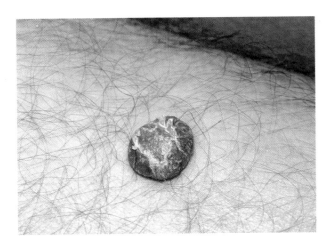

FIGURE 7–12

Sclerosing hemangioma. *(Courtesy of Jason L. Smith, MD.)*

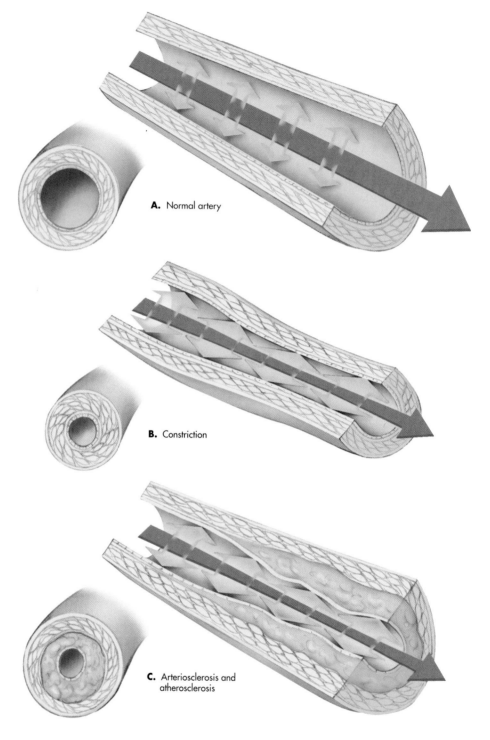

A. Normal artery

B. Constriction

C. Arteriosclerosis and
atherosclerosis

FIGURE 7–13

Blood vessels: **(A)** normal artery, **(B)** constriction, **(C)** arteriosclerosis and atherosclerosis.

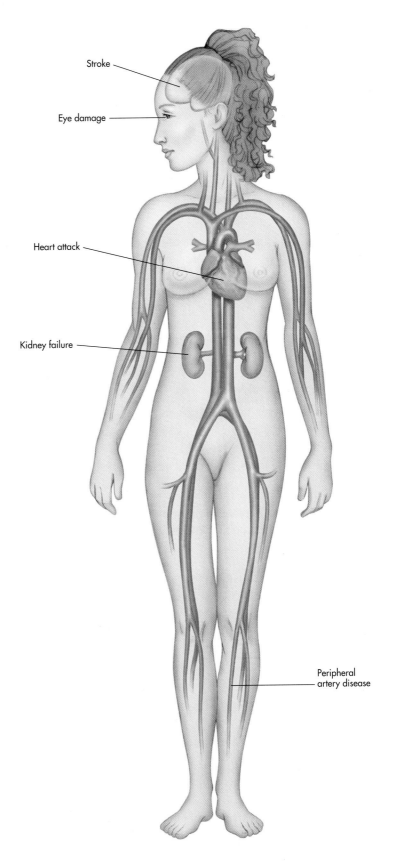

Stroke

Eye damage

Heart attack

Kidney failure

Peripheral
artery disease

FIGURE 7–14

Uncontrolled hypertension can lead to kidney failure, stroke, heart attack, peripheral artery disease, and eye damage.

VOCABULARY WORDS

Vocabulary words are terms that have not been divided into component parts. They are common words or specialized terms associated with the subject of this chapter. These words are provided to enhance your medical vocabulary.

WORD	DEFINITION
anastomosis (ă-năs″ tō-mō′ sĭs)	A surgical connection between blood vessels or the joining of one hollow or tubular organ to another
aneurysm (ăn′ ū-rĭzm)	A sac formed by a local widening of the wall of an artery or a vein; usually caused by injury or disease
artificial pacemaker (ăr″ tĭ-fĭsh′ ăl pās′ māk-ĕr)	An electronic device that stimulates impulse initiation within the heart
auscultation (ŏs″ kool-tā′ shŭn)	A method of physical assessment using a stethoscope to listen to sounds within the chest, abdomen, and other parts of the body
bruit (broot)	Noise, a sound of venous or arterial origin heard on auscultation
cardiocybernetics (kăr″ dē-ō-sī″ bĕr-nĕt′ ĭks)	An exercise program that combines a daily workout with relaxation therapy and guided imagery
cardiomyopathy (kăr″ dē-ō-mī-ŏp′ ă-thē)	Disease of the heart muscle that may be caused by a viral infection, a parasitic infection, or overconsumption of alcohol
catheterization (kăth″ ĕ-tĕr-ĭ-zā′ shŭn)	The process of inserting a catheter into the heart or the urinary bladder
cholesterol (kō-lĕs′ tĕr-ŏl)	A waxy, fat-like substance in the bloodstream of all animals. It is believed to be dangerous when it builds up on arterial walls and contributes to the risk of coronary heart disease.
circulation (sər″-kyə lā′ shən)	The process of moving the blood in the veins and arteries throughout the body
claudication (klaw-dĭ-kā′ shŭn)	The process of lameness, limping; may result from inadequate blood supply to the muscles in the leg
coronary bypass (kŏr′ ō-nă-rē bī′ păs)	A surgical procedure performed to increase blood flow to the myocardium by using a section of a saphenous vein or internal mammary artery to bypass the obstructed or occluded coronary artery

Vocabulary - continued

WORD	DEFINITION
diastole (dī-ăs′ tō-lē)	The relaxation phase of the heart cycle during which the heart muscle relaxes and the heart chambers fill with blood
dysrhythmia (dĭs-rĭth′ mē-ă)	An abnormal, difficult, or bad rhythm
echocardiography (ĕk″ ō-kăr″ dē-ŏg′ rah-fē)	A noninvasive ultrasound method for evaluating the heart for valvular or structural defects and coronary artery disease
extracorporeal circulation (ĕks-tră-kȯr-pōr′ ē-ăl sər″-kyə lā′ shən)	Pertaining to the circulation of the blood outside the body via a heart–lung machine or hemodialyzer
fibrillation (fĭ″ brĭl-ā′ shŭn)	Quivering of muscle fiber; may be atrial or ventricular
flutter (flŭt′ ər)	A condition of the heartbeat in which the contractions become extremely rapid
harvest (hăr′ vĭst)	To gather an organ and make it ready for transplantation
heart–lung transplant (hart-lŭng trăns′ plănt)	The surgical process of transferring the heart and lungs from a donor to a patient
heart transplant (hart trăns′ plănt)	The surgical process of transferring the heart from a donor to a patient
hemodynamic (hē″ mō-dī-năm′ ĭk)	Pertaining to the study of the heart's ability to function as a pump; the movement of the blood and its pressure
infarction (ĭn-fărk′ shŭn)	Process of development of an infarct, which is necrosis of tissue resulting from obstruction of blood flow
Korotkoff sounds (kor′ ŏt-kŏf sowndz)	Tapping sounds heard during auscultation of blood pressure
laser angioplasty (lā′ zĕr ăn′ jĭ-ō-plăs″ tē)	The use of light beams to clear a path through a blocked artery. Once the blockage is located, a laser probe is inserted into the blood vessel and advanced to the clogged area. The laser is activated by a qualified physician and, in an instant, the blockage is vaporized and blood flow is restored in the artery.

continued

Vocabulary - continued

WORD	DEFINITION
lipoproteins (lĭp-ō-prō′ tēns)	*Fat (lipid)* and *protein molecules* that are bound together. They are classified as: **VLDL**—very-low-density lipoproteins; **LDL**—low-density lipoproteins; and **HDL**—high-density lipoproteins. High levels of VLDL and LDL are associated with cholesterol and triglyceride deposits in arteries, which could lead to coronary heart disease, hypertension, and atherosclerosis. One's total cholesterol level should be below 200 mg/dL and HDL (good cholesterol) above 35 mg/dL. Elevated levels of LDL (bad cholesterol) is a risk factor associated with developing **coronary heart disease** *(CHD)* or **coronary artery disease** *(CAD).* The more risk factors that one has, the greater the possibility of developing coronary artery disease, a major cause of heart attacks. See Table 7–4 for associated coronary heart disease risk factors.
lubb-dupp (lŭb-dŭp)	The two separate heart sounds that can be heard with the use of a stethoscope
murmur (mər′ mər)	A soft blowing or rasping sound heard by auscultation of various parts of the body, especially in the region of the heart
occlusion (ŏ-kloo′ zhŭn)	The process or state of being closed
palpitation (păl-pĭ-tā′ shŭn)	Rapid throbbing or fluttering of the heart
percutaneous transluminal coronary angioplasty (pĕr″ kū-tā′ nē-ŭs trăns-lū′ mĭ-năl kŏr′ ō-nă-rē ăn′ jĭ-ō-plăs″ tē)	The use of a balloon-tipped catheter to compress fatty plaques against an artery wall. When successful, the plaques remain compressed, and this permits more blood to flow through the artery, thereby relieving the symptoms of heart disease.
Raynaud's phenomenon (rā-nōz fĕ-nŏm′ ĕ-nŏn)	A disorder that generally affects the blood vessels in the fingers and toes; it is characterized by intermittent attacks that cause the blood vessels in the digits to narrow. The attack is usually due to exposure to cold or occurs during emotional stress. Once the attack begins, the patient may experience pallor, cyanosis, and/or rubor in the affected part. See Figure 7–15.
rheumatic heart disease (roo-măt′ĭk hart dĭ-zēz′)	Endocarditis or valvular heart disease as a result of complications of acute rheumatic fever
septum (sĕp′ tŭm)	A wall or partition that divides or separates a body space or cavity

Vocabulary - continued

WORD	DEFINITION
shock (shŏk)	A state of disruption of oxygen supply to the tissues and a return of blood to the heart
spider veins (spī′dĕr vāns)	Hemangioma in which numerous telangiectatic vessels radiate from a central point. See Figure 7–16.
stroke (strōk)	A sudden severe attack such as a blockage or rupture of a blood vessel within the brain
systole (sĭs′ tō-lē)	The contractive phase of the heart cycle during which blood is forced into the aorta and the pulmonary artery
telangiectasis (tĕl-ăn″jĕ-ĕk-tă′sĭs)	A vascular lesion formed by dilatation of a group of small blood vessels; it may appear as a birthmark or be caused by long-term exposure to the sun. See Figure 7–17.
thrombophlebitis (thrŏm″bō-flē-bī′tĭs)	Inflammation of a vein associated with the formation of a thrombus. See Figure 7–18.
tissue plasminogen activator (tĭsh′ ū plăz-mĭn′ ŏ-jĕn ăk′ tĭ-vā″ tor)	A drug that is used within the first 6 hours of a myocardial infarction to dissolve fibrin clots. It reduces the chance of dying after a myocardial infarction by 50%. Examples are *Kabikinase (streptokinase)* and *Activase (alteplase recombinant)*.

TABLE 7–4   Risk Factors Associated With Developing Coronary Heart Disease

Male age 45 or older	Diabetes mellitus
Female age 55 or older	High-density lipoprotein (HDL) below 35 mg/dL
Female under age 55 with premature menopause and not on estrogen replacement therapy	Family history of early heart disease (parent or sibling; male less than 55, female less than 65)
Smoker	Obesity
Hypertension	

Note: To help lower cholesterol one should limit intake of foods that are high in saturated fat:

Wholemilk	Bacon
Dairy cream	Ribs
Cheese	Ground red meat
Butter	Cold cuts
Red meat, heavily marbled with fat	Poultry skin
Prime cuts	Coconut or palm oil
Sausage	Hydrogenated vegetable oil

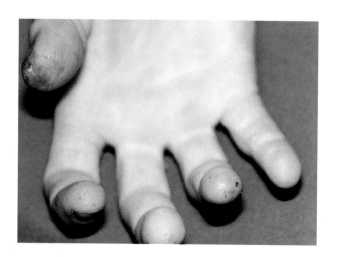

FIGURE 7–15

Raynaud's phenomenon. *(Courtesy of Jason L. Smith, MD.)*

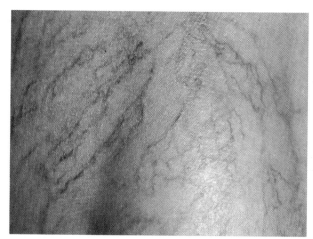

FIGURE 7–16

Spider veins. *(Courtesy of Jason L. Smith, MD.)*

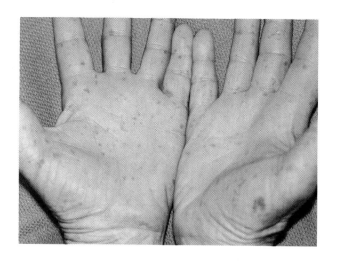

FIGURE 7–17

Telangiectasis. *(Courtesy of Jason L. Smith, MD.)*

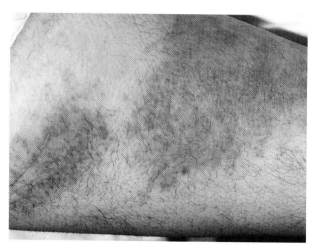

FIGURE 7–18

Thrombophlebitis. *(Courtesy of Jason L. Smith, MD.)*

ABBREVIATIONS

ACG	angiocardiography		IHSS	idiopathic hypertrophic subaortic stenosis
AI	aortic insufficiency		LA	left atrium
AMI	acute myocardial infarction		LBBB	left bundle branch block
AS	aortic stenosis		LD	lactic dehydrogenase
ASD	atrial septal defect		LDL	low-density lipoproteins
ASH	asymmetrical septal hypertrophy		LV	left ventricle
ASHD	arteriosclerotic heart disease		MI	myocardial infarction
AST	aspartate aminotransferase		MS	mitral stenosis
A-V, AV	atrioventricular		MVP	mitral valve prolapse
BBB	bundle branch block		OHS	open heart surgery
BP	blood pressure		PAT	paroxysmal atrial tachycardia
CAD	coronary artery disease		PMI	point of maximum impulse
CC	cardiac catheterization		PTCA	percutaneous transluminal coronary angioplasty
CCU	coronary care unit			
CHD	coronary heart disease		PVCs	premature ventricular contractions
CHF	congestive heart failure			
CK	creatine kinase		RA	right atrium
CO	cardiac output		RV	right ventricle
CPR	cardiopulmonary resuscitation		S-A, SA	sinoatrial
CVP	central venous pressure		SCD	sudden cardiac death
DVTs	deep vein thromboses		TEE	transesophageal echocardiography
ECC	extracorporeal circulation			
ECG	electrocardiogram		tPA	tissue plasminogen activator
EKG	electrocardiogram		VLDL	very-low-density lipoproteins
FHS	fetal heart sound		VSD	ventricular septal defect
HDL	high-density lipoproteins			
H&L	heart and lungs			

DRUG HIGHLIGHTS

Drugs that are generally used for cardiovascular diseases and disorders include digitalis preparations, antiarrhythmic agents, vasopressors, vasodilators, antihypertensive agents, and antilipemic agents.

Digitalis Drugs   Strengthen the heart muscle, increase the force and velocity of myocardial systolic contraction, slow the heart rate, and decrease conduction velocity through the atrioventricular (AV) node. These drugs are used in the treatment of congestive heart failure, atrial fibrillation, atrial flutter, and paroxysmal atrial tachycardia. With the administration of digitalis, toxicity may occur. The most common early symptoms of digitalis toxicity are anorexia, nausea, vomiting, and arrhythmias. *Examples: Crystodigin (digitoxin), Lanoxin (digoxin), and Cedilanid-D (deslanoside).*

Antiarrhythmic Agents

Used in the treatment of cardiac arrhythmias. *Examples: Tambocor (flecainide acetate), Tonocard (tocainide HCl), Inderal (propranolol HCl), and Calan (verapamil).*

Vasopressors

Cause contraction of the muscles associated with capillaries and arteries, thereby narrowing the space through which the blood circulates. This narrowing results in an elevation of blood pressure. Vasopressors are useful in the treatment of patients suffering from shock. *Examples: Intropin (dopamine HCl), Aramine (metaraminol bitartrate), and Levophed Bitartrate (norepinephrine).*

Vasodilators

Cause relaxation of blood vessels and lower blood pressure. Coronary vasodilators are used for the treatment of angina pectoris. *Examples: Sorbitrate (isosorbide dinitrate), nitroglycerin, amyl nitrate, and Cardilate (erythrityl tetranitrate).*

Antihypertensive Agents

Used in the treatment of hypertension. *Examples: Catapres (clonidine HCl), Aldomet (methyldopa), Lopressor (metoprolol tartrate), and Capoten (captopril).*

Antilipemic Agents

Used to lower abnormally high blood levels of fatty substances (lipids) when other treatment regimens fail. *Examples: Nicolar or Nicobid (niacin), Mevacor (lovastatin), Lopid (gemfibrozil), Atromid-S (clofibrate), and Questran (cholestyramine).*

 # DIAGNOSTIC AND LABORATORY TESTS

Test	Description
angiogram (ăn′ jē-ō-grăm)	A test used to determine the size and shape of arteries and veins of organs and tissues. A radiopaque substance is injected into the blood vessel, and x-rays are taken.
angiography (ăn″ jē-ŏg′ ră-fē)	The x-ray recording of a blood vessel after the injection of a radiopaque substance. Used to determine the condition of the blood vessels, organ, or tissue being studied. Types: aortic, cardiac, cerebral, coronary, digital subtraction (use of a computer technique), peripheral, pulmonary, selective, and vertebral.
cardiac catheterization (kăr′ dĭ-ăk kăth″ ĕ-tĕr-ĭ-zā′ shŭn)	A test used in diagnosis of heart disorders. A tiny catheter is inserted into an artery in the groin area of the patient and is fed through this artery to the

Test	Description
	heart. Dye is then pumped through the catheter, enabling the physician to locate by x-ray any blockages in the arteries supplying the heart.
cardiac enzymes (kar′ dĭ-ăk ĕn′- zīmz) **alanine aminotransferase (ALT)** **aspartate aminotransferase (AST)** **creatine phosphokinase (CPK)** **creatine kinase (CK)** **creatine kinase isoenzymes**	Blood tests performed to determine cardiac damage in an acute myocardial infarction. Levels begin to rise 6 to 10 hours after an MI and peak at 24 to 48 hours. Levels begin to rise 6 to 10 hours after an MI and peak at 24 to 48 hours. Used to detect area of damage. Level may be 5 to 8 times normal. Used to indicate area of damage; CK-MB heart muscle, CK-MM skeletal muscle, and CK-BB brain.
cholesterol (kōl-lĕs′ tĕr-ŏl)	A blood test to determine the level of cholesterol in the serum. Elevated levels may indicate an increased risk of coronary heart disease. Any level greater than 200 mg/dL is considered too high for good heart health.
electrophysiology (ē-lĕk″ trō-fĭz″ ĭ-ŏl′ ō-jē)	A cardiac procedure that maps the electrical activity of the heart from within the heart itself.
Holter monitor (hōlt′ ər mŏn′ ĭ-tər)	A method of recording a patient's ECG for 24 hours. The device is portable and small enough to be worn by the patient during normal activity.
lactic dehydrogenase (LDH) (lăk′ tĭk dē-hī-drŏj′ ĕ-nās)	Increased 6 to 12 hours after cardiac injury.
stress test (strĕs test)	A method of evaluating cardiovascular fitness. The ECG is monitored while the patient is subjected to increasing levels of work. A treadmill or ergometer is used for this test.
triglycerides (trī-glĭs′ ĕr-īds)	A blood test to determine the level of triglycerides in the serum. Elevated levels (greater than 200 mg/dL) may indicate an increased risk of coronary heart disease and diabetes mellitus.
ultrasonography (ŭl-tră-sŏn-ŏg′ ră-fē)	A test used to visualize an organ or tissue by using high-frequency sound waves. It may be used as a screening test or as a diagnostic tool to determine abnormalities of the aorta, arteries and veins, and the heart.

COMMUNICATION ENRICHMENT

This segment is provided for those who wish to enhance their ability to communicate in either English or Spanish.

► Related Terms

English	Spanish	English	Spanish
blood pressure	presión sanguinea (*prĕ*-sĭ-ōn săn-gĭ-nĕ-ă)	artery	arteria (ăr-*tĕ*-rĭ-ă)
cholesterol	colesterol (*kō*-lĕs-tĕ-rōl)	capillary	capilar (*că*-pĭ-lăr)
clot	coagulo (kō-*ă*-gŭ-lō)	vessel	vaso (*vă*-sō)
heart	corazón (*kō*-ră-zōn)	choke, suffocate	sofocar (sō-*fō*-kăr)
heart disease	enfermedad del corazón (ĕn-fĕr-*mĕ*-dăd dĕl *kō*-ră-zōn)	injection	inyeccion (*ĭn*-jĕc-sĭ-ōn)
		record	registro (*rĕ*-hĭs-trō)
high blood pressure	presion alta (*prĕ*-sĭ-ōn ăl-tă)	motion	moción (*mō*-sĭ-ōn)
murmur	murmullo (*mūr*-mū-jō)	inflammation	inflamación (ĭn-*flă*-mă-sĭ-ōn)
palpitations	palpitaciónes (*păl*-pĭ-tă-sĭ-ō-nĕs)	spasm	espasmo (ĕs-*păs*-mō)
pulse	pulso (*pūl*-sō)	oxygen	oxigeno (ōx-sĭ-*hĕ*-nō)
system	sistema (sĭs-*tĕ*-mă)	narrowing	estrecho (ĕs-*trĕ*-chō)
varicose veins	venas varicosas (*vĕ*-năs vă-rĭ-*kō*-săs)	puncture	pinchazo (pĭn-*chă*-sō)
veins	venas (*vĕ*-năs)	soften	ablandar (*ă*-blăn-dăr)
heartbeat	latidos del corazón (*lă*-tĭ-dōs dĕl kō-*ră*-zōn)	rhythm	ritmo (*rĭt*-mō)

STUDY AND REVIEW SECTION

LEARNING EXERCISES

▶ **Anatomy and Physiology**

Write your answers to the following questions. Do not refer back to the text.

1. The cardiovascular system includes:

    a. _____   b. _____

    c. _____   d. _____

2. Name the three layers of the heart.

    a. _____   b. _____

    c. _____

3. The heart weighs approximately _____ grams.

4. The _____ or upper chambers of the heart are separated by the

    _____ septum.

5. The _____ or lower chambers of the heart are separated by the

    _____ septum.

6. By listing each cardiovascular part in the proper order, trace the flow of blood through the heart, to the lungs, back to the heart, and on to the various body parts.

    a. _____   b. _____

    c. _____   d. _____

    e. _____   f. _____

    g. _____   h. _____

    i. _____   j. _____

    k. _____   l. _____

    m. _____   n. _____

7. The _____ _____ _____ controls the heart-beat.

8. The _____ _____ is called the pacemaker of the heart.

9. The _____ _____ includes the bundle of His and the peripheral fibers.

10. Name the three primary pulse points and state their locations on the body.

    a. _____   located _____

    b. _____   located _____

    c. _____   located _____

11. Define the following terms:

    a. Blood pressure _____

    b. Pulse pressure _____

12. The average adult heart is about the size of a _____ and normally beats

    at a pulse rate of _____ to _____ beats per minute.

13. The average adult usually has a systolic pressure between _____ and

    _____ mm Hg and a diastolic pressure between _____

    and _____ mm Hg.

14. Give the purpose and function of arteries. _____

    _____

15. Give the purpose and function of veins. _____

    _____

▶ Word Parts

1. In the spaces provided, write the definition of these prefixes, roots, combining forms, and suffixes. Do not refer to the listing of terminology words. Leave blank those terms you cannot define.

2. After completing as many as you can, refer back to the terminology word listings to check your work. For each word missed or left blank, write the term and its definition several times on the margins of these pages or on a separate sheet of paper.

3. To maximize the learning process, it is to your advantage to do the following exercises as directed. To refer to the terminology listings before completing these exercises invalidates the learning process.

Prefixes

Give the definitions of the following prefixes:

1. a- _____
2. bi- _____
3. brady- _____
4. con- _____
5. end- _____
6. endo- _____
7. extra- _____
8. hyper- _____
9. hypo- _____
10. peri- _____
11. pre- _____
12. semi- _____
13. tachy- _____
14. tri- _____

Roots and Combining Forms

Give the definitions of the following roots and combining forms:

1. angi _____
2. angin _____
3. angio _____
4. aort _____
5. aorto _____
6. arter _____
7. arteri _____
8. arterio _____
9. ather _____
10. athero _____
11. atri _____
12. atrio _____
13. card _____
14. cardi _____
15. cardio _____
16. cyan _____
17. dextro _____
18. dilat _____
19. electro _____
20. embol _____
21. glyc _____
22. hem _____
23. isch _____
24. kinet _____
25. log _____
26. lun _____
27. mano _____
28. mitr _____
29. myo _____
30. necr _____
31. oxy _____
32. phleb _____
33. phlebo _____
34. phono _____
35. pulmonar _____
36. rrhythm _____

37. scler _____   38. sino _____

39. sphygmo _____   40. sten _____

41. stetho _____   42. strict _____

43. systol _____   44. tens _____

45. thromb _____   46. ton _____

47. vascul _____   48. vaso _____

49. vector _____   50. veni _____

51. veno _____   52. ventricul _____

Suffixes

Give the definitions of the following suffixes:

1. -ac _____   2. -al _____

3. -ar _____   4. -blast _____

5. -centesis _____   6. -clysis _____

7. -cuspid _____   8. -dynia _____

9. -ectasis _____   10. -ectomy _____

11. -emia _____   12. -er _____

13. -gen _____   14. -gram _____

15. -graph _____   16. -graphy _____

17. -ia _____   18. -ic _____

19. -ide _____   20. -ion _____

21. -ism _____   22. -ist _____

23. -itis _____   24. -ive _____

25. -lith _____   26. -logy _____

27. -malacia _____   28. -megaly _____

29. -meter _____   30. -oma _____

31. -or _____   32. -osis _____

33. -pathy _____   34. -plasty _____

35. -plegia _____   36. -ptosis _____

37. -puncture _____   38. -rrhaphy _____

39. -scope _____   40. -spasm _____

41. -systole _____   42. -tome _____

43. -tomy _____   44. -tripsy _____

45. -um _____   46. -y _____

▶ **Identifying Medical Terms**

In the spaces provided, write the medical terms for the following meanings:

1. _____ A tumor of a blood vessel

2. _____ The germ cell from which blood vessels develop

3. _____ Surgical repair of a blood vessel or vessels

4. _____ A condition of narrowing of a blood vessel

5. _____ Surgical excision of an artery

6. _____ An arterial stone

7. _____ Incision into an artery

8. _____ Inflammation of an artery

9. _____ Having two points or cusps; pertaining to the mitral valve

10. _____ Pain in the heart

11. _____ One who specializes in the study of the heart

12. _____ Enlargement of the heart

13. _____ Pertaining to the heart and lungs

14. _____ The process of drawing together as in the narrowing of a vessel

15. _____ A condition in which a blood clot obstructs a blood vessel

16. _____ Inflammation of a vein

17. _____ A stone within a vein

18. _____ A fast heartbeat

19. _____ A widening of a blood vessel

▶ **Spelling**

In the spaces provided, write the correct spelling of these misspelled terms:

1. artrectomy _____
2. athrosclerosis _____
3. atriventrcular _____
4. endcarditis _____
5. extrsystole _____
6. iscemia _____
7. mycardial _____
8. oyxgen _____
9. phelebitis _____
10. persystolic _____

WORD PARTS STUDY SHEET

Word Parts	Give the Meaning
brady-	_____
endo-	_____
hyper-	_____
hypo-	_____
tachy-	_____
angin-	_____
angio-	_____
aorto-	_____
arter-, arteri-, arterio-	_____
ather-, athero-	_____
card-, cardi-, cardio-	_____
cyan-	_____
electro-	_____
embol-	_____
isch-	_____
lun-	_____
mano-	_____
mitr-	_____
phleb-	_____

pulmonar- _____

rrhythm- _____

scler- _____

sphygmo- _____

sten- _____

stetho- _____

tens- _____

thromb- _____

veni-, veno- _____

-dynia _____

-emia _____

-gram _____

-graphy _____

-ia, -ism, -osis, -y _____

-ion _____

-ist _____

-itis _____

-malacia _____

-megaly _____

-meter _____

-scope _____

-tripsy _____

REVIEW QUESTIONS

▶ Matching

Select the appropriate lettered meaning for each numbered line.

_____ 1. cholesterol

_____ 2. claudication

_____ 3. dysrhythmia

a. The two separate heart sounds that can be heard with the use of a stethocope

b. The use of light beams to clear a path through a blocked artery

_____ 4. harvest

_____ 5. laser angioplasty

_____ 6. lipoproteins

_____ 7. lubb-dupp

_____ 8. palpitation

_____ 9. percutaneous transluminal coronary angioplasty

_____ 10. tissue plasminogen activator

c. Fat and protein molecules that are bound together

d. A waxy, fat-like substance in the bloodstream of all animals

e. The process of lameness, limping

f. An abnormal, difficult, or bad rhythm

g. To gather an organ and make it ready for transplantation

h. A drug that is used within the first 6 hours of a myocardial infarction to dissolve fibrin clots

i. Rapid throbbing or fluttering of the heart

j. The use of a balloon-tipped catheter to compress fatty plaques against an artery wall

k. The process of being closed

▶ **Abbreviations**

Place the correct word, phrase, or abbreviation in the space provided.

1. acute myocardial infarction _____

2. atrioventricular _____

3. BP _____

4. CAD _____

5. cardiac catheterization _____

6. ECG, EKG _____

7. HDL _____

8. heart and lungs _____

9. MI _____

10. tPA _____

▶ **Diagnostic and Laboratory Test**

Select the best answer to each multiple choice question. Circle the letter of your choice.

1. _____ is a cardiac procedure that maps the electrical activity of the heart from within the heart itself.
   a. electrocardiogram
   b. electrocardiomyogram
   c. electrophysiology
   d. cardiac catheterization

2. Blood tests performed to determine cardiac damage in an acute myocardial infarction.
   a. cardiac enzymes
   b. cholesterol
   c. triglycerides
   d. angiogram

3. A method of recording a patient's ECG for 24 hours.
   a. stress test
   b. Holter monitor
   c. ultrasonography
   d. angiography

4. A test used to determine the size and shape of arteries and veins of organs and tissues.
   a. electrophysiology
   b. stress test
   c. angiogram
   d. cholesterol

5. The x-ray recording of a blood vessel after the injection of a radiopaque substance.
   a. angiogram
   b. angiography
   c. stress test
   d. cardiac catheterization

CRITICAL THINKING ACTIVITY

▶ Case Study

Angina Pectoris

Please read the following case study and then answer the questions that follow.

A 45-year-old male was seen by a cardiologist and the following is a synopsis of his visit.

Present History: The patient states that during a workout session he felt a tightness in his chest, became short of breath, and felt very apprehensive. He states that this uncomfortable sensation went away after he stopped exercising.

Signs and Symptoms: Chief complaint: tightness in his chest, dyspnea, apprehension.

Diagnosis: Angina pectoris. Diagnosis was determined by a complete physical examination, an electrocardiogram, and blood enzyme studies.

Treatment: Nitroglycerin sublingual tablets 0.4 mg as needed for chest pain. The patient is instructed to seek medical attention without delay, if the pain is not relieved by three tablets, taken one every 5 minutes over a 15-minute period.

Prevention: Teach the patient to avoid situations that precipitate angina attacks. Proper rest and diet, stress management, lifestyle changes, avoidance of alcohol and tobacco are recommended.

Critical Thinking Questions

1. Signs and symptoms of angina pectoris include tightness in the chest, _____ (shortness of breath), and apprehension.

2. The diagnosis of angina pectoris was determined by a complete physical examination, an

   _____, and blood enzyme studies.

3. The medication regimen prescribed included _____ 0.4 mg as needed for chest pain.

4. What should the patient do if the medication does not relieve the pain?

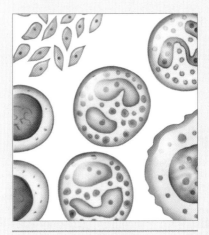

BLOOD AND THE LYMPHATIC SYSTEM

OBJECTIVES

On completion of this chapter, you should be able to:

- Describe the blood.

- Describe the formed elements in blood.

- Name the four blood types.

- Describe and state the functions of the lymphatic system.

- Describe the accessory organs of the lymphatic system.

- Describe the immune system/response.

- Analyze, build, spell, and pronounce medical words that relate to surgical procedures and pathology.

- Identify and give the meaning of selected vocabulary words.

- Identify and define selected abbreviations.

- Review Drug Highlights presented in this chapter.

- Provide the description of diagnostic and laboratory tests related to blood and the lymphatic system.

- Successfully complete the study and review section.

▶ ANATOMY AND PHYSIOLOGY OVERVIEW

Blood and lymph are two of the body's main fluids and are circulated through two separate but interconnected vessel systems. *Blood* is circulated, by the action of the heart, through the circulatory system consisting largely of arteries, veins, and capillaries. *Lymph* does not actually circulate. It is propelled in one direction, away from its source, through increasingly larger lymph vessels, to drain into large veins of the circulatory system located in the neck region. Numerous valves within the lymph vessels permit one-directional flow, opening and closing as a consequence of pressure caused by the massaging action of muscles on the vessels and the fluid they contain. The various organs and components of blood and the lymphatic system are described in this chapter.

▶ BLOOD

Blood is a fluid consisting of formed elements and plasma, both of which are continuously produced by the body for the purpose of transporting respiratory gases *(oxygen and carbon dioxide)*, chemical substances *(foods, salts, hormones)*, and cells that act to protect the body from foreign substances. The blood volume within an individual depends on body weight. An individual weighing 154 lb (70 kg) has a blood volume of about 5 qt or 5 L.

FORMED ELEMENTS

The formed elements in blood are the red blood cells or *erythrocytes, platelets* or *thrombocytes,* and white blood cells or *leukocytes.* Formed elements constitute about 45% of the total volume of blood and are sometimes referred to as whole blood (Table 8–1).

BLOOD AND THE LYMPHATIC SYSTEM

ORGAN/STRUCTURE	PRIMARY FUNCTIONS
Blood	Fluid consisting of formed elements and plasma that transport respiratory gases (oxygen and carbon dioxide), chemical substances (foods, salts, hormones), and cells that act to protect the body from foreign substances
Lymphatic System	A vessel system composed of lymph capillaries, lymphatic vessels, lymphatic ducts, and lymph nodes that convey lymph from the tissue to the blood. The three main functions of the lymphatic system are:
	1. It transports proteins and fluids, lost by capillary seepage, back to the bloodstream
	2. It protects the body against pathogens by phagocytosis and immune response
	3. It serves as a pathway for the absorption of fats from the small intestines into the bloodstream
Spleen	Major site of erythrocyte destruction; serves as a reservoir for blood; acts as a filter, removing microorganisms from the blood
Tonsils	Filter bacteria and aid in the formation of white blood cells
Thymus	Essential role in the formation of antibodies and the development of the immune response in the newborn; manufactures infection-fighting T cells and helps distinguish normal T cells from those that attack the body's own tissue

TABLE 8–1   Types of Blood Cells and Functions

Blood Cell	Function
Erythrocyte (red blood cell)	Transports oxygen and carbon dioxide
Thrombocyte (platelet)	Blood clotting
Leukocyte (white blood cell)	Body's main defense against invasion of pathogens
Types of leukocytes	
Neutrophil	Protection against infection, phagocytosis
Eosinophil	Destroys parasitic organisms, plays a key role in allergic reactions
Basophil	Key role in releasing histamine and other chemicals that act on blood vessels, essential to nonspecific immune response to inflammation
Monocyte	One of the first lines of defense in the inflammatory process, phagocytosis
Lymphocyte	Provides the body with immune capacity
B lymphocyte	Identifies foreign antigens and differentiates into antibody-producing plasma cells (source for immunoglobulins–antibodies)
T lymphocyte	Essential for the specific immune response of the body

Erythrocytes

Erythrocytes are doughnut-shaped cells without nuclei. They transport oxygen (most of which is bound to hemoglobin contained in the cell) and carbon dioxide. There are approximately 5 million erythrocytes per cubic millimeter, and they have a life span of 80 to 120 days. Erythrocytes are formed in the red bone marrow and are commonly called red blood cells (Fig. 8–1).

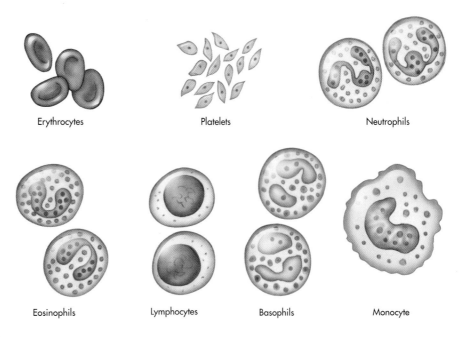

Erythrocytes   Platelets   Neutrophils

Eosinophils   Lymphocytes   Basophils   Monocyte

FIGURE 8–1

The formed elements of blood: erythrocytes, leukocytes (neutrophils, eosinophils, basophils, lymphocytes, and monocytes), and thrombocytes (platelets).

Thrombocytes

Thrombocytes are disk-shaped cells about half the size of erythrocytes. They play an important role in the clotting process by releasing *thrombokinase,* which, in the presence of calcium, reacts with *prothrombin* to form *thrombin.* There are approximately 200,000 to 500,000 thrombocytes per cubic millimeter. Thrombocytes are fragments of certain giant cells called megakaryocytes, which are formed in the red bone marrow. Thrombocytes are commonly called *platelets* (Fig. 8–1).

Leukocytes

Leukocytes are sphere-shaped cells containing nuclei of varying shapes and sizes. Leukocytes are the body's main defense against the invasion of *pathogens.* At the time pathogens enter the tissue, the leukocytes leave the blood vessels through their walls and move in an ameba-like motion to the area of infection, where they perform *phagocytosis.* There are approximately 8000 leukocytes per cubic millimeter. There are five types of leukocytes: *neutrophils, eosinophils, basophils, lymphocytes,* and *monocytes.*

Except for the lymphocytes, leukocytes are formed in the red bone marrow. Lymphocytes are formed in lymph nodes and other lymphoid tissue. Leukocytes are commonly called *white blood cells* (Fig. 8–1).

BLOOD GROUPING

There are four recognized *blood types,* and each is named for the *antigens* contained in the red cells. The four blood types identified are types A, B, AB, and O.

RH FACTOR

The presence of a substance called an *agglutinogen* in the red blood cells is responsible for what is known as the *Rh factor.* It was first discovered in the blood of the rhesus monkey from which the factor gets its name. About 85% of the population have the Rh factor and are called Rh positive. The other 15% lack the Rh factor and are designated Rh negative.

PLASMA

The fluid part of the blood is called *plasma.* It comprises about 55% of the total volume of blood, is clear and somewhat straw-colored, and is composed of water (91%) and chemical compounds (9%). Plasma is the medium for circulation of blood cells, it provides nutritive substances to various body structures, and it removes waste products of metabolism from body structures. There are four major plasma proteins: *albumin, globulin, fibrinogen,* and *prothrombin.*

▶ THE LYMPHATIC SYSTEM

The *lymphatic system* is a vessel system apart from, but connected to, the circulatory system. The lymphatic system returns fluids from tissue spaces to the bloodstream. The lymphatic system is composed of *lymph capillaries, lymphatic vessels, lymphatic ducts,* and *lymph nodes.* The system conveys lymph from the tissues to the blood. Lymph is a clear, colorless, alkaline fluid that is about 95% water. The principal component of lymph is fluid from plasma that has seeped out of capillary walls into spaces among the body tissues. Lymph contains white blood cells, particularly lymphocytes. Figure 8–2 shows the major lymphatics of the body. The three main functions of the lymphatic system are:

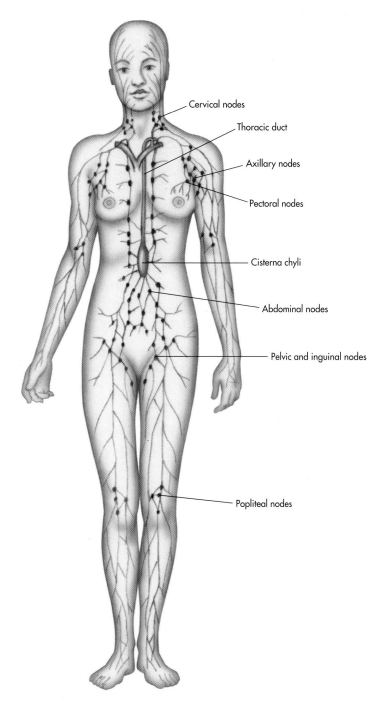

Cervical nodes

Thoracic duct

Axillary nodes

Pectoral nodes

Cisterna chyli

Abdominal nodes

Pelvic and inguinal nodes

Popliteal nodes

FIGURE 8–2

The lymphatic system.

1. It transports proteins and fluids, lost by capillary seepage, back to the bloodstream.
2. It protects the body against pathogens by phagocytosis and immune response.
3. It serves as the pathway for the absorption of fats from the small intestines into the bloodstream.

▶ ACCESSORY ORGANS

The *spleen,* the *tonsils,* and the *thymus* are not actually part of the lymphatic system; however, they are closely related to it in their functions. See Figure 8–3.

THE SPLEEN

The *spleen* is a soft, dark red oval body lying in the upper left quadrant of the abdomen. The spleen is the major site of erythrocyte destruction. It serves as a reservoir for blood. The spleen plays an essential role in the immune response and acts as a filter, removing microorganisms from the blood.

THE TONSILS

The *tonsils* are lymphoid masses located in depressions of the mucous membranes of the face and pharynx. They consist of the *palatine tonsil, pharyngeal tonsil* (adenoid), and the *lingual tonsil.* The tonsils filter bacteria and aid in the formation of white blood cells.

THE THYMUS

The *thymus* is considered one of the endocrine glands, but because of its function and appearance, it is a part of the lymphoid system. It is located in the mediastinal cavity. The thymus plays an essential role in the formation of antibodies and the development of the immune response in the newborn. It manufactures infection-fighting *T cells* and helps distinguish normal T cells from those that attack the body's own tissue. T cells are important in the body's cellular immune response.

The Immune System/Response

All of us live in a virtual "sea" of microorganisms, organisms so tiny that they cannot be seen with the naked eye. Many of these organisms are not harmful to humans, while others are *pathogenic,* capable of causing disease. Each day our bodies are faced with microorganisms, potentially harmful toxins in the environment, and even some of our own cells that may change into cancer. Fortunately, the average, healthy human body is equipped with natural defenses that assist the body in fighting off disease and cancer. These natural defenses are intact skin, the cleansing action of the body's secretions (such as tears, mucus), white blood cells, body chemicals (such as hormones, enzymes), and antibodies. As long as the immune system is intact and functioning properly, it can defend the body against invading foreign substances and cancer.

The *immune system* consists of the tissues, organs, and physiologic processes used by the body to identify abnormal cells, foreign substances, and foreign tissue cells that may have been transplanted into the body. Many of these tissues and organs are part of the lymphatic system.

The Immune Response

The *immune response* is the reaction of the body to foreign substances and the means by which it protects the body. The following is an overview of this response.

The immune response may be described as humoral immunity or antibody-mediated immunity, and cellular immunity or cell-mediated immunity.

Humoral (pertaining to body fluids or substances contained in them) *immunity* or *antibody-mediated immunity* involves the production of plasma lymphocytes (B cells) in response to antigen exposure with subsequent formation of antibodies. *Antibodies* are protein substances that are developed in response to a specific antigen. An *antigen* is a

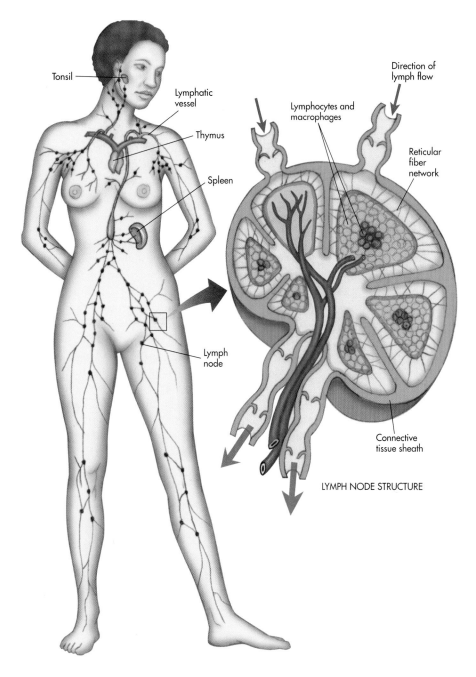

Tonsil

Lymphatic
vessel

Thymus

Spleen

Lymph
node

Direction of
lymph flow

Lymphocytes and
macrophages

Reticular
fiber
network

Connective
tissue sheath

LYMPH NODE STRUCTURE

FIGURE 8–3

The tonsils, lymph nodes, thymus, spleen, and lymphatic vessels with an expanded view of a lymph node.

substance such as bacteria, toxins, or certain allergens that induces the formation of antibodies. Humoral immunity is a major defense against bacterial infections.

Cellular immunity or *cell-mediated immunity* involves the production of lymphocytes (T cells) that responds to any form of injury and NK (natural killer) cells that attack foreign cells, normal cells infected with viruses, and cancer cells. Cellular immunity constitutes a major defense against infections caused by viruses, fungi, and a few bacteria, such as the tubercle bacillus that causes tuberculosis. It also helps defend against the formation of tumors, especially cancer.

There are four general phases associated with the body's immune response to a foreign substance and these are:

1. The first phase is the recognition of the foreign substance or the invader (enemy).
2. Activation of the body's defenses by producing more white blood cells that are designed to seek and destroy the invader(s), especially the macrophages that eat and engulf the foreign substances and lymphocytes, B cells, and T cells (see Table 8–2), constitutes the second phase.

    T cells of the helper type identify the enemy and rush to the spleen and lymph nodes, where they stimulate the production of other cells to aid in the fight of the foreign substance.

    T cells of the natural killer (NK) type are large granular lymphocytes that also specialize in killing cells of the body that have been invaded by foreign substances and fighting cells that have turned cancerous.

    The B cells reside in the spleen or lymph nodes and produce antibodies for specific antigens.
3. During the attack phase, the above defenders of the body produce antibodies and/or seek out to kill and/or remove the foreign invader. This is done by phagocytosis, where the macrophages squeeze out between the cells in the capillaries and crawl into the tissue to the site of the infection. Here they surround and eat the foreign substances that caused the infection. Other white blood cells respond to infection by producing antibodies. Antibodies are released into the bloodstream and carried to the site of the infection, where they surround and immobilize the invaders. Later, both antibody and invader may be eaten by the phagocytes.
4. In the slowdown phase, the number of defenders returns to normal, following victory over the foreign invader.

TABLE 8–2   Summary of Functions of Lymphocytes

Type of cell	Functions
T cells (thymus-dependent)	Cellular immunity
B cells (bone marrow-derived)	Humoral immunity
NK cells (natural killers)	Attack foreign cells, normal cells infected with viruses, and cancer cells

LIFE SPAN CONSIDERATIONS

▶ THE CHILD

In the embryo, plasma and blood cells are formed about the 2nd week of life. At approximately the 5th week of development, blood formation occurs in the liver and later in the spleen, thymus, lymphatic system, and bone marrow. At 12 weeks the fetus is 11.5 cm (4.5 inches) from crown to head and weighs 45 g (1.6 oz). The fetal **liver** is the chief producer of red blood cells, and **bile** is secreted by the gallbladder. At 16 weeks blood vessels are visible through the now-transparent skin. Fetal circulation provides oxygenation and nutrition to the fetus and disposes of carbon dioxide and other waste products.

The **thymus gland** plays an important role in the development of the immune response in the newborn. At birth, the average weight of the thymus is 10 to 15 g. It attains a weight of 40 g at puberty, after which it begins to undergo involution, with the thymus being replaced with adipose and connective tissue.

▶ THE OLDER ADULT

With advancing age, lymphatic tissue shrinks, the bone marrow becomes less productive, and the walls of peripheral vessels stiffen. There is also loss of elasticity in the peripheral vessels, which causes increases in peripheral resistance, impairs the flow of blood, and results in an increase in the workload of the left ventricle. As a result of these changes in the peripheral vascular system, the transportation of oxygen and nutrients to the tissues and the removal of wastes from the tissues are affected adversely. The transportation of oxygen may also be compromised by the decrease of **hemoglobin** of some older adults.

Immune response declines with age, limiting the body's ability to identify and fight foreign substances such as bacteria and viruses. With aging there is loss of the thymus cortex, which leads to a reduced production of T lymphocytes, including T cells, natural killer cells, and B lymphocytes. Persons at the extremes of the life span are more likely to develop immune-response problems than those in their middle years. Frequency and severity of infections are generally increased in elderly persons because of a decreased ability of the immune system to respond adequately to invading microorganisms. The incidence of **autoimmune diseases** also increases with aging, most likely due to a decreased ability of antibodies to differentiate between self and nonself. Failure of the immune response system to recognize mutant, or abnormal, cells may be the reason for the high incidence of cancer associated with increasing age.

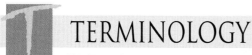

TERMINOLOGY

WITH SURGICAL PROCEDURES & PATHOLOGY

TERM	WORD PARTS			DEFINITION
agglutination (ă-gloo″ tĭ-nā′ shŭn)	agglutinat ion	R S	clumping process	The process of clumping together, as of blood cells that are incompatible
allergy (ăl′ ĕr-jē)	all ergy	R S	other work	Individual hypersensitivity to a substance that is usually harmless
anemia (ăn-nē′ mĭ-ă)	an emia	P S	lack of blood condition	A condition of a lack of red blood cells
angiology (ăn″ jĭ-ŏl′ ō-jē)	angio logy	CF S	vessel study of	The study of the blood vessels and the lymphatics
anisocytosis (ăn-ī″ sō-sī-tō′ sĭs)	aniso cyt osis	CF R S	unequal cell condition of	A condition in which the erythrocytes are unequal in size and shape
antibody (ăn′ tĭ-bŏd″ ē)	anti body	P S	against body	A protein substance produced in the body in response to an invading foreign substance *(antigen)*

TERMINOLOGY SPOTLIGHT

An **antibody** is also referred to as an immunoglobulin. It is a complex glycoprotein produced by B lymphocytes in response to the presence of an antigen. Antibodies neutralize or destroy antigens in several ways. They can initiate destruction of the antigen by activating the complement system, neutralizing toxins released by bacteria, opsonizing (coating) the antigen or forming a complex to stimulate phagocytosis, promoting antigen clumping, or preventing the antigen from adhering to host cells. See Table 8–3 for the five classes of antibodies: IgG, IgM, IgA, IgE, and IgD.

TABLE 8–3   Antibodies/Immunoglobulins

Antibody	Functions
IgG	Crosses placenta to provide passive immunity for the newborn Opsonizing (coating) microorganisms to enhance phagocytosis Activates complement system (a group of proteins in the blood) *Components of complement are labeled C1 through C9. Complement acts by directly killing organisms; by opsonizing an antigen; and by stimulating inflammation and the B-cell-mediated immune response.*

continued

Terminology - continued

TERM	WORD PARTS			DEFINITION

TABLE 8–3   continued

IgM	Activates complement		
	First antibody produced in response to bacterial and viral infections		
IgA	Protects epithelial surfaces		
	Activates complement		
	Passed to breast-feeding newborn via the colostrum		
IgE	Active in allergic reactions and some parasitic infections		
	Trigger mast cells to release histamine, serotonin, kinins, slow-reacting substance of anaphylaxis, and the neutrophil factor. These mediators produce allergic skin reaction, asthma, and hay fever.		
IgD	Role not clear, possibly influences B lymphocyte differentiation		

TERM	WORD PARTS			DEFINITION
anticoagulant (ăn″ tĭ-kō-ăg′ ū-lănt)	anti coagul ant	P R S	against clots forming	An agent that works against the formation of blood clots
antigen (ăn′ tĭ-jĕn)	anti gen	P S	against formation, produce	An invading foreign substance that induces the formation of antibodies
antihemophilic (ăn″ tĭ-hē″ mō-fĭl′ ĭk)	anti hemo phil ic	P CF S S	against blood attraction pertaining to	Pertaining to an agent that is effective against the bleeding tendency in hemophilia
antihemorrhagic (ăn″ tĭ-hĕm″ ō-răj′ ĭk)	anti hemo rrhag ic	P CF S S	against blood bursting forth pertaining to	Pertaining to an agent that prevents or arrests hemorrhage, the bursting forth of blood
autohemotherapy (ăw″ tō-hĕ″ mō-thĕr′ ăh-pē)	auto hemo therapy	P CF S	self blood treatment	Treatment of a patient by using the patient's own blood
basocyte (bā′ sō-sīt)	baso cyte	CF S	base cell	A base cell leukocyte
basophil (bā′ sō-fĭl)	baso phil	CF S	base attraction	A cell that has an attraction for a base dye
coagulable (kō-ăg′ ū-lăb-l)	coagul able	R S	to clot capable	Capable of forming a clot
creatinemia (krē″ ă-tĭn-ē′ mĭ-ă)	creatin emia	R S	flesh, creatine blood condition	A condition of excess creatine in the blood
dysemia (dĭs-ē′ mĕ-ăh)	dys emia	P S	bad blood condition	A bad blood condition A blood disease

continued

Terminology - continued

TERM	WORD PARTS			DEFINITION
dysglycemia (dĭs″ glī-sē′ mē-ăh)	dys glyc emia	P R S	bad sweet, sugar blood condition	A condition of abnormal blood sugar metabolism
eosinophil (ē″ŏ-sĭn′ ō-fĭl)	eosino phil	CF S	rose-colored attraction	A cell that stains readily with the acid stain; attraction for the rose-colored stain
erythroblast (ĕ-rĭth′ rō-blăst)	erythro blast	CF S	red immature cell, germ cell	An immature red blood cell
erythroclastic (ĕ-rĭth″ rō-klăs′ tĭk)	erythro clast ic	CF R S	red destruction pertaining to	Pertaining to the destruction of red blood cells
erythrocyte (ĕ-rĭth′ rō-sīt)	erythro cyte	CF S	red cell	A red blood cell
erythrocytosis (ĕ-rĭth″ rō-sī-tō′ sĭs)	erythro cyt osis	CF R	red cell condition of	An abnormal condition in which there is an increase in red blood cells
erythropathy (ĕ-rĭth″ rōp′ ă-thē)	erythro pathy	CF S	red disease	Disease of the red blood cells
erythropenia (ĕ-rĭth″ rō-pē′ nĭ-ă)	erythro penia	CF S	red lack of	Lack of red blood cells
erythropoiesis (ĕ-rĭth″ rō-poy-ē′ sĭs)	erythro poiesis	CF S	red formation	Formation of red blood cells
granulocyte (grăn′ ū-lō-sīt″)	granulo cyte	CF S	little grain, granular cell	A granular leukocyte
hematocele (hē″ mă-tō-sēl′)	hemato cele	CF S	blood hernia	A blood cyst, hernia
hematocrit (hē-măt′ ō-krĭt)	hemato crit	CF S	blood to separate	A blood test that separates solids from plasma in the blood by centrifuging the blood sample
hematologist (hē″ mă-tŏl′ ō-jĭst)	hemato log ist	CF R S	blood study of one who specializes	One who specializes in the study of the blood
hematology (hē″ mă-tŏl′ ō-jē)	hemato logy	CF S	blood study of	The study of the blood

Terminology - continued

TERM	WORD PARTS			DEFINITION
hematoma (hē″ mă-tō′ mă)	hemat oma	R S	blood tumor	A blood tumor. See Figure 8–4.
hemoglobin (hē″ mō-glō′ bĭn)	hemo globin	CF S	blood globe, protein	Blood protein; the iron-containing pigment of red blood cells
hemolysis (hē-mŏl′ ĭ-sĭs)	hemo lysis	CF S	blood destruction	Destruction of red blood cells
hemophilia (hē″ mō-fĭl′ ĭ-ă)	hemo philia	CF S	blood attraction	A hereditary blood disease characterized by prolonged coagulation and tendency to bleed
hemophobia (hē″ mō-fō′ bē-ă)	hemo phobia	CF S	blood fear	Fear of blood
hemopoiesis (hē″ mō-poy-ē′ sĭs)	hemo poiesis	CF S	blood formation	Formation of blood cells
hemorrhage (hĕm′ ĕ-rĭj)	hemo rrhage	CF S	blood bursting forth	Excessive bleeding; bursting forth of blood. See Figure 8–5.
hemostasis (hē-mŏs′ tā-sĭs)	hemo stasis	CF S	blood control, stopping	The control or stopping of bleeding
hypercalcemia (hī″ pĕr-kăl-sē′ mĭ-ă)	hyper calc emia	P R S	excessive lime, calcium blood condition	A condition of excessive amounts of calcium in the blood
hypercapnia (hī″ pĕr-kăp′ nē-ăh)	hyper capn ia	P R S	excessive smoke condition	A condition of excessive amounts of carbon dioxide in the blood
hyperglycemia (hī″ pĕr-glī-sē′ mĭ-ă)	hyper glyc emia	P R S	excessive sweet, sugar blood condition	A condition of excessive amounts of sugar in the blood
hyperlipemia (hī″ pĕr-lĭp-ē′ mĭ-ă)	hyper lip emia	P R S	excessive fat blood condition	A condition of excessive amounts of fat in the blood
hypoglycemia (hī″ pō-glī-sē′ mĭ-ă)	hypo glyc emia	P R S	deficient sweet, sugar blood condition	A condition of deficient amounts of sugar in the blood
leukapheresis (loo″ kă-fĕ-rē′ sĭs)	leuka pheresis	CF S	white removal	Removal of white blood cells from the circulation

continued

Terminology - continued

TERM	WORD PARTS			DEFINITION
leukemia (loo-kē′ mē-ă)	leuk emia	R S	white blood condition	A disease of the blood characterized by overproduction of leukocytes. The disease may be malignant, acute, or chronic
leukocyte (loo′ kō-sīt)	leuko cyte	CF S	white cell	A white blood cell
leukocytopenia (loo″ kō-sī″ tō-pē′ nĭ-ă)	leuko cyto penia	CF CF S	white cell lack of	A lack of white blood cells
lymphadenitis (lĭm-făd″ ĕn-ī′ tĭs)	lymph aden itis	R R S	lymph gland inflammation	Inflammation of the lymph glands
lymphadenotomy (lĭm-făd″ ĕ-nō tō-mē)	lymph adeno tomy	R CF S	lymph gland incision	Incision into a lymph gland
lymphangiology (lĭm-făn″ jē-ŏl′ ō-jē)	lymph angio logy	R CF S	lymph vessel study of	The study of the lymphatic vessels
lymphostasis (lĭm-fō′ stā-sĭs)	lympho stasis	CF S	lymph control, stopping	The control or stopping of the flow of lymph
macrocyte (măk′ rō-sīt)	macro cyte	CF S	large cell	An abnormally large erythrocyte
monocyte (mŏn′ ō-sīt)	mono cyte	P S	one cell	The largest leukocyte, which has one nucleus
mononucleosis (mŏn″ ō-nū″ klē-ō′ sĭs)	mono nucle osis	P R S	one kernel, nucleus condition	A condition of excessive amounts of mononuclear leukocytes in the blood
neutrophil (nū′ trō-fĭl)	neutro phil	CF S	neither attraction	A leukocyte that stains with neutral dyes
pancytopenia (păn″ sī-tō-pē′ nĭ-ă)	pan cyto penia	P CF S	all cell lack of	A lack of the cellular elements of the blood
phagocytosis (făg″ ō-sī-tō′ sĭs)	phago cyt osis	CF R S	eat, engulf cell condition of	A condition of the engulfing and eating of bacteria by the phagocytes

Terminology - continued

TERM	WORD PARTS			DEFINITION
plasmapheresis (plăz″ mă-fĕr-ē′ sĭs)	plasma pheresis	R S	a thing formed, plasma removal	Removal of blood from the body and centrifuging it to separate the plasma from the blood
polycythemia (pŏl″ ē-sī-thē′ mĭ-ă)	poly cyth emia	P R S	many cell blood condition	A condition of too many red blood cells
prothrombin (prō-thrŏm′ bĭn)	pro thromb in	P R S	before clot chemical	A chemical substance that interacts with calcium salts to produce thrombin
reticulocyte (rĕ-tĭk′ ū-lō-sīt)	reticulo cyte	CF S	net cell	A red blood cell containing a network of granules
septicemia (sĕp″ tĭ-sē′ mĭ-ă)	septic emia	R S	putrefying blood condition	A condition in which pathogenic bacteria are present in the blood
seroculture (sē′ rō-kŭl″ chūr)	sero culture	CF S	whey, serum cultivation	A bacterial culture of blood serum
serodiagnosis (sē″ rō-dī″ ăg-nō′ sĭs)	sero dia gnosis	CF P S	whey, serum through knowledge	Diagnosis of disease by observing the reactions of blood serum
serologist (sē-rŏl′ ō-jĭst)	sero log ist	CF R S	whey, serum study of one who specializes	One who specializes in the study of serum
serology (sē-rŏl′ ō-jē)	sero logy	CF S	whey, serum study of	The study of serum
sideropenia (sĭd″ ĕr-ō-pē′ nĭ-ă)	sidero penia	CF S	iron lack of	Lack of iron in the blood
splenemia (splē-nē′ mĭ-ă)	splen emia	R S	spleen blood condition	A condition in which the spleen is congested with blood
splenomegaly (splē″ nō-mĕg′ ă-lē)	spleno megaly	CF S	spleen enlargement	Enlargement of the spleen
splenopexy (splē′ nō-pĕk″ sē)	spleno pexy	CF S	spleen fixation	Surgical fixation of a movable spleen
thalassemia (thăl-ă-sē′ mĭ-ă)	thalass emia	R S	sea blood condition	Hereditary anemias occurring in populations bordering the Mediterranian Sea and in Southeast Asia

continued

Terminology - continued

TERM	WORD PARTS			DEFINITION
thrombectomy (thrŏm-bĕk′ tō-mē)	thromb ectomy	R S	clot excision	Surgical excision of a blood clot
thrombocyte (thrŏm′ bō-sīt)	thrombo cyte	CF S	clot cell	A clotting cell; *a blood platelet*
thrombogenic (thrŏm″ bō-jĕn′ ĭk)	thrombo genic	CF S	clot formation, produce	Formation of a blood clot
thrombolysis (thrŏm-bŏl′ ĭ-sĭs)	thrombo lysis	CF S	clot destruction	Destruction of a blood clot
thrombosis (thrŏm-bō′ sĭs)	thromb osis	R S	clot condition of	Condition of a blood clot
thymitis (thī-mī′ tĭs)	thym itis	R S	thymus inflammation	Inflammation of the thymus gland
thymocyte (thī′ mō-sīt)	thymo cyte	CF S	thymus cell	A lymphocyte derived from the thymus
thymoma (thī-mō′ mă)	thym oma	R S	thymus tumor	A tumor of the thymus
tonsillectomy (tŏn″ sĭl-ĕk′ tō-mē)	tonsill ectomy	R S	tonsil excision	Surgical excision of the tonsil

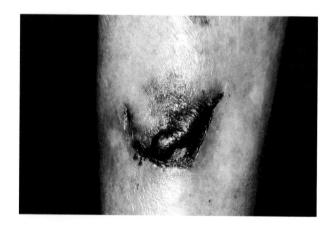

FIGURE 8–4

Traumatic hematoma. *(Courtesy of Jason L. Smith, MD.)*

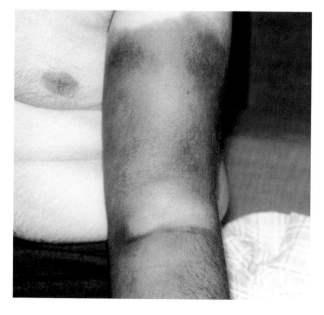

FIGURE 8–5

Hemorrhage, vein. *(Courtesy of Jason L. Smith, MD.)*

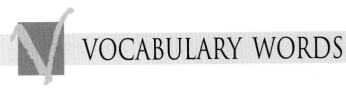

VOCABULARY WORDS

Vocabulary words are terms that have not been divided into component parts. They are common words or specialized terms associated with the subject of this chapter. These words are provided to enhance your medical vocabulary.

WORD	DEFINITION
acquired immune deficiency syndrome (AIDS) (ă-kwīrd ĭm″ ū-nē dĕ-fĭsh′ ĕn-sē sĭn-drōm)	AIDS is a disease caused by the human immunodeficiency virus (HIV). This virus is transmitted through sexual contact, through exposure to infected blood or blood components, and perinatally from mother to infant. The HIV virus invades the T4 lymphocytes, and as the disease progresses the body's immune system becomes paralyzed. The patient becomes severely weakened, and potentially fatal infections can occur. *Pneumocystis carinii* pneumonia and Kaposi's sarcoma account for many of the deaths of AIDS patients.
albumin (ăl-bū′ mĭn)	One of a group of simple proteins found in blood plasma and serum
autoimmune disease (aw″ tō-ĭm-mūn dĭ-zēz)	A condition in which the body's immune system becomes defective and produces antibodies against itself. Hemolytic anemia, rheumatoid arthritis, myasthenia gravis, and scleroderma are considered as autoimmune diseases.
autotransfusion (aw″ tō-trăns-fū′ zhŭn)	The process of reinfusing a patient's own blood. Methods used are: "harvesting" the blood 1 to 3 weeks before elective surgery; "salvaging" intraoperative blood; and collecting blood from trauma or selected surgical patients for reinfusion within 4 hours.
blood (blud)	The fluid that circulates through the heart, arteries, veins, and capillaries
corpuscle (kŏr′ pŭs-ĕl)	A blood cell
embolus (ĕm′ bō-lŭs)	A blood clot carried in the bloodstream
erythropoietin (ĕ-rĭth″ rō-poy′ ĕ-tĭn)	A hormone that stimulates the production of red blood cells
extravasation (ĕks-tră″ vă-sā′ shŭn)	The process whereby fluids and/or medications (IVs) escape into surrounding tissue
fibrin (fī′ brĭn)	An insoluble protein formed from fibrinogen by the action of thrombin in the blood-clotting process

continued

Vocabulary - continued

WORD	DEFINITION
fibrinogen (fĭ-brĭn′ ō-gĕn)	A blood protein converted to fibrin by the action of thrombin in the blood-clotting process
globulin (glŏb′ ū-lĭn)	An albuminous protein found in body fluids and cells
hemochromatosis (hē″ mō-krō″ mă-tō′ sĭs)	A disease condition in which iron is not metabolized properly and it accumulates in body tissues. The skin has a bronze hue, the liver becomes enlarged, and diabetes and cardiac failure may occur.
heparin (hĕp′ ă-rĭn)	A substance found in the liver, lungs, and other body tissues that inhibits blood clotting
immunoglobulin (Ig) (ĭm″ ū-nō-glŏb′ ū-lĭn)	A blood protein capable of acting as an antibody. The five major types are IgA, IgD, IgE, IgG, and IgM.
Kaposi's sarcoma (kăp′ō-sēz săr-kō′mă)	A malignant neoplasm that causes violaceous vascular lesions and general lymphadenopathy; it is the most common AIDS-related tumor. See Figures 8–6 and 8–7.
lymph (lĭmf)	A clear, colorless, alkaline fluid found in the lymphatic vessels
lymphangitis (lĭm″ făn-jī′tĭs)	Inflammation of lymphatic vessels. See Figure 8–8.
lymphedema (lĭmf-ĕ-dē′mă)	An abnormal accumulation of lymph in the interstitial spaces. See Figures 8–9 and 8–10.
lymphoma (lĭm-fō′mă)	A lymphoid neoplasm, usually malignant. See Figures 8–11 and 8–12.
opportunistic infection (ŏp″ ŏr-too-nĭs′ tĭk ĭn-fĕk′ shŭn)	A protozoal, fungal, viral, or bacterial infection that occurs when one's immune system is compromised. AIDS patients are very vulnerable and develop one or more opportunistic infections.
plasma (plăz′ mă)	The fluid part of the blood
Pneumocystis carinii (nū″ mō-sĭs′ tĭs kă-rī′ nē-ī)	A protozoan that causes pneumocystis carinii pneumonia (PCP)

Vocabulary - continued

WORD	DEFINITION
pneumocystis pneumonia (nū″ mō-sĭs′ tĭs nū-mō′ nē-ă)	An opportunistic infection that is prevalent in AIDS patients. If not treated, the mortality rate is high.
radioimmuno-assay (rā″ dē-ō-ĭm″ ū-nō-ăs′ ā)	A method of determining the concentration of protein-bound hormones in the blood plasma
serum (sē′ rŭm)	The clear, yellowish fluid that separates from the clot when blood clots
stem cell (stĕm sĕl)	A cell in the bone marrow that gives rise to various types of blood cells
thrombin (thrŏm′ bĭn)	A blood enzyme that causes clotting by forming fibrin
thromboplastin (thrŏm″ bō-plăs′ tĭn)	An essential factor in the production of thrombin and blood clotting
transfusion (trăns-fū″ zhŭn)	The process whereby blood is transferred from one individual to the vein of another
vasculitis (văs″ kū-lī′tĭs)	Inflammation of a lymph or blood vessel. See Figure 8–13.

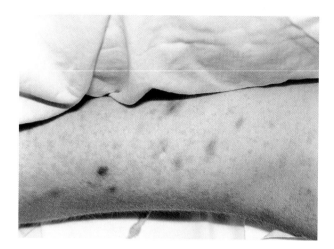

FIGURE 8–6

Kaposi's sarcoma. *(Courtesy of Jason L. Smith, MD.)*

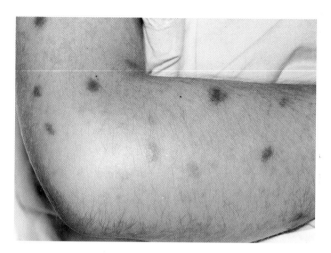

FIGURE 8–7

Kaposi's sarcoma. *(Courtesy of Jason L. Smith, MD.)*

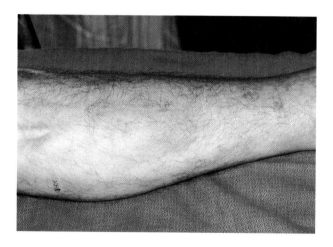

FIGURE 8–8

Lymphangitis. *(Courtesy of Jason L. Smith, MD.)*

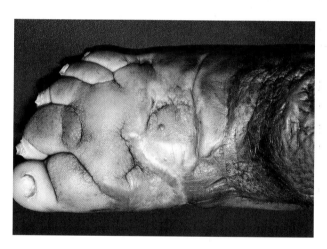

FIGURE 8–9

Congenital lymphedema. *(Courtesy of Jason L. Smith, MD.)*

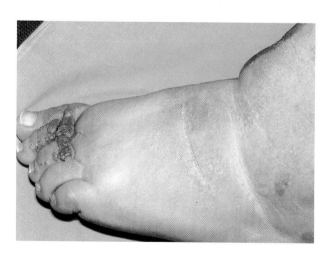

FIGURE 8–10

Chronic lymphedema. *(Courtesy of Jason L. Smith, MD.)*

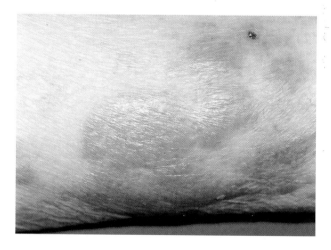

FIGURE 8–11

Lymphoma. *(Courtesy of Jason L. Smith, MD.)*

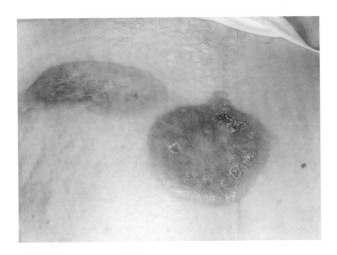

FIGURE 8–12

Cutaneous T-cell lymphoma. *(Courtesy of Jason L. Smith, MD.)*

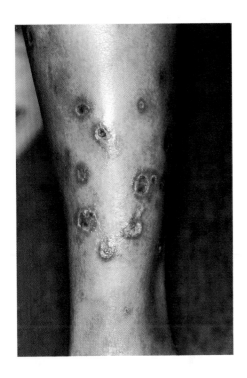

FIGURE 8–13

Vasculitis. *(Courtesy of Jason L. Smith, MD.)*

 ABBREVIATIONS

ABO	blood group	**Hct**	hematocrit
AHF	antihemophilic factor	**HIV**	human immunodeficiency virus
AIDS	acquired immune deficiency syndrome	**lymphs**	lymphocytes
		MCH	mean corpuscular hemoglobin
ALL	acute lymphocytic leukemia	**MCHC**	mean corpuscular hemoglobin concentration
BAC	blood alcohol concentration	**MCV**	mean corpuscular volume
baso	basophils	**mono**	monocyte
BSI	body systems isolation	**PCP**	pneumocystis carinii pneumonia
CBC	complete blood count	**PCV**	packed cell volume
CLL	chronic lymphocytic leukemia	**PMN**	polymorphonuclear neutrophil
CML	chronic myelogenous leukemia	**poly**	polymorphonuclear
diff	differential count	**PT**	prothrombin time
EBV	Epstein–Barr virus	**PTT**	partial thromboplastin time
ELISA	enzyme-linked immuno sorbent assay	**RBC**	red blood cell (count)
		Rh	Rhesus (factor)
eosins	eosinophils	**RIA**	radioimmunoassay
ESR	erythrocyte sedimentation rate	**segs**	segmented (mature RBCs)
Hb, Hgb	hemoglobin	**WBC**	white blood cell (count)

DRUG HIGHLIGHTS

Drugs that are generally used in blood and lymphatic diseases and disorders include anticoagulants, antiplatelet drug (aspirin), thrombolytic agents, hemostatic agents, hematinic agents, epoetin alfa, and drugs used in treating megaloblastic anemias.

Anticoagulants	Used in inhibiting or preventing a blood clot formation. Hemorrhage can occur at almost any site in patients on anticoagulant therapy. *Examples: heparin sodium, dicumarol, Coumadin Sodium (warfarin sodium), and Athrombin-K (warfarin potassium).*
Antiplatelet Drug *(aspirin)*	May be recommended by physicians to reduce the risk of a second heart attack and/or to reduce the risk of having a heart attack and/or stroke. It is generally recommended that an individual take aspirin 80, 160, or 320 mg per day to prevent thromboembolic disorders.
Thrombolytic Agents	Act to dissolve existing thrombus when administered soon after its occurrence. These agents dissolve the clot, reopen the artery, restore blood flow to the heart, and prevent further damage to the myocardium. Unless contraindicated, thrombolytic therapy is the treatment of choice for an acute myocardial infarction patient who reaches the hospital within 6 hours of the onset of chest pain. *Examples: Kabikinase or Streptase (streptokinase), Eminase (anistreplase [APSAC]), and Activase (alteplase).*
Hemostatic Agents	Used to control bleeding and may be administered systemically or topically. *Examples: Proplex (factor IX complement), Amicar (aminocaproic acid), vitamin K, and Surgicel (oxidized cellulose).*
Hematinic Agents *(irons)*	Used to treat iron deficiency anemia. Oral iron preparations interfere with the absorption of oral tetracycline antibiotics. These products should not be taken within 2 hours of each other. *Examples: Femiron, (ferrous fumarate), Fergon, Fertinic (ferrous gluconate), and Feosol (ferrous sulfate).*
Epoetin Alfa *(Epogen, Amgen)*	A genetically engineered hemopoietin that stimulates the production of red blood cells. It is a recombinant version of erythropoietin and is indicated for treating anemia in patients with chronic renal failure and AIDS patients taking zidovudine (AZT).
Agents	Used in treating megaloblastic anemias; include *Folvite (folic acid) and vitamin B$_{12}$ (cyanocobalamin).*

DIAGNOSTIC AND LABORATORY TESTS

Test	Description
antinuclear antibodies (ANA) (ăn″ tĭ-nū′ klē-ăr ăn′ tĭ-bŏd″ ēs)	A blood test to identify antigen–antibody reactions. ANA antibodies are present in a number of autoimmune diseases.
bleeding time (blēd′ ĭng tīm)	A puncture of the ear lobe or forearm to determine the time required for blood to stop flowing. Duke method (ear lobe) 1 to 3 minutes is the normal time, and with the Ivy (forearm), 1 to 9 minutes is the normal time for the flow of blood to cease. Times greater than these may indicate thrombocytopenia, aplastic anemia, leukemia, decreased platelet count, hemophilia, and potential hemorrhage. Anticoagulant drugs delay the bleeding time.
blood typing (ABO group and Rh factor) (blod tīp′ ĭng)	A blood test to determine an individual's blood type and Rh factor. Blood types are A, B, AB, and O. Rh factor may be negative or positive.
bone marrow aspiration (bōn măr′ ō ăs-pĭ-rā′ shŭn)	Removal of bone marrow for examination; may be performed to determine aplastic anemia, leukemia, certain cancers, and polycythemia.
complete blood count (CBC) (kom-plēt′ blod kount)	This blood test includes a hematocrit, hemoglobin, red and white blood cell count, and differential. This test is usually a part of a complete physical examination and a good indicator of hematologic system functioning.
hematocrit (Hct) (hē-măt′ ō-krĭt)	A blood test performed on whole blood to determine the percentage of red blood cells in the total blood volume.
hemoglobin (Hb, Hgb) (hē″ mō-glō′ bĭn)	A blood test to determine the amount of iron-containing pigment of the red blood cells.
immunoglobulins (Ig) (ĭm″ ū-nō-glŏb′ ū-lĭns)	A serum blood test to determine the presence of IgA, IgD, IgE, IgG, and/or IgM. Lymphocytes and plasma cells produce immunoglobulins in response to antigen exposure. Increased and/or decreased values may indicate certain disease conditions.
partial thromboplastin time (PTT) (păr′ shāl thrŏm″ bō-plăs′ tĭn tīm)	A test performed on blood plasma to determine how long it takes for fibrin clots to form; used to regulate heparin dosage and to detect clotting disorders.

Test	Description
platelet count (plāt′ lĕt kount)	A test performed on whole blood to determine the number of thrombocytes present. Increased and/or decreased amounts may indicate certain disease conditions.
prothrombin time (PT) (prō-thrŏm′ bĭn tīm)	A test performed on blood plasma to determine the time needed for oxalated plasma to clot; used to regulate anticoagulant drug therapy and to detect clotting disorders.
red blood count (RBC) (red blod kount)	A test performed on whole blood to determine the number of erythrocytes present. Increased and/or decreased amounts may indicate certain disease conditions.
sedimentation rate (ESR) (sĕd″ ĭ-mĕn-tā′ shŭn rāt)	A blood test to determine the rate at which red blood cells settle in a long, narrow tube. The distance the RBCs settle in 1 hour is the rate. Increased and/or decreased level may indicate certain disease conditions.
viral load (vī′ ral lōd)	A blood test that measures the amount of HIV in the blood. Results can range from 50 to over one million copies per milliliter (mL) of blood. Two tests that are used to measure viral load are bDNA and PCR.
white blood count (WBC) (hwīt blod kount)	A blood test to determine the number of leukocytes present. Increased level indicates infection and/or inflammation and decreased level indicates aplastic anemia, pernicious anemia, and malaria.

COMMUNICATION ENRICHMENT

This segment is provided for those who wish to enhance their ability to communicate in either English or Spanish.

▶ **Related Terms**

English	Spanish	English	Spanish
AIDS	SIDA (sĭ-dă)	bleeding tendency	tendencia a sangrar (tĕn-dĕn-sĭ-ă ă săn-grăr)
allergies	alergias (ă-lĕr-hĭ-ăs)	blood	sangre (săn-grĕ)
anemia	anemia (ă-nĕ-mĭ-ă)	blood test	prueda de sangre (prū-ĕ-bă de săn-grĕ)

English	Spanish	English	Spanish
blood transfusion	transfusión de sangre (trăns-*fū*-sĭ-ōn dĕ săn-*grĕ*)	lymphatic	linfático (lĭn-*fă*-tĭ-kō)
blood type	tipo de sangre (*tĭ*pō dĕ săn-*grĕ*)	lymph gland	ganglio linfático (găn-*glĭ*-ō lĭn-fă-tĭ-kō)
hematologic system	sistema hematologico (sĭs-*tĕ*-mă ĕ-*mă*-tō-lō-hĭ-kō)	lymph node	nódulo linfático (nō-*dū*-lō lĭn-*fă*-ti-kō)
hemorrhage	hemorragia (ĕ-mō-*ră*-hĭ-ă)	lymphocyte	linfocito (lĭn-*fō*-sĭ-tō)
immunization	inmunización (ĭn-*mū*-nĭ-ză-sĭ-ōn)	spleen	baso (*bă*-sō)
lymph	linfo (*lĭn*-fō)	tonsil	tonsila; amigdala (tōn-*sĭ*-lă; ă-mĭg-dă-lă)
lymphadenitis	linfadenitis (lĭn-*fă*-dĕ-nĭ-tĭs)	tonsillectomy	tonsilectómia (tōn-sĭ-*lĕc*-tō-mĭ-ă)
lymphangitis	linfangitis (lĭn-*făn*-hĭ-tĭs)	vaccination	vacunación (vă-*kū*-nă-sĭ-ōn)
		vaccine	vacuna (vă-*kū*-nă)

Have you had vaccinations for:	Le han puesto vacunación de: (¿Le *ăn* pū-*ĕs*-tō vă-*kū*-nă-sĭ-ōn dĕ)	Have you had vaccinations for:	Le han puesto vacunación de: (¿Le *ăn* pū-*ĕs*-tō vă-*kū*-nă-sĭ-ōn dĕ)
1. diphtheria?	1. difteria? (dĭf-*tĕ*-rĭ-ă)	7. cholera?	7. cólera? (*kō*-lĕ-ră)
2. whooping cough?	2. tosferina? (tōs-*fĕ*-rĭ-nă)	8. BCG?	8. BCG? (*bĕ*- sĕ- hĕ)
3. polio?	3. polio? (*pō*-lĭ-ō)	9. yellow fever?	9. fiebre amarilla? (fĭ-*ĕ*-brĕ ă-mă-rĭ-jă)
4. tetanus?	4. tétanos? (tĕ-*tă*-nōs)	10. measles?	10. sarampion? (să-*răm*-pĭ-ōn)
5. smallpox?	5. viruela? (vĭ-rū-*ĕ*-lă)	11. hepatitis?	11. hepatitis? (ĕ-*pă*-tĭ-tĭs)
6. typhoid fever?	6. fiebre tifoidea? (fĭ-*ĕ*-brĕ tĭ-fō-ĭ-dĕ-ă)	12. mumps?	12. paperas? (*pă*-pĕ-răs)

STUDY AND REVIEW SECTION

LEARNING EXERCISES

▶ **Anatomy and Physiology**

Write your answers to the following questions. Do not refer back to the text.

1. Name the three formed elements of blood.

   a. _____   b. _____

   c. _____

2. State the function of erythrocytes. _____

   _____

3. There are approximately _____ million erythrocytes per cubic millimeter of blood.

4. The life span of an erythrocyte is _____.

5. State the function of leukocytes. _____

   _____

6. There are approximately _____ thousand leukocytes per cubic millimeter of blood.

7. Name the five types of leukocytes.

   a. _____   b. _____

   c. _____   d. _____

   e. _____

8. State the function of thrombocytes. _____

   _____

9. There are approximately _____ thrombocytes per cubic millimeter of blood.

10. Name the four blood types.

   a. _____   b. _____

   c. _____   d. _____

11. State the three main functions of the lymphatic system.

a. _____

b. _____

c. _____

12. Name the three accessory organs of the lymphatic system.

a. _____

b. _____

c. _____

▶ Word Parts

1. In the spaces provided, write the definition of these prefixes, roots, combining forms, and suffixes. Do not refer to the listings of terminology words. Leave blank those terms you cannot define.

2. After completing as many as you can, refer back to the terminology word listings to check your work. For each word missed or left blank, write the term and its definition several times on the margins of these pages or on a separate sheet of paper.

3. To maximize the learning process, it is to your advantage to do the following exercises as directed. To refer to the terminology listings before completing these exercises invalidates the learning process.

Prefixes

Give the definitions of the following prefixes:

1. an- _____   2. anti- _____

3. auto- _____   4. dia- _____

5. dys- _____   6. hyper- _____

7. hypo- _____   8. mono- _____

9. pan- _____   10. poly- _____

11. pro- _____

Roots and Combining Forms

Give the definitions of the following roots and combining forms:

1. aden _____   2. adeno _____

3. agglutinat _____   4. all _____

5. angio _____

6. aniso _____

7. baso _____

8. calc _____

9. capn _____

10. clast _____

11. coagul _____

12. creatin _____

13. cyt _____

14. cyth _____

15. cyto _____

16. eosino _____

17. erythro _____

18. glyc _____

19. granulo _____

20. hemat _____

21. hemato _____

22. hemo _____

23. leuk _____

24. leuko _____

25. lip _____

26. log _____

27. lymph _____

28. lympho _____

29. macro _____

30. neutro _____

31. nucle _____

32. phago _____

33. plasma _____

34. reticulo _____

35. septic _____

36. sero _____

37. sidero _____

38. splen _____

39. spleno _____

40. thalass _____

41. thromb _____

42. thrombo _____

43. thym _____

44. thymo _____

45. tonsill _____

Suffixes

Give the definitions of the following suffixes:

1. -able _____

2. -ant _____

3. -blast _____

4. -body _____

5. -cele _____

6. -crit _____

7. -culture _____

8. -cyte _____

9. -ectomy _____

10. -emia _____

11. -ergy _____

12. -gen _____

13. -genic _____   14. -globin _____

15. -gnosis _____   16. -ia _____

17. -ic _____   18. -in _____

19. -ion _____   20. -ist _____

21. -itis _____   22. -logy _____

23. -lysis _____   24. -megaly _____

25. -oma _____   26. -osis _____

27. -pathy _____   28. -penia _____

29. -pexy _____   30. -pheresis _____

31. -phil _____   32. -philia _____

33. -phobia _____   34. -poiesis _____

35. -rrhag _____   36. -rrhage _____

37. -stasis _____   38. -therapy _____

39. -tomy _____

▶ Identifying Medical Terms

In the spaces provided, write the medical terms for the following meanings:

1. _____   Process of clumping together, as of blood cells that are incompatible

2. _____   Individual hypersensitivity to a substance that is usually harmless

3. _____   A protein substance produced in the body in response to an invading foreign substance

4. _____   An agent that works against the formation of blood clots

5. _____   An invading foreign substance that induces the formation of antibodies

6. _____   Pertaining to an agent that prevents or arrests hemorrhage

7. _____   A base cell, leukocyte

8. _____   Capable of forming a clot

9. _____   Excess of creatine in the blood

10. _____ A cell that readily stains with the acid stain

11. _____ Pertaining to the destruction of red blood cells

12. _____ A granular leukocyte

13. _____ One who specializes in the study of the blood

14. _____ Blood protein

15. _____ Excessive amounts of sugar in the blood

16. _____ Excessive amounts of fat in the blood

17. _____ A white blood cell

18. _____ The control or stopping of the flow of lymph

19. _____ Condition of excessive amounts of mononuclear leukocytes in the blood

20. _____ A chemical substance that interacts with calcium salts to produce thrombin

21. _____ Surgical fixation of a movable spleen

22. _____ A clotting cell; a blood platelet

23. _____ Formation of a blood clot

24. _____ Inflammation of the thymus

▶ Spelling

In the spaces provided, write the correct spelling of these misspelled terms:

1. allregy _____ 2. cretinemia _____

3. dyglycema _____ 4. erythcytosis _____

5. hemacele _____ 6. hemacrit _____

7. hemorhage _____ 8. lukemia _____

9. lymphadnotomy _____ 10. serlogy _____

WORD PARTS STUDY SHEET

Word Parts	Give the Meaning
an-	_____
auto-	_____
mono-	_____
pan-	_____
poly-	_____
angio-	_____
cyt-, cyth-	_____
eosino-	_____
erythro-	_____
granulo-	_____
hemat-, hemato-, hemo-	_____
leuk-, leuko-	_____
lymph-, lympho-	_____
macro-	_____
neutro-	_____
nucle-	_____
phago-	_____
splen-, spleno-	_____
thromb-, thrombo-	_____
thym-, thymo-	_____
tonsill-	_____
-blast	_____
-cele	_____
-crit	_____
-cyte	_____
-ectomy	_____
-emia	_____

-genic

_____

-globin

_____

-gnosis

_____

-logy

_____

-lysis

_____

-oma

_____

-penia

_____

-pexy

_____

-pheresis

_____

-philia

_____

-phobia

_____

-poiesis

_____

-rrhage

_____

-stasis

_____

REVIEW QUESTIONS

▶ Matching

Select the appropriate lettered meaning for each numbered line.

_____ 1. autotransfusion

_____ 2. erythrocyte

_____ 3. erythropoietin

_____ 4. extravasation

_____ 5. hemorrhage

_____ 6. immunoglobulin

_____ 7. hemochromatosis

_____ 8. radioimmunoassay

_____ 9. reticulocyte

_____ 10. thrombectomy

a. A method of determining the concentration of protein-bound hormones in the blood plasma
b. A disease condition in which iron is not metabolized properly and accumulates in body tissues
c. A blood protein capable of acting as an antibody
d. A red blood cell
e. A hormone that stimulates the production of red blood cells
f. Excessive bleeding
g. The process whereby fluids and/or medications escape into surrounding tissue
h. The process of reinfusing a patient's own blood
i. Surgical excision of a blood clot
j. A red blood cell containing a network of granules
k. A white blood cell

▶ Abbreviations

Place the correct word, phrase, or abbreviation in the space provided.

1. acquired immune deficiency syndrome _____

2. body systems isolation _____

3. CML _____

4. hemoglobin _____

5. Hct _____

6. human immunodeficiency virus _____

7. PCP _____

8. PT _____

9. RBC _____

10. radioimmunoassay _____

▶ Diagnostic and Laboratory Tests

Select the best answer to each multiple choice question. Circle the letter of your choice.

1. A blood test to identify antigen–antibody reactions.
   a. sedimentation rate
   b. hematocrit
   c. immunoglobulins
   d. antinuclear antibodies

2. This blood test includes a hematocrit, hemoglobin, red and white blood cell count, and differential.
   a. blood typing
   b. sedimentation rate
   c. CBC
   d. Hb, Hgb

3. A blood test performed on whole blood to determine the percentage of red blood cells in the total blood volume.
   a. RBC
   b. WBC
   c. Hct
   d. PTT

4. A blood test to determine the number of leukocytes present.
   a. RBC
   b. WBC
   c. Hct
   d. PTT

5. A puncture of the ear lobe or forearm to determine the time required for blood to stop flowing.
    a. bleeding time
    b. platelet count
    c. prothrombin time
    d. PTT

CRITICAL THINKING ACTIVITY

▶ **Case Study**

Acquired Immune Deficiency Syndrome (AIDS)

Please read the following case study and then answer the questions that follow.

A 52-year-old female was seen by a physician and the following is a synopsis of her visit. *Note: More than 10% of all AIDS cases in the United States have occurred in persons age 50 or older.*

Present History: The patient states that several months after the death of her husband she became sexually involved with a younger man. She states that they didn't use condoms, as they were not concerned about pregnancy, and now she has found out that he has AIDS. She is most anxious, and states that lately she has had "night sweats," weight loss for no apparent reason, constant fatigue, diarrhea, swollen lymph nodes, and unusual confusion.

Signs and Symptoms: Chief complaint: Night sweats, weight loss, fatigue, diarrhea, swollen lymph nodes, and unusual confusion.

Diagnosis: Acquired immune deficiency syndrome (AIDS). Diagnosis was determined by a complete medical and social history, a physical examination, CD_4 lymphocyte count, which was 400 cells/mm^3 (normal is 800 to 1050 cells/mm^3), and laboratory evidence of immune dysfunction, identification of HIV antibodies, and signs and symptoms.

Treatment: The regimen includes treating any associated condition with proper medical intervention, and starting the patient on a combination of antiretroviral therapy of three drugs: AZT—zidovudine; 3TC—lamiudine; and a protease inhibitor, Norvir—ritonavir. Drug therapy is carefully monitored for older adults, as they may have preexisting conditions, such as cardiac disease and/or renal insufficiency, that can make them less tolerant of drugs. Clinical evaluation and laboratory monitoring every 3 to 6 months and more frequently if needed. Provide for professional assistance as needed. Information on services available for the older adult with HIV infection and AIDS may be obtained by calling the CDC's AIDS Hotline at 1–800–342 AIDS.

Critical Thinking Questions

1. Signs and symptoms of AIDS include night sweats, weight loss, fatigue, _____, swollen lymph nodes, and confusion.

2. The diagnosis of AIDS was determined by a complete physical examination, laboratory evidence of _____ dysfunction, and a CD_4 lymphocyte count of 400 cells/mm^3.

3. _____ is an antiretroviral drug that is combined with two other drugs in the treatment of AIDS.

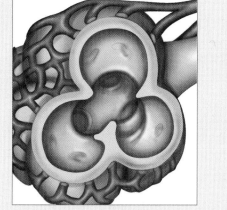

9

THE RESPIRATORY SYSTEM

OBJECTIVES

On completion of this chapter, you should be able to:

- Describe the organs of the respiratory system.

- State the functions of the organs of the respiratory system.

- Define terms that are used by physiologists and respiratory specialists to describe the volume of air exchanged in breathing.

- State the vital function of respiration.

- Provide the respiratory rates for some different age groups.

- Analyze, build, spell, and pronounce medical words that relate to surgical procedures and pathology.

- Identify and give the meaning of selected vocabulary words.

- Identify and define selected abbreviations.

- Review Drug Highlights presented in this chapter.

- Provide the description of diagnostic and laboratory tests related to the respiratory system.

- Successfully complete the study and review section.

▶ ANATOMY AND PHYSIOLOGY OVERVIEW

The respiratory system consists of the *nose, pharynx, larynx, trachea, bronchi,* and *lungs*. The primary function of the respiratory system is to furnish oxygen for use by individual tissue cells and to take away their gaseous waste product, carbon dioxide. See Figure 9–1. This process is accomplished through the act of *respiration*. Respiration consists of external and internal processes. *External respiration* is the process whereby the lungs are ventilated and oxygen and carbon dioxide are exchanged between the air in the lungs and the blood within capillaries of the alveoli. *Internal respiration* is the process whereby oxygen and carbon dioxide are exchanged between the blood in tissue capillaries and the cells of the body.

▶ THE NOSE

The *nose* is the projection in the center of the face and consists of an external and internal portion. The *external portion* is a triangle of cartilage and bone that is covered with skin and lined with mucous membrane. The external entrance of the nose is known as the *nostrils* or *anterior nares*. The *internal portion* of the nose is divided into two chambers by a partition, the *septum*, separating it into a right and a left cavity. These cavities are divided into three air passages: the *superior, middle,* and *inferior conchae*. These passages lead to the pharynx and are connected by openings with the paranasal sinuses, with the ears by the eustachian tube, and with the region of the eyes by the nasolacrimal ducts.

The *palatine bones* separate the nasal cavities from the mouth cavity. When the palatine bones fail to unite during fetal development, a congenital defect known as *cleft palate* occurs. This defect may be corrected by surgery. The nose, as well as the rest of the respiratory system, is lined with mucous membrane, which is covered with *cilia*. The nasal mucosa produces about 946 mL or 1 qt of mucus per day. Four pairs of paranasal sinuses drain into the nose. These are the *frontal, maxillary, ethmoidal,* and *sphenoidal* sinuses (Fig. 9–2).

FUNCTIONS OF THE NOSE

Five functions have been attributed to the nose. These functions are:

1. It serves as an air passageway.
2. It warms and moistens inhaled air.

THE RESPIRATORY SYSTEM

ORGAN/STRUCTURE	PRIMARY FUNCTIONS
The Nose	Serves as an air passageway; warms and moistens inhaled air; its cilia and mucous membrane trap dust, pollen, bacteria, and other foreign matter; contains olfactory receptors, which sort out odors; aids in phonation and the quality of voice
The Pharynx	Serves as a passageway for air and for food; aids in phonation by changing its shape
The Larynx	Production of vocal sounds
The Trachea	Provides an open passageway for air to the lungs
The Bronchi	Provide a passageway for air to and from the lungs
The Lungs	Bring air into intimate contact with blood so that oxygen and carbon dioxide can be exchanged in the alveoli

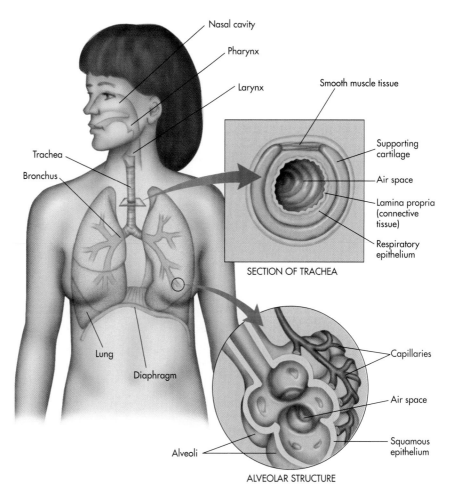

FIGURE 9-1

The respiratory system: nasal cavity, pharynx, larynx, trachea, bronchus, and lung with expanded views of the trachea and alveolar structure.

3. Its cilia and mucous membrane trap dust, pollen, bacteria, and other foreign matter.
4. It contains olfactory receptors, which sort out odors.
5. It aids in phonation and the quality of voice.

▶ THE PHARYNX

The *pharynx* or throat is a musculomembranous tube about 5 inches long that extends from the base of the skull, lies anterior to the cervical vertebrae, and becomes continuous with the esophagus. It is divided into three portions: the *nasopharynx* located behind the nose, the *oropharynx* located behind the mouth, and the *laryngopharynx* located behind the larynx. Seven openings are found in the pharynx: two openings from the eustachian tubes, two openings from the posterior nares into the nasopharynx, the fauces or opening from the mouth into the oropharynx, and the openings from the larynx and the esophagus into the laryngopharynx (Fig. 9–2). Associated with the pharynx are three pairs of lymphoid tissues, which are the *tonsils*. The nasopharynx contains the *adenoids* or *pharyngeal* tonsils. The oropharynx contains the *faucial* or *palatine* tonsils and the *lingual* tonsils. The tonsils are accessory organs of the lymphatic system and aid in filtering bacteria and other foreign substances from the circulating lymph.

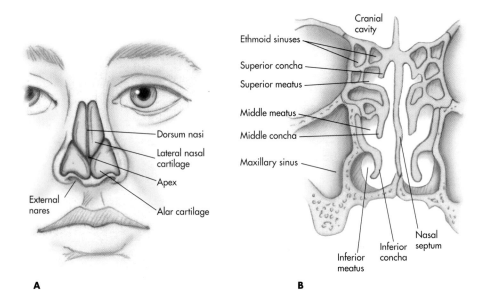

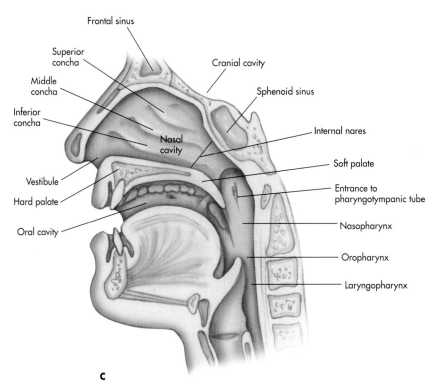

FIGURE 9-2

The nose, nasal cavity, and pharynx: **(A)** nasal cartilages and external structure, **(B)** meatuses and positions of the entrance to the ethmoid and maxillary sinuses, **(C)** sagittal section of the nasal cavity and pharynx.

FUNCTIONS OF THE PHARYNX

The following three functions are associated with the pharynx:

1. It serves as a passageway for air.
2. It serves as a passageway for food.
3. It aids in phonation by changing its shape.

▶ THE LARYNX

The *larynx* or voicebox is a muscular, cartilaginous structure lined with mucous membrane. It is the enlarged upper end of the trachea below the root of the tongue and hyoid bone (Fig. 9–1).

CARTILAGE OF THE LARYNX

The larynx is composed of nine cartilages bound together by muscles and ligaments. The three unpaired cartilages, each of which is described below, are the *thyroid, cricoid,* and *epiglottic,* and the three paired cartilages are the *arytenoid, cuneiform,* and *corniculate.*

The Thyroid Cartilage

The *thyroid cartilage* is the largest cartilage in the larynx and forms the structure commonly called the *"Adam's apple."* This structure is usually larger and more prominent in men than in women and contributes to the deeper male voice.

The Epiglottic Cartilage

The *epiglottic cartilage* is a small cartilage attached to the superior border of the thyroid cartilage. Known as the *epiglottis,* it covers the entrance of the larynx, and during swallowing, it acts as a lid to prevent aspiration of food into the trachea. When the epiglottis fails to cover the entrance to the larynx, food or liquid intended for the esophagus may enter, causing irritation, coughing, or in extreme cases, choking.

The Cricoid Cartilage

The *cricoid cartilage* is the lowermost cartilage of the larynx. It is shaped like a signet ring with the broad portion being posterior and the anterior portion forming the arch and resembling the ring's band.

   The cavity of the larynx contains a pair of *ventricular folds* (false vocal cords) and a pair of vocal folds or true vocal cords. The cavity is divided into three regions: the vestibule, the ventricle, and the entrance to the glottis. The *glottis* is a narrow slit at the opening between the true vocal folds.

FUNCTION OF THE LARYNX

The function of the larynx is the production of vocal sounds. High notes are formed by short, tense vocal cords. Low notes are produced by long, relaxed vocal cords. The nose, mouth, pharynx, and bony sinuses aid in phonation.

▶ THE TRACHEA

The *trachea* or windpipe is a cylindrical cartilaginous tube that is the air passageway extending from the pharynx and larynx to the main bronchi. It is about 1 inch wide and 4½ inches (11.3 cm) long. It is composed of smooth muscle that is reinforced at the front and sides by C-shaped rings of cartilage. Mucous membrane lining the trachea contains *cilia,* which sweep foreign matter out of the passageway. The function of the trachea is to provide an open passageway for air to the lungs (see Fig. 9–1).

▶ THE BRONCHI

The *bronchi* are the two main branches of the trachea, which provide the passageway for air to the lungs. The trachea divides into the *right bronchus* and the *left bronchus.* The right bronchus is larger and extends down in a more vertical direction than the left bronchus. When a foreign body is inhaled or aspirated, it frequently lodges in the right bronchus or enters the right lung. Each bronchus enters the lung at a depression, the *hilum.* They then subdivide into the bronchial tree composed of smaller bronchi, bronchioles, and alveolar ducts. The bronchial tree terminates in the *alveoli,* which are tiny air sacs supporting a network of capillaries from pulmonary blood vessels. The function of the bronchi is to provide a passageway for air to and from the lungs (see Fig. 9–1).

▶ THE LUNGS

The *lungs* are cone-shaped, spongy organs of respiration lying on either side of the heart within the pleural cavity of the thorax. They occupy a large portion of the thoracic cavity and are enclosed in the *pleura,* a serous membrane composed of several layers. The six layers of the pleura are the *costal, parietal, pericardiaca, phrenica, pulmonalis,* and *visceral.* The *parietal pleura* extends from the roots of the lungs and lines the walls of the thorax and the superior surface of the diaphragm. The *visceral pleura* covers the surface of the lungs and enters into and lines the interlobar fissures. The pleural cavity is a space between the parietal and visceral pleura and contains a serous fluid that lubricates and prevents friction caused by the rubbing together of the two layers. The thoracic cavity is separated from the abdominal cavity by a musculomembranous wall, the *diaphragm.* The central portion of the thoracic cavity, between the lungs, is a space called the *mediastinum,* containing the heart and other structures.

The lungs consist of elastic tissue filled with interlacing networks of tubes and sacs that carry air and with blood vessels carrying blood. The broad inferior surface of the lung is the *base,* which rests on the diaphragm, while the *apex,* or pointed upper margin, rises from 2.5 to 5 cm above the sternal end of the first rib. The lungs are divided into *lobes* with the right lung having three lobes and the left lung having only two lobes. The left lung has an indentation, the *cardiac depression,* for the normal placement of the heart. In an average adult male, the right lung weighs approximately 625 g and the left about 570 g. In an average adult male, the total lung capacity is 3.6 to 9.4 L, whereas in an average adult female it is 2.5 to 6.9 L. The lungs contain around 300 million *alveoli,* which are the air cells where the exchange of oxygen and carbon dioxide takes place. The main function of the lungs is to bring air into intimate contact with blood so that oxygen and carbon dioxide can be exchanged in the alveoli (see Fig. 9–3).

▶ RESPIRATION

VOLUME

The following terms are used by physiologists and respiratory specialists to describe the volume of air exchanged in breathing:

Tidal Volume. The amount of air in a single inspiration or expiration. In the average adult male, about 500 cc of air enters the respiratory tract during normal quiet breathing.

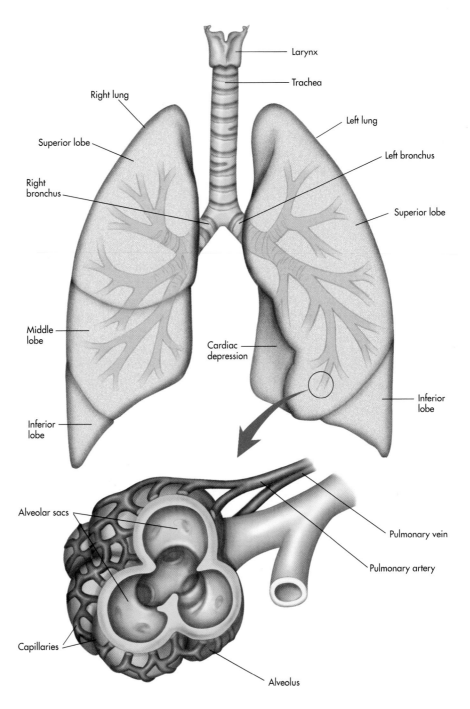

Larynx

Trachea

Right lung

Superior lobe

Left lung

Left bronchus

Right bronchus

Superior lobe

Middle lobe

Cardiac depression

Inferior lobe

Inferior lobe

Alveolar sacs

Pulmonary vein

Pulmonary artery

Capillaries

Alveolus

FIGURE 9–3

The larynx, trachea, bronchi, and lungs with an expanded view showing the structures of an alveolus and the pulmonary blood vessels.

Supplemental Air. The amount of air that may be forcibly expired after a normal quiet respiration. This is also the expiratory reserve volume and measures approximately 1600 cc.

Complemental Air. The amount of air that may be forcibly inspired over and above a normal inspiration. This is known as the inspiratory reserve volume.

Residual Volume. The amount of air remaining in the lungs after maximal expiration—about 1500 cc.

Minimal Air. The small amount of air that remains in the alveoli. After death, if the thorax is opened and the lungs collapse, the minimal air pressure will allow the lungs to float.

Vital Capacity. The volume of air that can be exhaled after a maximal inspiration. This amount equals the sum of the tidal air, complemental air, and the supplemental air.

Functional Residual Capacity. The volume of air that remains in the lungs at the end of a normal expiration.

Total Lung Capacity. The maximal volume of air in the lungs after a maximal inspiration.

THE VITAL FUNCTION OF RESPIRATION

Temperature, pulse, respiration, and *blood pressure* are the vital signs that are essential elements for determining an individual's state of health. A deviation from normal of one or all of the vital signs denotes a state of illness. Evaluation of an individual's response to changes occurring within the body can be measured by taking his or her vital signs. Through careful analysis of these changes in the vital signs, a physician may determine a diagnosis, a prognosis, and a plan of treatment for the patient. The variations of certain vital signs signify a typical disease process and its stages of development. For example, in a patient who has pneumonia the temperature is elevated to 101° to 106°F, and pulse and respiration increase to almost twice their normal rates. When the patient's temperature falls, he or she will perspire profusely and his or her pulse and respiration will begin to return to normal rates.

The process of *respiration* is interrelated with other systems of the body. The *medulla oblongata* and the *pons* of the central nervous system regulate and control respiration. The rate, rhythm, and depth of respiration are controlled by nerve impulses from the medulla oblongata and the pons via the spinal cord and nerves to the muscles of the diaphragm, abdomen, and rib cage.

RESPIRATORY RATES

Individuals of different ages breathe at different respiratory rates. *Respiratory rate* is regulated by the respiratory center located in the medulla oblongata. The following are respiratory rates for some different age groups:

Newborn	30 to 80 per minute
1st year	20 to 40 per minute
5th year	20 to 25 per minute
15th year	15 to 20 per minute
Adult	15 to 20 per minute

LIFE SPAN CONSIDERATIONS

▶ THE CHILD

At 12 weeks' gestation the lungs of the fetus have a definite shape. At 20 weeks the fetus is able to suck its thumb and swallow amniotic fluid. The cellular structure of the **alveoli** of the lungs are complete. At 24 weeks the nostrils open, respiratory movements occur, and alveoli begin the production of **surfactant.** Surfactant is a substance in the lung that regulates the amount of surface tension of the fluid lining the alveoli. In preterm infants the lack of surfactant contributes to respiratory distress syndrome.

During fetal life gaseous exchange occurs at the placental interface. The lungs do not function until birth. The respiratory rate of the newborn is 30 to 80 per minute. During the first year it is 20 to 40 per minute and at age 5 it is 20 to 25 per minute. Around the 15th year the respiratory rate is 15 to 20, the same as the average, healthy adult rate. Diaphragmatic abdominal breathing is common in infants. Accessory muscles of respiration are not as strong in infants as in older children and adults.

Oxygen consumption and metabolic rate are higher in children than in adults. Airway diameter is smaller in children, thereby increasing the potential for airway obstruction. The mucous membranes of children are vascular and susceptible to trauma, edema, and spasm.

▶ THE OLDER ADULT

With advancing age, the respiratory system is vulnerable to injuries caused by infections, environmental pollutants, and allergic reactions. Age-related changes include a decline in the protection normally provided by intact mucous barrier, a decrease in the effectiveness of the bronchial cilia, and changes in the composition of the connective tissues of the lungs and chest. Older adults rely more on the **diaphragm** for inspiration, and when lying down, breathing requires more effort. **Vital capacity** declines with age; there is a decline in the elastic recoil of the lungs and an increase in the stiffness of the chest wall. This makes it more difficult for the older adult to inspire or expire air.

In the pharynx and larynx muscle atrophy can occur, with slackening of the vocal cords and loss of elasticity of the laryngeal muscles and cartilages. These changes may cause a gravelly, softer voice with a rise in pitch, making communication more difficult, especially if there is impaired hearing.

TERMINOLOGY
WITH SURGICAL PROCEDURES & PATHOLOGY

TERM	WORD PARTS			DEFINITION
aerophore (air′ ō-for)	aero phore	CF S	air bearing	An apparatus for inflating the lungs of stillborn infants
aeropleura (air′ ō-ploo″ ră)	aero pleura	CF R	air pleura	Air in the pleural cavity
alveolus (ăl-vē′ ō-lŭs)	alveol us	R S	small, hollow air sac pertaining to	Pertaining to a small air sac in the lungs
anosmia (ăn-ŏz′ mĭ-ă)	an osm ia	P R S	lack of smell condition	A condition in which there is a lack of the sense of smell
anoxia (ăn-ŏks′ ĭ-ă)	an ox ia	P R S	lack of oxygen condition	A condition in which there is a lack of oxygen
anthracosis (ăn″ thră-kō′ sĭs)	anthrac osis	R S	coal condition of	Black lung; a lung condition caused by inhalation of coal dust and silica
aphonia (ă-fō′ nĭ-ă)	a phon ia	P R S	lack of voice condition	A condition of inability to produce vocal sounds
aphrasia (ă-frā-′ zĭ-ă)	a phras ia	P R S	lack of speech condition	A condition of inability to speak
apnea (ăp′ -nē ă)	a pnea	P S	lack of breathing	Temporary cessation of breathing

☼ TERMINOLOGY SPOTLIGHT

Apnea is defined as a temporary cessation of breathing. **Sleep apnea** is cessation of breathing during sleep. The disruption of sleep patterns due to an obstruction of airways affects about 10 million Americans. To be so classified, the apnea must last for at least 10 seconds and occurs 30 or more times during a 7-hour period of sleep. This definition may not apply to older adults in whom periods of sleep apnea are increased. Sleep apnea is classified according to the mechanism involved.

Terminology - continued

TERM	WORD PARTS			DEFINITION
atelectasis (ăt″ ĕ-lĕk′ tă-sĭs)	atel ectasis	R S	imperfect dilation, expansion	A condition of imperfect dilation of the lungs; the collapse of an alveolus, a lobule, or a larger lung unit
bronchiectasis (brŏng″ kĭ-ĕk′ tă-sĭs)	bronchi ectasis	CF S	bronchi dilation, expansion	Dilation of the bronchi
bronchiolitis (brŏng″ kĭ-ō-lī′ tĭs)	bronchiol itis	R S	bronchiole inflammation	Inflammation of the bronchioles
bronchitis (brŏng-kī′ tĭs)	bronch itis	R S	bronchi inflammation	Inflammation of the bronchi
bronchomycosis (brŏng″ kō-mī-kō′ sĭs)	broncho myc osis	CF R S	bronchi fungus condition of	A fungus condition of the bronchi
bronchoplasty (brŏng′ kō-plăs″ tē)	broncho plasty	CF S	bronchi surgical repair	Surgical repair of the bronchi
bronchoscope (brŏng′ kō-skōp)	broncho scope	CF S	bronchi instrument	An instrument used to examine the bronchi
cyanosis (sī″ ăn-ō′ -sĭs)	cyan osis	R S	dark blue condition of	A dark blue condition of the skin and mucous membrane caused by oxygen deficiency
diaphragmalgia (dī″ ă-frăg-măl′ jĭ-ă)	dia phragm algia	P R S	through partition pain	Pain in the diaphragm

- Obstructive apnea is caused by obstruction to the upper airway. This condition generally occurs in middle-aged men who are obese and have a history of excessive daytime sleepiness. It is associated with loud snorting, snoring, and gasping sounds.
- Central apnea is marked by absence of respiratory muscle activity. A person with this type of apnea may exhibit excessive daytime sleepiness, but the snorting and gasping sounds during sleep are absent.
- Mixed apnea begins with absence of respiratory effort followed by upper airway obstruction.

Sleep deprivation can make a person tired, sluggish, irritable, prone to accidents, and less productive. Although the amount of sleep needed is different for every person, adults need at least 7 hours of sleep in a 24-hour time period, children under the age of 10 need 11 to 13 hours of sleep, and teenagers need 10 to 12 hours of sleep.

continued

Terminology - continued

TERM	WORD PARTS			DEFINITION
diaphragmatocele (dī″ ă-frăg-măt′ ō-sēl)	dia phragmato cele	P CF S	through partition hernia	A hernia of the diaphragm
dysphonia (dĭs-fō′ nĭ-ă)	dys phon ia	P R S	difficult voice condition	A condition of difficulty in speaking
dyspnea (dĭsp-nē′ ă)	dys pnea	P S	difficult breathing	Difficulty in breathing
endotracheal (ĕn″ dō-trā′ kē-ăl)	endo trache al	P CF S	within trachea pertaining to	Pertaining to within the trachea
eupnea (ūp-nē′ ă)	eu pnea	P S	good, normal breathing	Good or normal breathing
exhalation (ĕks″ hə-lā′ shən)	ex halat ion	P R S	out breathe process	The process of breathing out
expectoration (ĕk-spĕk″ tə′ rā′ shən	ex pectorat ion	P R S	out breast process	The process by which saliva, mucus, or phlegm is expelled from the air passages
hemoptysis (hē-mŏp′ tĭ-sĭs)	hemo ptysis	CF S	blood to spit	The spitting up of blood
hemothorax (hē″ mō-thō-răks)	hemo thorax	CF R	blood chest	Blood in the chest cavity
hyperpnea (hī″ pĕrp-nē′ ă)	hyper pnea	P S	excessive breathing	Excessive or rapid breathing
hypoxia (hī-pŏks′ ĭ-ă)	hyp ox ia	P R S	below, deficient oxygen condition	A condition of deficient amounts of oxygen in the inspired air
inhalation (ĭn″ hă-lā′ shŭn)	in halat ion	P R S	in breathe process	The process of breathing in
laryngeal (lăr-ĭn′ jĭ-ăl)	larynge al	CF S	larynx pertaining to	Pertaining to the larynx
laryngectomy (lăr″ ĭn-jĕk′ tō-mē)	laryng ectomy	R S	larynx excision	Surgical excision of the larynx

Terminology - continued

TERM	WORD PARTS			DEFINITION
laryngitis (lăr″ ĭn-jī′ tĭs)	laryng itis	R S	larynx inflammation	Inflammation of the larynx
laryngoplasty (lăr-ĭn′ gō-plăs″ tē)	laryngo plasty	CF S	larynx surgical repair	Surgical repair of the larynx
laryngoscope (lăr-ĭn′ gō-skōp)	laryngo scope	CF S	larynx instrument	An instrument used to examine the larynx
laryngostenosis (lăr-ĭng″ gō-stĕ-nō′sĭs)	laryngo sten osis	CF R S	larynx narrowing condition of	A condition of narrowing of the larynx
laryngostomy (lăr″ ĭn-gŏs′ tō-mē)	laryngo stomy	CF S	larynx new opening	Establishing a new opening in the larynx
lobectomy (lō-bĕk′ tō-mē)	lob ectomy	R S	lobe excision	Surgical excision of a lobe of any organ or gland, such as the lung
nasomental (nā″ zō-mĕn′ tăl)	naso ment al	CF R S	nose chin pertaining to	Pertaining to the nose and chin
nasopharyngitis (nā″ zō-făr′ ĭn-jī′ tĭs)	naso pharyng itis	CF R S	nose pharynx inflammation	Inflammation of the nose and pharynx
orthopnea (or″ thŏp-nē′ ă)	ortho pnea	CF S	straight breathing	Inability to breathe unless in an upright or straight position
palatoplegia (păl″ ă-tō-plē′ jĭ-ā)	palato plegia	CF S	palate stroke, paralysis	Paralysis of the muscles of the soft palate
pharyngalgia (făr″ ĭn-găl′ jĭ-ă)	pharyng algia	R S	pharynx pain	Pain in the pharynx
pharyngitis (făr″ ĭn-jī′ tĭs)	pharyng itis	R S	pharynx inflammation	Inflammation of the pharynx
pleuritis (ploo-rī′ tĭs)	pleur itis	R S	pleura inflammation	Inflammation of the pleura
pleurodynia (ploo″ rō-dĭn′ ĭ-ă)	pleuro dynia	CF S	pleura pain	Pain in the pleura

continued

Terminology - continued

TERM	WORD PARTS			DEFINITION
pneumoconiosis (nū″ mō-kō″ nĭ-ō′ sĭs)	pneumo coni osis	CF R S	lung dust condition of	A condition of the lung caused by the inhalation of dust
pneumonitis (nū″ mō-nī′ tĭs)	pneumon itis	R S	lung inflammation	Inflammation of the lung
pneumothorax (nū″ mō-thō′ răks)	pneumo thorax	CF R	air chest	A collection of air in the chest cavity
pulmometer (pŭl-mŏm′ ĕ-tĕr)	pulmo meter	CF S	lung instrument to measure	An instrument used to measure lung capacity
pulmonectomy (pŭl″ mō-nĕk′ tō-mē)	pulmon ectomy	R S	lung excision	Surgical excision of the lung or a part of a lung
pyothorax (pī″ ō-thō′ răks)	pyo thorax	CF R	pus chest	Pus in the chest cavity
rhinoplasty (rī′ nō-plăs″ tē)	rhino plasty	CF S	nose surgical repair	Surgical repair of the nose
rhinorrhagia (rī″ nō-ră′ jĭ-ă)	rhino rrhagia	CF S	nose bursting forth	The bursting forth of blood from the nose
rhinorrhea (rī″ nō-rē′ ă)	rhino rrhea	CF S	nose flow, discharge	Discharge from the nose
rhinostenosis (rī″ nō-stĕn-ō′ sĭs)	rhino sten osis	CF R S	nose narrowing condition of	A condition of narrowing of the nasal passages
rhinotomy (rī-nŏt′ ō-mē)	rhino tomy	CF S	nose incision	Incision of the nose
sinusitis (sī″ nūs-ī′ tĭs)	sinus itis	R S	a curve, hollow inflammation	Inflammation of a sinus
spirogram (spī′ rō-grăm)	spiro gram	CF S	breath a mark, record	A record made by a spirograph showing respiratory movements
spirometer (spī-rŏm′ ĕt-ĕr)	spiro meter	CF S	breath instrument to measure	An instrument used to measure the volume of respired air

Terminology - continued

TERM	WORD PARTS			DEFINITION
tachypnea (tăk″ ĭp-nē′ ă)	tachy pnea	P S	fast breathing	Fast breathing
thoracocentesis (thō″ răk-ō-sĕn-tē′ sĭs)	thoraco centesis	CF S	chest surgical puncture	Surgical puncture of the chest for removal of fluid
thoracopathy (thō″ răk-ŏp′ ă-thē)	thoraco pathy	CF S	chest disease	Any disease of the chest
thoracoplasty (thō′ ră-kō-plăs″ tē)	thoraco plasty	CF S	chest surgical repair	Surgical repair of the chest
thoracotomy (thō″ răk-ŏt′ ō-mē)	thoraco tomy	CF S	chest incision	Incision of the chest
tonsillectomy (tŏn″ sĭl-ĕk′ tō-mē)	tonsill ectomy	R S	almond, tonsil excision	Surgical excision of the tonsils
tonsillitis (tŏn″ sĭl-ī′ tĭs)	tonsill itis	R S	almond, tonsil inflammation	Inflammation of the tonsils
tracheal (trā′ kē-ăl)	trache al	R S	trachea pertaining to	Pertaining to the trachea
trachealgia (trā″ kē-ăl′ jĭ-ă)	trache algia	R S	trachea pain	Pain in the trachea
tracheitis (trā″ kē-ī′ tĭs)	trache itis	R S	trachea inflammation	Inflammation of the trachea
tracheolaryngo- tomy (trā″ kē-ō-lăr″ ĭn-gŏt′ ō-mē)	tracheo laryngo tomy	CF CF S	trachea larynx incision	Incision into the larynx and trachea
tracheostomy (trā″ kē-ŏs′ tō-mē)	tracheo stomy	CF S	trachea new opening	New opening into the trachea

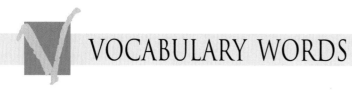

VOCABULARY WORDS

Vocabulary words are terms that have not been divided into component parts. They are common words or specialized terms associated with the subject of this chapter. These words are provided to enhance your medical vocabulary.

WORD	DEFINITION
artificial respiration (ăr″ tĭ-fĭsh′ ăl rĕs″ pĭr-ā′ shŭn)	The process of using artificial means to cause air to flow into and out of an individual's lungs when breathing is inadequate or ceases
asphyxia (ăs-fĭk′ sĭ-ă)	A condition in which there is a depletion of oxygen in the blood with an increase of carbon dioxide in the blood and tissues. First-aid treatment is by artificial respiration.
aspiration (ăs″ pĭ-rā′ shŭn)	The process of taking substances in or out by means of suction
asthma (ăz′ mă)	A disease of the bronchi characterized by wheezing, dyspnea, and a feeling of constriction in the chest
carbon dioxide (kăr bən dī-ŏk′ sīd)	A colorless, odorless gas used with oxygen to stimulate respiration
Cheyne-Stokes respiration (chān′ stōks′ rĕs″ pĭr-ā′ shŭn)	A rhythmic cycle of breathing with a gradual increase in respiration followed by apnea (which may last from 10 to 60 sec), then a repeat of the same cycle
coryza (kŏr-rī′ ză)	The common cold characterized by sneezing, nasal discharge, coughing, and malaise
cough (kawf)	Sudden, forceful expulsion of air from the lungs. It is an essential protective response that clears irritants, secretions, or foreign objects from the trachea, bronchi, and/or lungs.
croup (croop)	A respiratory disease characterized by a "barking" cough, dyspnea, hoarseness, and laryngeal spasm
cystic fibrosis (sĭs′ tĭk fĭ-brō′ sĭs)	An inherited disease that affects the pancreas, respiratory system, and sweat glands. The etiology is unknown, and the prognosis is generally poor.
emphysema (ĕm″ fĭ-sē′ mă)	A chronic pulmonary disease in which the bronchioles become obstructed with mucus

Vocabulary - continued

WORD	DEFINITION
empyema (ĕm″ pī-ē′ mă)	Pus in a body cavity, especially the pleural cavity
epistaxis (ĕp″ ĭ-stăk′ sĭs)	Nosebleed
Heimlich maneuver (hīm′ lĭk)	A technique for removing a foreign body (usually a bolus of food) that is blocking the trachea
hyperbaric oxygenation (hī″ pĕr-băr′ ĭk ŏk″ sĭ-jĕn-ā′ shŭn)	The process of administering oxygen in a closed chamber at a pressure greater than one and one-half to three times absolute atmospheric pressure
hyperventilation (hī″ pĕr-vĕn″ tĭ-lā′ shŭn)	The process of excessive ventilating, thereby increasing the air in the lungs beyond the normal limit
influenza (ĭn″ flū-ĕn′ ză)	An acute, contagious respiratory infection caused by a virus. Onset is usually sudden, and symptoms are fever, chills, headache, myalgia, cough, and sore throat.
Kussmaul's breathing (koos′ mowiz brēth′ ĭng)	A distressing, deep gasping type of breathing associated with metabolic acidosis and coma; also called air hunger
legionnaire's disease (lē jə naerz′ dĭ-zēz′)	A severe pulmonary pneumonia caused by *Legionella pneumophilia*
mesothelioma (mĕs″ ō-thē″ lĭ-ō′ mă)	A malignant tumor of mesothelium (serous membrane of the pleura) caused by the inhalation of asbestos
nares (nā′ rĕs)	The nostrils
olfaction (ŏl-făk′ shŭn)	The process of smelling
oropharynx (or″ ō-făr′ ĭnks)	The central portion of the throat that lies between the soft palate and upper portion of the epiglottis
palatopharyngoplasty (păl″ ăt-ō-făr″ ĭn′ gō-plăs″ tē)	A type of surgery that cures snoring and sleep apnea by removing the uvula and the tonsils and reshaping the lining at the back of the throat to enlarge the air passageway

continued

Vocabulary - continued

WORD	DEFINITION
pertussis (pĕr-tŭs′ ĭs)	An acute, infectious disease characterized by coryza, an explosive paroxysmal cough ending in a "crowing" or "whooping" sound; *also called whooping cough*
pleurisy (ploo′ rĭsē)	Inflammation of the pleura caused by injury, infection, or a tumor
pneumonia (nū-mō′ nĭ-ă)	Inflammation of the lung caused by bacteria, viruses, or chemical irritants
pollinosis (pŏl-ĭn-ō′ sĭs)	Hay fever; nasal congestion of mucous membranes caused by an allergic reaction to a pollen or pollens
polyp (pŏl′ ĭp)	A tumor with a stem; may occur where there are mucous membranes, such as the nose, ears, mouth, uterus, and intestines
rale (rahl)	An abnormal sound heard on auscultation of the chest; a crackling, rattling, or bubbling sound
respirator (rĕs′ pĭ-rā″ tor)	A type of machine used for prolonged artificial respiration
respiratory distress syndrome (hyaline membrane disease) (rĕs′ pĭ-ră-tō″ rē dĭs-trĕs′ sĭn′ drōm)	A condition that may occur in a premature infant in which the lungs are not matured to the point of manufacturing lecithin, a pulmonary surfactant. This results in collapse of the alveoli, which leads to cyanosis and hypoxia.
rhinovirus (rī″ nō-vī′ rŭs)	One of a subgroup of viruses that causes the common cold in humans
rhonchus (rŏng′ kŭs)	A rale or rattling sound in the throat or bronchial tubes caused by a partial obstruction
sarcoidosis (sar″ koyd-ō′ sĭs)	A chronic granulomatous condition that may involve almost any organ system of the body. The lungs are usually involved and this causes dyspnea on exertion. With multisystem involvement the patient may experience fatigue, fever, anorexia, weight loss, joint pain, and skin changes, including erythemanodosum, plaques, maculopapular eruptions, and subcutaneous nodules. See Figures 9–4 and 9–5.
sputum (spū′ tŭm)	Substance coughed up from the lungs; may be watery, thick, purulent, clear, or bloody and may contain microorganisms
stridor (strī′ dōr)	A high-pitched sound caused by obstruction of the air passageway

Vocabulary - continued

WORD	DEFINITION
tuberculosis (tū-bĕr″ kū-lō′ sĭs)	An infectious disease caused by the tubercle bacillus, *Mycobacterium tuberculosis*
wheeze (hwēz)	A whistling sound caused by obstruction of the air passageway

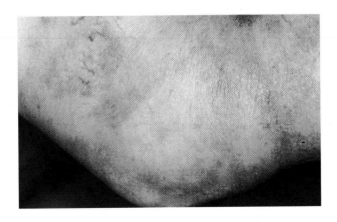

FIGURE 9–4

Sarcoidosis. *(Courtesy of Jason L. Smith, MD.)*

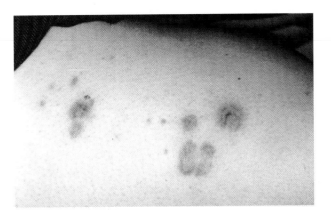

FIGURE 9–5

Sarcoidosis. *(Courtesy of Jason L. Smith, MD.)*

ABBREVIATIONS

ABGs	arterial blood gases	**IPPB**	intermittent positive-pressure breathing
AFB	acid-fast bacilli	**IRDS**	infant respiratory distress syndrome
ARD	acute respiratory disease	**IRV**	inspiratory reserve volume
ARDS	adult respiratory distress syndrome	**MBC**	maximal breathing capacity
CF	cystic fibrosis	**MV**	minute volume
CO₂	carbon dioxide	**MVV**	maximal voluntary ventilation
COLD	chronic obstructive lung disease	**O₂**	oxygen
COPD	chronic obstructive pulmonary disease	**PEEP**	positive end-expiratory pressure
CXR	chest x-ray	**PND**	postnasal drip
ENT	ear, nose, and throat	**PPD**	purified protein derivative
ERV	expiratory reserve volume	**R**	respiration
ET	endotracheal	**RD**	respiratory disease
FEF	forced expiratory flow	**RDS**	respiratory distress syndrome
FEV	forced expiratory volume	**SIDS**	sudden infant death syndrome
HBOT	hyperbaric oxygen therapy	**SOB**	shortness of breath
HMD	hyaline membrane disease	**T & A**	tonsillectomy and adenoidectomy

TB	tuberculosis	**URI**	upper respiratory infection
TLC	total lung capacity	**VC**	vital capacity
TV	tidal volume		

DRUG HIGHLIGHTS

Drugs that are generally used in respiratory system diseases and disorders include antihistamines, decongestants, antitussives, expectorants, mucolytics, bronchodilators, inhalational corticosteroids, and antituberculosis agents.

Antihistamines

Act to counter the effects of histamine by blocking histamine 1 (H_1) receptors. They are used in the treatment of allergy symptoms, for preventing or controlling motion sickness, and in combination with cold remedies to decrease mucus secretion and produce bedtime sedation.
Examples: Benadryl (diphenhydramine HCl), Hismanal (astemizole), and Dimetane (brompheniramine maleate).

Decongestants

Act to constrict dilated arterioles in the nasal mucosa. These agents are used for the temporary relief of nasal congestion associated with the common cold, hay fever, other upper respiratory allergies, and sinusitis.
Examples: Sudafed (pseudoephedrine HCl), Coricidin (phenylephrine HCl), Sinutab Long-Lasting Sinus Spray (xylometazoline HCl), and Afrin (oxymetazoline HCl).

Antitussives
Non-narcotic agents

May be classified as non-narcotic and narcotic.
Anesthetize the stretch receptors located in the respiratory passages, lungs, and pleura by dampening their activity and thereby reducing the cough reflex at its source.
Examples: Tessalon (benzonatate), Benylin (diphenhydramine HCl), and dextromethorphan hydrobromide.

Narcotic agents

Depress the cough center that is located in the medulla, thereby raising its threshold for incoming cough impulse.
Examples: codeine and Codimal (hydrocodone bitartrate).

Expectorants

Promote and facilitate the removal of mucus from the lower respiratory tract.
Examples: Robitussin (guaifenesin) and terpin hydrate.

Mucolytics

Break chemical bonds in mucus, thereby lowering its thickness.
Example: Mucomyst (acetylcysteine).

Bronchodilators

Are used to improve pulmonary airflow.
Examples: Adrenalin (epinephrine), Proventil (albuterol), ephedrine sulfate, aminophylline, and Tedral SA (theophylline).

Inhalational Corticosteroids

Used in the treatment of bronchial asthma, and in seasonal or perennial allergic conditions when other forms of treatment are not effective.
Examples: Decadron (dexamethasone phosphate), Beclovent (beclomethasone dipropionate), and Azmacort (triamcinolone acetonide).

Antituberculosis Agents

Used in the long-term treatment of tuberculosis (9 months to 1 year). They are often used in *combination of two or more drugs and the primary drug regimen for active tuberculosis combines the drugs Myambutol (ethambutol HCl); INH, Nydrazid (isoniazid); and Rifadin, Rimactane (rifampin).*

DIAGNOSTIC AND LABORATORY TESTS

Test	Description
acid-fast bacilli (AFB) (ăs ĭd-făst″ bă-sĭl′ ī)	A test performed on sputum to detect the presence of *Mycobacterium tuberculosis,* an acid-fast bacilli. Positive results indicate tuberculosis.
antistreptolysin O (ASO) (ăn″ tĭ-strĕp-tŏl′ ĭ-sĭn)	A test performed on blood serum to detect the presence of streptolysin enzyme O, which is secreted by beta-hemolytic streptococcus. Positive results indicate streptococcal infection.
arterial blood gases (ABGs) (ăr-tē′ rē-ăl blod găs′ ĕs)	A series of tests performed on arterial blood to establish acid–base balance. Important in determining respiratory acidosis and/or alkalosis, metabolic acidosis and/or alkalosis.
bronchoscopy (brŏng-kŏs′ kō-pē)	Visual examination of the larynx, trachea, and bronchi via a flexible bronchoscope. With the use of biopsy forceps, tissues and secretions can be removed for further analysis.
culture, sputum (kŭl′ tūr, spū′ tŭm)	Examination of the sputum to determine the presence of microorganisms. Abnormal results may indicate tuberculosis, bronchitis, pneumonia, bronchiectasis, and other infectious respiratory diseases.
culture, throat (kŭl′ tūr, thrōt)	A test done to identify the presence of microorganisms in the throat, especially beta-hemolytic streptococci.
laryngoscopy (lăr″ ĭn-gŏs′ kō-pē)	Visual examination of the larynx via a laryngoscope.
nasopharyngography (nă″ zō-făr-ĭn-ŏg′ ră-fē)	X-ray examination of the nasopharynx.
pulmonary function test (pŭl′ mō-nĕ-rē fŭng′ shŭn test)	A series of tests performed to determine the diffusion of oxygen and carbon dioxide across the cell membrane in the lungs. Tests included are: tidal volume (TV), vital capacity (VC), expiratory reserve volume (ERV), inspiratory capacity (IC), residual volume (RV), forced inspiratory volume (FIV), functional residual capacity (FRC), maximal voluntary ventilation (MVV), total lung capacity (TLC), and flow volume loop (F-V loop). Abnormal results may indicate various respiratory diseases and conditions.
rhinoscopy (rī-nŏs′ kō-pē)	Visual examination of the nasal passages.

COMMUNICATION ENRICHMENT

This segment is provided for those who wish to enhance their ability to communicate in either English or Spanish.

▶ **Related Terms**

English	Spanish	English	Spanish
asthma	asma (ăs-mă)	nosebleed	hemorragia nasal (ĕ-mōr-ră-hĭ-ă nă-săl)
breath	aliento; respiro (ă-lĭ-ĕn-tō; rĕs-pĭ-rō)	phlegm	flema (flĕ-mă)
bronchitis	bronquitis (brōn-kĭ-tĭs)	pneumonia	neumonía; pulmonía (nĕ-ū-mō-nĭ-ă; pūl-mō-nĭ-ă)
chest	pecho (pĕ-chō)	pollen	polen (pō-lĕn)
cough	tos (tōs)	throat	garganta (găr-găn-tă)
deep breath	rispire profundo (rĕs-pĭ-rĕ prō-fūn-dō)	sore throat	dolor de garganta (dō-lōr dĕ găr-găn-tă)
diaphragm	diafragma (dĭ-ă-frăg-mă)	tuberculosis	tuberculosis (tŭ-bĕr-kū-lōs-ĭs)
difficulty in breathing	dificultad en respirar (dĭ-fĭ-cŭl-tăd ĕn rĕs-pĭ-răr)	voice	voz (vōz)
dust	polvo (pōl-vō)	whooping cough	tosferina (tōs-fĕ-rĭ-nă)
hoarseness	ronquedad; ronquera (rōn-kĕ-dăd; rōn-kay-ră)	respiration	respiración (rĕs-pĭ-ră-sĭ-ōn)
lungs	pulmónes (pŭl-mō-nĕs)	thorax	tórax (tō-răx)
nose	nariz (nă-riz)	hoarse	ronco (rōn-kō)
		snore	ronquido (rōn-kĭ-dō)
		influenza	gripe (grĭ-pĕ)

English	Spanish	English	Spanish
pleurisy	pleuritis (plĕ-ū-rĭ-tĭs)	tonsillitis	tonsilitis; amigdalitis (tōn-sĭ-lĭ-tĭs; ˘a-mĭg-dă-lĭ-tĭs)
exhale	exhalar (ex-hă-lăr)	croup	crup (crūp)
inhale	inhalar (ĭn-hă-lăr)	aspiration	aspiración (ăs-pĭ-ră-sĭ-ōn)
larynx	laringe (lă-rĭn-hĕ)	asphyxia	asfixia (ăs-fix-ĭ-ă)
tonsil	tonsila; amigdala (tōn-sĭ-lă; ă-mĭg-dă-lă)	common cold	resfriado común (rĕs-frĭ-ă-dō cō-mūn)

STUDY AND REVIEW SECTION

LEARNING EXERCISES

▶ Anatomy and Physiology

Write your answers to the following questions. Do not refer back to the text.

1. List the organs of the respiratory system.

    a. _____   b. _____

    c. _____   d. _____

    e. _____   f. _____

2. State the primary function of the respiratory system. _____

    _____

3. Define external respiration. _____

4. Define internal respiration. _____

5. List the five functions of the nose.

    a. _____

    b. _____

    c. _____

d. _____

e. _____

6.   Name the three divisions of the pharynx.

a. _____   b. _____

c. _____

7.   List the three functions of the pharynx.

a. _____

b. _____

c. _____

8.   State the function of the epiglottis. _____

9.   Define glottis. _____

10.   State the function of the larynx. _____

11.   State the function of the trachea. _____

12.   The trachea divides into the _____ _____ and

the _____ _____.

13.   State the function of the bronchi. _____

14.   Give a brief description of the lungs. _____

_____

15.   Define pleura. _____

16.   The thoracic cavity is separated from the abdominal cavity by a musculomembra-

nous wall commonly known as the _____.

17.   The central portion of the thoracic cavity, between the lungs, is a space called the

_____.

18.   The right lung has _____ lobes and the left lung has _____ lobes.

19.   The air cells of the lungs are the _____.

20.   State the main function of the lungs. _____

_____.

21.   The vital signs, which are essential elements for determining an individual's state

of health, are _____, _____, _____,

and _____.

22. Define the following terms:

    a. Tidal volume _____

    b. Residual volume _____

    c. Vital capacity _____

23. The _____ _____ and the _____ of the central nervous system regulate and control respiration.

24. The respiratory rate for a newborn is _____ to _____ breaths per minute.

25. The respiratory rate for an adult is _____ to _____ breaths per minute.

▶ Word Parts

1. In the spaces provided, write the definition of these prefixes, roots, combining forms, and suffixes. Do not refer to the listings of terminology words. Leave blank those terms you cannot define.

2. After completing as many as you can, refer back to the terminology word listings to check your work. For each word missed or left blank, write the term and its definition several times on the margins of these pages or on a separate sheet of paper.

3. To maximize the learning process, it is to your advantage to do the following exercises as directed. To refer to the terminology listings before completing these exercises invalidates the learning process.

Prefixes

Give the definitions of the following prefixes:

1. a- _____   2. an- _____

3. dia- _____   4. dys- _____

5. endo- _____   6. eu- _____

7. ex- _____   8. hyp- _____

9. hyper- _____   10. in- _____

11. tachy- _____

Roots and Combining Forms

Give the definitions of the following roots and combining forms:

1. aero _____

2. alveol _____

3. anthrac _____

4. atel _____

5. bronch _____

6. bronchi _____

7. bronchiol _____

8. broncho _____

9. coni _____

10. cyan _____

11. halat _____

12. hemo _____

13. laryng _____

14. larynge _____

15. laryngo _____

16. lob _____

17. ment _____

18. myc _____

19. naso _____

20. ortho _____

21. osm _____

22. ox _____

23. palato _____

24. pectorat _____

25. pharyng _____

26. phon _____

27. phragm _____

28. phragmato _____

29. phras _____

30. pleur _____

31. pleura _____

32. pleuro _____

33. pneumo _____

34. pneumon _____

35. pulmo _____

36. pulmon _____

37. pyo _____

38. rhino _____

39. sinus _____

40. spiro _____

41. sten _____

42. thoraco _____

43. thorax _____

44. tonsill _____

45. trache _____

46. tracheo _____

Suffixes

Give the definitions of the following suffixes:

1. -al _____

2. -algia _____

3. -cele _____

4. -centesis _____

5. -dynia _____   6. -ectasis _____

7. -ectomy _____   8. -gram _____

9. -ia _____   10. -ion _____

11. -itis _____   12. -meter _____

13. -osis _____   14. -pathy _____

15. -phore _____   16. -plasty _____

17. -plegia _____   18. -pnea _____

19. -ptysis _____   20. -rrhagia _____

21. -rrhea _____   22. -scope _____

23. -stomy _____   24. -tomy _____

25. -us _____

▶ Identifying Medical Terms

In the spaces provided, write the medical terms for the following meanings:

1. _____ Air in the pleural cavity

2. _____ Pertaining to a small air sac in the lungs

3. _____ Inability to produce vocal sounds

4. _____ Dilation of the bronchi

5. _____ Inflammation of the bronchi

6. _____ Surgical repair of the bronchi

7. _____ Difficulty in speaking

8. _____ Good or normal breathing

9. _____ The spitting up of blood

10. _____ The process of breathing in

11. _____ Inflammation of the larynx

12. _____ A condition of narrowing of the larynx

13. _____ Pertaining to the nose and chin

14. _____ Pain in the pharynx

15. _____ A collection of air in the chest cavity

16. _____ Surgical repair of the nose

17. _____   Discharge from the nose

18. _____   Inflammation of a sinus

19. _____   Any disease of the chest

▶ Spelling

In the spaces provided, write the correct spelling of these misspelled terms:

1. bronchscope _____   2. diaphramatcele _____

3. expectorion _____   4. laryngal _____

5. orthpnea _____   6. peluritis _____

7. pulmnectomy _____   8. rhintomy _____

9. trachypnea _____   10. trachal _____

WORD PARTS STUDY SHEET

Word Parts	Give the Meaning
a-	
dys-	
eu-	
hyp-	
hyper-	
tachy-	
anthrac-	
atel-	
bronchi-, broncho-	
coni-	
cyan-	
laryng-, larynge-, laryngo-	
ment-	
myc-	
naso-, rhin-, rhino-	

ortho- _____

ox- _____

pharyng- _____

pneumo- _____

pneumon-, pulmo-, pulmon- _____

pyo- _____

sinus- _____

trache-, tracheo- _____

-al _____

-algia _____

-ectasis _____

-ia, -osis _____

-itis _____

-meter _____

-plasty _____

-pnea _____

-ptysis _____

-rrhagia _____

-rrhea _____

-scope _____

-stomy _____

-tomy _____

-us _____

REVIEW QUESTIONS

▶ Matching

Select the appropriate lettered meaning for each numbered line.

_____ 1. cough

_____ 2. cystic fibrosis

_____ 3. influenza

_____ 4. nares

_____ 5. olfaction

_____ 6. pollinosis

_____ 7. rhinovirus

_____ 8. sputum

_____ 9. tachypnea

_____ 10. thoracocentesis

a. Substance coughed up from the lungs
b. Hay fever
c. The process of smelling
d. One of a subgroup of viruses that causes the common cold in humans
e. Fast breathing
f. The nostrils
g. Surgical puncture of the chest for removal of fluid
h. Sudden, forceful expulsion of air from the lungs
i. An inherited disease that affects the pancreas, respiratory system, and sweat glands
j. Slow breathing
k. An acute, contagious respiratory infection caused by a virus

▶ Abbreviations

Place the correct word, phrase, or abbreviation in the space provided.

1. acid-fast bacilli _____

2. CF _____

3. Chest x-ray _____

4. chronic obstructive lung disease _____

5. ET _____

6. PND _____

7. respiration _____

8. SIDS _____

9. shortness of breath _____

10. TB _____

▶ Diagnostic and Laboratory Tests

Select the best answer to each multiple choice question. Circle the letter of your choice.

1. A test performed on sputum to detect the presence of *Mycobacterium tuberculosis*.
   a. antistreptolysin O
   b. acid-fast bacilli
   c. pulmonary function test
   d. bronchoscopy

2. The visual examination of the nasal passages.
   a. bronchoscopy
   b. laryngoscopy
   c. rhinoscopy
   d. nasopharyngography

3. _____ is/are important in determining respiratory acidosis and/or alkalosis, metabolic acidosis and/or alkalosis.
   a. Acid-fast bacilli
   b. Antistreptolysin O
   c. Arterial blood gases
   d. Pulmonary function test

4. A series of tests to determine the diffusion of oxygen and carbon dioxide across the cell membrane in the lungs.
   a. acid-fast bacilli
   b. antistreptolysin O
   c. arterial blood gases
   d. pulmonary function test

5. The visual examination of the larynx, trachea, and bronchi via a flexible scope.
   a. bronchoscopy
   b. laryngoscopy
   c. nasopharyngography
   d. rhinoscopy

CRITICAL THINKING ACTIVITY

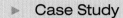

▶ Case Study

Pulmonary Tuberculosis

Please read the following case study and then answer the questions that follow.

A 28-year-old male was seen by a physician and the following is a synopsis of the visit.

Present History: The patient states that he has had a persistent cough for the past 3 weeks, is very tired, has lost 8 lb recently, doesn't have an appetite, and wakes up in the middle of the night soaked in sweat.

Signs and Symptoms: Chief complaint: chronic cough, fatigue, night sweats, weakness, anorexia, and weight loss.

Diagnosis: Pulmonary tuberculosis. The diagnosis was determined by a physical examination, a sputum culture that was positive for *Mycobacterium tuberculosis,* a positive PPD (purified protein derivative) test, and a chest x-ray that revealed lesions in the upper right lobe.

Treatment: The physician ordered a regimen of diet, rest, and a combination of three antituberculosis agents: isoniazid, rifampin, and ethambutol. The medication is to be taken as ordered for 9 months. A follow-up visit was scheduled for 2 weeks.

Prevention: Avoid exposure to *Mycobacterium tuberculosis* bacillus. The Centers for Disease Control and Prevention has published a booklet on *Guidelines for Preventing the Transmission of Tuberculosis in Health-Care Settings.* The following are specific actions to reduce the risk of tuberculosis transmission:

- Screening patients for active TB and TB infection
- Providing rapid diagnostic services
- Prescribing an appropriate curative and preventive therapy
- Maintaining physical measures to reduce microbial contamination of the air
- Providing isolation rooms for persons with, or suspected of having, infectious TB
- Screening health-care-facility personnel for TB infection
- Promptly investigating and controlling outbreaks

Critical Thinking Questions

1. Signs and symptoms of pulmonary tuberculosis include a chronic cough, fatigue, night sweats, weakness, _____, and weight loss.

2. The diagnosis was determined by a physical examination, a positive PPD test, and a positive sputum culture for _____ _____ bacillus.

3. Treatment included diet, rest, and a medication regimen of three antituberculosis agents: _____, rifampin, and ethambutol.

10

THE URINARY SYSTEM

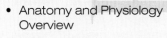

OBJECTIVES

On completion of this chapter, you should be able to:

- Describe the organs of the urinary system.

- State the vital function of the urinary system.

- Describe the formation of urine.

- Describe urinalysis.

- Identify the normal constituents of urine.

- Identify abnormal constituents of urine.

- Analyze, build, spell, and pronounce medical words that relate to surgical procedures and pathology.

- Identify and give the meaning of selected vocabulary words.

- Identify and define selected abbreviations.

- Review Drug Highlights presented in this chapter.

- Provide the description of diagnostic and laboratory tests related to the urinary system.

- Successfully complete the study and review section.

▶ ANATOMY AND PHYSIOLOGY OVERVIEW

The urinary system consists of two *kidneys*, two *ureters*, one *bladder*, and one *urethra* (Fig. 10–1). It may be referred to as the excretory system, genitourinary system, or urogenital system. The vital function of the urinary system is extraction of certain wastes from the bloodstream, conversion of these materials to urine, transport of the urine from the kidneys via the ureters to the bladder, and elimination of it at appropriate intervals via the urethra. Through this vital function, homeostasis of body fluids is maintained. See Figure 10–2.

▶ THE KIDNEYS

The *kidneys* are purplish-brown, bean-shaped organs located at the back of the abdominal cavity *(retroperitoneal area)*. They lie, one on each side of the spinal column, just above the waistline, against the muscles of the back. Each kidney is surrounded by three capsules; the *true capsule,* the *perirenal fat,* and the *renal fascia.* The true capsule is a smooth, fibrous connective membrane that is loosely adherent to the surface of the kidney. The perirenal fat is the adipose capsule that embeds each kidney in fatty tissue. The renal fascia is a sheath of fibrous tissue that helps to anchor the kidney to the surrounding structures and helps to maintain its normal position.

EXTERNAL STRUCTURE

Each kidney has a *concave* border and a *convex* border. The center of the concave border opens into a notch called the *hilum.* The renal artery and vein, nerves, and lymphatic vessels enter and leave through the hilum. The ureter enters the kidney through the hilum into a sac-like collecting portion called the *renal pelvis.*

INTERNAL STRUCTURE

When a cross section is made through the kidney, two distinct areas are seen comprising its anterior: the *cortex,* which is the outer layer, and the *medulla* or inner portion. The cortex contains the arteries, veins, convoluted tubules, and glomerular capsules. The medulla contains the renal pyramids, cone-like masses with papillae projecting into calyces of the pelvis.

MICROSCOPIC ANATOMY

Microscopic examination of the kidney reveals about 1 million *nephrons,* which are the structural and functional units of the organ. Each nephron consists of a *renal corpuscle*

THE URINARY SYSTEM

ORGAN/STRUCTURE	PRIMARY FUNCTIONS
Kidneys	Produce urine and help regulate body fluids
Ureters	Transport urine from the kidneys to the bladder
Urinary Bladder	Serves as a reservoir for urine
Urethra	Conveys urine to the outside of the body; in the male conveys both urine and semen

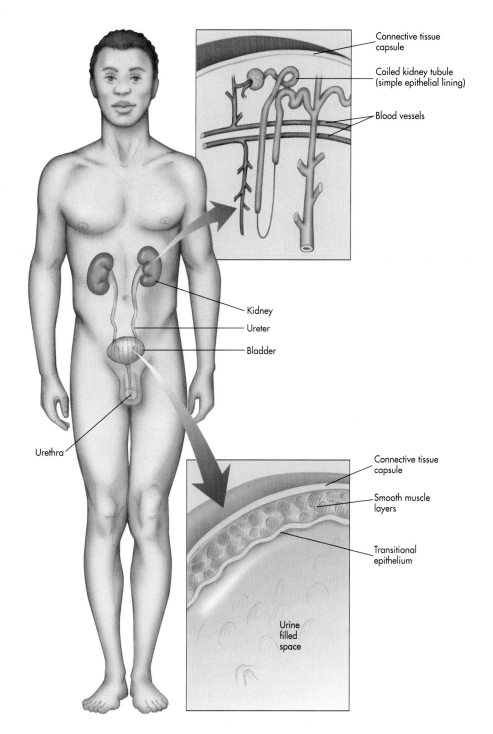

Connective tissue capsule

Coiled kidney tubule (simple epithelial lining)

Blood vessels

Kidney

Ureter

Bladder

Urethra

Connective tissue capsule

Smooth muscle layers

Transitional epithelium

Urine filled space

FIGURE 10–1

The urinary system: kidneys, ureters, bladder, and urethra with expanded view of a nephron and the urine-filled space within a bladder.

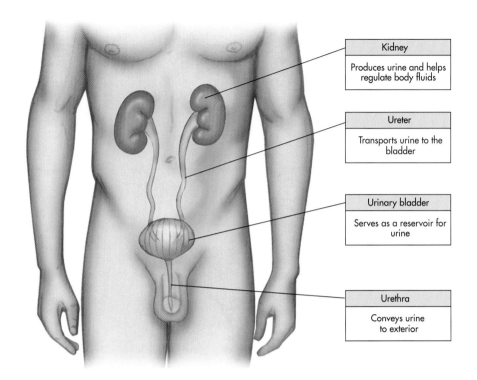

FIGURE 10–2

The organs of the urinary system with major functions.

and *tubule.* The renal corpuscle or malpighian corpuscle consists of a glomerulus and Bowman's capsule. Extending from each *Bowman's capsule* is a tubule consisting of the proximal convoluted portion, the loop of Henle, and a distal convoluted portion that opens into a collecting tubule.

THE NEPHRON

The vital function of the *nephron* is to remove the waste products of metabolism from the blood plasma. These waste products are urea, uric acid, and creatinine, plus any excess sodium, chloride, and potassium ions and ketone bodies. The nephron plays a vital role in the maintenance of normal fluid balance in the body by allowing for re-absorption of water and some electrolytes back into the blood. Approximately 1000 to 1200 mL of blood passes through the kidney per minute. At a rate of 1000 mL of blood per minute about 1.5 million mL pass through the kidney in each 24-hour day (Fig. 10–3).

▶ THE URETERS

There are two *ureters,* one for each kidney. They are narrow, muscular tubes that transport urine from the kidneys to the bladder. They are from 28 to 34 cm long and vary in diameter from 1 mm to 1 cm. The walls of the ureters consist of three layers: an inner coat of mucous membrane, a middle coat of smooth muscle, and an outer coat of fibrous tissue.

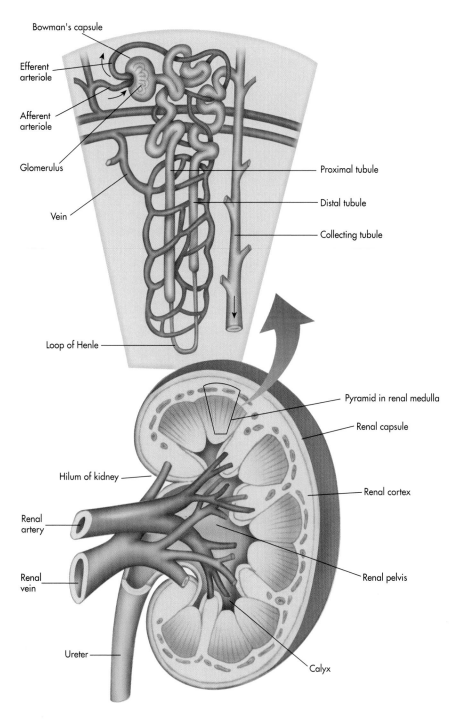

FIGURE 10–3

The kidney with an expanded view of a nephron.

▶ THE URINARY BLADDER

The *urinary bladder* is the muscular, membranous sac that serves as a reservoir for urine. It is located in the anterior portion of the pelvic cavity and consists of a lower portion, the *neck,* which is continuous with the urethra, and an upper portion, the *apex,* which is connected with the umbilicus by the median umbilical ligament. The *trigone* is a small triangular area near the base of the bladder. The wall of the bladder consists of four layers: an inner layer of epithelium, a muscular coat of smooth muscle, an outer layer comprised of longitudinal muscle *(detrusor urinae),* and a fibrous layer. An empty bladder feels firm as the muscular wall becomes thick. As the bladder fills with urine, the muscular wall becomes thinner and it distends according to the amount of urine present.

▶ THE URETHRA

The *urethra* is the musculomembranous tube extending from the bladder to the outside of the body. The external urinary opening is the *urinary meatus.* The male urethra is approximately 20 cm long and is divided into three sections: *prostatic, membranous,* and *penile.* It conveys both urine and semen. The female urethra is approximately 3 cm long. The urinary meatus is situated between the clitoris and the opening of the vagina. The female urethra conveys only urine.

▶ URINE

THE FORMATION OF URINE

Urine is formed by the process of *filtration* and *reabsorption* in the nephron. Blood enters the nephron via the afferent arteriole. As it passes through the glomerulus, water and dissolved substances are filtered through the glomerular membrane and collect in the Bowman's capsule. The glomerular filtrate passes through the proximal tubule, into the loop of Henle, into the distal tubule, and then into the collecting tubule. Water and some selected substances are reabsorbed into the capillaries surrounding the tubules. Substances such as uric acid and hydrogen ions, through the process of secretion, may be added to the fluid now known as urine. Urine consists of 95% water and 5% solid substances. It is secreted by the kidneys and transported by the ureters to the bladder, where it is stored before being discharged from the body via the urethra. An average normal adult feels the need to void when the bladder contains around 300 to 350 mL of urine. An average of 1000 to 1500 mL of urine is voided daily. Normal urine is clear, is yellow to amber in color, and has a faintly aromatic odor, a specific gravity of 1.015 to 1.025, and a slightly acid pH.

URINALYSIS

Urinalysis is a laboratory procedure that may involve the physical, chemical, and microscopic examination of urine. A freshly voided urine specimen will provide for more accurate test results as certain changes may occur in urine that is left standing. If the urinalysis cannot be performed on the specimen within 1 hour of the time voided, it should be refrigerated, with the time of collection written on the label of the container. Urine should be collected in a clean, dry container. A disposable container is preferred. When a bacteriologic culture is to be done on urine, the specimen is collected by *catheterization.*

Urinalysis is a valuable diagnostic tool, as abnormal conditions or diseases may be quickly and easily detected because of the fact that the physical and chemical constituents of normal urine are constant.

NORMAL CONSTITUENTS

The following are the normal constituents of urine as detected by various examinations of the specimen:

Under Physical Examination

- **Color**—should be yellow to amber in color because of the presence of the yellow pigment urochrome
- **Appearance**—normal urine is described as being clear
- **Reaction**—acid, between 5.0 and 7.0 pH with an average pH of 6.0
- **Specific gravity**—between 1.015 and 1.025
- **Odor**—faintly aromatic
- **Quantity**—around 1000 to 1500 mL per day

Under Chemical Examination

- **pH**—5.0 to 7.0
- **Protein**—negative
- **Glucose**—negative
- **Ketones**—negative
- **Bilirubin**—negative
- **Blood**—negative
- **Nitrites**—negative
- **Urobilinogen**—0.1 to 1.0

Under Microscopic Examination

- **Red blood cells**—not normally found in urine although they may be present as a result of menstrual contamination or trauma of catheterization
- **White blood cells**—usually present, especially in females; normal to find zero to five white blood cells per high-power field
- **Epithelial cells**—normally found in urine. There are three kinds of epithelial cells: renal from the renal cells of the kidney; transitional from the pelvis of the kidney, ureters, and bladder; and the third type, squamous, from the urethra and vagina
- **Yeast**—not normally found in urine
- **Urinary casts**—not normally found in urine. When present, they are highly diagnostic as they are molded in the shape of the kidney tubules in which they are formed and are seen in urine with a pH of 6.0 or less
- **Trichomonas**—not normally found in urine
- **Crystals**—not normally found in urine
- **Other features**—cotton fibers, powder, oil, spermatozoa, and hair may be seen in normal urine

ABNORMAL CONSTITUENTS

The following are the indications of abnormal constituents that may be found in urine during urinalysis:

Under Physical Examination

- **Color**—red or reddish tint may be caused by the presence of hemoglobin, dyes, or phenophthalein. Orange may be due to pyridum or santonin. Greenish-yellow to greenish-brown or black may be caused by bile pigments or thymol indigo. The color of urine darkens on standing
- **Appearance**—a milky appearance may be caused by fat globules, pus, or bacteria. A smoky appearance may be caused by blood cells. Haze or turbidity may be caused by refrigeration
- **Reaction**—high acidity: diabetic acidosis, fever, pulmonary emphysema, diarrhea, and dehydration
- **Alkalinity**—chronic cystitis, urinary tract infection, renal failure, pyloric obstruction, and salicylate intoxication; also may indicate an old urine specimen
- **Specific gravity**—low: dilute urine 1.001 to 1.010, diabetes insipidus; high: concentrated urine 1.025 to 1.030, diabetes mellitus, hepatic disease, congestive heart failure
- **Odor**—fruity sweet: acetone, associated with diabetes mellitus; unpleasant: decomposition of certain chemicals, drugs, foods, alcohol, or beer
- **Quantity**—high: diabetes mellitus, diabetes insipidus, nervousness, diuretics, excessive intake of fluids; low: acute nephritis, heart disease, fever, diarrhea, vomiting; none: uremia, acute nephritis, renal failure

Under Chemical Examination

- **Protein**—an important sign of renal disease, acute glomerulonephritis, pyelonephritis
- **Glucose**—diabetes mellitus, pain, excitement, acromegaly, liver damage
- **Ketones**—uncontrolled diabetes mellitus, an increase in metabolic needs as during a high-protein–low-carbohydrate diet, during vomiting, diarrhea, and starvation
- **Bilirubin**—liver disease, biliary obstruction, congestive heart failure
- **Blood**—renal disease or disorders, trauma
- **Nitrites**—bacteriuria
- **Urobilinogen**—absent: biliary obstruction; reduced: antibiotic therapy; increased: early warning of hepatic or hemolytic diseases

LIFE SPAN CONSIDERATIONS

▶ THE CHILD

Soon after implantation, the embryonic mass differentiates into three distinct layers of cells: the **ectoderm, mesoderm,** and **endoderm.** The urinary and reproductive organs originate from the mesoderm. At 10 weeks urine forms and enters the bladder. At about the 3rd month of gestation, the fetal kidneys begin to secrete urine. The amount increases gradually as the fetus matures. The newborn's kidneys are immature and lack the ability to concentrate urine. Glomerular filtration and absorption are relatively low until the child is 1 or 2 years of age. In the child the kidneys are more susceptible to trauma, because they usually do not have as much fat padding as in the adult. Infants are more prone to fluid volume changes, excess, and/or dehydration.

Urinary tract infections (UTIs) are common in children. The microorganisms *Escherichia coli, Klebsiella,* and *Proteus* cause most urinary tract infections seen in children. The signs and symptoms of urinary tract infection are age related. See Table 10–1.

▶ THE OLDER ADULT

With advancing age, the **kidneys** may lose mass as blood vessels degenerate. The loss of glomerular capillaries causes a decrease in glomerular filtration and the kidneys lose their ability to conserve water and sodium. Additionally, the tubules of the aging kidneys diminish in their capacity for conserving base and ridding the body of excess hydrogen ions. Because the renal system helps to regulate acid–base balance, fluid and electrolyte imbalances may occur quickly in the older adult. Additional changes noted in the urinary system of the older adult are loss of muscle tone in the **ureters, bladder,** and **urethra.** The bladder capacity may be reduced by half and the older adult may have to make frequent trips to the bathroom. **Urge incontinence** (or the inability to retain urine voluntarily) is a concern for older adults.

During the fourth decade the kidneys begin to decrease in size and function. By the eighth decade the kidneys have generally shrunk 30% and have lost a proportionate amount of function. If stressed, kidneys respond more slowly to changes in one's internal environment. Some causes of stressful situations that may cause the kidneys to respond more slowly and contribute to fluid and electrolyte imbalance are:

- vomiting and diarrhea
- surgery
- diuretics
- decreased fluid intake
- fever
- renal damage from medications

TABLE 10–1   Signs and Symptoms of Urinary Tract Infection in Children

Infants	Fever, loss of weight, nausea, vomiting, increased urination, foul-smelling urine, persistent diaper rash, failure to thrive
Older Child	Increased urination (frequency), pain during urination, abdominal pain, hematuria, fever, chills, bedwetting in a "trained" child

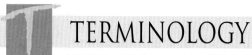

TERMINOLOGY

WITH SURGICAL PROCEDURES & PATHOLOGY

TERM	WORD PARTS			DEFINITION
albuminuria (ăl-bū″ mĭn-oo′rĭ-ă)	albumin uria	R S	protein urine	Presence of serum protein in the urine
antidiuretic (ăn″ tĭ-dī″ ū-rĕt′ĭk)	anti di(a) uret ic	P P R S	against through urine pertaining to	Pertaining to a medication that decreases urine secretion
anuria (ăn-ū′ rĭ-ă)	an uria	P S	without urine	Without the formation of urine
bacteriuria (băk-tē″ rĭ-ū′ rĭ-ă)	bacteri uria	R S	bacteria urine	Presence of bacteria in the urine
calciuria (kăl″ sĭ-ū′ rĭ-ă)	calci uria	R S	calcium urine	Presence of calcium in the urine
cystectasy (sĭs-tĕk′ tă-sē)	cyst ectasy	R S	bladder dilation	Dilation of the bladder
cystectomy (sĭs-tĕk′ tō-mē)	cyst ectomy	R S	bladder excision	Surgical excision of the bladder or part of the bladder
cystistaxis (sĭs″ tĭ-stăk′ sĭs)	cysti staxis	CF S	bladder dripping, trickling	The oozing of blood from the mucous membrane into the bladder
cystitis (sĭs-tī′ tĭs)	cyst itis	R S	bladder inflammation	Inflammation of the bladder

TERMINOLOGY SPOTLIGHT

Cystitis in men is usually secondary to some other type of infection such as epididymitis, prostatitis, gonorrhea, syphilis, and/or kidney stones. Left untreated, bladder and other urinary tract infections can travel into the kidneys and cause serious complications. Each year, approximately 10 million Americans seek treatment for urinary tract infections, with cystitis being most common. **Interstitial cystitis** (IC) is a painful inflammation of the bladder wall. Approximately 450,000 people suffer from this condition, of whom 90% are women. Symptoms can vary from mild to severe. The cause is unknown, and IC does not respond to antibiotic therapy.

See Table 10–2 for prevalence of urinary tract infections according to age and sex.

Terminology - continued

TERM	WORD PARTS			DEFINITION

TABLE 10-2 The Prevalence of Urinary Tract Infection According to Age and Sex

Age Group	Prevalence	Male:Female Ratio
Pre-school	2 to 3%	1:10
School age	1 to 2%	1:30
Reproductive years	25%	1:50
Elderly (65 to 70)	20%	1:10

TERM	WORD PARTS			DEFINITION
cystocele (sĭs′ tō-sēl)	cysto cele	CF S	bladder hernia	Hernia of the bladder that protrudes into the vagina
cystodynia (sĭs″ tō-dĭn′ ĭ-ă)	cysto dynia	CF S	bladder pain	Pain in the bladder
cystogram (sĭs′ tō-grăm)	cysto gram	CF S	bladder a mark, record	An x-ray record of the bladder
cystolithectomy (sĭs″ tō-lĭ-thĕk′ tō-mē)	cysto lith ectomy	CF S S	bladder stone excision	Surgical excision of a stone from the bladder
cystopexy (sĭs′ tō-pĕk″ sē)	cysto pexy	CF S	bladder fixation	Surgical fixation of the bladder to the abdominal wall
cystoplasty (sĭs′ tō-plăs″ tē)	cysto plasty	CF S	bladder surgical repair	Surgical repair of the bladder
cystoplegia (sĭs″ tō-plē′ jĭ-ă)	cysto plegia	CF S	bladder paralysis	Paralysis of the bladder
cystopyelitis (sĭs″ tō-pī″ ĕ-lī′ tĭs)	cysto pyel itis	CF R S	bladder renal pelvis inflammation	Inflammation of the bladder and renal pelvis
cystorrhagia (sĭs″ tō-rā′ jĭ-ă)	cysto rrhagia	CF S	bladder bursting forth	Bursting forth of blood from the bladder
cystorrhaphy (sĭst-ōr′ ā-fē)	cysto rrhaphy	CF S	bladder suture	Surgical suture of the bladder
cystoscope (sĭst′ ō-skōp)	cysto scope	CF S	bladder instrument	An instrument used for examination of the bladder

continued

Terminology - continued

TERM	WORD PARTS			DEFINITION
dialysis (dī-ăl′ ĭ-sĭs)	dia lysis	P S	through destruction, to separate	A procedure to separate waste material from the blood and to maintain fluid, electrolyte, and acid–base balance in impaired kidney function or in the absence of the kidney
diuresis (dī″ ū-rē′ sĭs)	di(a) ure sis	P R S	through urinate condition	A condition of increased or excessive flow of urine
dysuria (dĭs-ū′ rĭ-ă)	dys uria	P S	difficult, painful urine	Difficult or painful urination
enuresis (ĕn″ ū-rē′ sĭs)	en ure sis	P R S	within urinate condition of	A condition of involuntary emission of urine; *bedwetting*
glomerular (glō-mĕr′ ū-lăr)	glomerul ar	R S	glomerulus, little ball pertaining to	Pertaining to the glomerulus
glomerulitis (glō-mĕr″ ū-lī′ tĭs)	glomerul itis	R S	glomerulus, little ball inflammation	Inflammation of the renal glomeruli
glomerulone-phritis (glō-mĕr″ ū-lō-nĕ-frī′ tĭs)	glomerulo nephr itis	CF R S	glomerulus, little ball kidney inflammation	Inflammation of the kidney involving primarily the glomeruli
glycosuria (glī″ kō-soo′ rĭ-ă)	glycos uria	R S	sweet, sugar urine	Presence of glucose in the urine
hematuria (hē″ mă-tū′ rĭ-ă)	hemat uria	R S	blood urine	Presence of blood in the urine
hydronephrosis (hī″ drō-nĕf-rō′ sĭs)	hydro nephr osis	P R S	water kidney condition of	A condition in which urine collects in the renal pelvis because of an obstructed outflow
hypercalciuria (hī″ pĕr-kăl″ sĭ-ū′ rĭ-ă)	hyper calci uria	P R S	excessive calcium urine	An excessive amount of calcium in the urine
incontinence (ĭn-kən′ tĭn-əns)	in continence	P R	not to hold	The inability to hold urine

Terminology - continued

TERM	WORD PARTS			DEFINITION
ketonuria (kē″ tō-nū′ rĭ-ă)	keton uria	R S	ketone urine	Presence of ketones in the urine
meatal (mē″ā′ tăl)	meat al	R S	passage pertaining to	Pertaining to a passage
meatoscopy (mē″ ă-tŏs′ kō-pē)	meato scopy	CF S	passage to view, examine	Instrumental examination of the meatus of the urethra
meatotomy (mē″ ă-tŏt′ ō-mē)	meato tomy	CF S	passage incision	Incision of the urinary meatus to enlarge the opening
micturition (mĭk′ tū-rĭ′ shŭn)	micturit ion	R S	to urinate process	The process of urination
nephradenoma (nĕf″ răd-ĕ-nō′ mă)	nephr aden oma	R R S	kidney gland tumor	Glandular tumor of the kidney
nephratony (nĕ-frăt′ ō-nē)	nephr a tony	R P S	kidney not, lack of tension	Lack of normal kidney tone
nephrectasia (nĕf″ rĕk-tā′ zĭ-ă)	nephr ectasia	R S	kidney distention	Distention of the kidney
nephrectomy (nĕ-frĕk′ tō-mē)	nephr ectomy	R S	kidney excision	Surgical excision of a kidney
nephremia (nĕf-rē′ mĭ-ă)	nephr emia	R S	kidney blood condition	A condition in which the kidney is congested with blood
nephritis (nĕf-rī′ tĭs)	nephr itis	R S	kidney inflammation	Inflammation of the kidney
nephrocystitis (nĕf″ rō-sĭs′ tĭ′ tĭs)	nephro cyst itis	CF R S	kidney bladder inflammation	Inflammation of the bladder and the kidney
nephrohyper-trophy (nĕf″ rō-hī-pĕr′ trō-fē)	nephro hyper trophy	CF P S	kidney excessive nourishment, development	Excessive development of the kidney
nephrolith (nĕf′ rō-lĭth)	nephro lith	CF S	kidney stone, calculus	Kidney stone, calculus

continued

Terminology - continued

TERM	WORD PARTS			DEFINITION
nephrology (ně-frŏl′ ō-jē)	nephro logy	CF S	kidney study of	The study of the kidney
nephroma (ně-frō′ mă)	nephr oma	R S	kidney tumor	Kidney tumor
nephromalacia (něf″ rō-mă-lā′ sǐ-ă)	nephro malacia	CF S	kidney softening	Abnormal softening of the kidney
nephromegaly (něf″ rō-měg′ ă-lē)	nephro megaly	CF S	kidney enlargement	Enlargement of the kidney
nephropathy (ně-frŏp′ ă-thē)	nephro pathy	CF S	kidney disease	Disease of the kidney
nephropexy (něf′ rō-pěks″ ē)	nephro pexy	CF S	kidney fixation	Surgical fixation of a floating kidney
nephroptosis (něf″ rŏp-tō′ sǐs)	nephro ptosis	CF S	kidney prolapse, drooping	Prolapse of the kidney
nephropyosis (něf″ rō-pī-ō′ sǐs)	nephro py osis	CF R S	kidney pus condition of	A condition of pus in the kidney
nephrosclerosis (něf″ rō-sklē - rō′ sǐs)	nephro scler osis	CF R S	kidney hardening condition of	A condition of hardening of the kidney
nocturia (nŏk-tū′ rǐ-ă)	noct uria	R S	night urine	Excessive urination during the night
oliguria (ŏl-ǐg-ū′ rǐ-ă)	olig uria	P S	scanty urine	Scanty urination
paranephritis (păr″ ă-ně-frī′ tǐs)	para nephr itis	P R S	beside kidney inflammation	Inflammation of the suprarenal capsule
periureteritis (pěr″ ǐ-ū-rē″ těr-ī′ tǐs)	peri ureter itis	P R S	around ureter inflammation	Inflammation around the ureter
periurethral (pěr″ ǐ-ū-rē′ thrăl)	peri urethr al	P R S	around urethra pertaining to	Pertaining to around the urethra
polyuria (pŏl″ ē-ū′ rǐ-ă)	poly uria	P S	excessive urine	Excessive urination

Terminology - continued

TERM	WORD PARTS			DEFINITION
pyelocystitis (pī″ ĕ-lō-sĭs-tī′ tĭs)	pyelo cyst itis	CF R S	renal pelvis bladder inflammation	Inflammation of the bladder and renal pelvis
pyelocystosto-mosis (pī″ ĕ-lō-sĭs″ tō-stō-mō′ sĭs)	pyelo cysto stom osis	CF CF R S	renal pelvis bladder mouth condition of	Establishing a surgical opening between the renal pelvis and bladder
pyelolithotomy (pī″ ĕ-lō-lĭth-ŏt′ ō-mē)	pyelo litho tomy	CF CF S	renal pelvis stone incision	Surgical incision into the renal pelvis for removal of a stone
pyelonephritis (pī″ ĕ-lō-nĕ-frī′ tĭs)	pyelo nephr itis	CF R S	renal pelvis kidney inflammation	Inflammation of the kidney and renal pelvis
pyeloplication (pī″ ĕ-lō-plĭ-kā′ shŭn)	pyelo plicat ion	CF R S	renal pelvis to fold process	The process of shortening the wall of the renal pelvis by surgical folds
pyuria (pī-ū′ rĭ-ă)	py uria	R S	pus urine	Pus in the urine
renal (rē′ năl)	ren al	R S	kidney pertaining to	Pertaining to the kidney
trigonitis (trĭg″ ō-nī′ tĭs)	trigon itis	R S	trigone inflammation	Inflammation of the trigone of the bladder
ureagenetic (ū-rē″ă-jĕn-ĕt′ ĭk)	urea genet ic	R R S	urea producing pertaining to	Pertaining to producing urea
uremia (ū-rē′ mĭ-ă)	ur emia	R S	urine blood condition	A condition of excess urea and other nitrogenous waste in the blood
ureterocolostomy (ū-rē″ tĕr-ō-kō-lŏs′ tō-mē)	uretero colo stomy	CF CF S	ureter colon new opening	Surgical implantation of the ureter into the colon
ureteronephrec-tomy (ū-rē″ tĕr-ō-nĕf-rĕk′ tō-mē)	uretero nephr ectomy	CF R S	ureter kidney excision	Surgical excision of a kidney and its ureter
ureteropathy (ū-rē″ tĕr-ŏp′ ă-thē)	uretero pathy	CF S	ureter disease	Disease of the ureter

continued

Terminology - continued

TERM	WORD PARTS			DEFINITION
ureteroplasty (ū-rē′ těr-ō-plăs″ tē)	uretero plasty	CF S	ureter surgical repair	Surgical repair of the ureter
ureterorrhaphy (ū-rē″ těr-ōr′ ră-fē)	uretero rrhaphy	CF S	ureter suture	Suture of the ureter
ureterostenosis (ū-rē″ těr-ō-stěn-ŏ′ sĭs)	uretero sten osis	CF R S	ureter narrowing condition of	A condition of narrowing of the ureter
ureterovesical (ū-rě″ těr-ō-věs′ ĭ-kăl)	uretero vesic al	CF R S	ureter bladder pertaining to	Pertaining to a connection between the ureter and bladder
urethralgia (ū-rē-thrăl′ jĭ-ă)	urethr algia	R S	urethra pain	Pain in the urethra
urethropenile (ū-rē″ thrō-pē′ nīl)	urethro penile	CF R	urethra penis	Relating to the urethra and penis
urethroperineal (ū-rē″ thrō-pěr″ ĭ nē′ăl)	urethro perine al	CF R S	urethra perineum pertaining to	Pertaining to the urethra and perineum
urethropexy (ū-rēth′ rō-pěks-ě)	urethro pexy	CF S	urethra fixation	Surgical fixation of the urethra
urethrophraxis (ū-rē″ thrō-frăks′ ĭs)	urethro phraxis	CF S	urethra to obstruct	Obstruction of the urethra
urethrospasm (ū-rē′ thrō-spăzm)	urethro spasm	CF S	urethra tension, spasm	Urethral spasm
urethrotome (ū-rē′ thrō-tōm)	urethro tome	CF S	urethra instrument to cut	An instrument used to cut a urethral stricture
urethrovaginal (ū-rē″ thrō-văg′ ĭ-năl)	urethro vagin al	CF R S	urethra vagina pertaining to	Pertaining to the urethra and vagina
urinal (ū′ rĭn-ăl)	urin al	R S	urine pertaining to	A container, toilet, or bathroom fixture into which one urinates
urinalysis (ū′ rĭ-năl′ i-sĭs)	urin a lysis	R P S	urine apart destruction, to separate	Analysis of the urine; a separating of the urine for examination to determine the presence of abnormal elements

Terminology - continued

TERM	WORD PARTS			DEFINITION
urination (ū″ rĭ-nā′ shŭn)	urinat ion	R S	urine process	The process of voiding urine
urinometer (ū″ rĭ-nŏm′ ĕ-tĕr)	urino meter	CF S	urine instrument to measure	An instrument used to measure the specific gravity of urine
urobilin (ū″ rō-bī′ lĭn)	uro bil in	CF R S	urine bile chemical	A brown pigment formed by the oxidation of urobilinogen; may be formed in the urine after exposure to air
urologist (ū-rŏl′ ō-jĭst)	uro log ist	CF R S	urine study of one who specializes	One who specializes in the study of the urinary system
urology (ū-rŏl′ ō-jē)	uro logy	CF S	urine study of	The study of the urinary system
uropoiesis (ū″ rō-poy-ē′ sĭs)	uro poiesis	CF S	urine formation	Formation of urine by the kidneys
uroporphyrin (ū″ rō-por′ fĭ-rĭn)	uro porphyr in	CF R S	urine purple chemical	A reddish-purple pigment present in urine in cases of porphyria or certain drugs

 VOCABULARY WORDS

Vocabulary words are terms that have not been divided into component parts. They are common words or specialized terms associated with the subject of this chapter. These words are provided to enhance your medical vocabulary.

WORD	DEFINITION
catheter (kăth′ ĕ-tĕr)	A tube of elastic, elastic web, rubber, glass, metal, or plastic that is inserted into a body cavity to remove fluid or to inject fluid
edema (ĕ-dē′ mă)	An abnormal condition in which the body tissues contain an accumulation of fluid

continued

Vocabulary - continued

WORD	DEFINITION
excretory (ĕks′ krə-tō-rē)	Pertaining to the elimination of waste products from the body
extracorporeal shock-wave lithotriptor (ĕks″ tră-kor-por′ ē-ăl lĭth′ ō-trip″ tor)	A device used to crush kidney stones *(renal calculi)*. The patient is sedated and immersed in a water bath while shock waves pound the stones until they crumble into small pieces. These pieces are flushed out with urine.
hemodialysis (hē″ mō-dī-ăl′ ĭ-sĭs)	The use of an artificial kidney to separate waste from the blood. The blood is circulated through tubes made of semipermeable membranes, and these tubes are continually bathed by solutions that remove waste.
lithotripsy (lĭth′ ō trĭp″ sē)	The crushing of a kidney stone
meatus (mē-ā′ tŭs)	An opening or passage; the external opening of the urethra
nephron (nef′ rŏn)	The structural and functional unit of the kidney
percutaneous ultrasonic lithotripsy (pĕr″ kū-tā′ nē-ŭs)	The crushing of a kidney stone by using ultrasound. This is an invasive surgical procedure performed by using a nephroscope or fluoroscopy.
peritoneal dialysis (pĕr″ ĭ-tō-nē′ ăl dī-ăl′ ĭ-sĭs)	Separation of waste from the blood by using a peritoneal catheter and dialysis. Fluid is introduced into the peritoneal cavity, and wastes from the blood pass into this fluid. The fluid and waste are then removed from the body. Types of peritoneal dialysis are IPD—intermittent—and CAPD—continuous ambulatory.
renal colic (rē′ năl kŏl′ ĭk)	An acute pain that occurs in the kidney area and is caused by blockage during the passage of a stone
renal failure (rē′ năl fāl′ yŭr)	Cessation of proper functioning of the kidney
renal transplant (rē′ năl trăns′ plănt)	Surgical procedure to implant a donor kidney to a recipient
renin (rĕn′ ĭn)	An enzyme produced by the kidney
residual urine (rē-zĭd′ ŭ-ăl ū′ rĭn)	Urine that is left in the bladder after urination

Vocabulary - continued

WORD	DEFINITION
retention (rē-těn′ shŭn)	The holding back of a substance that should be excreted—urine, feces, or perspiration
sediment (sěd′ ĭ-měnt)	The substance that settles at the bottom of a liquid; a precipitate
specific gravity (spě-sĭf′ ĭk grăv′ ĭ-tē)	The weight of a substance compared with an equal amount of water. Urine has a specific gravity of 1.015 to 1.025.
specimen (spěs′ ĭ-měn)	A sample of tissue, blood, urine, or other material intended to show the nature of the whole
sterile (stěr′ ĭl)	A state of being free from living microorganisms; asepsis
stricture (strik′ chŭr)	An abnormal narrowing of a duct or passage such as the esophagus, ureter, or urethra
supernatant (sū″ pěr-nā′ tǎnt)	The liquid floating on the surface after a precipitate settles
urea (ū-rē′ ǎ)	The chief nitrogenous constituent of urine
urethral stricture (ū-rē′ thrǎl strĭk′ chŭr)	A narrowing or constriction of the urethra
urgency (ŭr-jěn′ sē)	The sudden need to void, urinate
uric acid (ū′ rĭk ǎs′ ĭd)	An end product of purine metabolism; a common component of urinary and renal stones
urine (ū′ rĭn)	A waste product of fluid and dissolved substances secreted by the kidneys, stored in the bladder, and excreted through the urethra
urochrome (ū′ rō-krōm)	The pigment that gives urine the normal yellow color
urolithiasis (ū″ rō-lĭ-thē″ ǎ-sĭs)	The formation of a urinary stone and its associated illness
void (voyd)	To empty the bladder

ABBREVIATIONS

ADH	antidiuretic hormone	**HCO₃**	bicarbonate
A/G	albumin/globulin ratio	**HD**	hemodialysis
AGN	acute glomerulonephritis	**H₂O**	water
ATN	acute tubular necrosis	**HPF**	high-power field
BUN	blood urea nitrogen	**I & O**	intake and output
CAPD	continuous ambulatory peritoneal dialysis	**IPD**	intermittent peritoneal dialysis
CC	clean catch	**IVP**	intravenous pyelogram
CGN	chronic glomerulonephritis	**IVU**	intravenous urogram
CRF	chronic renal failure	**K**	potassium
Cl	chloride	**KUB**	kidney, ureter, bladder
CMG	cystometrogram	**LPF**	low-power field
C & S	culture and sensitivity	**Na**	sodium
cysto	cystoscopic examination	**PD**	peritoneal dialysis
ECF	extracellular fluid	**pH**	potential of hydrogen
ECSL	extracorporeal shockwave lithotriptor	**PKU**	phenylketonuria
		PSP	phenolsulfonphthalein
ESRD	end-stage renal disease	**PUL**	percutaneous ultrasonic lithotripsy
ESWL	extracorporeal shockwave lithotripsy		
GBM	glomerular basement membrane	**RP**	retrograde pyelogram
		UA	urinalysis
GFR	glomerular filtration rate	**UTI**	urinary tract infection
GU	genitourinary	**VCUG**	voiding cystourethrogram

DRUG HIGHLIGHTS

Drugs that are generally used for urinary system diseases and disorders include diuretics, urinary tract antibacterials and antiseptics, and other drugs.

Diuretics

Decrease reabsorption of sodium chloride by the kidneys, thereby increasing the amount of salt and water excreted in the urine. This action reduces the amount of fluid retained in the body and prevents edema. Diuretics are classified according to site and mechanism of action.

Thiazide

Appear to act by inhibiting sodium and chloride reabsorption in the early portion of the distal tubule.
Examples: Naturetin (bendroflumethiazide), Diuril (chlorothiazide), HydroDiuril (hydrochlorothiazide), and Renese (polythiazide).

Loop	Act by inhibiting the reabsorption of sodium and chloride in the ascending loop of Henle. *Examples: Bumex (bumetanide) and Lasix (furosemide).*
Potassium-sparing	Act by inhibiting the exchange of sodium for potassium in the distal tubule. They inhibit potassium excretion. *Examples: Aldactone (spironolactone) and Dyrenium (triamterene).*
Osmotic	Are capable of being filtered by the glomerulus, but have a limited capability of being reabsorbed into the bloodstream. *Example: Osmitrol (mannitol).*
Carbonic anhydrase inhibitor	Act to increase the excretion of bicarbonate ion, which carries out sodium, water, and potassium. *Example: Diamox (acetazolamide).*
Urinary Tract Antibacterials	Sulfonamides are generally the drugs of choice for treating acute, uncomplicated urinary tract infections, especially those caused by *Escherichia coli* and *Proteus mirabilis* bacterial strains. They exert a bacteriostatic effect against a wide range of gram-positive and gram-negative microorganisms. *Examples: Thiosulfil (sulfamethizole), Gantrisin (sulfisoxazole), Gantanol (sulfamethoxazole), Microsulfon (sulfadiazine), and Bactrim and Septra, which are mixtures of trimethoprim and sulfamethoxazole.*
Urinary Tract Antiseptics	May inhibit the growth of microorganisms by bactericidal, bacteriostatic, anti-infective, and/or antibacterial action. *Examples: NegGram (nalidixic acid), Furadanton and Macrodantin (nitrofurantoin), Mandelamine and Hiprex (methenamine), and Cipro (ciprofloxacin HCl).*
Other Drugs	Disorders of the lower urinary tract may be treated with drugs that either stimulate or inhibit smooth muscle activity, thereby improving urinary bladder functions. These functions are the storage of urine and its subsequent excretion from the body. *Examples: Cystospaz-M and Levsin (hyoscyamine sulfate), Urispas (flavoxate HCl), and Urecholine (bethanechol chloride).*
Rimso-50 (dimethyl sulfoxide)	Used in the treatment of interstitial cystitis.
Pyridium (phenazopyridine HCl)	Analgesic, anesthetic action on the urinary tract mucosa. This medication causes the urine to turn an orange color.

DIAGNOSTIC AND LABORATORY TESTS

Test	Description
blood urea nitrogen (BUN) (blod ū-rē′ ă nĭ′ trō-jĕn)	A blood test to determine the amount of urea that is excreted by the kidneys. Abnormal results indicate urinary tract disease.
creatinine (krē′ ă-tĭn ēn)	A blood test to determine the amount of creatinine present. Abnormal results indicate kidney disease.
creatinine clearance (krē′ ă-tĭn ēn klir′ ăns)	A urine test to determine the glomerular filtration rate (GFR). Abnormal results indicate kidney disease.
culture, urine (kūl′ tūr, ū′ rĭn)	A urine test to determine the presence of microorganisms. Abnormal results indicate urinary tract infection.
cystoscopy (sĭs-tŏs′ kō-pĕ)	Visual examination of the bladder and urethra via a lighted cystoscope. Abnormal results may indicate the presence of renal calculi, a tumor, prostatic hyperplasia, and/or bleeding.
intravenous pyelography (pyelogram) (ĭn-tră-vē′ nŭs pĭ″ ĕ-lŏg′ rā-fē)	A test to visualize the kidneys, ureters, and bladder. A radiopaque substance is intravenously injected, and x-rays are taken. Abnormal results may indicate renal calculi, kidney or bladder tumors, and kidney disease.
kidney, ureter, bladder (KUB) (kĭd′ nē, ū′ rĕ-tĕr, blăd′ dĕr)	A flat-plate x-ray is taken of the abdomen to indicate the size and position of the kidneys, ureters, and bladder.
renal biopsy (rē′ năl bī′ ŏp-sē)	The removal of tissue from the kidney. Abnormal results may indicate kidney cancer, kidney transplant rejection, and glomerulonephritis.
ultrasonography, kidneys (ŭ-tră-sŏn-ŏg′ ră-fē, kĭd′ nēs)	The use of high-frequency sound waves to visualize the kidneys. The sound waves (echoes) are recorded on an oscilloscope and film. Abnormal results may indicate kidney tumors, cysts, abscess, and kidney disease.

COMMUNICATION ENRICHMENT

This segment is provided for those who wish to enhance their ability to communicate in either English or Spanish.

▶ Related Terms

English	Spanish	English	Spanish
bladder	vejiga (vĕ-hĭ-gă)	urethral	uretral (ū-rĕ-trăl)
burning	ardiente (ăr-dĭ-ĕn-tĕ)	urethritis	uretritis (ū-rĕ-trĭ-tĭs)
dialysis	diálisis (dĭ-ă-lĭs-ĭs)	urethroscope	uretroscopio (ū-rĕ-trō-scō-pĭ-ō)
dysuria	disuria (dĭ-sŭ-rĭ-ă)	urethroscopy	uretroscopia (ū-rĕ-trō-scō-pĭ-ă)
kidney	riñón (rĭn-yōn)	urinalysis	urinálisis (ū-rĭ-nă-lĭs-ĭs)
kidney stone	cálculo renal (căl-cŭ-lō rĕ-năl)	urinary	urinario (ū-rĭ-nă-rĭ-ō)
urethral discharge	descargar uretral (dĕs-căr-găr ŭ-rĕ-trăl)	urinary calculus	cálculo urinario (căl-cŭ-lō ū-rĭ-nă-rĭ-ō)
urinate	orinar (ō-rĭ-năr)	urinary tract	vías urinarias (vĭ-ăs ū-rĭ-nă-rĭ-ăs)
urine	orine (ō-rĭ-nĕ)	urination	urinación (ū-rĭ-nă-sĭ-ōn)
cloudy	nublado (nŭ-blă-dō)	urogenital	urogenital (ū-rō-hĕ-nĭ-tăl)
pink	rosado (rō-să-dō)	urolith	urolito (ū-rō-lĭ-tō)
loss of bladder control	perdida de control vejiga (per-dĭ-dă dĕ cōn-trōl vĕ-hē-gā)	urolithiasis	urolitiasis (ū-rō-lĭ-tĭ-ăs-ĭs)
		urologic	urológico (ū-rō-lō-hĭ-kō)
fever	fiebre (fĭ-ĕ-brĕ)	urologist	urólogo (ū-rō-lō-hō)
urgent	urgente (ūr-hĕn-tĕ)	urology	urología (ū-rō-lō-hĭ-ă)
urethra	uretra (ū-rĕ-tra)		

STUDY AND REVIEW SECTION

LEARNING EXERCISES

▶ **Anatomy and Physiology**

....

Write your answers to the following questions. Do not refer back to the text.

1. List the organs of the urinary system.

   a. _____   b. _____

   c. _____   d. _____

2. State the vital function of the urinary system. _____

   _____

3. Name the three capsules that surround each kidney.

   a. _____   b. _____

   c. _____

4. Define hilum. _____

5. Define renal pelvis. _____

6. The cortex of the kidney contains the _____, _____,

   _____ _____, and _____ _____.

7. The medulla is the _____ portion of the kidney.

8. Define nephron. _____

9. Each nephron consists of a _____ _____ and

   a _____.

10. The malpighian corpuscle consists of _____ and

    _____ _____.

11. State the vital function of the nephron. _____

    _____

12. Urine is formed by the process of _____ and

    _____ in the nephron.

13. Urine consists of _____ percent water and _____ percent solid substances.

14. An average of _____ to _____ mL of urine is voided daily.

15. Describe the ureters and state their function. _____

_____

16. Describe the urinary bladder and state its function. _____

_____

17. Define trigone. _____

18. State the function of the male urethra. _____

19. State the function of the female urethra. _____

20. The external urinary opening is the _____ _____.

21. Define urinalysis. _____

_____

22. Give the normal constituents for the physical examination of urine.

    a. Color _____   b. Appearance _____

    c. Reaction _____   d. Specific gravity _____

    e. Odor _____   f. Quantity _____

23. Name the three types of epithelial cells that may be found in urine.

    a. _____   b. _____

    c. _____

24. A urine that has a fruity sweet odor may indicate _____

    _____.

25. Under chemical examination, the presence of protein in urine is an important

    sign of _____

    _____.

▶ Word Parts

....

1. In the spaces provided, write the definition of these prefixes, roots, combining forms, and suffixes. Do not refer to the listings of terminology words. Leave blank those terms you cannot define.

2. After completing as many as you can, refer back to the terminology word listings to check your work. For each word missed or left blank, write the term and its definition several times on the margins of these pages or on a separate sheet of paper.

3. To maximize the learning process, it is to your advantage to do the following exercises as directed. To refer to the terminology listings before completing these exercises invalidates the learning process.

Prefixes

Give the definitions of the following prefixes:

1. a- _____
2. an- _____
3. anti- _____
4. di(a)- _____
5. dia- _____
6. dys- _____
7. en- _____
8. hydro- _____
9. hyper- _____
10. in- _____
11. olig- _____
12. para- _____
13. peri- _____
14. poly- _____

Roots and Combining Forms

Give the definitions of the following roots and combining forms:

1. aden _____
2. albumin _____
3. bacteri _____
4. bil _____
5. calci _____
6. colo _____
7. continence _____
8. cyst _____
9. cysti _____
10. cysto _____
11. genet _____
12. glomerul _____
13. glomerulo _____
14. glycos _____
15. hemat _____
16. keton _____
17. litho _____
18. log _____
19. meat _____
20. meato _____
21. micturit _____
22. nephr _____
23. nephro _____
24. noct _____
25. penile _____
26. perine _____
27. plicat _____
28. porphyr _____
29. py _____
30. pyel _____

31. pyelo _____

32. ren _____

33. scler _____

34. sten _____

35. stom _____

36. trigon _____

37. ur _____

38. ure _____

39. urea _____

40. uret _____

41. ureter _____

42. uretero _____

43. urethr _____

44. urethro _____

45. urin _____

46. urinat _____

47. urino _____

48. uro _____

49. vagin _____

50. vesic _____

Suffixes

Give the definitions of the following suffixes:

1. -al _____

2. -algia _____

3. -ar _____

4. -cele _____

5. -dynia _____

6. -ectasia _____

7. -ectasy _____

8. -ectomy _____

9. -emia _____

10. -gram _____

11. -ic _____

12. -in _____

13. -ion _____

14. -ist _____

15. -itis _____

16. -lith _____

17. -logy _____

18. -lysis _____

19. -malacia _____

20. -megaly _____

21. -meter _____

22. -oma _____

23. -osis _____

24. -pathy _____

25. -pexy _____

26. -phraxis _____

27. -plasty _____

28. -plegia _____

29. -poiesis _____

30. -ptosis _____

31. -rrhagia _____

32. -rrhaphy _____

33. -scope _____

34. -scopy _____

35. -sis _____   36. -spasm _____

37. -staxis _____   38. -stomy _____

39. -tome _____   40. -tomy _____

41. -tony _____   42. -trophy _____

43. -uria _____

▶ **Identifying Medical Terms**

In the spaces provided, write the medical terms for the following meanings:

1. _____ Pertaining to a medication that decreases urine secretion

2. _____ Surgical excision of the bladder or part of the bladder

3. _____ Inflammation of the bladder

4. _____ Surgical fixation of the bladder to the abdominal wall

5. _____ Surgical suture of the bladder

6. _____ Difficult or painful urination

7. _____ Inflammation of the renal glomeruli

8. _____ An excessive amount of calcium in the urine

9. _____ Pertaining to a passage

10. _____ The process of urinating

11. _____ Lack of normal kidney tone

12. _____ Kidney stone

13. _____ Enlargement of the kidney

14. _____ Pertaining to around the urethra

15. _____ Pus in the urine

16. _____ Disease of the ureter

17. _____ Suture of the ureter

18. _____ Pain in the urethra

19. _____ Urethral spasm

20. _____ One who specializes in the study of the urinary system

► **Spelling**

In the spaces provided, write the correct spelling of these misspelled terms:

1. cystplasty _____
2. cystorhagia _____
3. euresis _____
4. glycouria _____
5. hemauria _____
6. incontence _____
7. nephemia _____
8. nephrcysitis _____
9. nephrmalaca _____
10. nephrtosis _____
11. nocuria _____
12. ueteroplasty _____
13. urethropraxis _____
14. urinalsis _____
15. urbilin _____
16. uropioesis _____

WORD PARTS STUDY SHEET

Word Parts	Give the Meaning
an-	_____
di(a)-	_____
dys-	_____
en-	_____
hydro-	_____
in-	_____
olig-	_____
poly-	_____
albumin-	_____
bacteri-	_____
calci-	_____
cyst-, vesic-, cysti-, cysto-	_____
glomerul-, glomerulo-	_____
glycos-	_____
hemat-	_____
keton-	_____

litho- _____

nephr-, nephro-, ren- _____

noct- _____

penile- _____

py- _____

pyelo- _____

sten- _____

ureter-, uretero- _____

urethr-, urethro- _____

urin-, urinat-, urino-, uro- _____

-al, -ar _____

-cele _____

-ectasy _____

-ectomy _____

-malacia _____

-megaly _____

-meter _____

-oma _____

-phraxis _____

-plasty _____

-ptosis _____

-rrhaphy _____

-staxis _____

-stomy _____

-tony _____

REVIEW QUESTIONS

▶ Matching

Select the appropriate lettered meaning for each numbered line.

_____ 1. lithotriptor

_____ 2. hemodialysis

_____ 3. lithotripsy

_____ 4. peritoneal dialysis

_____ 5. renal colic

_____ 6. urethral stricture

_____ 7. urgency

_____ 8. urination

_____ 9. urolithiasis

_____ 10. urinometer

a. An acute pain that occurs in the kidney area and is caused by blockage during the passage of a stone
b. The crushing of a kidney stone
c. The process of voiding urine
d. A device used to crush kidney stones
e. The use of an artificial kidney to separate waste from the blood
f. Separation of waste from the blood by using a peritoneal catheter and dialysis
g. A narrowing or constriction of the urethra
h. Formation of a urinary stone and its associated illness
i. An instrument used to measure the specific gravity of urine
j. The sudden need to void, urinate
k. Analysis of the urine

▶ Abbreviations

Place the correct word, phrase, or abbreviation in the space provided.

1. antidiuretic hormone _____

2. BUN _____

3. chronic renal failure _____

4. cysto _____

5. GU _____

6. HD _____

7. intravenous pyelogram _____

8. PD _____

9. pH _____

10. urinalysis _____

► **Diagnostic and Laboratory Tests**

Select the best answer to each multiple choice question. Circle the letter of your choice.

1. A urine test to determine the glomerular filtration rate.
   a. BUN
   b. creatinine
   c. creatinine clearance
   d. KUB

2. A urine test to determine the presence of microorganisms.
   a. BUN
   b. creatinine
   c. urine culture
   d. KUB

3. A test to visualize the kidneys, ureters, and bladder.
   a. cystoscopy
   b. intravenous pyelography
   c. KUB
   d. renal biopsy

4. The use of high-frequency sound waves to visualize the kidneys.
   a. retrograde pyelography
   b. intravenous pyelography
   c. ultrasonography
   d. cystoscopy

5. A flat-plate x-ray of the abdomen to indicate the size and position of the kidneys, ureters, and bladder.
   a. cystoscopy
   b. KUB
   c. BUN
   d. retrograde pyelography

CRITICAL THINKING ACTIVITY

► Case Study

Acute Cystitis

Please read the following case study and then answer the questions that follow.

A 21-year-old female was seen by a physician and the following is a synopsis of the visit.

Present History: The patient states that she goes to the bathroom a lot and that it "burns" and "hurts." She also has chills and fever.

Signs and Symptoms: Chief complaint: Frequency, burning sensation and pain during urination, chills, and fever.

Diagnosis: Acute cystitis. The diagnosis was determined by a history of the symptoms, a complete urinalysis (physical, chemical, and microscopic) that revealed red blood cells, white blood cells, and bacteria.

Treatment: The physician ordered a sulfonamide, Pyridium, and provided her with written Guidelines to Help Avoid Cystitis (female).

Prevention: In the United States, approximately 10 million people seek treatment for urinary tract infection each year, with cystitis being the most common. Cystitis is most often caused by an ascending infection from the urethra and it is more common in the female, because of the short length of the urethra, which promotes the transmission of bacteria from the skin and genitals to the internal bladder. The most common type of bacteria that causes cystitis in females is *Escherichia coli (E. coli)*, the colon bacillus.

Guidelines to Help Avoid Cystitis (Female)

- Drink 8 glasses or more of water/day.
- Females should wipe themselves from front to back after a bowel movement to avoid contaminating the urinary meatus.
- Have sexual partner wear a condom.
- Do not use vaginal deodorants, bubble baths, colored toilet paper, and other substances that could cause irritation to the urinary meatus.
- Wear cotton underclothes and keep the genital area dry.

Critical Thinking Questions

1. Signs and symptoms of cystitis include frequency, burning _____ and pain during urination, chills, and fever.

2. The diagnosis was determined by a history of the symptoms, a complete _____ that revealed red blood cells, white blood cells, and bacteria.

3. Treatment included a _____, Pyridium, and written Guidelines to Help Avoid Cystitis.

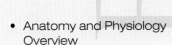

11

THE ENDOCRINE SYSTEM

- Anatomy and Physiology Overview
- The Pituitary Gland
- The Pineal Gland
- The Thyroid Gland
- The Parathyroid Glands
- The Pancreas
- The Adrenal Glands
- The Ovaries
- The Testes
- The Placenta
- The Gastrointestinal Mucosa
- The Thymus
- Life Span Considerations
- Terminology With Surgical Procedures & Pathology
- Vocabulary Words
- Abbreviations
- Drug Highlights
- Diagnostic and Laboratory Tests
- Communication Enrichment
- Study and Review Section

   Learning Exercises

   Word Parts Study Sheet

   Review Questions

   Critical Thinking Activity

OBJECTIVES

On completion of this chapter, you should be able to:

- Describe the primary glands of the endocrine system.

- State the primary functions of the endocrine glands.

- Describe the secondary glands of the endocrine system.

- State the vital function of the endocrine system.

- Identify and state the functions of the various hormones secreted by the endocrine glands.

- Analyze, build, spell, and pronounce medical words that relate to surgical procedures and pathology.

- Identify and give the meaning of selected vocabulary words.

- Identify and define selected abbreviations.

- Review Drug Highlights presented in this chapter.

- Provide the description of diagnostic and laboratory tests related to the endocrine system.

- Successfully complete the study and review section.

► ANATOMY AND PHYSIOLOGY OVERVIEW

The endocrine system consists of primary and secondary glands of internal secretion. The primary glands are the *pituitary (hypophysis), pineal, thyroid, parathyroid, pancreas, adrenals (suprarenals), ovaries* and *testes.* The secondary glands of the endocrine system are the thymus, the placenta during pregnancy, and the gastrointestinal mucosa. The endocrine glands are ductless and secrete their hormones directly into the bloodstream. The vital function of the endocrine system involves the production and regulation of chemical substances called *hormones,* which play an essential role in maintaining homeostasis (Fig. 11–1 and Table 11–1).

The word *hormone* is derived from the Greek language and means *to excite* or *to urge on.* A hormone is a chemical transmitter that is released in small amounts and transported via the bloodstream to a target organ or other cells. There are many hormones in the body, and their release is controlled by nerve stimulation. The release of hormones is either stimulated or retarded according to the feedback system regulating supply and demand. Hormones are either proteins, peptides, derivatives of amino acids, or steroids that are synthesized from cholesterol.

The endocrine system and the nervous system closely interact with each other. The *hypothalamus,* located in the brain, plays a vital role in regulating endocrine functions as it synthesizes and secretes releasing hormones such as thyrotropin-releasing hormone (TRH) and gonadotropin-releasing hormone (GnRH) and releasing factors such as corticotropin-releasing factor (CRF), growth hormone-releasing factor (GHRF), prolactin-

THE ENDOCRINE SYSTEM

GLAND	PRIMARY FUNCTIONS
Pituitary (Hypophysis)	Master gland; regulatory effects on other endocrine glands
Anterior lobe	Influences growth and sexual development, thyroid function, adrenocortical function; regulates skin pigmentation
Posterior lobe	Stimulates the reabsorption of water and elevates blood pressure; stimulates the release of milk and the uterus to contract during labor, delivery, and parturition
Pineal	Helps regulate the release of gonadotropin and controls body pigmentation
Thyroid	Vital role in metabolism and regulates the body's metabolic processes, influences bone and calcium metabolism, helps maintain plasma calcium homeostasis
Parathyroid	Maintenance of a normal serum calcium level, plays a role in the metabolism of phosphorus
Pancreas (Islets of Langerhans)	Regulates blood glucose levels and plays a vital role in metabolism of carbohydrates, proteins, and fats
Adrenals (Suprarenals)	
Adrenal cortex	Regulates carbohydrate metabolism, anti-inflammatory effect; helps body cope during stress; regulates electrolyte and water balance; promotes development of male characteristics
Adrenal medulla	Synthesizes, secretes, and stores catecholamines (dopamine, epinephrine, norepinephrine)
Ovaries	Promote growth, development, and maintenance of female sex organs
Testes	Promote growth, development, and maintenance of male sex organs

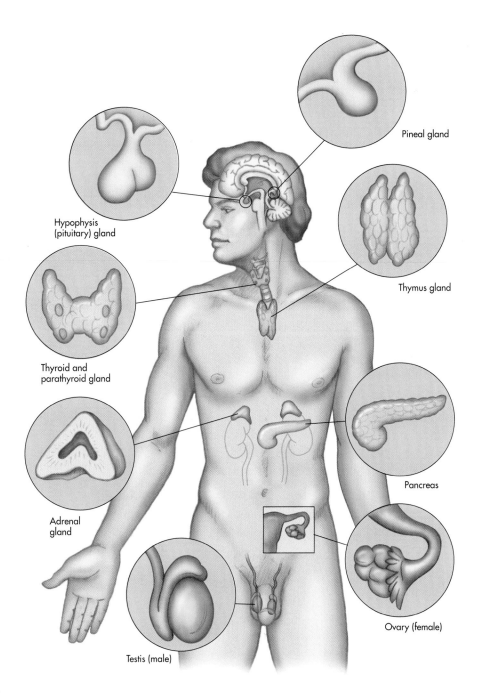

FIGURE 11–1

The primary glands of the endocrine system.

releasing factor (PRF), and melanocyte-stimulating hormone-releasing factor (MRF). The hypothalamus also synthesizes and secretes release-inhibiting hormones such as growth hormone release-inhibiting hormone. It also produces release-inhibiting factors such as prolactin release-inhibiting factor (PIF) and melanocyte-stimulating hormone release-inhibiting factor (MIF). The hypothalamus also exerts direct nervous control over the anterior pituitary and the adrenal medulla and controls the secretion of the hormones epinephrine and norepinephrine.

TABLE 11–1   Summary of the Endocrine Glands, Hormones, and Hormonal Functions

Endocrine Glands	Hormones	Hormonal Functions
Pituitary Gland		
Anterior lobe	Growth hormone (GH)	Growth and development of bones, muscles, and other organs
	Adrenocorticotropin hormone (ACTH)	Growth and development of the adrenal cortex
	Thyroid-stimulating hormone (TSH)	Growth and development of the thyroid gland
	Follicle-stimulating hormone (FSH)	Stimulates the growth of ovarian follicles in the female and sperm in the male
	Luteinizing hormone (LH)	Stimulates the development of the corpus luteum in the female and the production of testosterone in the male
	Prolactin hormone (PRL)	Stimulates the mammary glands to produce milk after childbirth
	Melanocyte-stimulating hormone (MSH)	Regulates skin pigmentation and promotes the deposit of melanin in the skin after exposure to sunlight
Posterior lobe	Antidiuretic hormone (ADH)	Stimulates the reabsorption of water by the renal tubules and has a pressor effect that elevates the blood pressure
	Oxytocin	Acts on the mammary glands to stimulate the release of milk and stimulates the uterus to contract during labor, delivery, and parturition
Pineal Gland	Melatonin	Helps regulate the release of gonadotropin and influences the body's internal clock
	Serotonin	Neurotransmitter, vasoconstrictor, and smooth muscle stimulant; acts to inhibit gastric secretion
Thyroid Gland	Thyroxine	Maintenance and regulation of the basal metabolic rate (BMR)
	Triiodothyronine	Influences the basal metabolic rate
	Calcitonin	Influences calcium metabolism
Parathyroid Glands	Parathormone hormone (PTH)	Plays a role in maintenance of a normal serum calcium level and in the metabolism of phosphorus
Islets of Langerhans	Glucagon	Facilitates the breakdown of glycogen to glucose
	Insulin	Plays a role in maintenance of normal blood sugar
	Somatostatin	Suppresses the release of glucagon and insulin
Adrenal Glands		
Cortex	Cortisol	Principal steroid hormone. Regulates carbohydrate, protein, and fat metabolism; gluconeogenesis; increases blood sugar level; anti-inflammatory effect; helps body cope during times of stress.
	Corticosterone	Steroid hormone. Essential for normal use of carbohydrates, the absorption of glucose, and gluconeogenesis. Also influences potassium and sodium metabolism.
	Aldosterone	Principal mineralocorticoid. Essential in regulating electrolyte and water balance.
	Testosterone	Development of male secondary sex characteristics
	Androsterone	Development of male secondary sex characteristics

continued

TABLE 11–1   continued

Endocrine Glands	Hormones	Hormonal Functions
Adrenal Glands (cont.)		
Medulla	Dopamine	Dilates systemic arteries, elevates systolic blood pressure, increases cardiac output, increases urinary output
	Epinephrine (adrenaline)	Vasoconstrictor, vasopressor, cardiac stimulant, antispasmodic, and sympathomimetic
	Norepinephrine	Vasoconstrictor, vasopressor, and neurotransmitter
Ovaries	Estrogens (estradiol, estrone, and estriol)	Female sex hormones. Essential for the growth, development, and maintenance of female sex organs and secondary sex characteristics. Promotes the development of the mammary glands, and plays a vital role in a woman's emotional well-being and sexual drive.
	Progesterone	Prepares the uterus for pregnancy
Testes	Testosterone	Essential for normal growth and development of the male accessory sex organs. Plays a vital role in the erection process of the penis and, thus, is necessary for the reproductive act, copulation.
Thymus Gland	Thymosin	Promotes the maturation process of T lymphocytes
	Thymopoietin	Influences the production of lymphocyte precursors and aids in their process of becoming T lymphocytes
Gastrointestinal Mucosa	Gastrin	Stimulates gastric acid secretion
	Secretin	Stimulates pancreatic juice, bile, and intestinal secretion
	Pancreozymin	Stimulates the pancreas to produce pancreatic juice
	Cholecystokinin	Contraction and emptying of the gallbladder
	Enterogastrone	Regulates gastric secretions

▶ THE PITUITARY GLAND (HYPOPHYSIS)

The *pituitary gland* is a small gray gland located at the base of the brain. It lies or rests in a shallow depression of the sphenoid bone known as the *sella turcica*. It is attached by the infundibulum stalk to the hypothalamus. The pituitary is approximately 1 cm in diameter and weighs approximately 0.6 g. It is divided into the anterior lobe or adenohypophysis and the posterior lobe or neurohypophysis. The pituitary is called the *master gland* of the body because of its regulatory effects on the other endocrine glands (see Fig. 11–1).

THE ANTERIOR LOBE

The *adenohypophysis* or anterior lobe secretes several hormones that are essential for the growth and development of bones, muscles, other organs, sex glands, the thyroid gland, and the adrenal cortex. The hormones secreted by the anterior lobe and their functions are described below and shown in Figure 11–2.

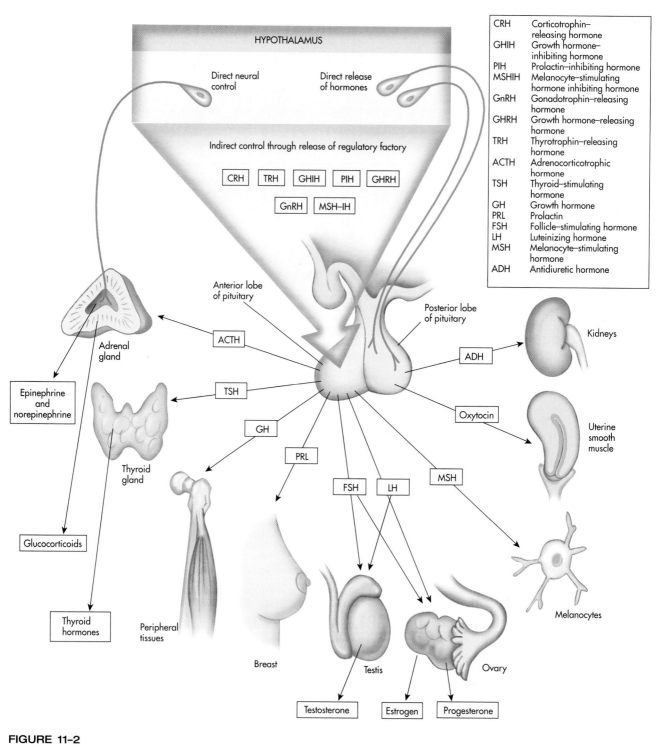

FIGURE 11-2

The pituitary hormones and their target cells, tissues, and/or organs.

GROWTH HORMONE (GH)

Growth hormone, also called somatotropin hormone (STH), is essential for the growth and development of bones, muscles, and other organs. It also enhances protein synthesis, decreases the use of glucose, and promotes fat destruction (lipolysis). Hyposecretion of this hormone may result in *dwarfism* and *Simmonds' disease.* Hypersecretion of the hormone may result in *gigantism* during early life and *acromegaly* in adults.

Adrenocorticotropin (ACTH)

Adrenocorticotropin is essential for growth and development of the middle and inner zones of the adrenal cortex. The adrenal cortex secretes the glucocorticoids cortisol and corticosterone.

Thyroid-Stimulating Hormone (TSH)

Thyroid-stimulating hormone is essential for the growth and development of the thyroid gland. It stimulates the production of thyroxine and triiodothyronine. It also influences the body's metabolic processes and plays an important role in metabolism.

Follicle-Stimulating Hormone (FSH)

Follicle-stimulating hormone is a gonadotropic hormone that is essential in stimulating the growth of ovarian follicles in the female and the production of sperm in the male.

Luteinizing Hormone (LH)

Luteinizing hormone is a gonadotropic hormone that is essential in the maturation process of the ovarian follicles and stimulates the development of the corpus luteum in the female and the production of testosterone in the male.

Prolactin (PRL)

Prolactin is also known as *lactogenic hormone* (LTH). It is a gonadotropic hormone that stimulates the mammary glands to produce milk after childbirth.

Melanocyte-Stimulating Hormone (MSH)

Melanocyte-stimulating hormone regulates skin pigmentation and promotes the deposit of melanin in the skin after exposure to sunlight.

THE POSTERIOR LOBE

The *neurohypophysis* or posterior lobe secretes two known hormones: antidiuretic hormone and oxytocin (see Fig. 11–2). The following is a description of the functions of these hormones.

Antidiuretic Hormone (ADH)

Antidiuretic hormone is also known as *vasopressin* (VP). It stimulates the reabsorption of water by the renal tubules and has a pressor effect that elevates blood pressure. Hyposecretion of this hormone may result in *diabetes insipidus.*

Oxytocin

Oxytocin acts on the mammary glands to stimulate the release of milk and stimulates the uterus to contract during labor, delivery, and parturition.

▶ THE PINEAL GLAND (BODY)

The *pineal gland* is a small, pine cone–shaped gland located near the posterior end of the corpus callosum. It is less than 1 cm in diameter and weighs approximately 0.1 g (see Fig. 11–1). The pineal gland secretes *melatonin* and *serotonin*. Melatonin is a hormone that may be released at night to help regulate the release of gonadotropin. Serotonin is a hormone that is a neurotransmitter, vasoconstrictor, and smooth muscle stimulant and acts to inhibit gastric secretion.

▶ THE THYROID GLAND

The *thyroid gland* is a large, bilobed gland located in the neck. It is anterior to the trachea and just below the thyroid cartilage. The thyroid is approximately 5 cm long and 3 cm wide and weighs approximately 30 g (see Fig. 11–1). It plays a vital role in metabolism and regulates the body's metabolic processes. The hormones described below are stored and secreted by the thyroid gland.

Thyroxine (T$_4$)

Thyroxine is essential for the maintenance and regulation of the *basal metabolic rate* (BMR). It contains four iodine atoms, which are attached to its nucleus. Thyroxine influences growth and development, both physical and mental, and the metabolism of fats, proteins, carbohydrates, water, vitamins, and minerals. It can be synthetically produced or extracted from animal thyroid glands in crystalline form to be used in the treatment of thyroid dysfunction, especially cretinism, myxedema, and Hashimoto's disease.

Triiodothyronine (T$_3$)

Triiodothyronine is an effective thyroid hormone that contains three iodine atoms. It influences the basal metabolic rate and is more biologically active than thyroxine.

Calcitonin

Also known as thyrocalcitonin, *calcitonin* is a thyroid hormone that influences bone and calcium metabolism. It helps maintain plasma calcium homeostasis.

Hyposecretion of the thyroid hormones T$_3$ and T$_4$ results in *cretinism* during infancy, *myxedema* during adulthood, and *Hashimoto's disease*, which is a chronic thyroid disease. Hypersecretion of the thyroid hormones T$_3$ and T$_4$ results in *hyperthyroidism*, which is also called *thyrotoxicosis*, and *Graves' disease, exophthalmic goiter, toxic goiter,* or *Basedow's disease.* Simple or endemic goiter is an enlargement of the thyroid gland caused by a deficiency of iodine in the diet.

▶ THE PARATHYROID GLANDS

The *parathyroid glands* are small, yellowish-brown bodies occurring as two pairs and located on the dorsal surface and lower aspect of the thyroid gland. Each parathyroid gland is approximately 6 mm in diameter and weighs approximately 0.033 g (Fig. 11–1). The hormone secreted by the parathyroids is *parathormone* (PTH). This hormone is essential for the maintenance of a normal serum calcium level. It also plays a role in the metabolism of phosphorus. Hyposecretion of PTH may result in *hypoparathyroidism,* which may result in *tetany.* Hypersecretion of PTH may result in *hyperparathyroidism,* which may result in *osteoporosis, kidney stones,* and *hypercalcemia.*

▶ THE PANCREAS (THE ISLETS OF LANGERHANS)

The *islets of Langerhans* are small clusters of cells located on the surface of the pancreas (see Fig. 11–1). They are composed of three major types of cells: *alpha, beta,* and *delta.* The alpha cells secrete the hormone glucagon, which facilitates the breakdown of glycogen to glucose, thereby elevating blood sugar. The beta cells secrete the hormone insulin, which is essential for the maintenance of normal blood sugar (70–110 mg/100 mL of blood). Insulin is essential to life. It promotes the use of glucose in cells, thereby lowering the blood glucose level, and plays a vital role in carbohydrate, protein, and fat metabolism. Insulin can be synthetically produced in various types and was first discovered and used successfully by Sir F. G. Banting. Hyposecretion or inadequate use of insulin may result in *diabetes mellitus.* Hypersecretion of insulin may result in *hyperinsulinism.* The delta cells secrete a hormone, *somatostatin,* that suppresses the release of glucagon and insulin.

▶ THE ADRENAL GLANDS (SUPRARENALS)

The *adrenal glands* are two small, triangular-shaped glands located on top of each kidney. Each gland weighs about 5 g and consists of an outer portion or *cortex* and an inner portion called the *medulla* (Fig. 11–1).

THE ADRENAL CORTEX

The *cortex* is essential to life as it secretes a group of hormones, the glucocorticoids, the mineralocorticoids, and the androgens. These hormones and their effects on the body are described below.

The Glucocorticoids

The two glucocorticoid hormones are *cortisol* and *corticosterone.*

Cortisol. *Cortisol* (hydrocortisone) is the principal steroid hormone secreted by the cortex. The following are some of the known influences and functions of this hormone:

- It regulates carbohydrate, protein, and fat metabolism.
- It stimulates output of glucose from the liver (gluconeogenesis).
- It increases the blood sugar level.
- It regulates other physiologic body processes.
- It promotes the transport of amino acids into extracellular tissue, thereby making them available for energy.
- It influences the effectiveness of catecholamines such as dopamine, epinephrine, and norepinephrine.
- It has an anti-inflammatory effect.
- It helps the body cope during times of stress.

Hyposecretion of this hormone may result in *Addison's disease.* Hypersecretion of cortisol may result in *Cushing's disease.*

Corticosterone. *Corticosterone* is a steroid hormone secreted by the adrenal cortex. It is essential for the normal use of carbohydrates, the absorption of glucose, and the process known as *gluconeogenesis.* It also influences potassium and sodium metabolism.

The Mineralocorticoids

Aldosterone is the principal *mineralocorticoid* secreted by the adrenal cortex. It is essential in regulating electrolyte and water balance by promoting sodium and chloride retention and potassium excretion. Hyposecretion of this hormone may result in a *reduced plasma volume.* Hypersecretion of this hormone may result in a condition known as *primary aldosteronism.*

The Androgens

Androgen refers to a substance or hormone that promotes the development of male characteristics. The two main androgen hormones are *testosterone* and *androsterone*. These hormones are essential for the development of the male secondary sex characteristics.

THE ADRENAL MEDULLA

The *medulla* synthesizes, secretes, and stores catecholamines, specifically, dopamine, epinephrine, and norepinephrine. A discussion of these substances and their effects on the body follows.

Dopamine

Dopamine acts to dilate systemic arteries, elevates systolic blood pressure, increases cardiac output, and increases urinary output. It is used in the treatment of shock and is a neurotransmitter in the nervous system.

Epinephrine

Epinephrine (Adrenalin, adrenaline) acts as a vasoconstrictor, vasopressor, cardiac stimulant, antispasmodic, and sympathomimetic. Its main function is to assist in the regulation of the sympathetic branch of the autonomic nervous system. It can be synthetically produced and may be administered parenterally *(by an injection),* topically *(on a local area of the skin),* or by inhalation *(by nose or mouth).* The following are some of the known influences and functions of this hormone:

- It elevates the systolic blood pressure.
- It increases the heart rate and cardiac output.
- It increases glycogenolysis, thereby hastening the release of glucose from the liver. This action elevates the blood sugar level and provides the body with a spurt of energy; referred to as the "fight-or-flight" syndrome.
- It dilates the bronchial tubes and relaxes air passageways.
- It dilates the pupils so that one can see more clearly.

Norepinephrine

Norepinephrine (noradrenalin) acts as a vasoconstrictor, vasopressor, and neurotransmitter. It elevates systolic and diastolic blood pressure, increases the heart rate and cardiac output, and increases glycogenolysis.

▶ THE OVARIES

The *ovaries* produce *estrogens (estradiol, estrone,* and *estriol)* and *progesterone.* Estrogen is the female sex hormone secreted by the graafian follicles of the ovaries. Progesterone is a steroid hormone secreted by the corpus luteum. These hormones are essential for promoting the growth, development, and maintenance of secondary female sex organs and characteristics. They also prepare the uterus for pregnancy, promote development of the mammary glands, and play a vital role in a woman's emotional well-being and her sexual drive (see Fig. 11–1).

▶ THE TESTES

The *testes* produce the male sex hormone *testosterone,* which is essential for normal growth and development of the male accessory sex organs. Testosterone plays a vital role in the erection process of the penis and, thus, is necessary for the reproductive act, copulation (see Fig. 11–1).

▶ THE PLACENTA

During pregnancy the *placenta,* a spongy structure joining mother and child, serves as an endocrine gland. It produces chorionic gonadotropin hormone, estrogen, and progesterone.

▶ THE GASTROINTESTINAL MUCOSA

The *mucosa* of the pyloric area of the stomach secretes the hormone *gastrin,* which stimulates gastric acid secretion. Gastrin also affects the gallbladder, pancreas, and small intestine secretory activities.

The mucosa of the duodenum and jejunum secretes the hormone *secretin,* which stimulates pancreatic juice, bile, and intestinal secretion. The mucosa of the duodenum also secretes *pancreozymin-cholecystokinin,* which stimulates the pancreas. *Enterogastrone,* a hormone that regulates gastric secretions, is also secreted by the duodenal mucosa.

▶ THE THYMUS

The *thymus* is a bilobed body located in the mediastinal cavity in front of and above the heart (Fig. 11–3). It is composed of lymphoid tissue and is a part of the lymphoid system. It is a ductless gland-like body and secretes the hormones *thymosin* and *thymopoietin.* Thymosin promotes the maturation process of T lymphocytes (thymus-dependent). Thymopoietin is a hormone that influences the production of lymphocyte precursors and aids in their process of becoming T lymphocytes.

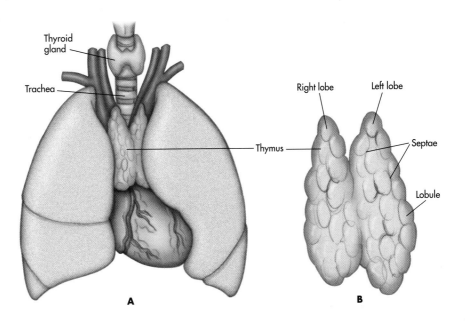

FIGURE 11-3

The thymus gland. **(A)** Appearance and position, **(B)** with anatomic structures.

LIFE SPAN CONSIDERATIONS

▶ THE CHILD

Most of the structures and glands of the endocrine system develop during the first 3 months of pregnancy. The endocrine system of the newborn is supplemented by hormones that cross the placental barrier. Both male and female newborns may have swelling of the breast and genitalia from maternal hormones.

Either excessively high or insufficient production of growth hormone (GH) by the anterior lobe of the pituitary gland can cause abnormal growth patterns. Excessive production of GH can cause **gigantism.** Insufficient production of GH can cause **dwarfism.**

Type I—**insulin-dependent diabetes mellitus** (IDDM)—is the most common endocrine system disorder of childhood. The rate of occurrence is highest among 5–7-year-olds and 11–13-year-olds. The classic symptoms of diabetes mellitus—**polyuria, polydipsia,** and **polyphagia**—appear more rapidly in children. Other symptoms seen during childhood are weakness, loss of weight, lethargy, anorexia, irritability, dry skin, vaginal yeast infections in the female child and/or recurrent infections, and abdominal cramps. The management of diabetes mellitus during childhood is very difficult, because diet, exercise, and medication have to be adjusted and regulated according to the various stages of growth and development of the child.

▶ THE OLDER ADULT

With aging, **hormonal changes** vary with each individual. Generally the number of tissue receptors decreases, thus diminishing the body's response to hormones. This is especially the case with older adults who develop Type II—**non-insulin-dependent diabetes mellitus** (NIDDM). In this condition sufficient insulin is produced, but because the number of cell receptors is reduced, glucose does not enter the cells.

An older adult may not be diagnosed with diabetes until he or she goes in for a regular eye exam and the ophthalmologist discovers a problem and/or one goes in for a physical examination and the blood test indicates an elevated blood glucose level. There are multiple risk factors associated with the older adult and the development of diabetes; these are:

- Age-related decreased insulin production
- Age-related insulin resistance
- Heredity
- Decreased physical activity
- Multiple diseases
- Polypharmacy
- Obesity
- New stressors in life

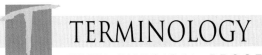

TERMINOLOGY
WITH SURGICAL PROCEDURES & PATHOLOGY

TERM	WORD PARTS			DEFINITION
acidosis (ăs″ ĭ-dō′ sĭs)	acid osis	R S	acid condition of	A condition of excessive acidity of body fluids
acromegaly (ăk″ rō-měg′ ă-lē)	acro megaly	CF S	extremity enlargement, large	Enlargement of the extremities caused by excessive growth hormone
adenalgia (ăd″ ēn -ăl′ jĭ-ă)	aden algia	R S	gland pain	Pain in a gland
adenectomy (ăd″ ĕn-ĕk′ tō-mē)	aden ectomy	R S	gland excision	Surgical excision of a gland
adenoma (ăd″ ĕ-nō′ mă)	aden oma	R S	gland tumor	A tumor of a gland
adenomalacia (ăd″ ĕ-nō-mă-lā′ shĭ-ă	adeno malacia	CF S	gland softening	A softening of a gland
adenosclerosis (ăd″ ĕ-nō-sklĕ-rō′ sĭs)	adeno scler osis	CF R S	gland hardening condition of	A condition of hardening of a gland
adenosis (ăd″ ĕ-nō′ sĭs)	aden osis	R S	gland condition of	Any disease condition of a gland
adrenal (ăd-rē′ năl)	ad ren al	P R S	toward kidney pertaining to	Pertaining to toward the kidney
adrenalectomy (ăd-rē″ năl-ĕk′ tō-mē)	ad ren al ectomy	P R S S	toward kidney pertaining to excision	Surgical excision of the adrenal gland
adrenopathy (ăd″ rĕn-ŏp′ ă-thē)	ad reno pathy	P CF S	toward kidney disease	Any disease of the adrenal gland
adrenotropic (ăd-rē″ nō-trōp′ ĭk)	ad reno trop ic	P CF R S	toward kidney nourishment pertaining to	Pertaining to the nourishment of the adrenal glands

continued

Terminology - continued

TERM	WORD PARTS			DEFINITION
cretinism (krē′ tĭn-ĭzm)	cretin ism	R S	cretin condition of	A congenital deficiency in secretion of the thyroid hormones T$_3$ and T$_4$
diabetes (dī″ ă-bē′ tēz)	dia betes	P S	through to go	A disease characterized by excessive discharge of urine

 TERMINOLOGY SPOTLIGHT

Diabetes mellitus is a complex disorder of metabolism. It affects 14 million Americans, with care and treatment costing $20 billion annually.

The National Diabetes Data Group of the National Institutes of Health has categorized the various forms of diabetes mellitus: Type I—insulin-dependent diabetes mellitus (IDDM); Type II—non-insulin-dependent diabetes mellitus (NIDDM); Type III—women who have developed glucose intolerance in association with pregnancy; and Type IV—diabetes associated with pancreatic disease, hormonal changes, the adverse effects of drugs, and other anomalies. One in 10 people who have diabetes are Type I diabetics and must take insulin on a regular basis.

The American Diabetes Association estimates that 7 million American have diabetes and do not know it. Are you at risk for diabetes? Do you have any, some, or many of the signs and symptoms of diabetes? See Table 11–2 for the warning signs and symptoms of diabetes mellitus.

TABLE 11–2   Warning Signs and Symptoms of Diabetes Mellitus

Type I IDDM	Type II NIDDM
Frequent urination (polyuria) Excessive thirst (polydipsia) Extreme hunger (polyphagia) Unexplained weight loss Extreme fatigue Blurred vision	Any Type I symptom Tingling or numbing in the feet Frequent vaginal or skin infection

TERM	WORD PARTS			DEFINITION
dwarfism (dwar′ fizm)	dwarf ism	R S	small condition of	A condition of being abnormally small
endocrine (ĕn′ dō-krĭn)	endo crine	P R	within to secrete	A ductless gland that produces an internal secretion
endocrinologist (ĕn″ dō-krĭn-ŏl′ ō-gĭst)	endo crino log ist	P CF R S	within to secrete study of one who specializes	One who specializes in the study of the endocrine glands
endocrinology (ĕn″ dō-krĭn-ŏl′ ō-jē)	endo crino logy	P CF S	within to secrete study of	The study of the endocrine glands

Terminology - continued

TERM	WORD PARTS			DEFINITION
endocrinopathy (ĕn″ dō-krĭn-ŏp′ ă-thē)	endo crino pathy	P CF S	within to secrete disease	A disease of an endocrine gland or glands
endocrino-therapy (ĕn″ dō-krĭn″ ō-thĕr′ ă-pē)	endo crino therapy	P CF S	within to secrete treatment	Treatment with endocrine preparations
euthyroid (ū-thī′ royd)	eu thyr oid	P R S	good, normal thyroid, shield resemble	Normal activity of the thyroid gland
exocrine (ĕks′ ō-krĭn)	exo crine	P R	out, away from to secrete	External secretion of a gland
exophthalmic (ĕks″ ŏf-thăl′ mĭk)	ex ophthalm ic	P R S	out, away from eye pertaining to	Pertaining to an abnormal protrusion of the eye
galactorrhea (gă-lăk″ tō-rĭ′ ă)	galacto rrhea	CF S	milk flow, discharge	Excessive secretion of milk after cessation of nursing
gigantism (jī′ găn-tĭzm)	gigant ism	R S	giant condition of	A condition of being abnormally large
glandular (glăn′ dū-lăr)	glandul ar	R S	little acorn pertaining to	Pertaining to a gland
glucocorticoid (glū″ kō-kŏrt′ ĭ-koyd)	gluco cortic oid	CF R S	sweet, sugar cortex resemble	A general classification of the adrenal cortical hormones
hirsutism (hŭr′ sūt-ĭzm)	hirsut ism	R S	hairy condition of	An abnormal condition characterized by excessive growth of hair, especially in women. See Figure 11–4.
hypergonadism (hī″ pĕr-gō′ năd-ĭzm)	hyper gonad ism	P R S	excessive seed condition of	A condition of excessive secretion of the sex glands
hyperinsulinism (hī″ pĕr-ĭn′ sū-lĭn-ĭzm)	hyper insulin ism	P R S	excessive insulin condition of	A condition of excessive amounts of insulin in the blood
hyperkalemia (hī″ pĕr-kă-lē′ mĭ-ă)	hyper kal emia	P R S	excessive potassium (K) blood condition	A condition of excessive amounts of potassium in the blood

continued

Terminology - continued

TERM	WORD PARTS			DEFINITION
hyperthyroidism (hī″ pĕr-thī′ royd-ĭzm)	hyper thyr oid ism	P R S S	excessive thyroid, shield resemble condition of	A condition caused by excessive secretion of the thyroid gland
hypocrinism (hī″ pō-krĭ′ nĭzm)	hypo crin ism	P R S	deficient to secrete condition of	A condition caused by deficient secretion of any gland
hypogonadism (hī″ pō-gō′ năd-ĭzm)	hypo gonad ism	P R S	deficient seed condition of	A condition caused by deficient internal secretion of the gonads
hypoparathyroid-ism (hī″ pō-păr″ ă-thī′ royd-ĭzm)	hypo para thyr oid ism	P P R S S	deficient beside thyroid, shield resemble condition of	Deficient internal secretion of the parathyroid glands
hypophysis (hī-pŏf′ ĭ-sĭs)	hypo physis	P S	deficient, under growth	Any undergrowth; the pituitary body
hypothyroidism (hī″ pō-thī′ royd-ĭzm)	hypo thyr oid ism	P R S S	deficient thyroid, shield resemble condition of	Deficient secretion of the thyroid gland
insulinogenic (ĭn″ sū-lĭn″ ō-jĕn′ ĭk)	insulino genic	CF S	insulin formation produce	The formation or production of insulin
insulinoid (ĭn′ sū-lĭn-oyd″)	insulin oid	R S	insulin resemble	Resembling insulin
insuloma (ĭn′ sū-lō″ mă)	insul oma	R S	insulin tumor	A tumor of the islets of Langerhans
lethargic (lĕ-thar′ jĭk)	letharg ic	R S	drowsiness pertaining to	Pertaining to drowsiness, sluggish
myxedema (mĭks″ ĕ-dē′ mă)	myx edema	R S	mucus swelling	A condition of mucus swelling resulting from hypofunction of the thyroid gland. See Figure 11–5.
pancreatic (păn″ krē-ăt′ ĭk)	pan creat ic	P R S	all flesh pertaining to	Pertaining to the pancreas

Terminology - continued

TERM	WORD PARTS			DEFINITION
parathyroid (păr″ ă-thī′ royd)	para	P	beside	An endocrine gland located beside the thyroid gland
	thyr	R	thyroid, shield	
	oid	S	resemble	
pineal (pĭn′ ē-ăl)	pine	R	pine cone	An endocrine gland that is shaped like a small pine cone
	al	S	pertaining to	
pinealectomy (pĭn″ ē-ăl-ĕk′ tō-mē)	pineal	R	pineal body	Surgical excision of the pineal body
	ectomy	S	excision	
pinealoma (pĭn″ ē-ă-lō′ mă)	pineal	R	pineal body	A tumor of the pineal body
	oma	S	tumor	
pituitarism (pĭt-ū′ ĭ-tă-rĭzm)	pituitar	R	phlegm	Any condition of the pituitary gland
	ism	S	condition	
pituitary (pĭ-tū′ ĭ-tăr″ ē)	pituitar	R	phlegm	Pertaining to phlegm; the pituitary body or gland, the hypophysis
	y	S	pertaining to	
progeria (prō-jē′ rĭ-ă)	pro	P	before	A condition of premature old age occurring in childhood
	ger	R	old age	
	ia	S	condition	
thymectomy (thī-mĕk′ tō-mē)	thym	R	thymus	Surgical excision of the thymus gland
	ectomy	S	excision	
thymitis (thī-mī′ tĭs)	thym	R	thymus	Inflammation of the thymus gland
	itis	S	inflammation	
thymopexy (thī′ mō-pĕks″ ē)	thymo	CF	thymus	Surgical fixation of an enlarged thymus in a new position
	pexy	S	fixation	
thyroid (thī′ royd)	thyr	R	thyroid, shield	Resembling a shield; one of the endocrine glands
	oid	S	resemble	
thyroidectomy (thī″ royd-ĕk′ tō-mē)	thyr	R	thyroid, shield	Surgical excision of the thyroid gland
	oid	S	resemble	
	ectomy	S	excision	
thyroiditis (thī″ royd′ī′ tĭs)	thyr	R	thyroid, shield	Inflammation of the thyroid gland
	oid	S	resemble	
	itis	S	inflammation	
thyroptosis (thī″ rŏp-tō′ sĭs)	thyro	CF	thyroid, shield	Downward drooping of the thyroid into the thorax
	ptosis	S	drooping	
thyrosis (thī-rō′ sĭs)	thyr	R	thyroid, shield	Any condition of abnormal functioning of the thyroid
	osis	S	condition of	

continued

Terminology - continued

TERM	WORD PARTS			DEFINITION
thyrotherapy (thī″ rō-thĕr′ ă-pē)	thyro therapy	CF S	thyroid, shield treatment	Pertaining to the treatment using thyroid gland extracts
thyrotome (thī″ rō-tōm)	thyro tome	CF S	thyroid, shield instrument to cut	An instrument used to cut the thyroid cartilage
thyrotoxicosis (thī″ rō-tŏks″ ĭ-kō′ sĭs)	thyro toxic osis	CF R S	thyroid, shield poison condition of	A poisonous condition of the thyroid gland caused by hyperactivity
virilism (vĭr′ ĭl-ĭzm)	viril ism	R S	masculine condition of	The condition of masculinity developed in a woman

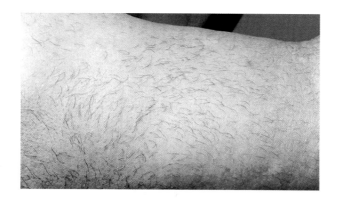

FIGURE 11–4

Hirsutism. *(Courtesy of Jason L. Smith, MD.)*

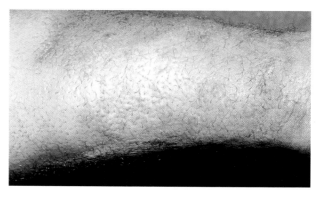

FIGURE 11–5

Pretibial myxedema. *(Courtesy of Jason L. Smith, MD.)*

 VOCABULARY WORDS

Vocabulary words are terms that have not been divided into component parts. They are common words or specialized terms associated with the subject of this chapter. These words are provided to enhance your medical vocabulary.

WORD	DEFINITION
aldosterone (ăl-dŏs′ tĕr-ōn)	A mineralocorticoid hormone secreted by the adrenal cortex that helps regulate metabolism of sodium, chloride, and potassium

Vocabulary - continued

WORD	DEFINITION
androgen (ăn′ drō-jĕn)	Hormones that produce or stimulate the development of male characteristics. The two major androgens are testosterone and androsterone.
catecholamines (kăt″ ĕ-kōl′ ăm-ēns)	Biochemical substances, epinephrine, norepinephrine, and dopamine
cortisone (kŏr′ tĭ-sōn)	A glucocorticoid hormone that is isolated from the adrenal cortex; *used as an anti-inflammatory agent*
dopamine (dō′ pă-mēn)	An intermediate substance in the synthesis of norepinephrine; used in the treatment of shock as it acts to elevate blood pressure and increase urinary output
epinephrine (ĕp″ ĭ-nĕf′ rĭn)	A hormone produced by the adrenal medulla; used as a vasoconstrictor, as a cardiac stimulant, to relax bronchospasm, and to relieve allergic symptoms; *also called adrenaline, Adrenalin*
estrogen (ĕs′ trō-jĕn)	Hormones produced by the ovaries, including estradiol, estrone, and estriol; female sex hormones important in the development of secondary sex characteristics and regulation of the menstrual cycle
hormone (hor′ mōn)	A chemical substance produced by the endocrine glands
hydrocortisone (hī″ drō-kŏr′ tĭ-sōn)	A glucocorticoid hormone produced by the adrenal cortex; *used as an anti-inflammatory agent*
insulin (in′ sū-lĭn)	A hormone produced by the beta cells of the islets of Langerhans of the pancreas; essential for the metabolism of carbohydrates and fats; *used in the management of diabetes mellitus*
iodine (ī′ ō-dīn)	A trace mineral that aids in the development and functioning of the thyroid gland
necrobiosis lipoidica diabeticorum (nĕk-rō-bī-ō′sĭs lĭp-oyd′īcă dī-ă-bĕt′īk′-ō″rŭm)	A skin disease commonly found in diabetics; it is marked by gradual degeneration and swelling of connective and elastic tissue; the lesions have a central yellowish area surrounded by a brownish border and are usually present on the anterior surface of the legs. See Figures 11–6 and 11–7.
norepinephrine (nŏr-ĕp″ ĭ-nĕf′ rĭn)	A hormone produced by the adrenal medulla; used as a vasoconstrictor of peripheral blood vessels in acute hypotensive states
oxytocin (ŏk″ sĭ-tō′ sĭn)	A hormone produced by the pituitary gland that stimulates uterine contraction during childbirth and stimulates the release of milk during nursing

continued

Vocabulary - continued

WORD	DEFINITION
progesterone (prō-jĕs′ tĕr-ōn)	A hormone produced by the corpus luteum of the ovary, the adrenal cortex, or the placenta; released during the second half of the menstrual cycle
somatotropin (sō-măt′ ō-trō″ pĭn)	Growth-stimulating hormone produced by the anterior lobe of the pituitary gland
steroids (stĕr′ oydz)	A group of chemical substances that includes hormones, vitamins, sterols, cardiac glycosides, and certain drugs
testosterone (tĕs-tŏs′ tĕr-ōn)	A hormone produced by the testes; male sex hormone important in the development of secondary sex characteristics and masculinization
thyroxine (thī-rŏks′ ēn)	A hormone produced by the thyroid gland; important in growth and development and regulation of the body's metabolic rate and metabolism of carbohydrates, fats, and proteins
vasopressin (văs″ ō-prĕs′ ĭn)	A hormone produced by the hypothalamus and stored in the posterior lobe of the pituitary gland; also called antidiuretic hormone, ADH

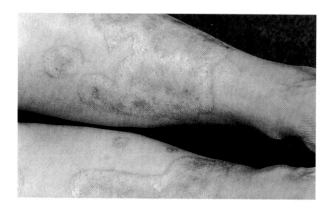

FIGURE 11–6

Necrobiosis lipoidica diabeticorum. *(Courtesy of Jason L. Smith, MD.)*

FIGURE 11–7

Necrobiosis lipoidica diabeticorum. *(Courtesy of Jason L. Smith, MD.)*

 # ABBREVIATIONS

ACTH	adrenocorticotropic hormone	**CRF**	corticotropin-releasing factor
ADA	American Diabetes Association	**DI**	diabetes insipidus
ADH	antidiuretic hormone	**DM**	diabetes mellitus
BG, bG	blood glucose	**FBS**	fasting blood sugar
BMR	basal metabolic rate	**FSH**	follicle-stimulating hormone

GH	growth hormone	PBI	protein-bound iodine
GHb	glycosylated hemoglobin	PIF	prolactin release-inhibiting factor
GHRF	glycosylated hemoglobin-releasing factor	PRF	prolactin-releasing factor
		PTH	parathormone
GnRF	gonadotropin-releasing factor	RAIU	radioactive iodine uptake
GTT	glucose tolerance test	RIA	radioimmunoassay
IDDM	insulin-dependent diabetes mellitus	SMBG	self-monitoring of blood glucose
		STH	somatotropin hormone
K	potassium	T_3	triiodothyronine
LH	luteinizing hormone	T_3RU	triiodothyronine resin uptake
LTH	lactogenic hormone	T_4	thyroxine
MIF	melanocyte-stimulating hormone release-inhibiting factor	TFS	thyroid function studies
		TSH	thyroid-stimulating hormone
MSH	melanocyte-stimulating hormone	VMA	vanillylmandelic acid
NIDDM	non-insulin-dependent diabetes mellitus	VP	vasopressin

DRUG HIGHLIGHTS

Drugs that are generally used for endocrine system diseases and disorders include thyroid hormones, antithyroid hormones, insulin, and oral hypoglycemic agents.

Thyroid Hormones	Increase metabolic rate, cardiac output, oxygen consumption, body temperature, respiratory rate, blood volume, and carbohydrate, fat, and protein metabolism, and influence growth and development at cellular level. Thyroid hormones are used as supplements or replacement therapy in hypothyroidism, myxedema, and cretinism. *Examples: Levothroid and Synthroid (levothyroxine sodium), Cytomel (liothyronine sodium), Euthroid and Thyrolar (liotrix), and thyroid, USP.*
Antithyroid Hormones	Inhibit the synthesis of thyroid hormones by decreasing iodine use in manufacture of thyroglobin and iodothyronine. They do not inactivate or inhibit thyroxine or triiodothyronine. They are used in the treatment of hyperthyroidism. *Example: Tapazole (methimazole), potassium iodide solution, Lugol's solution (strong iodine solution), and Iodotope I-131 (sodium iodide).*
Insulin	Stimulates carbohydrate metabolism by increasing the movement of glucose and other monosaccharides into cells. It also influences fat and carbohydrate metabolism in the liver and adipose cells. It decreases blood sugar, phosphate, and potassium, and increases blood pyruvate and lactate. *Insulin* is used in the treatment of insulin-dependent diabetes mellitus (Type I—IDDM), non-insulin-dependent diabetes mellitus (Type II—NIDDM) when other regimens are not effective, and to treat ketoacidosis.
Insulin Preparations	Insulin is given by subcutaneous injection and is available in rapid-acting, intermediate-acting, and long-acting preparations.
Rapid-acting	*Examples: Regular Novolin R, Humulin R, and Velosulin BR* Onset of Action ½ hour Appearance—clear

Intermediate-acting	*Examples: NPH, Novolin N, Humulin L, Iletin II, Lente Insulin, and Novolin L.*
	Onset of Action 1–1½ hours Appearance—cloudy
Long-acting	*Examples: Ultralente and Humulin U*
	Onset of Action 4–8 hours Appearance—cloudy

Oral Hypoglycemic Agents

Are agents of the sulfonylurea class and are used to stimulate insulin secretion from pancreatic cells in non-insulin-dependent diabetics with some pancreatic function. *Examples: Dymelor (acetohexamide), Diabinese (chlorpropamide), Glucotrol (glipizide), DiaBeta and Micronase (glyburide), Tolinase (tolazamide), and Orinase (tolbutamide).*

DIAGNOSTIC AND LABORATORY TESTS

Test	Description
catecholamines (kăt″ ĕ-kōl′ ă-mēns)	A test performed on urine to determine the amount of epinephrine and norepinephrine present. These adrenal hormones increase in times of stress.
corticotropin, corticotropin-releasing factor (CRF) (kor″ tĭ-kō-trō′ pin)	A test performed on blood plasma to determine the amount of corticotropin present. Increased levels may indicate stress, adrenal cortical hypofunction, and/or pituitary tumors. Decreased levels may indicate adrenal neoplasms and/or Cushing's syndrome.
fasting blood sugar (FBS) (făs-tĭng blod shoog′ ar)	A test performed on blood to determine the level of sugar in the bloodstream. Increased levels may indicate diabetes mellitus, diabetic acidosis, and many other conditions. Decreased levels may indicate hypoglycemia, hyperinsulinism, and many other conditions.
glucose tolerance test (GTT) (gloo′ kōs tŏl′ ĕr-ăns test)	A blood sugar test performed at specified intervals after the patient has been given a certain amount of glucose. Blood samples are drawn, and the blood glucose level of each sample is determined. It is more accurate than other blood sugar tests, and it is used to diagnose diabetes mellitus.
17-hydroxycorticosteroids (17-OHCS) (hī-drŏk″ sē-kor″ tĭ-kō-stĕr′ oyd)	A test performed on urine to identify adrenocorticosteroid hormones. It is used to determine adrenal cortical function.
17-ketosteroids (17-KS) (kē″ tō-stĕr′ oyd)	A test performed on urine to determine the amount of 17-KS present. 17-KS is the end product of androgens and is secreted from the adrenal glands and testes. It is used in the diagnosing of adrenal tumors.

Test	Description
protein-bound iodine (PBI) (prō′ tēn bound ī′ ō-dīn)	A test performed on serum to indicate the amount of iodine that is attached to serum protein. It may be used to indicate thyroid function.
radioactive iodine uptake (RAIU) (rā″ dē-ō-ăk′ tīv ī′ ō-dīn ŭp′ tāk)	A test to measure the ability of the thyroid gland to concentrate ingested iodine. Increased level may indicate hyperthyroidism, cirrhosis, and/or thyroiditis. Decreased level may indicate hypothyroidism.
radioimmunoassay (rā″ dē-ō-ĭm″ū-nō-ăs′ā)	A standard assay method that is used for the measurement of minute quantities of specific antibodies and/or antigens. It may be used for clinical laboratory measurements of hormones, therapeutic drug monitoring, and substance abuse screening.
thyroid scan (thī′ royd skăn)	A test to detect tumors of the thyroid gland. The patient is given radioactive iodine 131, which localizes in the thyroid gland, and the gland is then visualized with a scanner device.
thyroxine (T_4) (thī-rōks′ ĭn)	A test performed on blood serum to determine the amount of thyroxine present. Increased levels may indicate hyperthyroidism. Decreased levels may indicate hypothyroidism.
triiodothyronine uptake (T_3) (trī″ ī-ō″ dō-thī′ rō-nĭn ŭp′ tāk)	A test performed on blood serum to determine the amount of triiodothyronine present. Increased levels may indicate thyrotoxicosis, toxic adenoma, and/or Hashimoto's struma. Decreased levels may indicate starvation, severe infection, and severe trauma.
total calcium (tōt′ l kăl′ sē-ŭm)	A test performed on blood serum to determine the amount of calcium present. Increased levels may indicate hyperparathyroidism. Decreased levels may indicate hypoparathyroidism.
ultrasonography (ŭl-tră-sŏn-ŏg′ ră-fē)	The use of high-frequency sound waves to visualize the structure being studied. May be used to visualize the pancreas, thyroid, and any other gland. It is used as a screening test or as a diagnostic tool.

COMMUNICATION ENRICHMENT

This segment is provided for those who wish to enhance their ability to communicate in either English or Spanish.

▶ Related Terms

English	Spanish	English	Spanish
adrenal	adrenal (ă-*drĕ*-năl)	harden	endurecer (ĕn-*dŭ*-rĕ-sĕr)
diabetes	diabetes (dĭ-ă-*bĕ*-tĕs)	small	pequeño (pĕ-*kĕ*-ñō)
endocrine system	sistema endocrino (sĭs-*tĕ*-mă ĕn-dō-crĭ-nō)	large	grande (*grănd*-ĕ)
		giant	gigante (hĭ-*găn*-tĕ)
gland	glándula (glăn-*dŭ*-lă)	thyroidectomy	tiroidectomía (tĭ-rō-ĭ-dĕc-tō-mĭ-ă)
goiter	bocio (*bŏ*-sĭ-ō)		
insulin	insulina (ĭn-sŭ-*lĭ*-nă)	thyroxine	tiroxina (tĭ-rōx-*sĭ*-nă)
pancreas	pancreas (păn-*krĕ*-ăs)	hairy	peludo (pĕ-*lŭ*-dō)
parathyroids	paratiroides (pă-*ră*-tĭ-rō-ĭ-dĕs)	sweet	dulce (*dŭl*-sĕ)
pituitary	pituitario (pĭ-tŭ-ĭ-*tă*-rĭ-ō)	excessive	excesivo (ĕx-sĕ-*sĭ*-vō)
thyroid	tiroides (tĭ-rō-ĭ-*dĕs*)	seed	semilla (*sĕ*-mĭ-jă)
adrenalin	adrenalina (ă-*drĕ*-nă-lĭ-nă)	potassium	potasio (pō-*tă*-sĭ-ō)
hormone	hormona (*ōr*-mō-nă)	deficient	deficiente (dĕ-fĭ-sĭ-*ĕn*-tĕ)
iodine	iodo (ĭ-*ō*-dō)	phlegm	flema (*flĕ*-mă)
acidosis	acidismo (*ă*-sĭ-dĭs-mō)	masculine	masculino (*măs*-kŭ-lĭ-nō)
extremity	extremidad (ĕx-trĕ-*mĭ*-dăd)	within	dentro (*dĕn*-trō)
soften	ablandar (*ă*-blăn-dăr)		

STUDY AND REVIEW SECTION

LEARNING EXERCISES

▶ **Anatomy and Physiology**

Write your answers to the following questions. Do not refer back to the text.

1. Name the primary glands of the endocrine system.

   a. _____   b. _____

   c. _____   d. _____

   e. _____   f. _____

   g. _____   h. _____

2. Name the secondary glands of the endocrine system.

   a. _____   b. _____

   c. _____

3. State the vital function of the endocrine system. _____

   _____

4. Define hormone. _____

5. State the vital role of the hypothalamus in regulating endocrine functions.

   _____

   _____

   _____

6. Why is the pituitary gland known as the master gland of the body? _____

   _____

7. Name the hormones secreted by the adenohypophysis.

   a. _____   b. _____

   c. _____   d. _____

   e. _____   f. _____

   g. _____

8. Name the hormones secreted by the neurohypophysis.

   a. _____   b. _____

9. The pineal gland secretes the hormones _____

   and _____.

10. State the vital role of the thyroid gland. _____

   _____

11. Name the hormones stored and secreted by the thyroid gland.

   a. _____   b. _____

   c. _____

12. Parathormone is essential for the maintenance of a normal level of _____

   _____ and also plays a role in the metabolism of _____.

13. Insulin is essential for the maintenance of a normal level of _____.

14. The adrenal cortex secretes a group of hormones known as the _____,

   the _____, and the _____.

15. Name four functions of cortisol.

   a. _____   b. _____

   c. _____   d. _____

16. Name four functions of corticosterone.

   a. _____   b. _____

   c. _____   d. _____

17. _____ is the principal mineralocorticoid secreted by the adrenal cortex.

18. Define androgen. _____

   _____

19. Name the three main catecholamines synthesized, secreted, and stored by the adrenal medulla.

   a. _____   b. _____

   c. _____

20. Name three functions of the hormone epinephrine.

   a. _____

   b. _____

   c. _____

21. The ovaries produce the hormones _____ and _____.

22. The testes produce the hormone _____.

23. Name the two hormones secreted by the thymus.

   a. _____   b. _____

24. Name the four hormones secreted by the gastrointestinal mucosa.

   a. _____   b. _____

   c. _____   d. _____

▶ Word Parts

1. In the spaces provided, write the definitions of these prefixes, roots, combining forms, and suffixes. Do not refer to the listings of terminology words. Leave blank those terms you cannot define.

2. After completing as many as you can, refer back to the terminology word listings to check your work. For each word missed or left blank, write the term and its definition several times on the margins of these pages or on a separate sheet of paper.

3. To maximize the learning process, it is to your advantage to do the following exercises as directed. To refer to the terminology listings before completing these exercises invalidates the learning process.

Prefixes

Give the definitions of the following prefixes:

1. ad- _____   2. dia- _____

3. endo- _____   4. eu- _____

5. ex- _____   6. exo- _____

7. hyper- _____   8. hypo- _____

9. pan- _____   10. para- _____

11. pro- _____

Roots and Combining Forms

Give the definitions of the following roots and combining forms:

1. acid _____   2. acro _____

3. aden _____   4. adeno _____

5. cortic _____   6. creat _____

7. cretin _____   8. crin _____

9. crine _____   10. crino _____

11. dwarf _____   12. galacto _____

13. ger _____   14. gigant _____

15. glandul _____   16. gluco _____

17. gonad _____   18. hirsut _____

19. insul _____   20. insulin _____

21. insulino _____   22. kal _____

23. letharg _____   24. log _____

25. myx _____   26. ophthalm _____

27. pine _____   28. pineal _____

29. pituitar _____   30. ren _____

31. reno _____   32. scler _____

33. thym _____   34. thymo _____

35. thyr _____   36. thyro _____

37. toxic _____   38. trop _____

39. viril _____

Suffixes

Give the definitions of the following suffixes:

1. -al _____   2. -algia _____

3. -ar _____   4. -betes _____

5. -ectomy _____   6. -edema _____

7. -emia _____   8. -genic _____

9. -ia _____   10. -ic _____

11. -ism _____   12. -ist _____

13. -itis _____   14. -logy _____

15. -malacia _____   16. -megaly _____

17. -oid _____   18. -oma _____

19. -osis _____   20. -pathy _____

21. -pexy _____   22. -physis _____

23. -ptosis _____   24. -rrhea _____

25. -therapy _____   26. -tome _____

27. -y _____

▶ Identifying Medical Terms

In the spaces provided, write the medical terms for the following meanings:

1. _____   Any disease condition of a gland

2. _____   A congenital deficiency in secretion of the thyroid hormone

3. _____   A disease characterized by excessive discharge of urine

4. _____   The study of the endocrine system

5. _____   Normal activity of the thyroid gland

6. _____   External secretion of a gland

7. _____   A condition of being abnormally large

8. _____   A general classification of the adrenal cortex hormones

9. _____   An excessive amount of potassium in the blood

10. _____   Deficient secretion of any gland

11. _____   Deficient internal secretion of the gonads

12. _____   Pertaining to drowsiness; sluggishness

13. _____   A tumor of the pineal body

14. _____   Inflammation of the thymus

▶ Spelling

In the spaces provided, write the correct spelling of these misspelled terms:

1. adensclrosis _____   2. crtinism _____

3. exopthalmic _____   4. hypthyoidism _____

5. myexdema _____   6. pinael _____

7. pitutary _____   8. thyoid _____

9. thyrtome _____   10. virlism _____

WORD PARTS STUDY SHEET

Word Parts	Give the Meaning
endo-	
eu-	
ex-, exo-	
hyper-	
hypo-	
pan-	
pro-	
acro-	
aden-, adeno-	
creat-	
crin-, crine-, crino-	
dwarf-	
ger-	
gigant-	
insul-, insulin-, insulino-	
letharg-	
myx-	
pine-	
pituitar-	
ren-	
scler-	
thym-, thymo-	
thyr-, thyro-	
trop-	
viril-	
-betes	
-edema	

-emia   _____

-genic   _____

-ia, -ism, -osis   _____

-malacia   _____

-megaly   _____

-oid   _____

-oma   _____

-pathy   _____

-pexy   _____

-physis   _____

-ptosis   _____

-rrhea   _____

-therapy   _____

REVIEW QUESTIONS

▶ Matching

Select the appropriate lettered meaning for each numbered line.

_____ 1. aldosterone

_____ 2. androgen

_____ 3. catecholamines

_____ 4. cortisone

_____ 5. dopamine

_____ 6. epinephrine

_____ 7. insulin

_____ 8. iodine

_____ 9. thyroxine

_____ 10. vasopressin

a. Also called antidiuretic hormone, ADH

b. Biochemical substances, epinephrine, norepinephrine, and dopamine

c. A hormone essential for the metabolism of carbohydrates and fats

d. A hormone produced by the thyroid gland

e. The principal mineralocorticoid secreted by the adrenal cortex

f. Hormones that produce or stimulate the development of male characteristics

g. A glucocorticoid hormone used as an anti-inflammatory agent

h. An intermediate substance in the synthesis of norepinephrine

i. Also called adrenaline, Adrenalin

j. A trace mineral that aids in the development and functioning of the thyroid gland

k. A hormone produced by the testes

▶ Abbreviations

Place the correct word, phrase, or abbreviation in the space provided.

1. basal metabolic rate _____

2. diabetes mellitus _____

3. FBS _____

4. GTT _____

5. protein-bound iodine _____

6. PTH _____

7. RIA _____

8. somatotropin hormone _____

9. TFS _____

10. VP _____

▶ Diagnostic and Laboratory Tests

Select the best answer to each multiple choice question. Circle the letter of your choice.

1. A test performed on urine to determine the amount of epinephrine and
    norepinephrine present.
    a. catecholamines
    b. corticotropin
    c. protein-bound iodine
    d. total calcium

2. Increased levels may indicate diabetes mellitus, diabetes acidosis, and many other
    conditions.
    a. protein-bound iodine
    b. total calcium
    c. fasting blood sugar
    d. thyroid scan

3. A test used to detect tumors of the thyroid gland.
    a. thyroxine
    b. total calcium
    c. thyroid scan
    d. protein-bound iodine

4. A blood sugar test performed at specific intervals after the patient has been given a
    certain amount of glucose.
    a. fasting blood sugar
    b. glucose tolerance test
    c. protein-bound iodine
    d. corticotropin

5. A test used in the diagnosing of adrenal tumors.
    a. 17-HCS
    b. 17-OHCS
    c. 17-KS
    d. 17-HDL

CRITICAL THINKING ACTIVITY

▶ **Case Study**

Diabetes Mellitus Type I—IDDM

Please read the following case study and then answer the questions that follow.

A 20-year-old female was seen by a physician and the following is a synopsis of the visit.

Present History: The patient states that she has been very thirsty and hungry and urinating a lot. She says that diabetes runs in her family, and she is concerned that she may be developing the disease.

Signs and Symptoms: Chief complaints: polydipsia, polyphagia, polyuria.

Diagnosis: Diabetes mellitus Type I—IDDM. The diagnosis was determined by the characteristic symptoms, family history, a blood glucose test, and a glucose tolerance test.

Treatment: The management of diabetes mellitus Type I is based on trying to normalize insulin activity and blood glucose levels to reduce the development of complications of the disease. The patient was instructed in insulin therapy, diet therapy, an exercise program, and lifestyle modifications. The patient was taught how to properly administer insulin, with dosage based on her blood glucose test performed before breakfast, lunch, and dinner. A follow-up visit was scheduled for 2 weeks with instructions to call if there were any questions or problems.

Critical Thinking Questions

1. Signs and symptoms of diabetes mellitus Type I include _____, polyphagia, and polyuria.

2. The diagnosis was determined by the characteristic symptoms, family history, a blood glucose test, and a _____ tolerance test.

3. Treatment for diabetes mellitus Type I includes insulin therapy, _____ therapy, an exercise program, and lifestyle changes.

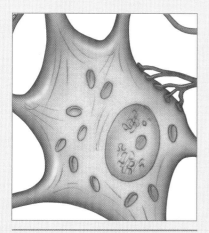

12

THE NERVOUS SYSTEM

OBJECTIVES

On completion of this chapter, you should be able to:

- Describe the tissues of the nervous system.
- Describe nerve fibers, nerves, and tracts.
- Describe the transmission of nerve impulses.
- Describe the central nervous system.
- Describe the peripheral nervous system.
- Describe the autonomic nervous system.
- Analyze, build, spell, and pronounce medical words that relate to surgical procedures and pathology.
- Identify and give the meaning of selected vocabulary words.
- Identify and define selected abbreviations.
- Review Drug Highlights presented in this chapter.
- Provide the description of diagnostic and laboratory tests related to the nervous system.
- Successfully complete the study and review section.

▶ ANATOMY AND PHYSIOLOGY OVERVIEW

The nervous system is usually described as having two interconnected divisions: the CNS or *central nervous system* and the PNS or *peripheral nervous system*. The CNS includes the brain and spinal cord. It is enclosed by the bones of the skull and spinal column. The PNS consists of the network of nerves and neural tissues branching throughout the body from 12 pairs of cranial nerves and 31 pairs of spinal nerves. See Figure 12–1. A general description of the nervous system and its functions is provided in this overview.

▶ TISSUES OF THE NERVOUS SYSTEM

There are two principal tissue types in the nervous system. These tissues are made up of *neurons* or nerve cells and their supporting tissues, collectively called *neuroglia*. Neurons are the structural and functional units of the nervous system. These cells are specialized conductors of impulses that enable the body to interact with its internal and external environments. There are several types of neurons, three of which are described for you.

MOTOR NEURONS

Motor neurons cause contractions in muscles and secretions from glands and organs. They also act to inhibit the actions of glands and organs, thereby controlling most of the body's functions. Motor neurons may be described as being *efferent* processes as they transmit impulses away from the neural cell body to the muscles or organs to be innervated. Motor neurons consist of a nucleated cell body with protoplasmic processes extending away from it in several directions. These processes are known as the *axon* and *dendrites*. Most axons are long and are covered with a fatty substance, the myelin sheath,

THE NERVOUS SYSTEM

ORGAN/STRUCTURE	PRIMARY FUNCTIONS
Neurons (nerve cells)	Structural and functional units of the nervous system. Specialized conductors of impulses that enable the body to interact with its internal and external environments
Neuroglia	Supporting tissue
Nerve Fibers and Tracts	Conduct impulses from one location to another
Central Nervous System	Receives impulses from throughout the body, processes the information, and responds with an appropriate action
Brain	Governs sensory perception, emotions, consciousness, memory, and voluntary movements
Spinal cord	Conduct sensory impulses to the brain; conduct motor impulses from the brain to body parts, and serves as a reflex center for impulses entering and leaving the spinal cord without involvement of the brain
Peripheral Nervous System	Links the central nervous system with other parts of the body
Cranial nerves (12 pairs)	Provide sensory input and motor control, or a combination of these
Spinal nerves (31 pairs)	Carry impulses to the spinal cord and to muscles, organs, and glands
Autonomic Nervous System	Controls involuntary bodily functions such as sweating and arterial blood pressure

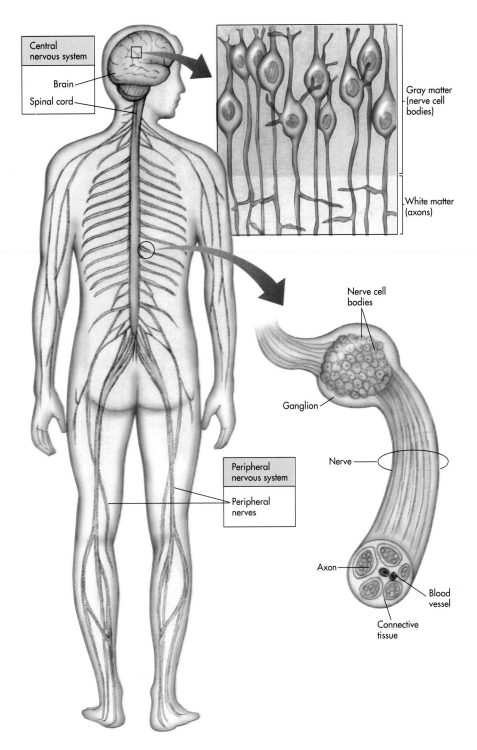

FIGURE 12–1

The nervous system is described as having two interconnected divisions: the central nervous system (CNS) consisting of the brain and spinal cord, and the peripheral nervous system (PNS) consisting of peripheral nerves.

that acts as an insulator and increases the transmission velocity of the nerve fiber it surrounds. Axons may be as long as several feet and reach from the cell body to the area to be activated. Dendrites resemble the branches of a tree, are short, or unsheathed, and transmit impulses to the cell body. Neurons usually have several dendrites and only one axon (Fig. 12–2).

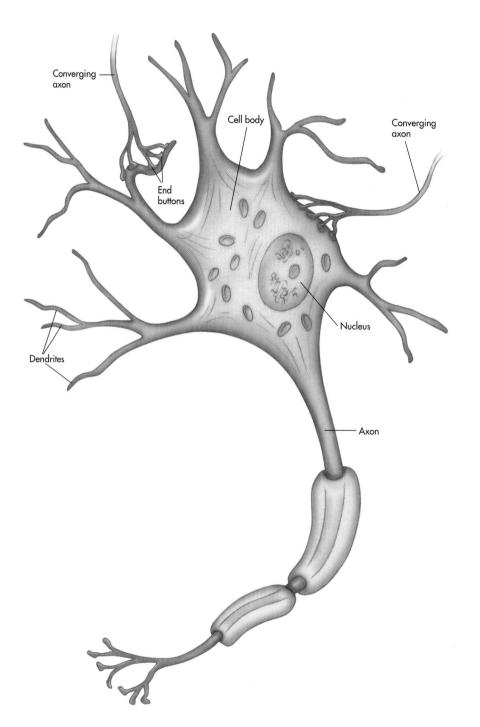

FIGURE 12–2

A neuron (nerve cell) with two converging axons.

SENSORY NEURONS

Sensory neurons differ in structure from motor neurons because they do not have true dendrites. The processes transmitting sensory information to the cell bodies of these neurons are called peripheral processes, are sheathed, and resemble axons. They are attached to sensory receptors and transmit impulses to the central nervous system (CNS). In turn, the CNS may stimulate motor neurons in response to this sensory information. Sensory neurons are sometimes referred to as *afferent nerves* as they carry impulses to the cell body and the central nervous system.

INTERNEURONS

Interneurons are sometimes called *central* or *associative neurons* and are located entirely within the central nervous system. They function to mediate impulses between sensory and motor neurons.

▶ NERVE FIBERS, NERVES, AND TRACTS

The terms *nerve fiber, nerve,* and *tract* are used to describe neuronal processes conducting impulses from one location to another. Each term is defined.

NERVE FIBER

A single elongated process, usually a long axon or a peripheral process from a sensory neuron, is called a *nerve fiber.* Each peripheral nerve fiber is wrapped by a protective membrane called a *sheath.* There are two types of sheaths, *myelinated (thick)* and *unmyelinated (thin),* formed by accessory cells. Some nerve fibers have only the unmyelinated sheath or neurilemma composed of *Schwann cells.* Myelinated fibers have an inner sheath of myelin, a thick fatty substance, and an outer sheath, the *neurilemma.* Nerve fibers of the central nervous system *(within the brain and spinal cord)* do not contain Schwann cells, which are necessary for the regeneration of a damaged nerve fiber. Therefore, damage to fibers of the CNS is permanent, whereas damage to a peripheral nerve may be reversible.

NERVE

A *nerve* is a bundle of nerve fibers, located outside the brain and spinal cord, that connects to various parts of the body. Nerves are usually described as being *afferent (conducting to the CNS)* or *efferent (conducting to muscles, organs, and glands).* Some nerves contain a mixture of afferent and efferent fibers and are called *mixed nerves.* Nerves are also referred to as sensory *(afferent)* and motor *(efferent).*

TRACTS

Groups of nerve fibers within the central nervous system are sometimes referred to as *tracts* when they have the same origin, function, and termination. The spinal cord contains afferent sensory tracts ascending to the brain and efferent motor tracts descending from the brain. The brain itself contains numerous tracts, the largest of which is the *corpus callosum* joining the left and right hemispheres.

▶ TRANSMISSION OF NERVE IMPULSES

Stimulation of a nerve occurs at a *receptor.* Sensory receptors are of different types, ranging from the simplest, which are free nerve endings for pain, to the most complex, as in the retina of the eye for vision. Receptors are generally specialized to specific types of stimulation such as heat, cold, light, pressure, or pain and react by initiating a chemical change or impulse. The transmission of an impulse by a nerve fiber is based on the *all-or-none principle.* This means that no transmission occurs until the stimulus reaches a set minimum strength, which may vary with different receptors. Once the minimum stimulus or threshold is reached, a maximum impulse is produced. A stimulation that is stronger than the minimum needed does not produce a larger impulse. Impulses travel from receptors, through dendrites or peripheral processes, to the neural cell bodies and on to an axon that terminates in several specialized knob-like branch endings. At this point, called a *synapse,* the impulse is transmitted, with the help of certain chemical agents, across a space separating the axon's end knobs from the dendrites of the next neuron or from a motor end plate attached to a muscle. This space is called a *synaptic cleft,* and the chemical agents released are called *neurotransmitters.* They are discharged into the synaptic cleft and alter the permeability of the postsynaptic membrane in which the cleft is located. This alternation may have an excitatory effect or, in some cases, an inhibitory effect, depending on the chemical reaction that occurs when the neurotransmitter crosses the synaptic cleft.

▶ THE CENTRAL NERVOUS SYSTEM (CNS)

Consisting of the brain and spinal cord, the *central nervous system* receives impulses from throughout the body, processes the information, and responds with an appropriate action. This activity may be at the conscious or unconscious level, depending on the source of the sensory stimulus. Both the brain and spinal cord can be divided into *gray* and *white matter.* The gray matter consists of unsheathed cell bodies and true dendrites. The white matter is composed of myelinated nerve fibers. In the spinal cord, the arrangement of white and gray matter results in an H-shaped core of gray cell bodies surrounded by tracts of nerve fibers interconnected to the brain. The reverse is generally true of the brain where the surface layer or cortex is gray matter and most of the internal structures are white matter.

THE BRAIN

The nervous tissue of the *brain* consists of millions of nerve cells and fibers. It is the largest mass of nervous tissue in the body, weighing about 1380 g in the male and 1250 g in the female. When fully developed, the brain fills the cranial cavity and is enclosed by three membranes known collectively as the *meninges.* From the outside in, these are the *dura mater, arachnoid,* and *pia mater.* The major substructures or divisions of the brain are the *cerebrum, diencephalon, midbrain, cerebellum, pons, medulla oblongata,* and the *reticular formation* (Fig. 12–3).

The Cerebrum

Representing seven eighths of the brain's total weight, the *cerebrum* contains nerve centers that govern all sensory and motor activity, including sensory perception, emotions, consciousness, memory, and voluntary movements. See Table 12–1. It is divided by the longitudinal fissure into two cerebral hemispheres, the right and left, that are joined by large fiber tracts *(the corpus callosum)* that allow information to pass from one hemisphere to the other. The surface or *cortex* of each hemisphere is arranged in folds creat-

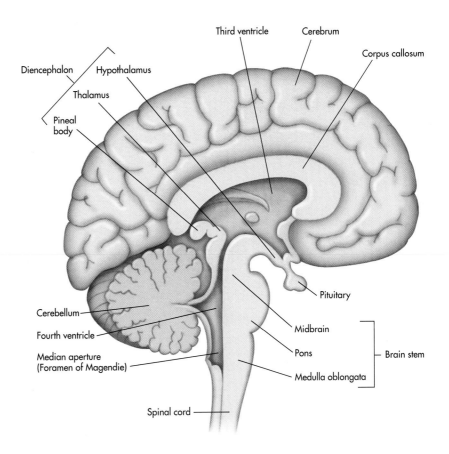

FIGURE 12-3

The major divisions of the brain.

ing bulges and shallow furrows. Each bulge is called a *gyrus* or *convolution*. A furrow is known as a *sulcus*. This surface is composed of gray, unmyelinated cell bodies and is known as the *cerebral cortex*. The cortex has been divided into lobes as a means of identifying certain locations. These lobes correspond to the overlying bones of the skull and are the *frontal lobe, parietal lobe, temporal lobe,* and *occipital lobe.*

Another reference system for locating areas of the cerebral cortex is by way of *fissures* and *sulci.* As noted earlier, the cerebrum is divided by a deep longitudinal fissure. Each hemisphere, thus created, contains *six major sulci.* The two most often used as reference points are the lateral and central sulci. The lateral sulcus lies below the frontal and parietal lobes and forms the upper border of the temporal lobe. The central sulcus runs from the longitudinal fissure to the lateral sulcus and separates the frontal lobe from the parietal lobe. The occipital lobe is the lower rear part of the cerebrum beneath the parietal lobe and posterior to the temporal lobe (Fig. 12–4).

Electrical stimulation of the various areas of the cortex during neurosurgery has identified specialized cell activity within the different lobes. The *frontal lobe* has been identified as the brain's major motor area. The *parietal lobe* contains centers for sensory input from all parts of the body and is known as the somesthetic area. Temperature, pressure, touch, and an awareness of muscle control are some of the sensory activities centered in this area. The *temporal lobe* contains centers for auditory and language input, and the *occipital lobe* is considered to be the primary sensory area for vision.

Throughout the cortex are areas known to integrate and store information. These memory or association areas comprise more than three fourths of the cerebral cortex. Below the cortex are masses of nerve fibers, the white matter, that interconnect areas

TABLE 12–1   Major Divisions of the Brain and Their Functions

Brain Area	Functions
Cerebrum	Governs all sensory and motor activity; sensory perception, emotions, consciousness, memory, and voluntary movements.
Diencephalon	
Thalamus	Relay center for all sensory impulses (except olfactory) being transmitted to the sensory areas of the cortex. Also relays motor impulses from the cerebellum and the basal ganglia to motor areas of the cortex. Thought to be involved with emotions and arousal mechanisms.
Hypothalamus	Principal regulator of autonomic nervous activity that is associated with behavior and expression. It also produces neurosecretions for the control of water balance, sugar and fat metabolism, regulation of body temperature, sleep-cycle control, appetite, and sexual arousal. Additionally, the hypothalamus produces hormones for the posterior pituitary gland.
Midbrain	Two-way conduction pathway; relay center for visual and auditory impulses. Contains afferent and efferent pathways connecting major motor areas of the forebrain and hindbrain, thereby serving as a two-way conduction pathway. Also found in the midbrain are four small masses of gray cells known collectively as the corpora quadrigemina. The upper two, called the superior colliculi, are associated with visual reflexes. The lower two, or inferior colliculi, are involved with the sense of hearing.
The Hindbrain	
Cerebellum	Coordination of voluntary movement.
Pons	Links the cerebellum and medulla to higher cortical areas; two-way conduction pathway between areas of the brain and other areas of the body; influences respiration.
Medulla oblongata	Cardiac, respiratory, and vasomotor control center. Regulation and control of breathing, swallowing, coughing, sneezing, and vomiting. Also regulates arterial blood pressure, thereby exerting control over the circulation of blood.
Recticular formation	Exerts control over or influences wakefulness, sleep, and certain reflex activities of the spinal nerves.

within the brain and lead to the spinal cord. Four paired masses of gray matter, the *dorsal ganglia,* have been found embedded within the white fibers. The dorsal ganglia function in the control of motor activity and an injury or a disease in this area can result in a loss of motor control.

The Diencephalon

The word *diencephalon* means "second portion of the brain" and refers to the thalamus and hypothalamus.

The Thalamus.   The *thalamus* is the largest of the two divisions of the diencephalon and is actually two large masses of gray cell bodies joined by a third or intermediate mass. The thalamus serves as a relay center for all sensory impulses *(except olfactory)* being transmitted to the sensory areas of the cortex. Besides its sensory function, the thalamus also relays motor impulses from the cerebellum and the basal ganglia to motor areas of the cortex. Some impulses related to emotional behavior are also passed from the hypothalamus, through the thalamus, to the cerebral cortex. See Table 12–1.

The Hypothalamus.   The *hypothalamus* lies beneath the thalamus and is a principal regulator of autonomic nervous activity that is associated with behavior and emotional

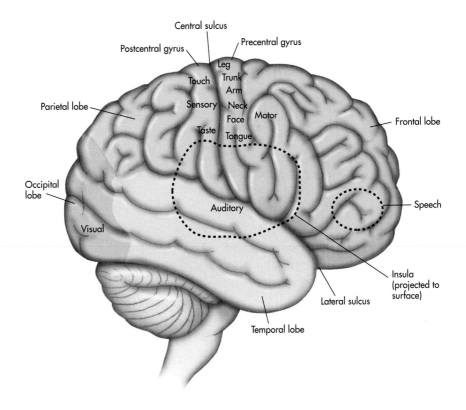

FIGURE 12–4

The brain, its lobes, and principal sulci. The location of certain sensory and motor areas are shown.

expression. It also produces neurosecretions for the control of water balance, sugar and fat metabolism, regulation of body temperature, and other metabolic activities. Additionally, the hypothalamus produces hormones for the posterior pituitary gland and exerts control over secretions from both the anterior and posterior pituitary. See Table 12–1. The pituitary gland is attached to the hypothalamus by a narrow stalk, the *infundibulum.*

The Midbrain

Located between the forebrain, which has just been described, and the hindbrain, the *midbrain* contains a number of large afferent and efferent pathways connecting major motor areas of the fore- and hindbrain. Also found in the midbrain are four small masses of gray cells known collectively as the *corpora quadrigemina.* The upper two, called the *superior colliculi,* are associated with visual reflexes such as the tracking movements of the eyes. The lower two, or *inferior colliculi,* are involved with the sense of hearing. See Table 12–1.

The Hindbrain

The *hindbrain* consists of the cerebellum, the pons, the medulla oblongata, and the recticular formation.

The Cerebellum.   The largest part of the hindbrain is the *cerebellum.* It occupies a space in the back of the skull, inferior to the cerebrum and dorsal to the pons and medulla oblongata. The cerebellum is oval in shape and divided into lobes by deep fissures. The surface of the cerebellum has a cortex of gray cell bodies, and its interior contains nerve fibers, white matter, connecting it to every part of the central nervous system. The cerebellum plays an important part in the coordination of voluntary movement. See Table 12–1.

The Pons.   The *pons* is a broad band of white matter located anterior to the cerebellum and between the midbrain and the medulla oblongata. The pons contains fiber tracts linking the cerebellum and medulla to higher cortical areas. See Table 12–1.

The Medulla Oblongata.   That part of the brain stem that connects the pons and the rest of the brain to the spinal cord is called the *medulla oblongata.* All the afferent and efferent tracts from the spinal cord either pass through or terminate in the medulla oblongata. The medulla also contains nerve centers instrumental to the regulation and control of breathing, swallowing, coughing, sneezing, and vomiting. Other centers in the medulla regulate arterial blood pressure, thereby exerting control over the circulation of blood. See Table 12–1.

The Reticular Formation.   The *reticular formation* is a diffuse network, consisting of small groups of cell bodies and their processes, located in the area of the brain stem. The reticular formation exerts control over or influences wakefulness, sleep, and certain reflex activities of the spinal nerves. See Table 12–1.

THE SPINAL CORD

As previously mentioned, the *spinal cord* has an H-shaped gray area of cell bodies encircled by an outer region of white matter. The white matter consists of nerve tracts and fibers providing sensory input to the brain and conducting motor impulses from the brain to spinal neurons. Other fibers connect nerve cells within the spinal cord with other areas of the cord. The spinal cord is about 44 cm long and extends down the vertebral canal from the medulla to terminate near the junction of the first and second lumbar vertebrae. The functions of the spinal cord are to conduct sensory impulses to the brain, to conduct motor impulses from the brain, and to serve as a reflex center for impulses entering and leaving the spinal cord without involvement of the brain (Fig. 12–5).

THE CEREBROSPINAL FLUID

The brain and spinal cord are surrounded by *cerebrospinal fluid.* This colorless fluid is produced by the *choroid plexuses* within the *ventricles* of the brain. There are four cavities or ventricles within the brain that are interconnected and are continuous with a small central canal that extends through the length of the spinal cord. Cerebrospinal fluid circulates through the ventricles, the central canal, and the subarachnoid space. This is a thin space between the arachnoid membrane and the pia mater, which is the membrane covering the surface of the brain and spinal cord. Cerebrospinal fluid is removed from circulation by the *arachnoid villi,* which are small projections of the arachnoid membrane that penetrate the tough outer membrane, the dura mater. The arachnoid villi allow the fluid to drain into the superior sagittal sinus. The normal adult will have between 120 and 150 mL of cerebrospinal fluid in circulation. The fluid serves to cushion the brain and cord from shocks that might cause injury. It also helps to support the brain by allowing it to float within the supporting liquid. It also contains neurotransmitters such as monoamines, acetylcholine, and neuropeptides.

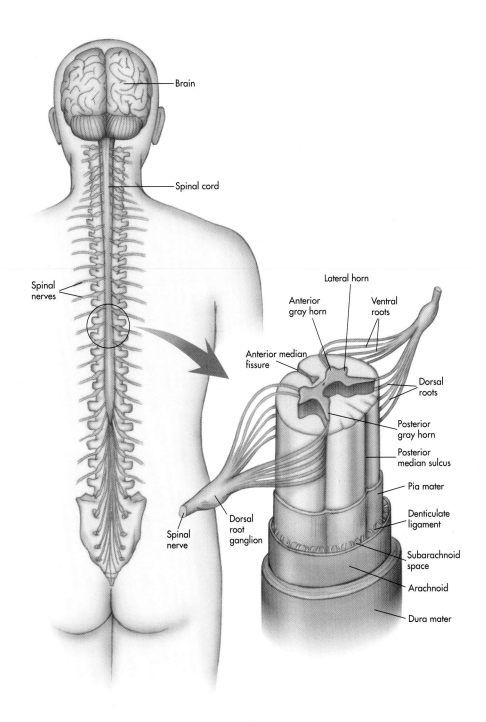

FIGURE 12-5

The brain, spinal cord, and spinal nerves. An expanded view of a spinal nerve is shown.

► THE PERIPHERAL NERVOUS SYSTEM (PNS)

The network of nerves branching throughout the body from the brain and spinal cord is known as the *peripheral nervous system*. There are 12 pairs of cranial nerves that attach to the brain and 31 pairs of spinal nerves connected to the spinal cord.

THE CRANIAL NERVES

The nerves described below attach to the brain and provide sensory input, motor control, or a combination of these functions. They are arranged symmetrically, 12 to each side of the brain, and generally are named for the area or function they serve (Fig. 12–6 and Table 12–2).

The Olfactory Nerve (I)

The *olfactory nerve* provides sensory input only and carries impulses for smell to the brain. The cell bodies of these nerve fibers are located in the nasal mucous membrane and serve as receptors for the sense of smell.

The Optic Nerve (II)

The *optic nerve* provides sensory input only and carries impulses for vision to the brain. The rods and cones of the eyes are receptors and transmit images through the cells of the retina to processes that form the optic nerve. The optic nerves from each eye unite after entering the cranial cavity to form the optic chiasm from which tracts, carrying images from both eyes, connect to the brain.

The Oculomotor Nerve (III)

The *oculomotor nerve* conducts motor impulses to four of the six external muscles of the eye and to the muscle that raises the eyelid. The cell bodies of motor nerves are located in the brain.

The Trochlear Nerve (IV)

The *trochlear nerve* conducts motor impulses to control the superior oblique muscle of the eyeball.

The Trigeminal Nerve (V)

The *trigeminal nerve* has both sensory and motor fibers. Its fibers form three sensory divisions, the ophthalmic, maxillary, and mandibular. These fibers provide sensory input from the face, nose, mouth, forehead, and top of the head. The mandibular division also contains motor fibers to the muscles of the jaw.

The Abducens Nerve (VI)

The *abducens nerve* conducts motor impulses to the lateral rectus muscle of the eyeball.

The Facial Nerve (VII)

The *facial nerve* has both sensory and motor fibers. Its motor fibers control the muscles of the face and scalp, thereby providing for facial expression. It also provides efferent fibers to control the lacrimal glands of the eyes as well as the submandibular and sublingual salivary glands. Sensory fibers of the facial nerve provide input from the forward two thirds of the tongue for the sense of taste.

The Acoustic Nerve (VIII)

Sometimes called the vestibulocochlear or auditory nerve, the *acoustic nerve* provides sensory input for hearing and equilibrium. Fibers of the cochlear division connect with receptors in the cochlea of the ear for hearing. Fibers of the vestibular division connect to receptors in the semicircular canals and vestibule located in the ear for the sense of equilibrium.

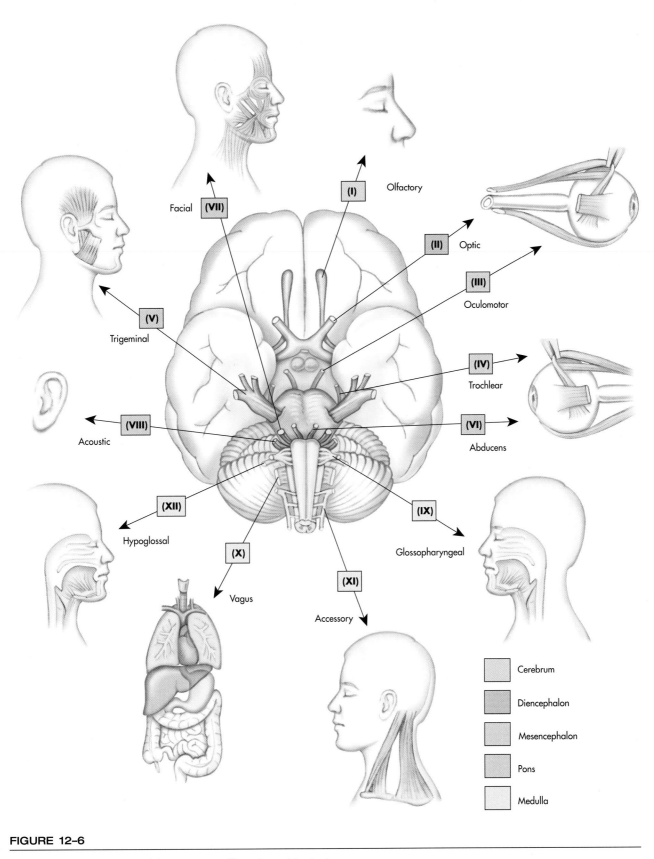

FIGURE 12–6

The relationship of the 12 cranial nerves to specific regions of the brain.

TABLE 12–2   Cranial Nerves and Functions

Nerve/Number	Function
Olfactory (I)	Sense of smell
Optic (II)	Vision
Oculomotor (III)	Motor impulses to four of the six external muscles of the eye and to the muscle that raises the eyelid
Trochlear (IV)	Motor impulses to control the superior oblique muscle of the eyeball
Trigeminal (V)	Provide sensory input from the face, nose, mouth, forehead, and top of the head; motor fibers to the muscles of the jaw (chewing)
Abducens (VI)	Conducts motor impulses to the lateral rectus muscle of the eyeball
Facial (VII)	Controls the muscles of the face and scalp; controls the lacrimal glands of the eye and the submandibular and sublingual salivary glands; input from the tongue for the sense of taste
Acoustic (VIII)	Input for hearing and equilibrium
Glossopharyngeal (IX)	General sense of taste; swallowing; control secretion of saliva
Vagus (X)	Controls muscles of the pharynx and larynx and of the thoracic and abdominal organs; swallowing, voice production, slowing of heartbeat, acceleration of peristalsis
Accessory (XI)	Control of the trapezius and sternocleidomastoid muscles, permitting movement of the head and shoulders
Hypoglossal (XII)	Control of the tongue; tongue movements

The Glossopharyngeal Nerve (IX)

The *glossopharyngeal nerve* has both sensory and motor fibers. The sensory fibers provide for the general sense of taste and attach to the back of the tongue and pharynx. Motor fibers innervate the stylopharyngeus muscle and are important to the act of the swallowing. Other efferent fibers control the secretion of saliva from the parotid gland.

The Vagus Nerve (X)

The *vagus nerve* contains both sensory and motor fibers and is the longest of the cranial nerves. The motor fibers control muscles of the pharynx and larynx. The sensory fibers provide input from the autonomic control of most of the organs in the thoracic and abdominal cavities.

The Accessory Nerve (XI)

The *accessory nerve* conducts motor impulses for the control of the trapezius and sternocleidomastoid muscles, permitting movement of the head and shoulders.

The Hypoglossal Nerve (XII)

The *hypoglossal nerve* conducts motor impulses for control of the muscles of the tongue.

THE SPINAL NERVES

There are 31 pairs of *spinal nerves* distributed along the length of the spinal cord and emerging from the vertebral canal on either side through the intervertebral foramina. At the point of attachment, each nerve is divided into *two roots* (see Fig. 12–5). The *dorsal* or *sensory root* is composed of afferent fibers carrying impulses to the cord, and the *ventral root* contains motor fibers carrying efferent impulses to muscles and organs. The cell bodies of the motor fibers lie in the gray matter of the spinal cord. The cell bodies for the sensory fibers are clustered just outside the spinal cord in small enlargements on each dorsal root. These enlargements are called the *spinal ganglia.* Named for the region of the vertebral column from which they exit, there are 8 pairs of *cervical spinal nerves,* 12 pairs of *thoracic spinal nerves,* 5 pairs of *lumbar spinal nerves,* 5 pairs of *sacral spinal nerves,* and 1 pair of *coccygeal spinal nerves.* A short distance from the cord, the fibers of the two roots unite to form a spinal nerve. Having formed a single nerve composed of afferent and efferent fibers, each spinal nerve then branches into several smaller nerves. The two primary branches from each spinal nerve are the *dorsal* and *ventral rami. (branches)* The dorsal rami *(branches)* carry motor and sensory fibers to the muscles and skin of the back and serve an area from the back of the head to the coccyx. The ventral rami, serving a much larger area, carry both motor and sensory fibers to the muscles and organs of the body, including the arms, legs, hands, and feet. The following describes the origin and purpose of the ventral branches of the 31 pairs of spinal nerves.

The ventral fibers from the first four cervical nerves form a network of interlaced nerve fibers called a *plexus,* which gives rise to peripheral nerves. Located in the neck, the *cervical plexus* innervates the muscles and skin of the neck and back of the head. The phrenic nerve, serving the diaphragm, also arises from the cervical plexus. Ventral fibers of cervical nerves 4 through 8 and the first thoracic nerve interlace to form the *brachial plexus.* Located in the area of the shoulder, the peripheral nerves from the brachial plexus innervate the shoulder, arm, forearm, wrist, and hand. The ventral rami of thoracic nerves 1 through 12 form the intercostal *(between the ribs)* nerves and the subcostal *(below the ribs)* nerves. Fibers of these nerves serve the muscles and skin of the thorax and upper abdomen. Ventral fibers of the first three and most of the fourth lumbar nerves interlace to form the *lumbar plexus.* Peripheral nerves from the lumbar plexus serve the muscles of the thigh and leg and the skin of the hip, scrotum, thigh, and leg. The ventral rami of the fourth and fifth lumbar together with those of the five sacral nerves interlace to form the *sacral plexus.* Peripheral nerves from the sacral plexus innervate the skin and muscles of the leg, foot, and external genitalia. Part of the fifth sacral and the entire coccygeal nerve are of limited importance and innervate the coccygeus muscle and the skin over the coccyx.

▶ THE AUTONOMIC NERVOUS SYSTEM (ANS)

Actually a part of the peripheral nervous system, the *autonomic nervous system* controls involuntary bodily functions such as sweating, secretions of glands, arterial blood pressure, smooth muscle tissue, and the heart. The autonomic nervous system is primarily composed of efferent fibers from certain cranial and spinal nerves and can be functionally divided into two divisions, the *sympathetic* and *parasympathetic.* These two divisions counteract each other's activity to keep the body in a state of homeostasis.

THE SYMPATHETIC DIVISION

Branches from the ventral roots of the 12 thoracic and the first 3 lumbar spinal nerves form the first part of the *sympathetic division.* The cell bodies of these nerve fibers are located in the *gray matter* of the spinal cord. Just outside the spinal cord, axons of these nerve cells leave the spinal nerves and enter almost immediately into masses of nerve cell bodies, the *sympathetic ganglia,* which form a chain that runs next to the vertebral column. This chain of about 23 ganglia runs from the base of the head to the coccyx and is known as the *sympathetic trunk.* Within the ganglia of the sympathetic trunk, fibers from the spinal nerves synapse with ganglionic nerve cell bodies. These ganglionic neurons produce long axons that reach to the parts of the body to be innervated. This arrangement, characteristic of autonomic nerves, creates a two-neuron chain as opposed to single-neuron control of regular motor nerves (Fig. 12–7).

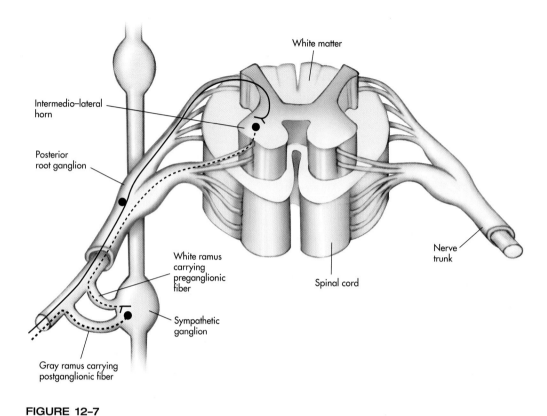

FIGURE 12-7

The origin of sympathetic neurons of the autonomic nervous system.

Because of the arrangement whereby *sympathetic fibers* from spinal nerves synapse with many cell bodies in the sympathetic ganglia, they tend to produce widespread innervation when activated. This condition has been described as preparing the individual for "fight or flight." On the other hand, fibers from the *parasympathetic division* have only the two-neuron chain and do not interact with as many cell bodies; therefore, their transmissions result in localized responses.

THE PARASYMPATHETIC DIVISION

Very long fibers branching from cranial nerves 3, 7, 9, and 10 along with long fibers of sacral nerves 2, 3, and 4 form the first stage of the *parasympathetic division*. Cell bodies for these long fibers are located in the brain and spinal cord. These long fibers extend to ganglia located close by the organs to be innervated. Fibers of *cranial* and *sacral nerves* synapse with ganglionic cell bodies, which then conduct impulses over short axons to the gland, smooth muscle tissue, or organ to be innervated. Fibers from the cranial nerves serve the iris and ciliary muscles of the eye, lacrimal glands, and salivary glands through four ganglia located in the head. Cranial nerve fibers extend via the vagus nerve to ganglia serving the thoracic, abdominal, and pelvic viscera. The fibers of the sacral spinal nerves form the pelvic nerve, which branches to synapse with small ganglia near or within the organs to be innervated. The cell bodies of these ganglia serve the lower colon, rectum, bladder, and reproductive organs. The *hypothalamus* is instrumental in the control of parasympathetic and sympathetic activity and is discussed elsewhere in this chapter and in Chapter 11, The Endocrine System.

LIFE SPAN CONSIDERATIONS

▶ THE CHILD

Neural tube development occurs about the third to fourth week of fetal life. This development becomes the **central nervous system.** At 6 weeks a developing baby's brain waves are measurable. At 28 weeks the fetal nervous system begins some regulatory functions. At 32 weeks the fetal nervous system is continuing to mature, so that rhythmic respirations and regulation of body temperature are possible if delivery of the fetus occurs at this time. Brain and nerve cell growth are most rapid from birth until about 4 years of age.

A baby's **brain** has three main structural parts: the **cerebrum,** the **cerebellum,** and the **brain stem.** The cerebrum serves as a control center as it receives, process, and acts on information. The cerebellum helps coordinate muscle activities and maintains posture and balance. The brain stem maintains vital body functions, such as breathing, heartbeat, blood pressure, digestion, and swallowing. While an infant's brain resembles an adult's, there is one area that is relatively unrefined. In an infant, the right and left hemispheres of the brain have not yet developed their own specific tasks. By the time a child is 3 years old, the two sides of the brain are well on their way to becoming specialized in different tasks.

While a baby is still in the womb, the brain is forging connections in the cerebellum, and the kicks and twitches that the fetus delivers to the mother are proof of this. At about four to six weeks of life, motor function is the main connection taking place in the brain. The initial movements characteristics of an infant soon give way to the repetition of smoother, deliberate ones as the brain's motor cortex process new signals and strengthens connections. Over the next 12 months, a baby's brain focuses first on gross-motor skills, such as holding up the head, rolling over, pushing up to a seated position, crawling, using the pincer grasp to pick up food. Between 2 and 4 years, the child will learn to run and kick a ball.

▶ THE OLDER ADULT

With aging, the number of nerve cells decrease, and there is a reduction in brain mass. Loss may occur in different areas of the brain and to varying degrees. In many older adults there is very little change in function, because a person has more nerve cells than needed. There is a decreasing levels of **neurotransmitters,** or chemicals communicating in synapse between nerve cells. This generally affects short-term memory, motor coordination, and control. The older adult has slower response time and decreased reflexes. Loss of cells in the brainstem changes sleep patterns. The older adult generally does not sleep as long or as well as a younger person. As one ages, the learning of new information and skills continues.

TERMINOLOGY

WITH SURGICAL PROCEDURES & PATHOLOGY

TERM	WORD PARTS			DEFINITION
acrophobia (ăk″ rō-fō′ bĭ-ă)	acro phobia	CF S	extremity fear	An abnormal fear of high places
akinesia (ă″ kĭ-nē′ zĭ-ă)	a kinesia	P S	lack of motion	A loss or lack of the power of voluntary motion
amentia (ă-mĕn′ shē-ah)	a ment ia	P R S	lack of mind condition	A congenital condition of mental retardation; *also called dementia*
amnesia (ăm-nē′ zĭ-ă)	a mnes ia	P R S	lack of memory condition	A condition in which there is a loss or lack of memory
analgesia (ăn″ ăl-jē′ zĭ-ă)	an algesia	P S	lack of pain	A lack of the sense of pain
anencephaly (ăn″ ĕn-sĕf′ ăl-ē)	an encephal y	P R S	lack of brain condition	A congenital condition in which there is a lack of development of the brain
anesthesia (ăn″ ĕs-thē′ zĭ-ă)	an esthesia	P S	lack of feeling	A loss or lack of the sense of feeling
anesthesiologist (ăn″ ĕs-thē″ zĭ-ŏl′ ō-jĭst)	an esthesio log ist	P CF R S	lack of feeling study of one who specializes	A physician who specializes in the science of anesthesia
aphagia (ă-fā′ jĭ-ă)	a phagia	P S	lack of to eat	A loss or lack of the ability to eat or swallow
aphasia (ă-fā′ zĭ-ă)	a phasia	P S	lack of to speak	A loss or lack of the ability to speak
apraxia (ă-prăks′ ĭ-ă)	a praxia	P S	lack of action	A loss or lack of the ability to use objects properly
arachnitis (ă″ răk-nī′ tĭs)	arachn itis	R S	spider inflammation	Inflammation of the arachnoid membrane
asthenia (ăs-thē′ nĭ-ă)	a sthenia	P S	lack of strength	A loss or lack of strength

Terminology - continued

TERM	WORD PARTS			DEFINITION
astrocyte (ăs′ trō-sīt)	astro cyte	P S	star-shaped cell	A star-shaped neuroglial cell with many branching processes
astrocytoma (ăs″ trō-sī-tō′ mă)	astro cyt oma	P R S	star-shaped cell tumor	A tumor composed of astrocytes
ataxia (ă-tăks′ ĭ-ă)	a taxia	P S	lack of order	A loss or lack of muscular coordination
atelencephalia (ăt-ĕl″ ĕn-sĭ-fā′ lĭ-ă)	atel encephal ia	R R S	imperfect brain condition	A congenital condition of imperfect development of the brain
atelomyelia (ăt″ ĕ-lō-mī-ē′ lĭ-ă)	atelo myel ia	CF R S	imperfect spinal cord condition	A condition of imperfect development of the spinal cord
bradykinesia (brăd″ ĭ-kĭ-nē′ sĭ-ă)	brady kinesia	P S	slow motion	An abnormal slowness of motion
bradylalia (brăd″ ĭ-lā′ lĭ-ă)	brady lalia	P S	slow to talk	An abnormal slowness of speech
cephalalgia (sĕf″ ă-lăl′ jĭ-ă)	cephal algia	R S	head pain	Head pain; *headache*
cephalohemo-meter (sĕf″ă-lō-hē-mōm′ ĕ-tĕr)	cephalo hemo meter	CF CF S	head blood instrument to measure	An instrument used to measure the intracranial blood pressure
cerebellar (sĕr″ ĕ-bĕl′ ăr)	cerebell ar	R S	little brain pertaining to	Pertaining to the cerebellum
cerebellospinal (sĕr″ ĕ-bĕl″ ō-spī′ năl)	cerebello spin al	CF R S	little brain a thorn, spine pertaining to	Pertaining to the cerebellum and spinal cord
cerebromalacia (sĕr″ ĕ-brō″ mă-lā′ shĭ-ă)	cerebro malacia	CF S	cerebrum softening	A softening of the cerebrum
cerebrospinal (sĕr″ ĕ-brō-spī′ năl)	cerebro spin al	CF R S	cerebrum a thorn, spine pertaining to	Pertaining to the cerebrum and the spinal cord
cordotomy (kŏr-dŏt′ ō-mē)	cordo tomy	CF S	cord incision	Surgical incision into the spinal cord, the anterolateral tracts, for relief of pain

continued

Terminology - continued

TERM	WORD PARTS			DEFINITION
craniectomy (krā″ nĭ-ĕk′ tō-mē)	crani ectomy	R S	skull excision	Surgical excision of a portion of the skull
craniocele (krā′ nĭ-ō-sēl)	cranio cele	CF S	skull hernia	Herniation of the brain substances through the skull
cranioplasty (krā′ nĭ-ō-plăs″ tē)	cranio plasty	CF S	skull surgical repair	Surgical repair of the skull
craniotomy (krā″ nĭ-ŏt′ ō-mē)	cranio tomy	CF S	skull incision	Surgical incision of the skull
diplegia (dī-plē′ jĭ-ă)	di(s) plegia	P S	two stroke, paralysis	Paralysis of identical parts on both sides of the body
diskectomy (dĭs-kĕk′ tō-mē)	disk ectomy	R S	a disk excision	Surgical excision of an intervertebral disk

 TERMINOLOGY SPOTLIGHT

Diskectomy is defined as surgical excision of an intervertebral disk. It is generally indicated when a disk ruptures. A ruptured disk occurs when the fiber-like outer lining of the disk degenerates. The center of the disk becomes mushy and essentially "squirts" out through the broken-down fibers. When this happens, the ruptured disk can pinch the spinal nerve root and press against the vertebra. A ruptured disk occurs most often from wear and tear on the disk. A pinched spinal nerve can cause leg pain, limiting daily activities; weakness in legs and feet; numbness in extremities; and impaired bowel and/or bladder functions.

A new procedure that may be used for a ruptured disk is called **microendoscopic diskectomy.** In this procedure a tiny camera, called an endoscope, is used to show the area around the ruptured disk on a monitor. The procedure requires a smaller incision than other surgical techniques and speeds up recovery time, which is about 3 weeks. During microendoscopic diskectomy surgery, a half-inch incision is made in the back and a tube is inserted into the incision. The tube allows the neurosurgeon to probe the area with the camera and insert surgical instruments. Once the muscle fibers are dilated, an opening is drilled through the spine and the endoscope is passed through the tube. Once the physician has the endoscope in place, he is able to find the nerve and the herniated part of the disk. He then removes the fragmented disk from the nerve.

Not everyone with a ruptured disk is a candidate for microendoscopic diskectomy. It is not recommended for extremely overweight people or for those whose disks have ruptured in an area that would make it difficult to use the endoscope.

dyslexia (dĭs-lĕks′ ĭ-ă)	dys lexia	P S	difficult diction	A condition in which an individual has difficulty in comprehending written language

Terminology - continued

TERM	WORD PARTS			DEFINITION
dysphasia (dĭs-fā′ zĭ-ă)	dys phasia	P S	difficult speak	Impairment of speech caused by a brain lesion
dysthymia (dĭs-thī′ mē-ă)	dys thym ia	P R S	difficult mind, emotion condition	A condition of mental disorder or disease
egocentric (ē″ gō-sĕn′ trĭk)	ego centr ic	CF R S	I, self center pertaining to	Pertaining to being self-centered
electroencephalo-graph (ē-lĕk″ trō-ĕn-sĕf′ ă-lō-grăf)	electro encephalo graph	CF CF S	electricity brain to write	An instrument used to record the electrical activity of the brain
electromyo-graphy (ē-lĕk″ trō-mī-ŏg′ ră-fē)	electro myo graphy	CF CF S	electricity muscle recording	The recording of the contraction of a skeletal muscle as a result of electrical stimulation; used in diagnosing disorders of nerves supplying muscles
encephalitis (ĕn-sĕf″ă-lī′ tĭs)	encephal itis	R S	brain inflammation	Inflammation of the brain
encephalocele (ĕn-sĕf′ ă-lō-sēl)	encephalo cele	CF S	brain hernia	Herniation of the brain via a congenital or traumatic opening of the skull
encephalomal-acia (ĕn-sĕf″ ă-lō-mă-lā′ sĭ-ă)	encephalo malacia	CF S	brain softening	A softening of the brain
encephalopathy (ĕn-sĕf″ă-lŏp′ ă-thē)	encephalo pathy	CF S	brain disease	Pertaining to any disease of the brain
epidural (ĕp″ ĭ-dū′ răl)	epi dur al	P R S	upon dura, hard pertaining to	Pertaining to situated upon the dura mater
foraminotomy (fō-răm″ ĭ-nŏt′ ō-mē)	foramino tomy	CF S	foramen incision	Surgical incision into the intervertebral foramen
ganglionectomy (gang″ lĭ-ō-nĕk′ tō-mē)	ganglion ectomy	R S	knot excision	Surgical excision of a ganglion (a mass of nerve tissue outside the brain and spinal cord)

continued

Terminology - continued

TERM	WORD PARTS			DEFINITION
glioma (glī-ō′ mă)	gli oma	R S	glue tumor	A tumor composed of neuroglial tissue
hemianopsia (hĕm″ ĭ-ă-nŏp′ sĭ-ă)	hemi an opsia	P P S	half lack of eye, vision	A condition of blindness of half the field of vision in one or both eyes
hemiparesis (hĕm″ ĭ-păr′ ĕ-sĭs)	hemi paresis	P S	half weakness	Slight paralysis that affects one side of the body
hemiplegia (hĕm″ ĭ-plē′ jĭ-ă)	hemi plegia	P S	half stroke, paralysis	Paralysis that affects one half of the body
hydrocephalus (hī″ drō-sĕf′ ă-lŭs)	hydro cephal us	P R S	water head pertaining to	Pertaining to an increased amount of cerebrospinal fluid within the brain
hyperesthesia (hī″ pĕr-ĕs-thē′ zĭ-ă)	hyper esthesia	P S	excessive feeling	Excessive feelings of sensory stimuli, such as pain, touch, or sound
hyperkinesis (hī″ pĕr-kĭn-ē′ sĭs)	hyper kinesis	P S	excessive motion	Excessive muscular movement and motion; inability to be still; *also known as hyperactivity*
hypermnesia (hī″ pĕrm-nē′ zĭ-ă)	hyper mnesia	P S	excessive memory	A state of excellent memory for names, dates, and details; may occur with psychosis, during neurosurgical procedures, or with brain injuries
hypnology (hĭp-nŏl′ ō-jē)	hypno logy	CF S	sleep study of	The scientific study of sleep
hypnosis (hĭp-nō′ sĭs)	hypn osis	R S	sleep condition of	An artificially induced condition of sleep
infratentorial (in″ frăh-tĕn-tō′ rĕ-ăl)	infra tentori al	P CF S	below tentorium, tent pertaining to	Pertaining to below the tentorium of the cerebellum
intracranial (ĭn″ trăh-krā′ nĕ-ăl)	intra crani al	P R S	within skull pertaining to	Pertaining to within the skull

Terminology - continued

TERM	WORD PARTS			DEFINITION
laminectomy (lăm″ ĭ-něk′ tō-mē)	lamin ectomy	R S	thin plate excision	Surgical excision of a vertebral posterior arch
lobotomy (lō-bŏt′ ō-mē)	lobo tomy	CF S	lobe incision	Surgical incision into the prefrontal or frontal lobe of the brain
logomania (lŏg″ ō-mā′ nĭ-ă)	logo mania	CF S	word madness	An excessive, repetitious, continuous flow of speech seen in monomania, a form of mental illness
macrocephalia (măk″ rō-sĕ-fā′ lĭ-ă)	macro cephal ia	CF R S	large head condition	A condition in which the head is abnormally large
meningioma (měn-ĭn″ jĭ-ō′ mă)	meningi oma	CF S	membrane tumor	A tumor of the meninges that originates in the arachnoidal tissue
meningitis (měn″ ĭn-jī′ tĭs)	mening itis	R S	membrane inflammation	Inflammation of the meninges of the spinal cord or brain
meningocele (měn-ĭn-gō-sēl)	meningo cele	CF S	membrane hernia	Congenital herniation of the skull or spinal column in which the meninges protrude through an opening
meningoence- **phalitis** (měn-ĭn″ gō-ĕn-sěf″ ă-lī′ tĭs)	meningo encephal itis	CF R S	membrane brain inflammation	Inflammation of the brain and its meninges
meningomyelo- **cele** (měn-ĭn″ gō-mī-ĕl′ ō-sēl)	meningo myelo cele	CF CF S	membrane spinal cord hernia	Congenital herniation of the spinal cord and meninges through a defect in the vertebral column
meningopathy (měn″ ĭn-gŏp′ă-thē)	meningo pathy	CF S	membrane disease	Any disease of the meninges
microcephalus (mī″ krō-sĕf′ ă-lŭs)	micro cephal us	P R S	small head pertaining to	Pertaining to an individual with a very small head
myelitis (mī″ ĕ-lī′ tĭs)	myel itis	R S	spinal cord inflammation	Inflammation of the spinal cord
myelodysplasia (mī″ ĕl-ō-dĭs-plā′ zĭ-ă)	myelo dys plasia	CF P S	spinal cord difficult formation	Difficult or defective formation of the spinal cord

continued

Terminology - continued

TERM	WORD PARTS			DEFINITION
myelography (mī″ ĕ-lŏg′ ră-fē)	myelo graphy	CF S	spinal cord recording	An x-ray recording of the spinal cord after injection of a radiopaque medium into the spinal canal
myelophthisis (mī″ ĕ-lŏf′ thĭ-sĭs)	myelo phthisis	CF S	spinal cord a wasting	Atrophy or a wasting away of the spinal cord
myelotome (mī-ĕl′ ō-tōm)	myelo tome	CF S	spinal cord instrument to cut	An instrument used to cut or dissect the spinal cord
neuralgia (nū-răl′ jĭ-ă)	neur algia	R S	nerve pain	Pain in a nerve or nerves
neurasthenia (nū″ răs-thē′ nĭ-ă)	neur asthenia	R S	nerve weakness	Nervous weakness, exhaustion, prostration common after depressed states
neurectomy (nū-rĕk′ tō-mē)	neur ectomy	R S	nerve excision	Surgical excision of a nerve
neurilemma (nū′ rĭ-lĕm″ mă)	neuri lemma	CF S	nerve a sheath, husk, rind	A thin membranous sheath that envelops a nerve fiber; *also called sheath of Schwann or neurolemma*
neuritis (nū-rī′ tĭs)	neur itis	R S	nerve inflammation	Inflammation of a nerve
neuroblast (nū′ rō-blăst)	neuro blast	CF S	nerve germ cell	The germ cell from which nervous tissue is formed
neuroblastoma (nū″ rō-blăs-tō′ mă)	neuro blast oma	CF S S	nerve germ cell tumor	A malignant tumor composed chiefly of neuroblast; occurs mostly in infants and children
neurocyte (nū′ rō-sīt)	neuro cyte	CF S	nerve cell	A nerve cell, a neuron
neuroglia (nū-rŏg′ lĭ-ă)	neuro glia	CF S	nerve glue	The supporting elements of the nervous system *(astrocytes, oligodendrocytes, and macroglia)*
neurologist (nū-rŏl′ ō-jĭst)	neuro log ist	CF R S	nerve study of one who specializes	One who specializes in the study of the nervous system

Terminology - continued

TERM	WORD PARTS			DEFINITION
neurology (nū-rŏl′ ō-jē)	neuro logy	CF S	nerve study of	The study of the nervous system
neurolysis (nū-rŏl′ ĭs-ĭs)	neuro lysis	CF S	nerve destruction	Destruction of nerve tissue
neuroma (nū-rō′ mă)	neur oma	R S	nerve tumor	A tumor of nerve cells and nerve fibers
neuromyelitis (nū″ rō-mī″ ĕl-ī′ tĭs)	neuro myel itis	CF R S	nerve spinal cord inflammation	Inflammation of the nerves and spinal cord
neuropathy (nū-rŏp′ ă-thē)	neuro pathy	CF S	nerve disease	Any nerve disease
neuroplasty (nū′ rō-plăs″ tē)	neuro plasty	CF S	nerve surgical repair	Surgical repair of a nerve or nerves
neurorrhaphy (nū-rōr′ ă-fē)	neuro rrhaphy	CF S	nerve suture	Suture of the ends of a severed nerve
neurosclerosis (nū″ rō-sklĕ-rō′ sĭs)	neuro scler osis	CF R S	nerve hardening condition of	A condition of hardening of nerve tissue
neurosis (nū-rō′ sĭs)	neur osis	R S	nerve condition of	An emotional condition or disorder
neurotomy (nū-rŏt′ ō-mē)	neuro tomy	CF S	nerve incision	Surgical incision or dissection of a nerve
neurotripsy (nū′ rō-trĭp″ sē)	neuro tripsy	CF S	nerve crushing	Surgical crushing of a nerve
oligodendroglio-ma (ŏl″ ĭ-gō-dĕn″ drō-glĭ-ō′ mă)	oligo dendro gli oma	P CF R S	little tree glue tumor	A malignant tumor derived and composed of oligodendroglia
papilledema (păp″ ĭl-ĕ-dē′ mă)	papill edema	R S	papilla swelling	Swelling of the optical disk, usually caused by increased intracranial pressure; also called choked disk
paranoia (păr″ ă-noy′ ă)	para noia	P S	beside mind	A mental disorder

continued

Terminology - continued

TERM	WORD PARTS			DEFINITION
paraplegia (păr″ă-plē′ jĭ-ă)	para plegia	P S	beside stroke, paralysis	Paralysis of both legs and, in some cases, the lower portion of the body
paresthesia (păr″ ĕs-thē′ zĭ-ă)	par esthesia	P S	beside feeling	An abnormal sensation, feeling of numbness, prickling or tingling
phagomania (făg″ ō-mā′ nĭ-ă)	phago mania	CF S	to eat madness	A madness for food
pheochromocy- toma (fē-ō-krō″ mō-sī-tō′ mă)	pheo chromo cyt oma	CF CF R S	dusky color cell tumor	A chromaffin cell tumor of the adrenal medulla or of the sympathetic nervous system
poliomyelitis (pōl″ ĭ-ō-mī″ ĕl-ī′ tĭs)	polio myel itis	CF R S	gray spinal cord inflammation	Inflammation of the gray matter of the spinal cord
polyneuritis (pŏl″ē nū-rī′ tĭs)	poly neur itis	P R S	many nerve inflammation	Inflammation of many nerves
psychologist (sī-kŏl′ ō-jĭst)	psycho log ist	CF R S	mind study of one who specializes	One who specializes in the study of the mind
psychology (sī-kŏl′ ō-jē)	psycho logy	CF S	mind study of	The study of the mind
psychosis (sī-kō′ sĭs)	psych osis	R S	mind condition of	An abnormal condition of the mind
psychosomatic (si″ kō-sō-măt′ĭk)	psycho somat ic	CF R S	mind body pertaining to	Pertaining to the interrelationship of the mind and the body
pyromania (pī″ rō-mā′ nĭ-ă)	pyro mania	P S	fire madness	A madness for fire
quadriplegia (kwŏd″ rĭ plē′ jĭ-ă)	quadri plegia	P S	four stroke, paralysis	Paralysis of all four extremities
rachiomyelitis (rā″ kĭ-ō-mī″ ĕ-lī′ tĭs)	rachio myel itis	CF R S	spine spinal cord inflammation	Inflammation of the spinal cord

Terminology - continued

TERM	WORD PARTS			DEFINITION
radicotomy (răd″ i-kŏt′ ō-mē)	radico tomy	CF S	root incision	A division or section of spinal nerve roots; *also called rhizotomy*
radiculitis (ră-dĭk″ ū-li′ tĭs)	radicul itis	R S	root inflammation	Inflammation of spinal nerve roots
somnambulism (sŏm-năm′ bū-lĭzm)	somn ambul ism	R R S	sleep to walk condition of	A condition of sleepwalking
spondylosyn-desis (spŏn″ dĭ-lō-sĭn′ dĕ-sĭs)	spondylo syn desis	CF P S	vertebra together binding	A surgical procedure to bind vertebra after removal of a herniated disk; *also called, spinal fusion*
subdural (sŭb-dū′ răl)	sub dur al	P R S	below dura, hard pertaining to	Pertaining to below the dura mater
supratentorial (sū″ pră-tĕn-tō′ rĭ-ăl)	supra tentori al	P R S	above tentorium, tent pertaining to	Pertaining to above the tentorium
sympathectomy (sĭm″ pă-thĕk′ tō-mē)	sympath ectomy	R S	sympathy excision	Surgical excision of a portion of the sympathetic nervous system
sympathomime-tic (sĭm″ pă-thō-mĭm-ĕt′ ĭk)	sympatho mimetic	CF S	sympathy imitating	Imitating effects of the sympathetic nervous system
trephination (trĕf″ ĭn-ā′ shŭn)	trephinat ion	R S	a bore, a hole process	The process of using a cylindrical saw to cut a circular piece of bone out of the skull
vagotomy (vā-gŏt′ ō-mē)	vago tomy	CF S	vagus, wandering incision	Surgical incision of the vagus nerve
ventriculocister-nostomy (vĕn-trĭk″ ū-lō-sĭs″tĕr-nōs′ tō-mē)	ventriculo cisterno stomy	CF CF S	little belly reservoir, cavity new opening	Surgical creation of an opening between the third ventricle and the interpeduncular cistern for drainage of cerebrospinal fluid
ventriculometry (vĕn-trĭk″ ū-lōm′ ĕ trē)	ventriculo metry	CF S	little belly measurement	Measurement of intracranial pressure

VOCABULARY WORDS

Vocabulary words are terms that have not been divided into component parts. They are common words or specialized terms associated with the subject of this chapter. These words are provided to enhance your medical vocabulary.

WORD	DEFINITION
acetylcholine (ACh) (ăs″ ĕ-tĭl-kō′ lēn)	A cholinergic neurotransmitter that occurs in various tissues and organs of the body. It is thought to play an important role in the transmission of nerve impulses at synapses and myoneural junctions.
agoraphobia (ăg″ ō-ră-fō′ bĭ ă)	Abnormal fear of being alone in public places; an anxiety syndrome and panic disorder
akathisia (ăk″ ă-thĭ′ zĭ ă)	The inability to remain still, motor restlessness, and anxiety
Alzheimer's disease (ahlts′ hĭ-merz dĭ-zēz ′)	A severe form of senile dementia that may be due to some defect in the neurotransmitter system. There is cortical destruction that causes variable degrees of confusion, memory loss, and other cognitive defects.
amyotrophic lateral sclerosis (ALS) (ă-mī″ ō-trŏf′ ĭk lăt′ ĕr-ăl sklĕ-rō′ sĭs)	Muscular weakness, atrophy, with spasticity caused by degeneration of motor neurons of the spinal cord, medulla, and cortex; *also called Lou Gehrig's disease*
anorexia nervosa (ăn″ ō-rĕks′ ĭ-ă ner-vō′ să)	A complex psychological disorder in which the individual refuses to eat or has an aberrant eating pattern
apoplexy (ăp′ ō-plĕk″ sē)	A sudden loss of consciousness caused by an embolus, a thrombus, or rupture of an artery in the brain; *also called a stroke or CVA (cerebrovascular accident)*
autism (ŏ′ tĭzm)	A mental disorder in which the individual is self-absorbed, inaccessible, and unable to relate to others and has language disturbances. A syndrome usually beginning in infancy and becoming apparent in the first or second year of life.
biogenic amines (bī″ ō-jĕn′ ĭk ăm′ ēns)	Chemical substances *(neurotransmitters)* that alter cerebral and vascular functions; epinephrine, norepinephrine, acetylcholine, dopamine, and serotonin
bulimia (bū-lĭm′ ĭ-ă)	A condition of episodic binge eating with or without self-induced vomiting

Vocabulary - continued

WORD	DEFINITION
chemonucleo-lysis (kĕm″ ō-nŭ-klē-ŏl′ ĭ-sĭs)	A method of dissolving a herniated nucleus pulposis by injection of a chemolytic agent
chorea (kō-rē′ ă)	A condition of rapid, jerky involuntary muscular movements of the limbs or face
coma (kō′ mă)	An unconscious state or stupor from which the patient cannot be aroused
concussion (brain) (kōn-kŭsh′ ŭn)	A loss of consciousness, temporary or prolonged, caused by a blow to the head
delirium (dē-lĭr′ ĭ-ŭm)	A state of mental confusion marked by illusions, hallucinations, excitement, restlessness, delusions, and speech incoherence
dorsal cord stimulation (DCS) (dōr-săl kōrd stĭm′ ū-lā′ shŭn)	A procedure used to relieve pain of the spinal cord by electric stimulation
endorphins (ĕn-dor′ fĭns)	Chemical substances produced in the brain that act as natural analgesics *(opiates)*
enkephalins (ĕn-kĕf′ ă-lĭns)	Chemical substances produced in the brain that act as natural analgesics *(opiates)*. They bind to opiate receptor sites involved in pain perception.
epilepsy (ĕp′ ĭ-lĕp″ sē)	A disorder of cerebral function resulting from abnormal electrical activity or malfunctioning of the chemical substances of the brain
evoked potentials (ē-vōkd′ pō-tĕn′ shăls)	Changes in electrical activity of the nervous system that are elicited by a physical stimulus or psychological event. They are used for evaluation of sensory function, localization of brain lesions, and evaluation of higher nervous function.
herpes zoster (hĕr′ pēz zŏs′ tĕr)	An acute viral disease characterized by painful vesicular eruptions along the segment of the spinal or cranial nerves; *also called shingles*. See Figures 12–8 and 12–9.
lyssa (līs′ să)	An acute infectious disease of the central nervous system transmitted to humans through the bite of a rabid animal; *also called rabies, hydrophobia*
multiple sclerosis (mŭl′ tĭ-pl sklē′ -rō′ sĭs)	A chronic disease of the central nervous system marked by damage to the myelin sheath. Plaques occur in the brain and spinal cord causing tremor, weakness, incoordination, paresthesia, and disturbances in vision and speech.

continued

Vocabulary - continued

WORD	DEFINITION
myasthenia gravis (mĭ-ăs-thē′ nĭ-ă gră′ vĭs)	A chronic disease caused by a defect in the myoneural conduction system. It is characterized by progressive muscular weakness, primarily of the face and neck. Secondarily, it may involve the muscles of the trunk and extremities.
narcolepsy (nar′ kō-lĕp″ sē)	A chronic condition in which there are recurrent attacks of uncontrollable drowsiness and sleep
nerve transposition (nerv trăns″ pō-zĭ′ shŭn)	The surgical process of dissecting and transposing the ulnar nerve
neurofibroma (nū″rō-fĭ-brō′mă)	A fibrous connective tissue tumor, especially involving the Schwann cells of a nerve. See Figure 12–10.
neuroleptic (nŭ″ rō-lĕp′ tĭk)	Medicine that produces psychomotor slowing, emotional quieting, and extrapyramidal effects; also called antipsychotic
neuropeptide (nū″ rō-pĕp′ tīd)	Biochemical units of emotion
neurotransmitter (nū″ rō-trăns′ mĭt-ĕr)	Substances within neurons and the cerebrospinal fluid that allow nerve cells to communicate with one another
nucleotome (nū″ klē-ō-tōm)	An instrument *(probe)* used to remove fluid from a herniated, slipped, or ruptured disk
palsy (pawl′ zē)	A loss of sensation or an impairment of motor function; *also called paralysis.* There are many types of palsy
paresis (păr′ ē-sĭs)	A slight, partial, or incomplete paralysis
Parkinson's disease (păr′ kĭn-sŭnz dĭ-zēz′)	A chronic disease of the nervous system. It is characterized by a loss of equilibrium and by salivation, frustration, nausea, dryness of the mouth, and muscular tremors; also called paralysis agitans, shaking palsy.
paroxysm (păr′ ok-sĭzm)	A sudden recurrence of the symptoms of a disease, an exacerbation; *also means a spasm or seizure*
percutaneous diskectomy (pĕr″ kū-tā′ nē-ŭs dĭs-kĕk′ tō-mē)	A surgical procedure that can be done on an outpatient basis for slipped or herniated disks. With the use of fluoroscopy, the surgeon inserts a nucleotome into the middle of the affected spinal disk and removes the thick, sticky nucleus of the disk. This allows the disk to soften and contract, thereby relieving the pressure on the spinal nerve that caused the severe pain of the low back and leg.

Vocabulary - continued

WORD	DEFINITION
plethysmography (plē″ thĭz-mōg′ ră-fē)	A noninvasive neurovascular examination technique
receptor (rē-sĕp′ tōr)	A sensory nerve ending that receives and relays responses to stimuli
Reye's syndrome (rīz sĭn′ drōm)	An acute disease that causes edema of the brain and increased intracranial pressure, hypoglycemia, and fatty infiltration of the liver and other vital organs. Occurs in children and has a relation to aspirin administration. May be viral in origin.
rhizotomy (rī-zŏt′ ō-mē)	Surgical incision and sectioning of a nerve root
sciatica (sī-ăt′ ĭ-kă)	Severe pain along the course of the sciatic nerve
sleep (slēp)	A state of rest for the body and mind. There are two distinct types: REM for rapid eye movement, sometimes called dream sleep, and NREM for no rapid eye movement.
syncope (sĭn′ kŭ-pē)	A temporary loss of consciousness caused by a lack of blood supply to the brain; *also called fainting*
tactile (tăk′ tĭl)	Pertaining to the sense of touch
Tay-Sachs disease (tā săks′ dĭ-zēz′)	An inherited disease that predominantly affects Jewish children of Ashkenazi origin. It is a progressive disease marked by degeneration of brain tissue.
transcutaneous electrical nerve stimulations (TENS) (trăns-kū-tā′ nē-ŭs nerv stĭm′ ū-lā′ shŭn)	The use of mild electrical stimulation to interfere with the transmission of painful stimuli. It has proved useful in relieving pain in some patients.
ventriculostomy (vĕn-trĭk″ ū-lŏs′ tō-mē)	The surgical creation of an opening between the third ventricle and the interpeduncular cistern for the relief of hydrocephalus; also used to monitor intracranial pressure (ICP) following head injury

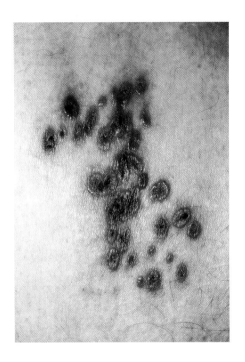

FIGURE 12-8

Herpes zoster. *(Courtesy of Jason L. Smith, MD.)*

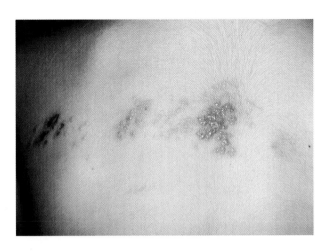

FIGURE 12-9

Herpes zoster. *(Courtesy of Jason L. Smith, MD.)*

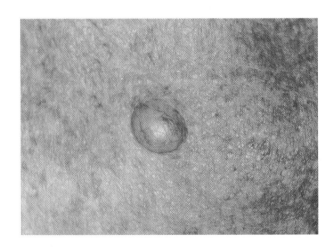

FIGURE 12-10

Neurofibroma. *(Courtesy of Jason L. Smith, MD.)*

ABBREVIATIONS

ACh	acetylcholine		**CP**	cerebral palsy
AD	Alzheimer's disease		**CSF**	cerebrospinal fluid
ALS	amyotrophic lateral sclerosis		**CT**	computerized tomography
ANS	autonomic nervous system		**CVA**	cerebrovascular accident
CBS	chronic brain syndrome		**DCS**	dorsal cord stimulation
CNS	central nervous system		**EEG**	electroencephalogram

EST	electric shock therapy	**MS**	multiple sclerosis
HDS	herniated disk syndrome	**NCV**	nerve conduction velocity
HNP	herniated nucleus pulposus	**PET**	positron emission tomography
ICP	intracranial pressure	**PNS**	peripheral nervous system
IVC	intraventricular catheter	**TENS**	transcutaneous electrical nerve stimulation
LP	lumbar puncture	**TIA**	transient ischemic attack
MR	mental retardation	**TNS**	transcutaneous nerve stimulation

DRUG HIGHLIGHTS

Drugs that are generally used for nervous system diseases and disorders include analgesics, analgesic-antipyretics, sedatives and hypnotics, antiparkinsonism drugs, anticonvulsants, and anesthetics.

Analgesics	Inhibit ascending pain pathways in the central nervous system. They increase pain threshold and alter pain perception.
Narcotic	*Examples: codeine phosphate, codeine sulfate, Dilaudid (hydromorphone HCl), Demerol (meperidine HCl), Darvon-N (propoxyphene napsylate), and morphine sulfate.*
Non-narcotic	*Examples: Stadol (butorphanol tartrate), Levorprome (methotrimeprazine), and Nubain (nalbuphine HCl).*
Analgesics-Antipyretics	Act to relieve pain (analgesic effect) and reduce fever (antipyretic effect). *Examples: Tylenol (acetaminophen); Bayer aspirin; Advil, Motrin, Nuprin (ibuprofen); and Naprosyn (naproxen).*
Sedatives and Hypnotics	Depress the central nervous system by interfering with the transmission of nerve impulses. Depending upon the dosage, barbiturates, benzodiazepines, and certain other drugs can produce either a sedative or a hypnotic effect. When used as a sedative, the dosage is designed to produce a calming effect without causing sleep. Used as a hypnotic, the dosage is sufficient to cause sleep.
Barbiturates	*Examples: Amytal (amobarbital), Butisol (butabarbital sodium), Nembutal (pentobarbital), Seconal (secobarbital), and Luminal (phenobarbital).*
Nonbarbiturates	*Examples: Noctec (chloral hydrate), Placidyl (ethchlorvynol), Dalmane (flurazepam HCl), Restoril (temazepam), and Halcion (triazolam).*
Antiparkinsonism Drugs	Exert an inhibitory effect upon the parasympathetic nervous system. They prolong the action of dopamine by blocking its uptake into presynaptic neurons in the central nervous system. *Examples: Symmetrel (amantadine HCl), Dopar (levodopa), Artane (trihexyphenidyl HCl), and Cogentin (benztropine mesylate).*
Anticonvulsants	Inhibit the spread of seizure activity in the motor cortex. *Examples: Dilantin (phenytoin), Tridione (trimethadione), Depakene (valproic acid), Mesantoin (mephenytoin), and Diamox (acetazolamide).*
Anesthetics	Interfere with the conduction of nerve impulses and are used to produce loss of sensation, muscle relaxation, and/or complete loss of consciousness. Block nerve transmission in the area to which they are applied.

Local	Block nerve transmission in the area to which they are applied. *Examples: Solarcaine (benzocaine), Nupercainal (dibucaine), Novocain (procaine HCl), Xylocaine (lidocaine HCl), and Tronothane (pramoxine HCl).*
General	Affect the central nervous system and produce either partial or complete loss of consciousness. They also produce analgesia, skeletal muscle relaxation, and reduction of reflex activity. *Examples: Pentothal (thiopental sodium), Fluothane (halothane), Penthrane (methoxyflurane), and nitrous oxide.*

DIAGNOSTIC AND LABORATORY TESTS

Test	Description
cerebral angiography (sĕr′ ĕ-brăl ăn″ jĭ-ŏg′ ră-fē)	The process of making an x-ray record of the cerebral arterial system. A radiopaque substance is injected into an artery of the arm or neck, and x-ray films of the head are taken. Cerebral aneurysms, tumors, or ruptured blood vessels may be visualized.
cerebrospinal fluid (CSF) analysis (sĕr″ ĕ-brō-spī′ năl floo′ ĭd ă-năl′ ĭ-sĭs)	Examination of spinal fluid for color, pressure, pH, and the level of protein, glucose, and leukocytes. Abnormal results may indicate hemorrhage, a tumor, and various disease processes.
computed tomography (CT) (kŏm-pū′ tĕd tō-mŏg″ ră-fē)	A diagnostic procedure used to study the structure of the brain. Computerized three-dimensional x-ray images allow the radiologist to differentiate between intracranial tumors, cysts, edema, and hemorrhage.
echoencephalography (ĕk″ ō-ĕn-sĕf′ ă-lŏg′ ră-fē)	The process of using ultrasound to determine the presence of a centrally located mass in the brain.
electroencephalography (EEG) (ē-lĕk-trō-ĕn-sĕf′ ă-lŏg′ ră-fē)	The process of determining the electrical activity of the brain via an electroencephalograph. Abnormal results may indicate epilepsy, brain tumor, infection, abscess, hemorrhage, and/or coma. Also brain "death" may be determined by an EEG.
lumbar puncture (lŭm′ băr pŭnk′ chūr)	Insertion of a needle into the lumbar subarachnoid space for removal of spinal fluid. The fluid is examined for color, pressure, and the level of protein, chloride, glucose, and leukocytes.
myelogram (mī′ ĕ-lō-grăm)	The x-ray of the spinal canal after the injection of a radiopaque dye. Useful in diagnosing spinal lesions, cysts, herniated disks, tumors, and nerve root damage.

Test	Description
neurologic examination (nū″-rō-lŏj′ ĭk ĕks-ăm″ ĭ-nā′ shŭn)	Assessment of a patient's vision, hearing, sense of taste, smell, touch and pain, position, temperature, gait, muscle strength, coordination, and reflex action. Used to determine a patient's neurologic status.
positron emission tomography (PET) (pŏz′ ĭ-trŏn ē-mĭsh′ ŭn tō-mŏg″ ră-fē)	A computer-based nuclear imaging procedure that can produce three-dimensional pictures of actual organ functioning. Useful in locating a brain lesion, in identifying blood flow and oxygen metabolism in stroke patients, in showing metabolic changes in Alzheimer's disease, and in studying biochemical changes associated with mental illness.
ultrasonography, brain (ŭl-tră-sŏn-ŏg′ ră-fē, brān)	The use of high-frequency sound waves to record echoes on an oscilloscope and film. Used as screening test or diagnostic tool.

COMMUNICATION ENRICHMENT

This segment is provided for those who wish to enhance their ability to communicate in either English or Spanish.

▶ Related Terms

English	Spanish
anxiety	ansiedad (ăn-sĭ-ĕ-dăd)
confused	confundido (cōn-fūn-dĭ-dō)
conscious	consciente (cōns-sĭ-ĕn-tĕ)
consciousness, loss of	perdida de consciencia (pĕr-dĭ-dă dĕ cōns-sĭ-ĕn-sĭ-ă)
convulsion	convulsión (cōn-vūl-sĭ-ōn)
coordination, loss of	perdida de coordinación (pĕr-dĭ-dă dĕ coor-dĭ-nă-sĭ-ōn)
cranial nerves	nervio craneal (nĕr-vĭ-ō kră-nĕ-ăl)

English	Spanish
depression	depresión (dĕ-prĕ-sĭ-ōn)
disorientation	desorientación (dē-sō-rĭ-ĕn-tă-sĭ-ōn)
emotional problems	problemas emocionales (prō-blĕ-măs ĕ-mō-sĭ-ō-nă-lĕs)
fainting	desmayo (dĕs-mă-yō)
headache	dolor de cabeza (dō-lōr dĕ kă-bĕ-ză)
insomnia	insomnio (ĭn-sōm-nĭ-ō)
loss of memory	perdida de memoria (pĕr-dĭ-dă dĕ mĕ-mō-rĭ-ă)
nervous	nervioso (nĕr-vĭ-ō-sō)
nervous system	sistema nervioso (sĭs-tĕ-mă nĕr-vĭ-ō-sō)
paralysis	parálisis (pă-ră-lĭ-sĭs)
polio	polio (pō-lĭ-ō)
psychiatric problem	problema psiquiatrico (prō-blĕ-mă sĭ-kĭă-trĭ-kō)
sensation, loss of	perdida de sensación (pĕr-dĭ-dă dĕ sĕn-să-sĭ-ōn)
stress	tensión (tĕn-sĭ-ōn)
stroke	latido (lă-tĭ-dō)
tremor	temblor (tĕm-blōr)
unconscious	inconsciente (ĭn-cōns-sĭ-ĕn-tĕ)
confuse	confundir (cōn-fūn-dĭr)

English	Spanish
nerve	nervio (*nĕr*-vĭ-ō)
knowledge	conocimiento (cō-*nō*-cĭ-mĭ-ĕn-tō)
cranium	cráneo (*kră*-nĕ-ō)
craniotomy	craneotomia (*kră*-nĕ-ō-tō-mĭ-ă)
nerve cell	neurona (nĕ-ū-*rō*-nă)
nerve fiber	fibra nerviosa (*fĭ*-bră *nĕr*-vĭ-ō-să)
concussion	concusión (cōn-*kū*-sĭ-ōn)
epilepsy	epilepsia (ĕ-pĭ-*lĕp*-sĭ-ă)
sleep	sueño (sū-*ĕ*-ñō)
fight	lucha (*lū*-chă)
flight	vuelo (*vū*-ĕ-lō)
"fight or flight"	"lucha o vuelo" (lū-chă ō vū-ĕ-lō)
hypnosis	hipnosis (*ĭp*-nō-sĭs)
neurology	neurología (nĕ-ū-rō-*lō*-hĭ-ă)
psychology	psicología (sĭ-kō-*lō*-hĭ-ă)

STUDY AND REVIEW SECTION

LEARNING EXERCISES

▶ Anatomy and Physiology

Write your answers to the following questions. Do not refer back to the text.

1. Name the two interconnected divisions of the nervous system.

   a. _____   b. _____

2. _____ are the structural and functional units of the nervous system.

3. State the three actions of motor neurons.

   a. _____

   b. _____

   c. _____

4. Describe an axon. _____

5. Describe a dendrite. _____

6. State an action of sensory nerves. _____

   _____

7. _____ function to mediate impulses between sensory and motor neurons.

8. Define the following terms:

   a. Nerve fiber _____

   b. Nerve _____

   c. Tracts _____

9. The central nervous system consists of the _____ and the

   _____ _____.

10. State three functions of the central nervous system.

    a. _____   b. _____

    c. _____

11. Name the three meninges enclosing the brain.

a. _____ b. _____ c. _____

12. Name the seven major divisions of the brain.

a. _____ b. _____

c. _____ d. _____

e. _____ f. _____

g. _____

13. The _____ _____ has been identified as the brain's major motor area.

14. The parietal lobe is also known as the _____ _____.

15. The temporal lobe contains centers for _____ and

_____ input.

16. The occipital lobe is the primary area for _____.

17. State the functions of the thalamus.

a. _____ b. _____

18. State three functions of the hypothalamus.

a. _____ b. _____

c. _____

19. The cerebellum plays an important part in the _____ of

_____ _____.

20. State five functions of the medulla oblongata.

a. _____ b. _____

c. _____ d. _____

e. _____

21. State the three functions of the spinal cord.

a. _____ b. _____

c. _____

22. The normal adult will have between _____ and

_____ mL of cerebrospinal fluid in circulation.

23. Name the 12 pairs of cranial nerves.

    a. _____   b. _____   c. _____

    d. _____   e. _____   f. _____

    g. _____   h. _____   i. _____

    j. _____   k. _____   l. _____

24. Name the four plexuses that are formed from the spinal nerves.

    a. _____   b. _____

    c. _____   d. _____

25. State four functions of the autonomic nervous system.

    a. _____   b. _____

    c. _____   d. _____

26. Name the two divisions of the autonomic nervous system.

    a. _____   b. _____

▶ Word Parts

1. In the spaces provided, write the definitions of these prefixes, roots, combining forms, and suffixes. Do not refer to the listings of terminology words. Leave blank those terms you cannot define.

2. After completing as many as you can, refer back to the terminology word listings to check your work. For each word missed or left blank, write the term and its definition several times on the margins of these pages or on a separate sheet of paper.

3. To maximize the learning process, it is to your advantage to do the following exercises as directed. To refer to the terminology listings before completing these exercises invalidates the learning process.

Prefixes

Give the definitions of the following prefixes:

1. a- _____   2. an- _____

3. astro- _____   4. brady- _____

5. di(s)- _____   6. dys- _____

7. epi- _____   8. hemi- _____

9. hydro- _____   10. hyper- _____

11. infra- _____

12. intra- _____

13. micro- _____

14. oligo- _____

15. par- _____

16. para- _____

17. poly- _____

18. pyro- _____

19. quadri- _____

20. sub- _____

21. supra- _____

22. syn- _____

Roots and Combining Forms

Give the definitions of the following roots and combining forms:

1. acro _____

2. ambul _____

3. arachn _____

4. atel _____

5. atelo _____

6. centr _____

7. cephal _____

8. cephalo _____

9. cerebell _____

10. cerebello _____

11. cerebro _____

12. chromo _____

13. cisterno _____

14. cordo _____

15. crani _____

16. cranio _____

17. cyt _____

18. dendro _____

19. disk _____

20. dur _____

21. ego _____

22. electro _____

23. encephal _____

24. encephalo _____

25. esthesio _____

26. foramino _____

27. ganglion _____

28. gli _____

29. hemo _____

30. hypn _____

31. hypno _____

32. lamin _____

33. lobo _____

34. log _____

35. logo _____

36. macro _____

37. mening _____

38. meningi _____

39. meningo _____

40. ment _____

41. mnes _____

42. myel _____

43. myelo _____
44. myo _____
45. neur _____
46. neuri _____
47. neuro _____
48. papill _____
49. phago _____
50. pheo _____
51. polio _____
52. psych _____
53. psycho _____
54. rachio _____
55. radico _____
56. radicul _____
57. scler _____
58. spin _____
59. spondylo _____
60. somat _____
61. somn _____
62. sympath _____
63. sympatho _____
64. tentori _____
65. thym _____
66. trephinat _____
67. vago _____
68. ventriculo _____

Suffixes

Give the definitions of the following suffixes:

1. -al _____
2. -algesia _____
3. -algia _____
4. -ar _____
5. -asthenia _____
6. -blast _____
7. -cele _____
8. -cyte _____
9. -desis _____
10. -ectomy _____
11. -edema _____
12. -esthesia _____
13. -glia _____
14. -gram _____
15. -graph _____
16. -graphy _____
17. -ia _____
18. -ic _____
19. -ion _____
20. -ism _____
21. -ist _____
22. -itis _____
23. -kinesia _____
24. -kinesis _____
25. -lalia _____
26. -lemma _____
27. -lexia _____
28. -logy _____

29. -lysis _____

30. -malacia _____

31. -mania _____

32. -meter _____

33. -metry _____

34. -mimetic _____

35. -mnesia _____

36. -noia _____

37. -oma _____

38. -opsia _____

39. -osis _____

40. -paresis _____

41. -pathy _____

42. -phagia _____

43. -phasia _____

44. -phobia _____

45. -phthisis _____

46. -plasia _____

47. -plasty _____

48. -plegia _____

49. -praxia _____

50. -rrhapy _____

51. -sthenia _____

52. -stomy _____

53. -taxia _____

54. -tome _____

55. -tomy _____

56. -tripsy _____

57. -us _____

58. -y _____

▶ **Identifying Medical Terms**

....

In the spaces provided, write the medical terms for the following meanings:

1. _____   A condition in which there is a loss or lack of memory

2. _____   A lack of the sense of pain

3. _____   A loss or lack of the ability to eat or swallow

4. _____   Inflammation of the arachnoid membrane

5. _____   A loss or lack of muscular coordination

6. _____   Head pain; headache

7. _____   Pertaining to the cerebellum

8. _____   Surgical excision of a portion of the skull

9. _____   A condition in which an individual has difficulty in comprehending written language

10. _____   Inflammation of the brain

11. _____ Pertaining to situated on the dura mater

12. _____ Paralysis that affects one side of the body

13. _____ The scientific study of sleep

14. _____ A condition in which the head is abnormally large

15. _____ Inflammation of the meninges of the spinal cord or brain

16. _____ Any disease of the meninges

17. _____ An instrument used to cut or dissect the spinal cord

18. _____ Pain in a nerve or nerves

19. _____ Inflammation of a nerve

20. _____ A nerve cell, a neuron

21. _____ The study of the nervous system

22. _____ A tumor of nerve cells and nerve fibers

23. _____ Surgical repair of a nerve or nerves

24. _____ An emotional condition or disorder

25. _____ A madness for food

26. _____ Inflammation of many nerves

27. _____ The study of the mind

28. _____ Inflammation of spinal nerve roots

29. _____ Surgical incision of the vagus nerve

30. _____ Measurement of intracranial pressure

▶ Spelling
....

In the spaces provided, write the correct spelling of these misspelled terms.

1. anestesia _____   2. atelomylia _____

3. cerebospinal _____   4. cranitomy _____

5. encephaocele _____   6. meningoma _____

7. meningmyelcele _____   8. neurpathy _____

9. polomyelitis _____   10. ventriulometry _____

WORD PARTS STUDY SHEET

Word Parts	Give the Meaning
astro-	_____
brady-	_____
hemi-	_____
hydro-	_____
infra-	_____
intra-	_____
micro-	_____
oligo-	_____
atel-, atelo-	_____
cephal-, cephalo-	_____
cerebell-, cerebello-	_____
cerebro-	_____
crani-, cranio-	_____
electro-	_____
encephal-, encephalo-	_____
foramino-	_____
hypn-	_____
lobo-	_____
logo-	_____
mening-, meningi-, meningo-	_____
myel-, myelo-	_____
neur-, neuri-, neuro-	_____
pheo-	_____
polio-	_____
rachio-	_____
radico-	_____
spin-	_____

-asthenia   _____

-cele   _____

-esthesia   _____

-graphy   _____

-kinesia, -kinesis _____

-mania   _____

-paresis   _____

-pathy   _____

-phobia   _____

-plegia   _____

-taxia   _____

-tome   _____

-tripsy   _____

REVIEW QUESTIONS

▶ Matching

Select the appropriate lettered meaning for each numbered line.

_____ 1. acetylcholine

_____ 2. Alzheimer's disease

_____ 3. apoplexy

_____ 4. endorphins

_____ 5. epilepsy

_____ 6. palsy

_____ 7. percutaneous diskectomy

_____ 8. neuropeptide

_____ 9. nucleotome

_____ 10. sciatica

a. An instrument used to remove fluid from a herniated, slipped, or ruptured disk

b. Chemical substances produced in the brain that act as natural analgesics

c. A stroke

d. A severe form of senile dementia

e. A disorder of cerebral function resulting from abnormal electrical activity or malfunctioning of the chemical substances of the brain

f. Biochemical units of emotion

g. A cholinergic neurotransmitter that occurs in various tissues and organs of the body

h. A loss of sensation or an impairment of motor function

i. Severe pain along the course of the sciatic nerve

j. A surgical procedure that can be done on an outpatient basis for slipped disk

k. An anxiety syndrome and panic disorder

▶ **Abbreviations**

Place the correct word, phrase, or abbreviation in the space provided.

1. Alzheimer's disease _____

2. amyotrophic lateral sclerosis _____

3. CNS _____

4. CP _____

5. computerized tomography _____

6. herniated disk syndrome _____

7. ICP _____

8. LP _____

9. MS _____

10. positron emission tomography _____

▶ **Diagnostic and Laboratory Tests**

Select the best answer to each multiple choice question. Circle the letter of your choice.

1. A diagnostic procedure used to study the structure of the brain.
   a. computed tomography
   b. echoencephalography
   c. electroencephalography
   d. myelogram

2. The process of using ultrasound to determine the presence of a centrally located mass in the brain.
   a. computed tomography
   b. echoencephalography
   c. electroencephalography
   d. myelogram

3. The x-ray of the spinal canal after the injection of a radiopaque dye.
   a. cerebral angiography
   b. computed tomography
   c. myelogram
   d. ultrasonography

4. A computer-based nuclear imaging procedure that can produce three-dimensional pictures of actual organ functioning.
   a. electroencephalography
   b. myelogram
   c. ultrasonography
   d. positron emission tomography

5. The use of high-frequency sound waves to record echoes on an oscilloscope and film.
    a. electroencephalography
    b. myelogram
    c. ultrasonography
    d. positron emission tomography

CRITICAL THINKING ACTIVITY

► **Case Study**

Alzheimer's Disease

Please read the following case study and then answer the questions that follow.

A 68-year-old female was seen by a physician and the following is a synopsis of the visit.

Present History: The husband states that he is very concerned about his wife. He has noticed that she has become confused and forgets where she puts things, and even puts things in the wrong place. Last Monday she put the iron in the freezer. The patient had very little to say about herself.

Signs and Symptoms: Chief complaint: Confusion, memory loss, and inappropriate placing of iron in the freezer.

Diagnosis: Alzheimer's. The diagnosis was determined by a complete physical examination, a medical history, neuropsychological testing, an electroencephalogram (EEG), and a computerized tomography (CT) scan.

Treatment: At this time there is no treatment available to stop or reverse the mental deterioration of Alzheimer's disease. Cognex (tacrine hydrochloride) capsules were approved by the FDA in 1993 for the treatment of mild to moderate dementia of the Alzheimer's type. The potential risks and benefits of the drug were discussed with the patient and her husband, and they decided not to try the medication at this time. Management of a patient with Alzheimer's involves support and assistance to the patient and her family. For more information you may call the Alzheimer's Association at 1–800–272–3900.

Prevention: There is no known prevention.

Critical Thinking Questions

1. Signs and symptoms of Alzheimer's disease include confusion, _____ loss, and the inappropriate placing of an object.

2. The diagnosis was determined by the a complete physical examination, a medical history, neuropsychological testing, an _____, and a computerized tomography scan.

3. Management of Alzheimer's involves support and _____.

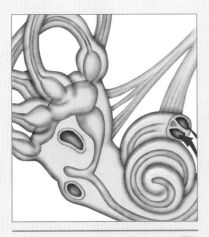

OUTLINE

13

SPECIAL SENSES: THE EAR

OBJECTIVES

On completion of this chapter, you should be able to:

- Describe the antomical structures of the ear.
- Describe the external ear.
- Describe the middle ear.
- Describe the inner ear.
- Analyze, build, spell, and pronounce medical words that relate to surgical procedures and pathology.
- Identify and give the meaning of selected vocabulary words.
- Identify and define selected abbreviations.
- Review Drug Highlights presented in this chapter.
- Provide the description of diagnostic and laboratory tests related to the ear.
- Successfully complete the study and review section

► ANATOMY AND PHYSIOLOGY OVERVIEW

The *ear* is the site of *hearing* and *equilibrium*. It contains specially designed anatomical structures that receive sound vibrations, are sensitive to the force of gravity, and react to the movements of the head. These anatomical structures are connected to sensory areas of the brain by specialized fibers from the eighth cranial nerve. The ear is generally described as having three distinct divisions: the *external ear*, the *middle ear*, and the *inner ear*. The following is a listing of the major components of the ear and some of their functions.

► THE EXTERNAL EAR

The *external ear* is the appendage on the side of the head consisting of the *auricle* or *pinna*, the *external acoustic meatus* or *auditory canal*, and the *tympanic membrane* or *eardrum*. The auricle collects sound waves that then pass through the auditory canal to vibrate the tympanic membrane that separates the external ear from the middle ear. The auditory canal is an S-shaped tubular structure about 2.5 cm long. Numerous glands line the canal and secrete *cerumen* or *earwax* to lubricate and protect the ear (Fig. 13–1).

SPECIAL SENSES: THE EAR

ORGAN/STRUCTURE	PRIMARY FUNCTIONS
The External Ear	
Auricle (pinna)	Collects and directs sound waves into the auditory canal and then into the tympanic membrane
Auditory canal (external acoustic meatus)	Numerous glands line the canal and secrete earwax to lubricate and protect the ear
Tympanic membrane (eardrum)	Separates the external ear from the middle ear
The Middle Ear	
Contains the ossicles: malleus, incus, and stapes; has five openings, and is lined with mucous membrane	Transmits sound vibrations Equalizes external/internal air pressure on the tympanic membrane Exerts control over potentially damaging or disruptive loud sounds
The Inner Ear	
Cochlea	Contains the organ of Corti, the organ of hearing
Vestibule	Contains the utricle and saccule, membranous pouches containing perilymph. The utricle communicates with the semicircular canals and contains hair cell sensory receptors connected to fibers from the eighth cranial nerve. These hair cells react to the force of gravity and movement and are a part of the sense of equilibrium.
The semicircular canals	Contains nerve endings in the form of hair cells that note changes in the position of the head and reports such movement to the brain through fibers leading to the eighth cranial nerve.

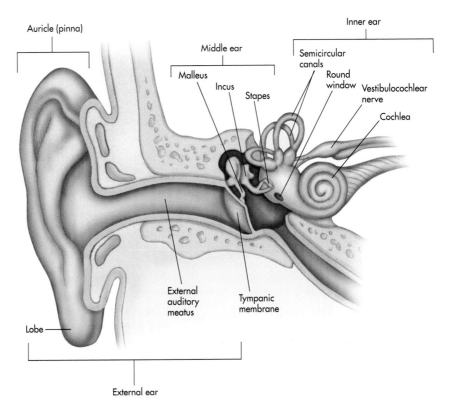

FIGURE 13–1

The ear and its anatomic structures.

▶ THE MIDDLE EAR

Beyond the tympanic membrane is a tiny cavity in the temporal bone of the skull. This cavity contains three small bones or *ossicles* instrumental to the hearing process. These ossicles are the *malleus, incus,* and *stapes.* Sometimes referred to as the *hammer, anvil,* and *stirrup* because of their shapes, these bones mechanically transmit sound vibrations from the tympanic membrane, to which the malleus is attached, through the incus to the stapes, which attaches to a thin membrane covering a small opening, the oval window, that marks the beginning of the inner ear. During transmission, tympanic vibrations may be amplified as much as 22 times their original force.

The cavity of the middle ear has five openings, one covered by the tympanic membrane, another to the auditory or eustachian tube, a third to the mastoid cells, and two openings to the inner ear, the oval and round windows (Fig. 13–1). The cavity is lined by mucous membrane that is continuous with that found in the mastoid air cells, the eustachian tube, and the throat. The spread of infection from the throat along this membrane to the middle ear is called otitis media. The continued spread of infection to the mastoid air cells is called mastoiditis.

Three functions have been attributed to the middle ear:

- It transmits sound vibrations.
- It equalizes external/internal air pressure on the tympanic membrane.
- It exerts control over potentially damaging or disruptive loud sounds through reflex contractions of the stapedius and tensor tympani muscles, which are attached to the stapes and the malleus, respectively.

► THE INNER EAR

The *inner ear* consists of a membranous labyrinth or maze located within a bony labyrinth. These structures are called *labyrinths* because of their complicated shapes. The bony labyrinth, located in the temporal bone, consists of the *cochlea, vestibule,* and *three semicircular canals.* Within the bony labyrinth, but separated from it by a fluid called *perilymph,* is the membranous labyrinth. It has much the same shape as the bony labyrinth and has three distinct divisions: the *cochlear duct* inside the cochlea, the *semicircular ducts* within the semicircular canals, and two sac-like structures, the *utricle* and *saccule,* located in the vestibule. Nerve endings in the form of hair cells located in various parts of the inner ear serve as receptors for the senses of *hearing* and *equilibrium.*

THE COCHLEA

The *cochlea* is a spiral-shaped bony structure containing the cochlear duct and so named because it resembles a snail shell. The spiral cavity of the bony cochlea is partitioned into three tube-like channels that run the entire length of the spiral. Two membranes form these tube-like areas. The *basilar membrane* forms the lower channel or *scala tympani,* and the *vestibular membrane (Reissner's membrane)* forms the upper channel, which is called the *scala vestibuli.* Between the two scala is a space, the *cochlear duct,* formed by the vestibular membrane on top and the basilar membrane as a floor. Located on the basilar membrane is the *organ of Corti* containing hair cell sensory receptors for the sense of hearing. A pale fluid, *perilymph,* fills the scala vestibuli and scala tympani. A different fluid, *endolymph,* fills the cochlear duct (Fig. 13–2).

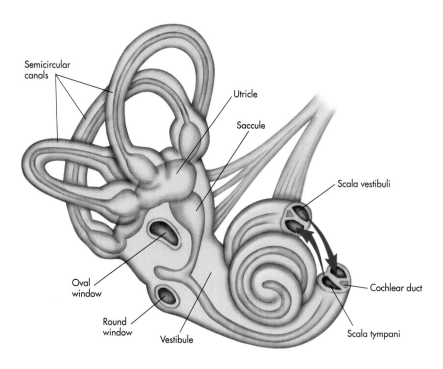

FIGURE 13–2

The cochlea.

The Hearing Process in the Inner Ear

The scala vestibuli and scala tympani open to the middle ear through the oval and round windows, respectively. The stapes fits into the round window and causes vibration of the perilymph, which, in turn, vibrates the basilar membrane and endolymph of the cochlear duct, thereby exciting the nerve endings contained on the *organ of Corti*. These nerve endings transmit the sounds, via the *eighth cranial nerve*, to the auditory areas of the brain. The sound waves, having excited the fluid of the cochlear duct, then pass on to the perilymph of the scala tympani and are dissipated against the membrane covering the round window.

THE VESTIBULE

The *vestibule* is a bony structure located between the cochlea and the three semicircular canals. The bony vestibule contains the *utricle* and *saccule,* membranous pouches containing perilymph. The utricle communicates with the semicircular canals and contains hair cell sensory receptors connected to fibers from the eighth cranial nerve. These hair cells react to the forces of gravity and movement and are a part of the sense of *equilibrium.*

THE SEMICIRCULAR CANALS

Located at right angles to each other, there are the superior, posterior, and inferior *semicircular canals.* Within the bony canals are the membranous semicircular ducts containing endolymph. At the base of each canal is an enlargement called an *ampulla* containing nerve endings in the form of hair cells. Changes in the position of the head causes the fluid in the canals to move against these sensory receptors, which, in turn, report such movement to the brain through fibers leading to the eighth cranial nerve. *Dizziness* and motion sickness are associated with rapid or erratic movement and the resulting sensory sensation in these areas.

LIFE SPAN CONSIDERATIONS

▶ THE CHILD

At 36 weeks the identifying characteristics of the fetus are soft ear lobes, few creases on the soles of the foot, ample vernix caseosa, and diminishing lanugo. At 40 weeks there are firm **ear lobes.** In newborns the walls of the ear canal is pliable because of underdeveloped cartilage and bone. The **eustachian tube** in infants is shorter and straighter than in older children and adults.

Babies respond to "mother-ese" and "parent-ese," whose melodic sounds actually provide a tutorial in the sounds that make up language. It is recommended that parents should sing and talk to even the youngest infants, because verbal stimulation is crucial to how well a child develops thinking and language skills later. According to Dr. William Staso, an expert in neurologic development, different kinds of stimulation should be emphasized at different ages.

First Month	A low level of stimulation reduces stress and increases the infant's wakefulness and alertness.
1 to 3 Months	The brain starts to discriminate among acoustic patterns of language, like intonation and pitch.
3 to 5 Months	Infants rely primarily on vision to acquire information about the world.
6 to 7 Months	Infants become alert to relationships such as cause and effect, the location of objects, and the function of objects.
7 to 8 Months	The brain is oriented to make association between sound and some meaningful activity or object.
9 to 12 Months	Learning adds up to a new level of awareness of the environment and increased interest in exploration; sensory and motor skills coordinate in a more mature fashion.

▶ THE OLDER ADULT

With aging, changes occur in the **external, middle,** and **inner ear.** The skin of the **auricle** may become dry and wrinkled. Production of **cerumen** declines and it is drier. There is also dryness of the external canal, which causes itching. Hairs in the external canal become coarser and longer, especially in males. The eardrum thickens and the bony joints in the middle ear degenerate.

Changes in the inner ear affect sensitivity to sound, understanding of speech, and balance. Degenerative changes include atrophy of the cochlea, the cochlear nerve cells, and the organ of Corti. These changes lead to the hearing loss, **presbycusis,** that is common in the older adult. Noisy surroundings make it difficult for older adults to discriminate between sounds, thereby impairing communication and socialization.

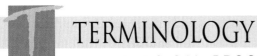

TERMINOLOGY

WITH SURGICAL PROCEDURES & PATHOLOGY

TERM	WORD PARTS			DEFINITION
acoustic (ă-koos′ tĭk)	acoust ic	R S	hearing pertaining to	Pertaining to the sense of hearing
audiogram (ŏ′ dĭ-ō-grăm″)	audio gram	CF S	to hear a mark, record	A record of hearing by audiometry
audiologist (ŏ″ dĭ-ŏl′ ō-jĭst)	audio log ist	CF R S	to hear study of one who specializes	One who specializes in disorders of hearing
audiology (ŏ″ dĭ-ŏl′ ō-jĭ)	audio logy	CF S	to hear study of	The study of hearing disorders

 TERMINOLOGY SPOTLIGHT

Audiology is the study of hearing disorders. Sustained noise over 85 decibels can cause permanent hearing loss. Risk doubles with each 5-decibel increase. About 2 in every 10 teens have lost some of their hearing ability from exposure to noise and are not aware of it, according to a study at the University of Florida. Standard hearing tests given to middle and high school students identified some hearing loss in 17% of the students. High-pitched sounds are the first to be affected by noise exposure. As hearing loss progresses, one can start to have difficulty hearing, particularly when there is noise in the background. Excessive noise can permanently damage the hair cell sensory receptors of the organ of Corti. These receptors are instrumental in transmitting sound to the brain.

In a study at the University of Florida, Alice Holmes, associate professor of communicative disorders, and her colleagues gave 342 students ages 10 to 20 audiologic exams that tested their ability to hear pure tones. Seventeen percent of the students did not hear one or more of the sounds in at least one ear.

Are you harming your hearing?	**Above 85 decibels**
Firecracker at 10 feet	160 decibels
Rock concert	125 decibels
Stereo headset, volume at six	115 decibels
Subway	100 decibels
Car horn	100 decibels
Garbage disposal	95 decibels
City traffic	90 decibels
Jet taking off at close range	120 decibels

Noise can get in the way of learning and cause stress. Research shows that noise can cause anger, aggression, poor performance, and insomnia. It may also be a factor in hypertension and cardiovascular and digestive problems. One study, at Germany's Max Planck Institute,

continued

Terminology - continued

TERM	WORD PARTS			DEFINITION
showed that consistent exposure to 70 decibels of noise caused vascular constriction, a condition that can be dangerous for people with coronary artery disease. It is recommended that one wear earplugs or other sound protection when mowing the lawn, working with noisy equipment, riding a motorcycle, or attending a rock concert. If the noise around you is so loud that you have to raise your voice, then it is loud enough to hurt your hearing.				
audiometer (ŏ″ dĭ-ŏm′ ĕ-tĕr)	audio meter	CF S	to hear instrument to measure	An instrument used to measure hearing
audiometry (ŏ″ dĭ-ŏm′ ĕ-trē)	audio metry	CF S	to hear measurement	Measurement of the hearing sense
audiphone (ŏ′ dĭ-fōn)	audi phone	CF R	to hear voice	An instrument that conveys sound to the auditory nerve through teeth or bone
auditory (ŏ′ dĭ-tō″ rē)	auditor y	R S	hearing pertaining to	Pertaining to the sense of hearing
aural (ŏ′ răl)	aur al	R S	the ear pertaining to	Pertaining to the ear
cholesteatoma (kō″ lē- stē″ ă-tō′ mă)	chole steat oma	CF R S	gall or bile fat tumor	A tumor-like mass filled with epithelial cells and cholesterol
electrocochleo- graphy (ē- lĕk″ trō-kŏk″ lē-ŏg′ ră-fē)	electro cochleo graphy	CF CF S	electricity land snail recording	A recording of the electrical activity produced when the cochlea is stimulated
endaural (ĕn′ dŏ″ ral)	end aur al	P R S	within ear pertaining to	Pertaining to within the ear
endolymph (ĕn′ dō-lĭmf)	endo lymph	P S	within serum, clear fluid	The clear fluid contained within the labyrinth of the ear
labyrinthectomy (lăb″ ĭ-rĭn-thĕk′ tō-mē)	labyrinth ectomy	R S	maze excision	Surgical excision of the labyrinth
labyrinthitis (lăb″ ĭ-rĭn-thī′ tĭs)	labyrinth itis	R S	maze inflammation	Inflammation of the labyrinth

Terminology - continued

TERM	WORD PARTS			DEFINITION
labyrinthotomy (lăb″ ĭ-rĭn-thŏt′ ō-mē)	labyrintho tomy	CF S	maze incision	Incision of the labyrinth
mastoidalgia (măs″ toyd-ăl′ jĭ-ă)	mast oid algia	R S S	breast form pain	Pain in the mastoid
mastoiditis (măs″ toyd-ī′ tĭs)	mast oid itis	R S S	breast form inflammation	Inflammation of the mastoid
myringectomy (mĭr-ĭn-jĕk′ tō-mē)	myring ectomy	R S	drum membrane excision	Surgical excision of the tympanic membrane
myringoplasty (mĭr-ĭn′ gō-plăst″ ē)	myringo plasty	CF S	drum membrane surgical repair	Surgical repair of the tympanic membrane
myringoscope (mĭr-ĭn′ gō-skōp)	myringo scope	CF S	drum membrane instrument	An instrument used to examine the eardrum
myringotome (mĭ-rĭn′ gō-tō)	myringo tome	CF S	drum membrane instrument to cut	An instrument used for cutting the eardrum
otic (ō′ tĭk)	ot ic	R S	ear pertaining to	Pertaining to the ear
otitis (ō-tī′ tĭs)	ot itis	R S	ear inflammation	Inflammation of the ear
otodynia (ō″ tō-dĭn′ ĭ-ă)	oto dynia	CF S	ear pain	Pain in the ear, earache
otolaryngologist (ō″ tō-lar″ ĭn-gŏl″ ō-jĭst)	oto laryngo log ist	CF CF R S	ear larynx study of one who specializes	One who specializes in the study of the ear and larynx
otolaryngology (ō″ tō-lar″ ĭn-gŏl′ ō-jē)	oto laryngo logy	CF CF S	ear larynx study of	The study of the ear and larynx

continued

Terminology - continued

TERM	WORD PARTS			DEFINITION
otolith (ō′ tō-lĭth)	oto lith	CF S	ear stone	Ear stone
otomycosis (ō″ tō-mī-kō′ sĭs)	oto myc osis	CF R S	ear fungus condition of	A fungus condition of the ear
otoneurology (ō″ tō-nū-rŏl′ ō-jē)	oto neuro logy	CF CF S	ear nerve study of	The study of ear conditions with nerve complications
otopharyngeal (ō″ tō-far-ĭn′ jē- āl)	oto pharynge al	CF CF S	ear pharynx pertaining to	Pertaining to the ear and pharynx
otoplasty (ō′ tō-plăs″ tē)	oto plasty	CF S	ear surgical repair	Surgical repair of the ear
otopyorrhea (ō″ tō-pī″ ō-rē′ ă)	oto pyo rrhea	CF CF S	ear pus flow	Flow of pus from the ear
otorhinolaryn-gology (ō″ tō-rī″ nō-lăr″ ĭn-gŏl′ ō-jē)	oto rhino laryngo logy	CF CF CF S	ear nose larynx study of	The study of the ear, nose, and larynx
otosclerosis (ō″ tō-sklē- rō′ sĭs)	oto scler osis	CF R S	ear hardening condition of	A hardening condition of the ear characterized by progressive deafness
otoscope (ō′ tō-skōp)	oto scope	CF S	ear instrument	An instrument used to examine the ear
perilymph (pĕr′ ĭ-lĭmf)	peri lymph	P S	around serum, pale fluid	Serum fluid of the inner ear
presbycusis (prĕz″ bĭ-kū′ sĭs)	presby cusis	R S	old hearing	Impairment of hearing in old age
stapedectomy (stā″ pē- dĕk′ tō-mē)	staped ectomy	R S	stirrup excision	Surgical excision of the stapes in the ear
tinnitus (tĭn-ī′ tŭs)	tinnit us	R S	a jingling pertaining to	A ringing or jingling sound in the ear
tympanectomy (tĭm″ păn-ĕk tō-mē)	tympan ectomy	R S	drum excision	Surgical excision of the tympanic membrane

Terminology - continued

TERM	WORD PARTS		DEFINITION
tympanic (tĭm-păn′ ĭk)	tympan ic	R S	drum pertaining to	Pertaining to the eardrum
tympanitis (tĭm-păn-ī′ tĭs)	tympan itis	R S	drum inflammation	Inflammation of the eardrum

VOCABULARY WORDS

Vocabulary words are terms that have not been divided into component parts. They are common words or specialized terms associated with the subject of this chapter. These words are provided to enhance your medical vocabulary.

WORD	DEFINITION
auricle (ŏ′ rĭ-kl)	The external portion of the ear, known as the flap of the ear; *the pinna* (pin′ na)
binaural (bīn-aw′ răl)	Pertaining to both ears
cerumen (sē- roo′ měn)	Earwax, the yellowish substance secreted by the glands in the canal of the external ear
cochlea (kŏk′ lē-ă)	A portion of the inner ear shaped like a snail shell; contains the organ of hearing referred to as the organ of Corti
deafness (děf′ něs)	Complete or partial loss of the ability to hear
ear (ēr)	Organ of hearing and equilibrium
equilibrium (ē″ kwĭ-lĭb′ rē-ŭm)	A state of balance. In the inner ear, the semicircular canals are the site of the organs of balance
eustachian tube (yoo-stā′ shən tūb)	A narrow tube between the middle ear and the throat that serves to equalize pressure on both sides of the eardrum
fenestration (fĕn″ ĕs-trā′ shŭn)	Surgical operation in which a new opening is made in the labyrinth of the inner ear for restoration of hearing
incus (ing′ kŭs)	The anvil, the middle of the three ossicles

continued

Vocabulary - continued

WORD	DEFINITION
labyrinth (lăb′ ĭ-rĭnth)	The inner ear; *made up of the vestibule, cochlea, and semicircular canals*
malleus (măl′ ē-ŭs)	The hammer, the largest of the three ossicles
Ménière's disease (mān″ ē- ā rz)	A disease of the inner ear *(labyrinth)* that presents a group of symptoms that recur. In acute attacks, bedrest is recommended. Vertigo and dizziness are the classic symptoms, and the patient experiences nausea, tinnitus, and a sensation of fullness or pressure in the ears. Deafness can occur.
monaural (mŏn-aw′ răl)	Pertaining to one ear
myringotomy (mĭr-ĭn-gŏt′ ō-mē)	Surgical incision of the tympanic membrane. It is used to remove unwanted fluids from the ear
ossicle (ŏs′ ĭ-kl)	Small bone. Any one of the three bones of the middle ear: the malleus, the incus, or the stapes
oval window (ō′ văl wĭn′ dō)	Membrane in the middle ear into which fits the footplate of the stapes
Rinne test (rĭn′ nē test)	A hearing test made with a tuning fork to compare bone conduction hearing with air conduction
stapes (stā′ pēz)	The stirrup, the innermost of the ossicles
tympanic thermometer (tĭm-păn′ĭk thĕr-mŏm′ĕ-tĕr)	An electronic thermometer that is used to determine core body temperature by measuring it from the tympanic membrane and its surrounding tissues See Figure 13–3.
tympanoplasty (tĭm″ păn-ō-plăs′ tē)	Surgical repair of the tympanic membrane
utricle (ū′ trĭk-l)	A small, sac-like structure of the labyrinth of the inner ear
vertigo (ver′ tĭ-gō)	A feeling of dizziness, light-headedness, caused by a disturbance of the equilibrium organs in the labyrinth

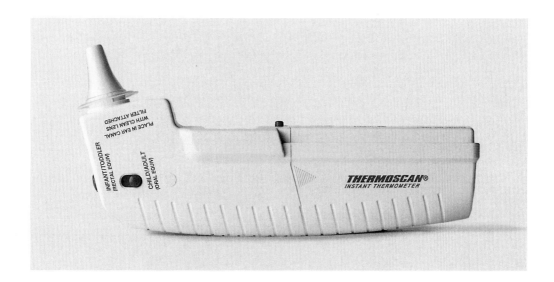

FIGURE 13-3

The Thermoscan Instant Thermometer. *(Courtesy of Thermoscan, Inc., San Diego, CA.)*

ABBREVIATIONS

AC	air conduction	**EENT**	eyes, ears, nose, throat
AD	auris dexter (right ear)	**ETF**	eustachian tube function
AS	auris sinistra (left ear)	**HD**	hearing distance
AU	auris unitas (both ears)	**OM**	otitis media
BC	bone conduction	**Oto**	otology
CPS	cycles per second	**PE tube**	polyethylene tube
db, dB	decibel	**SOM**	serous otitis media
ENG	electronystagmography	**UCHD**	usual childhood diseases
ENT	ear, nose, and throat		

DRUG HIGHLIGHTS

Drugs that are generally used for ear diseases and disorders include antibiotics and those used for vertigo.

Antibiotics   Used to treat infectious diseases. They may be natural or synthetic substances that inhibit the growth of or destroy microorganisms, especially bacteria.

Penicillins	Act by interfering with bacterial cell wall synthesis among newly formed bacterial cells. Penicillins are contraindicated in patients who are known to be allergic or hypersensitive to any of its varieties, or to any of the cephalosporins. *Examples: penicillin G, ampicillin, penicillin V, piperacillin, and amoxicillin.*
Cephalosporins	Are chemically and pharmacologically related to the penicillins. They act by inhibiting bacterial cell wall synthesis, thereby promoting the death of the developing microorganisms. Hypersensitivity to cephalosporins and/or penicillins may result in an allergic reaction. *Examples: Ancef (cefazolin sodium), Mandol (cefamandole nafate), Precef (ceforanide), Ceclor (cefaclor), Keflex (cephalexin), and Suprax (cefixime).*
Tetracyclines	Primarily bacteriostatic, and are active against a wide range of gram-negative and gram-positive microorganisms. They inhibit protein synthesis in the bacterial cell. Contraindicated in children 8 years of age and younger. These drugs cause permanent discoloration of tooth enamel. *Examples: Terramycin, (oxytetracycline); Achromycin, Sumycin, Tetracyn (tetracycline hydrochloride); and minocycline (Minocin).*
Erythromycin	Works by inhibiting protein synthesis in susceptible bacteria. These drugs may be used for patients who are allergic to penicillin. *Examples: E-Mycin, Ilotycin, Ilosone, E.E.S., Pediamycin, and Erypar.*
Drugs Used in Vertigo	Vertigo is an illusion of movement. It may be caused by a lesion or other process affecting the brain, the eighth cranial nerve, or the labyrinthine system of the ear. Drugs that are used for vertigo may include anticholinergics, antihistamines, and antidopamines. *Examples: Dramamine (dimenhydrinate), Benadryl (diphenhydramine HCl), Antivert (meclizine HCl), and Torecan (thiethylperazine maleate).*

DIAGNOSTIC AND LABORATORY TESTS

Test	Description
auditory evoked response (aw′ dĭ-tō″ rē ĕ-vō kd′ rē- spŏns)	The response to auditory stimuli (sound) that can be measured independent of the patient's subjective response. By using an electroencephalograph, the intensity of sound and presence of response can be determined. This test is useful for testing the hearing of children who are too young for standard tests, autistic, hyperkinetic, and/or retarded.
electronystagmography (ē-lĕk″ trō-nĭs″ tăg-mŏg′ ră-fē)	A recording of eye movement in response to specific stimuli, such as sound. It is used to determine the presence and location of a lesion in the vestibule of the ear, to help diagnose unilateral hearing loss of unknown origin, and to help identify the cause of vertigo, tinnitus, and dizziness.

falling test
(fă′ lĭng test)

A test to observe the patient for marked swaying or falling. With eyes open, the patient is asked to stand on one foot, stand heel to toe, and then to walk forward. The patient is asked to repeat each of the above with the eyes closed. Marked swaying or falling may indicate vestibular and cerebellar dysfunction.

past-pointing test
(păst-poynt′ ĭng test)

The patient is instructed to reach out and touch the examiner's index finger, which is held at shoulder level, then to lower the arm, close the eyes, and touch the finger again. The test is repeated using the finger of the examiner's opposite hand. The degree and direction of past-pointing is observed.

otoscopy
(ō-tŏs′ kō-pē)

Visual examination of the external auditory canal and the tympanic membrane via an otoscope.

tuning fork test
(tūn′ ĭng fork test)

A method of testing hearing by the use of a tuning fork. Two types of hearing loss (conductive and perceptive) may be distinguished through the use of this test.

tympanometry
(tīm″ păn-nŏm′ ĕ-trē)

Measurement of the movement of the tympanic membrane and pressure in the middle ear. It is used for detecting middle ear disorders.

COMMUNICATION ENRICHMENT

This segment is provided for those who wish to enhance their ability to communicate in either English or Spanish.

▶ Related Terms

English	Spanish
balance, loss of	pérdida de equilibrio (*pĕr*-dĭ-dă dĕ ĕ-kĭ-lĭ-brĭ-ō)
deaf	sordo (*sōr*-dō)
dizziness	vértigo (*vĕr*-tĭ-gō)
drops	gotas (*gō*-tăs)
earache	dolor de oído (dō-*lōr* dĕ o-*ĕ*-dō)

English	Spanish
ear	oído (o-*ē*-dō)
hear; listen	oír; escuchar (ō-*ĭr*; ĕs-kū-*chăr*)
hearing, difficulty in	dificultad de escuchar (*dĭ*-fĭ-cūl-tăd dĕ ĕs-kū-*chăr*)
hearing, loss of	pérdida de oído (*pĕr*-dĭ-dă dĕ o-*ē*-dō)
infection	infección (*ĭn*-fĕk-sĭ-ōn)
inflammation	inflamación (ĭn-flă-*mă*-sĭ-ōn)
loud	fuerte (*fū*-ĕr-tĕ)
left	izquierdo (iz-kū-*ĕr*-dō)
right	derecho (dĕ-*rĕ*-chō)
deafness	sordera (sōr-*dĕ*-ră)
wax	cera (*sĕ*-ra)
hearing	oir (*ō*-*ĭr*)
buzz, hum	zumbido (zūm-*bĭ*-dō)
temperature	temperatura (tĕm-pĕ-ră-*tū*-ră)
thermometer	termómetro (tĕr-*mō*-mĕ-trō)
equilibrium	equilibrio (ĕ-kĭ-lĭ-brĭ-ō)
air	aire (ă-ĭ-rĕ)
both	ambos (*ăm*-bōs)

English	Spanish
nose	nariz (*nă*-rĭz)
throat	garganta (găr-*găn*-tă)
eye	ojo (*ō*-hō)
middle	medio (*me*-dĭ-ō)
inner	interior (ĭn-*tĕ*-rĭ-ōr)
vibration	vibración (vĭ-*bră*-sĭ-ōn)
external	externo (ĕx-*tĕr*-nō)
internal	interno (ĭn-*tĕr*-nō)
ring	timbre (*tĭm*-brĕ)

STUDY AND REVIEW SECTION

LEARNING EXERCISES

▶ **Anatomy and Physiology**

Write your answers to the following questions. Do not refer back to the text.

1. The ear is the site of the senses of _____ and _____.

2. Name the three divisions of the ear.

    a. _____   b. _____

    c. _____

3. The external ear consists of the a. _____, the b. _____,

    and the c. _____.

4. Which structure of the external ear collects sound waves? _____

5. State the two functions of cerumen.

   a. _____   b. _____

6. Name the three ossicles of the middle ear.

   a. _____   b. _____

   c. _____

7. State the function of the ossicles. _____

   _____

8. State the three functions of the middle ear.

   a. _____   b. _____

   c. _____

9. The bony labyrinth of the inner ear consists of the _____,

   _____, and the _____.

10. Name the three divisions of the membranous labyrinth.

    a. _____   b. _____

    c. _____

11. Located on the basilar membrane is the _____, containing hair cell
    sensory receptors for the sense of hearing.

12. The _____ is a bony structure located between the cochlea and the three
    semicircular canals.

13. The auditory nerve is also known as the _____.

14. The hair cells located in each ampulla of the semicircular canals sense changes
    in _____ and report this information to the brain.

15. Name the two types of fluid found in the ear.

    a. _____   b. _____

▶ Word Parts

1. In the spaces provided, write the definitions of these prefixes, roots, combining
   forms, and suffixes. Do not refer to the listings of terminology words. Leave blank
   those terms you cannot define.

2. After completing as many as you can, refer back to the terminology word listings to
   check your work. For each word missed or left blank, write the term and its
   definition several times on the margins of these pages or on a separate sheet of
   paper.

3. To maximize the learning process, it is to your advantage to do the following exercises as directed. To refer to the terminology listings before completing these exercises invalidates the learning process.

Prefixes

Give the definitions of the following prefixes:

1. end- _____
2. endo- _____
3. peri- _____

Roots and Combining Forms

Give the definitions of the following roots and combining forms:

1. acoust _____
2. audi _____
3. audio _____
4. auditor _____
5. aur _____
6. chole _____
7. cochleo _____
8. electro _____
9. labyrinth _____
10. labyrintho _____
11. laryngo _____
12. log _____
13. mast _____
14. myc _____
15. myring _____
16. myringo _____
17. neuro _____
18. ot _____
19. oto _____
20. pharynge _____
21. phone _____
22. presby _____
23. pyo _____
24. rhino _____
25. scler _____
26. staped _____
27. steat _____
28. tinnit _____
29. tympan _____

Suffixes

Give the definitions of the following suffixes:

1. -al _____
2. -algia _____
3. -cusis _____
4. -dynia _____
5. -ectomy _____
6. -gram _____

7. -graphy _____   8. -ic _____

9. -ist _____   10. -itis _____

11. -lith _____   12. -logy _____

13. -lymph _____   14. -meter _____

15. -metry _____   16. -oid _____

17. -oma _____   18. -osis _____

19. -plasty _____   20. -rrhea _____

21. -scope _____   22. -tome _____

23. -tomy _____   24. -us _____

25. -y _____

▶ Identifying Medical Terms

In the spaces provided, write the medical terms for the following meanings:

1. _____   One who specializes in disorders of hearing

2. _____   Measurement of the hearing sense

3. _____   Pertaining to the sense of hearing

4. _____   Pertaining to within the ear

5. _____   Inflammation of the labyrinth

6. _____   Surgical repair of the tympanic membrane

7. _____   An instrument used for cutting the eardrum

8. _____   Pain in the ear, earache

9. _____   The study of the ear and larynx

10. _____   Pertaining to the ear and pharynx

11. _____   An instrument used to examine the ear

12. _____   Serum fluid of the inner ear

13. _____   Surgical excision of the stapes of the ear

14. _____   Surgical excision of the tympanic membrane

15. _____   A ringing or jingling sound in the ear

▶ **Spelling**

In the spaces provided, write the correct spelling of these misspelled terms:

1. acostic _____
2. audilogy _____
3. cholestoma _____
4. electrochleography _____
5. labrinthitis _____
6. myringplasty _____
7. otomcosis _____
8. otosterosis _____
9. typanic _____
10. typanitis _____

WORD PARTS STUDY SHEET

Word Parts	Give the Meaning
end-, endo-	_____
peri-	_____
acoust-	_____
audi-, audio-	_____
auditor-	_____
aur-	_____
cochleo-	_____
labyrinth-, labyrintho-	_____
mast-	_____
myc-	_____
myring-, myringo-	_____
ot-, oto-	_____
pharynge-	_____
phone-	_____
presby-	_____
pyo-	_____
rhino-	_____

scler- _____

staped- _____

steat- _____

tinnit- _____

tympan- _____

-cusis _____

-dynia _____

-gram _____

-graphy _____

-lith _____

-lymph _____

-meter _____

-metry _____

-oid _____

-oma _____

-osis _____

-plasty _____

-rrhea _____

-scope _____

-tome _____

-tomy _____

-us _____

-y _____

REVIEW QUESTIONS

▶ Matching

Select the appropriate lettered meaning for each numbered line.

_____ 1. auricle

_____ 2. binaural

_____ 3. cerumen

_____ 4. equilibrium

_____ 5. fenestration

_____ 6. labyrinth

_____ 7. myringotomy

_____ 8. ossicle

_____ 9. tympanoplasty

_____ 10. vertigo

a. A state of balance
b. The inner ear
c. Small bone
d. Surgical repair of the tympanic membrane
e. Pertaining to both ears
f. A feeling of dizziness
g. Surgical operation in which a new opening is made in the labyrinth
h. The external portion of the ear
i. Earwax
j. Surgical incision of the tympanic membrane
k. Organ of hearing

▶ Abbreviations

Place the correct word, phrase, or abbreviation in the space provided.

1. air conduction _____

2. right ear _____

3. AS _____

4. both ears _____

5. ENT _____

6. EENT _____

7. hearing distance _____

8. otology _____

9. SOM _____

10. usual childhood diseases _____

► **Diagnostic and Laboratory Tests**

Select the best answer to each multiple choice question. Circle the letter of your choice.

1. The response to auditory stimuli that can be measured independent of the patient's subjective response.
    a. auditory evoked response
    b. electronystagmography
    c. falling test
    d. otoscopy

2. A recording of eye movement in response to specific stimuli.
    a. auditory evoked response
    b. electronystagmography
    c. falling test
    d. otoscopy

3. A test to observe the patient for marked swaying.
    a. auditory evoked response
    b. electronystagmography
    c. falling test
    d. past-pointing test

4. The visual examination of the external auditory canal and the tympanic membrane.
    a. tuning fork test
    b. tympanometry
    c. electronystagmography
    d. otoscopy

5. The measurement of the movement of the tympanic membrane.
    a. tuning fork tests
    b. tympanometry
    c. otoscopy
    d. past-pointing test

CRITICAL THINKING ACTIVITY

▶ Case Study

Acute Otitis Media

Please read the following case study and then answer the questions that follow.

A 4-year-old female was seen by a physician and the following is a synopsis of the visit.

Present History: The mother states that her daughter has been complaining of an earache, ringing in the ears, and has been running a fever. She is irritable and doesn't want to eat.

Signs and Symptoms: Chief complaint: otodynia (otalgia), tinnitus, fever, irritability, and anorexia.

Diagnosis: Otitis media acute. The diagnosis was determined by a physical examination of the ear (otoscopy). A culture of the fluid taken from the ear showed the presence of bacteria—*Streptococcus pneumoniae.*

Treatment: The physician ordered an analgesic for pain (Tylenol) and an antibiotic (amoxicillin) for the infection.

Prevention: Since most middle ear infections are caused by an upper respiratory infection that has spread through the eustachian tube, URIs should be treated promptly.

Critical Thinking Questions

1. Signs and symptoms of otitis media include otodynia, _____ (ringing in the ears), fever, irritability, and anorexia.

2. The diagnosis was determined by a physical examination of the ear called an _____ and a culture of the fluid taken from the ear.

3. Treatment included an analgesic (Tylenol) and an _____ (amoxicillin).

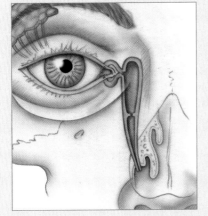

14

SPECIAL SENSES: THE EYE

OBJECTIVES

On completion of this chapter, you should be able to:

- Describe the anatomical structures of the eye.
- Describe the external structures of the eye.
- Describe the internal structures of the eye.
- Analyze, build, spell, and pronounce medical words that relate to surgical procedures and pathology.
- Identify and give the meaning of selected vocabulary words.
- Identify and define selected abbreviations.
- Review Drug Highlights presented in this chapter.
- Provide the description of diagnostic and laboratory tests related to the eye.
- Successfully complete the study and review section.

► ANATOMY AND PHYSIOLOGY OVERVIEW

In this overview of the anatomy and physiology of the eye, a general description is offered as an aid to those learning the terminology associated with the functions of the eye.

The *eye* is composed of special anatomical structures that work together to facilitate sight. Light passes through the cornea, pupil, lens, and the vitreous body to stimulate sensory receptors *(rods and cones)* on the *retina* or innermost layer of the eye. *Vision* is made possible through the coordinated actions of nerves that control the movement of the eyeball, the amount of light admitted by the pupil, the focusing of that light on the retina by the lens, and the transmission of the resulting sensory impulses to the brain by the optic nerve.

► EXTERNAL STRUCTURES

The orbit, the muscles of the eye, the eyelids, the conjunctiva, and the lacrimal apparatus make up the external structures of the eye.

THE ORBIT

The *orbit* is a cone-shaped cavity in the front of the skull that contains the *eyeball*. Formed by the combination of several bones, this cavity is lined with fatty tissue that cushions the eyeball and has several openings or *foramina* through which blood vessels and nerves pass. The largest of these is the optic foramen for the optic nerve and ophthalmic artery.

THE MUSCLES OF THE EYE

Connecting the eyeball to the orbital cavity are *six short muscles* that provide it with support and rotary movement. Of the six, four are straight *(rectus)* muscles and two are slanted *(oblique)* muscles.

SPECIAL SENSES: THE EYE

ORGAN/STRUCTURE	PRIMARY FUNCTIONS
The Orbit	Contains the eyeball. Cavity is lined with fatty tissue that cushions the eyeball and has several openings through which blood vessels and nerves pass
The Muscles of the Eye	Six short muscles provide support and rotary movement of the eyeball
The Eyelids	Protect the eyeballs from intense light, foreign particles, and impact
The Conjunctiva	Acts as a protective covering for the exposed surface of the eyeball
The Lacrimal Apparatus	Produces, stores, and removes tears that cleanse and lubricate the eye
The Eyeball	Organ of vision
Sclera	The outer layer known as the "white" of the eye consists of the cornea, which bends light rays and helps to focus them on the surface of the retina
Choroid	Pigmented vascular membrane that prevents internal reflection of light
Ciliary body	Smooth muscle forming a part of the ciliary body that governs the convexity of the lens. The ciliary body secretes nutrient fluids that nourish the cornea, the lens, and surrounding tissues
Iris	Colored membrane attached to the ciliary body. It has a circular opening in its center, the pupil, and two muscles that contract to regulate the amount of light admitted by the pupil
Retina	Innermost layer. Contains photoreceptive cells that translate light waves focused on its surface into nerve impulses
The lens	Sharpens the focus of light on the retina (accommodation)

THE EYELIDS

Each eye has a pair of *eyelids* that protect the eyeball from intense light, foreign particles, and impact. Known as the *superior* and *inferior plapebrae,* those movable "curtains" join to form a *canthus* or angle at either corner of the eye. The slit between the eyelids is called the *palpebral fissure,* through which light reaches the inner eye. The edges of the eyelids contain *eyelashes* and *sebaceous glands,* which secrete an oily substance onto the eyelids.

THE CONJUNCTIVA

Lining the underside of each eyelid and reflected onto the anterior portion of the eyeball is a mucous membrane known as the *conjunctiva.* This membrane acts as a protective covering for the exposed surface of the eyeball.

THE LACRIMAL APPARATUS

Included in the *lacrimal apparatus* are those structures that produce, store, and remove the tears that cleanse and lubricate the eye. These structures are the lacrimal gland, its ducts, the lacrimal canaliculi, the lacrimal sac, and the nasolacrimal duct, which empties into the nasal cavity (Fig. 14–1).

The Lacrimal Gland

Located above the outer corner of the eye, the *lacrimal gland* secretes tears through approximately 12 ducts onto the surface of the conjunctiva of the upper lid. This fluid washes across the anterior surface of the eye and is collected by the *lacrimal canaliculi.*

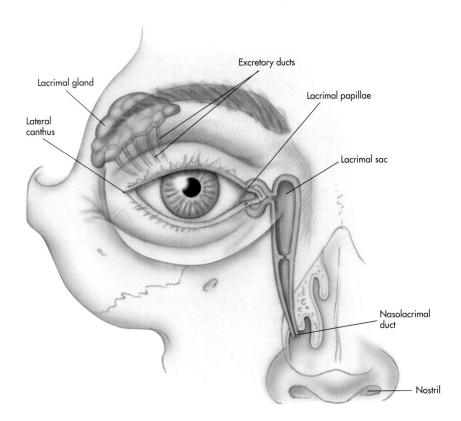

FIGURE 14–1

The lacrimal apparatus and its anatomic structure.

The Lacrimal Canaliculi

The *lacrimal canaliculi* are the two ducts *(superior and inferior)* at the inner corner of the eye that collect tears and drain into the lacrimal sac.

The Lacrimal Sac

The enlargement of the upper portion of the lacrimal duct is known as the *lacrimal sac.* Tears secreted by the lacrimal glands are pulled into this sac and subsequently forced into the nasolacrimal duct by the blinking action of the eyelids. The sac is dilated and pulls in fluid as the muscles associated with blinking close the lids. The sac constricts, forcing the fluid down the nasolacrimal duct, as the lids are opened.

The Nasolacrimal Duct

The passageway draining lacrimal fluid into the nose is known as the *nasolacrimal duct.* The lacrimal sac is the enlarged upper portion of this duct.

▶ INTERNAL STRUCTURES

The eyeball, its various structures, and the nerve fibers connecting it to the brain make up the internal eye (Fig. 14–2).

THE EYEBALL

The *eyeball* is the organ of vision. It is globe shaped and divided into two cavities. The space in front of the lens, called the *ocular cavity,* is further divided by the iris into *anterior* and *posterior chambers,* both filled with a watery fluid known as the *aqueous humor.* Behind the lens is a much larger cavity filled with a jelly-like material, the *vitreous humor,* which maintains the eyeball's spherical shape. The three layers forming the outer, middle, and inner surfaces of the eyeball are discussed, along with the lens and its functions.

The Outer Layer

The eyeball's outer layer is composed of the *sclera* or white of the eye and the *cornea* or anterior transparent portion of the eye's fibrous outer surface. The curved surface of the cornea is important in that it bends light rays and helps to focus them on the surface of the retina.

The Middle Layer

Known as the *uvea,* the middle layer of the eyeball, lying just below the sclera, consists of the *iris,* the *ciliary body,* and the *choroid* or pigmented vascular membrane that prevents internal reflection of light.

The Ciliary Body. The *ciliary body* is a thickened portion of the vascular membrane to which the iris is attached. Smooth muscle forming a part of the ciliary body governs the convexity of the lens. The ciliary body secretes nutrient fluids (the *aqueous humor*) that nourish the cornea, the lens, and the surrounding tissues.

The Iris. The *iris* is a colored membrane attached to the ciliary body and suspended between the lens and the cornea in the aqueous humor. It has a circular opening in its center, the *pupil,* and two muscles that contract or dilate to regulate the amount of light admitted by the pupil.

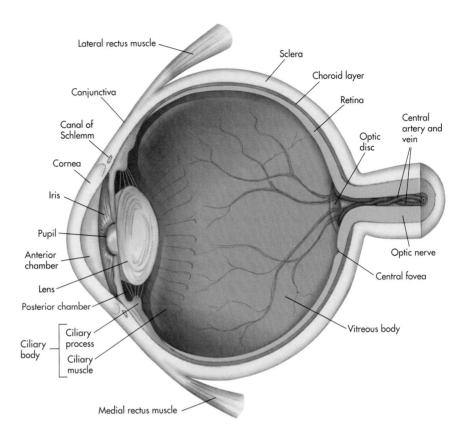

Lateral rectus muscle

Sclera

Choroid layer

Conjunctiva

Retina

Canal of
Schlemm

Central
artery and
vein

Cornea

Optic
disc

Iris

Pupil

Anterior
chamber

Optic nerve

Lens

Central fovea

Posterior chamber

Ciliary
process

Vitreous body

Ciliary
body

Ciliary
muscle

Medial rectus muscle

FIGURE 14-2

The eyeball and its anatomic structures.

The Inner Layer

The innermost layer, or *retina*, contains photoreceptive cells that translate light waves focused on its surface into nerve impulses. The photosensitive cells of the retina are the *rods* and *cones*. Most of the approximately 6 million cone cells are grouped into a small area called the *macula lutea*. In the center of the macula lutea is a small depression, the *fovea centralis*, containing only cone cells, which is the central focusing point within the eye. The eye contains approximately 120 million rods that are sensitive to dim light. They contain *rhodopsin*, a pigment necessary for night vision. The point at which nerve fibers from the retina converge to form the optic nerve is known as the *optic disk*. At this point, fibers of the optic nerve extend, through the optic chiasm, to the thalamus and on to the visual cortical areas of the brain. The absence of rods and cones in the area of the optic disk creates a blind spot in the visual field.

The Lens

A colorless crystalline body, biconvex in shape and enclosed in a transparent capsule, the *lens* is suspended by ligaments just behind the iris. Contraction and relaxation of the ciliary muscle control the tension of the suspensory ligaments to change the shape of the lens. The function of the lens is to sharpen the focus of light on the retina. This process, called *accommodation*, is reflexive in nature and combines changes in the size of the pupil, the curvature of the lens, and the convergence of the optic axes to keep the image in the same place on both retinae. Accommodation occurs for both near and distant vision.

LIFE SPAN CONSIDERATIONS

▶ THE CHILD

The **eyes** begin to develop as an outgrowth of the forebrain in the 4-week-old embryo. At 24 weeks the eyes are structurally complete. At 28 weeks eyebrows and eyelashes are present, and the eyelids open. The newborn can see, and **visual acuity** is estimated to be around 20/400. Most newborns appear cross-eyed because their eye muscles are not fully developed. At first, the eyes appear to be blue or gray. Permanent coloring becomes fixed between 6 and 12 months of age. Tears do not appear until approximately 1 to 3 months, because the lacrimal gland ducts are immature. Depth perception begins to develop around 9 months of age.

Visual acuity improves with age and by the age of 2 or 3 years, it is around 20/30 or 20/20. Children are farsighted until about 5 years of age.

Every minute that an infant is awake he or she is taking in the sights, sounds, smells, and feel of the surrounding world. For the 1- to 3-month-old, the human face is a favorite sight. By the second month, the baby's eye coordination has improved enough to follow something moving from one side of his or her face to the other. By the end of 3 months, brightly colored wall hangings or toys are favored.

▶ THE OLDER ADULT

Sensory decline alters one's perception of the world. Smells become harder to distinguish and detect. Eyes may need corrective lenses to adjust for decreasing ability to focus. As the ciliary muscles weaken, pupil size is decreased, reducing light to the retina. The lens become stiff, thicker, and more opaque and begin to yellow. These changes make the older adult sensitive to glare, and the ability to focus is impaired; therefore, farsightedness, **presbyopia,** is common in the older adult. Night vision is impaired and driving at night is often very difficult for the older adult. The lens eventually may become opaque as **cataracts** develop. Vascular degeneration may affect the **retina,** which contains nerve cells for receiving images, and this condition causes permanent visual loss.

The leading cause of new cases of blindness in the older adult is age-related **macular degeneration,** a disease that affects the macula, the part of the eye that is responsible for sharp central vision. For the first time, researchers have linked gene defects to macular degeneration. The discovery may lead to identification of people at high risk for the disorder and perhaps ways to treat or prevent vision loss.

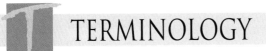

TERMINOLOGY

WITH SURGICAL PROCEDURES & PATHOLOGY

TERM	WORD PARTS			DEFINITION
amblyopia (ăm″ blĭ-ō′ pĭ-ă)	ambly opia	R S	dull vision	Dullness of vision
ametropia (ă″ mĕ-trō′ pĭ-ă)	ametr opia	R S	dispropor- tionate eye, vision	A defect in the refractive powers of the eye in which images fail to come to focus on the retina
anisocoria (ăn-ī″ sō-kō′ rĭă)	aniso cor ia	CF R S	unequal pupil condition	A condition in which the pupils are unequal
aphakia (ă-fā′kĭ-ă)	a phak ia	P R S	lack of, without lentil, lens condition	A condition in which the crystalline lens is absent
astigmatism (ă-stĭg′mă-tĭzm	a stigmat ism	P R S	lack of, without point condition of	A defect in the refractive powers of the eye in which a ray of light is not focused on the retina but is spread over an area
bifocal (bī-fō′kăl)	bi foc al	P R S	two focus pertaining to	Pertaining to having two foci, as in bifocal glasses
blepharitis (blĕf′ăr-ī′tĭs)	blephar itis	R S	eyelid inflammation	Inflammation of the edges of the eyelids
blepharoptosis (blĕf″ă-rō-tō′ sĭs)	blepharo ptosis	CF S	eyelid prolapse, drooping	A drooping of the upper eyelid(s)
choroiditis (kō″royd-ī′tĭs)	choroid itis	R S	choroid inflammation	Inflammation of the vascular coat of the eye
choroidoretinitis (kō″royd-ō-rĕt″ ĭn-ī′tĭs)	choroido retin itis	CF R S	choroid retina inflammation	Inflammation of the choroid and retina
corneal (kŏr′ nēəl)	corne al	R S	cornea pertaining to	Pertaining to the cornea

continued

Terminology - continued

TERM	WORD PARTS			DEFINITION
cycloplegia (sī″klō-plē′jĭ-ă)	cyclo plegia	CF S	ciliary body stroke, paralysis	Paralysis of the ciliary muscle
dacryocystitis (dăk″ rĭ-ō-sĭs-tī′ tĭs)	dacryo cyst itis	CF R S	tear sac inflammation	Inflammation of the tear sac(s)
dacryoma (dăk‴rĭ-ō′ mă)	dacry oma	R S	tear tumor	A tumor-like swelling caused by obstruction of the tear duct(s)
diplopia (dĭp-lō′ pĭ-ă)	dipl opia	P S	double eye, vision	Double vision
ectropion (ĕk-trō′ pĭ-ŏn)	ec trop ion	P R S	out turn process	A process of turning outward, as the edge of an eyelid(s)
electroretinogram (ē- lĕk″ trō-rĕt′ ĭ-nō-grăm)	electro retino gram	CF CF S	electricity retina mark, record	A record of the electrical response of the retina to light stimulation
emmetropia (ĕm″ ĕ-trō′ pĭ-ă)	em metr opia	P R S	in measure eye, vision	Normal or perfect vision
esotropia (ĕs″ ō-trō′ pĭ-ă)	eso trop ia	P R S	inward turn condition	A condition in which the eye or eyes turn inward; *crossed eyes*
gonioscope (gō′ nĭ-ō-skōp)	gonio scope	CF S	angle instrument	An instrument used to examine the angle of the anterior chamber of the eye
hyperopia (hī‴ pĕr-ō′ pĭ-ă)	hyper opia	P S	beyond eye, vision	A defect in vision in which parallel rays come to a focus beyond the retina; *farsightedness*
intraocular (ĭn″trăh-ŏk′ ū-lăr)	intra ocul ar	P R S	within eye pertaining to	Pertaining to within the eye

TERMINOLOGY SPOTLIGHT

Intraocular means pertaining to within the eye. **Glaucoma** is a group of eye diseases characterized by increased intraocular pressure (IOP). The three major categories of glaucoma are: closed-angle (acute) glaucoma; open-angle (chronic) glaucoma; and congenital glaucoma.

Terminology - continued

TERM	WORD PARTS			DEFINITION

Glaucoma occurs when the intraocular fluid accumulates in the anterior chamber of the eye and drains too slowly from the aqueous humor. This causes a buildup of intraocular pressure that is too high for the proper functioning of the optic nerve. When glaucoma is diagnosed early and managed properly, blindness may be prevented.

Glaucoma is the leading cause of blindness in the United States. Approximately 80,000 people are totally blind from glaucoma with approximately 250,000 people being blind in one eye and approximately 1.2 million more with some degree of visual loss from glaucoma. About 2% of the population aged 40 to 50 and 8% over age 70 have elevated intraocular pressure. Some 20 million people in the United States are susceptible to developing glaucoma. Glaucoma affects people of all ages and all races. Most patients have no symptoms from glaucoma; therefore, it is important to know the factors that predispose someone to glaucoma.

The predisposing factors for developing glaucoma include:

- Over 60 years of age
- African ancestry
- Someone in family has glaucoma or diabetes
- Previous eye injury
- Taking steroid medication

- Myopia
- Thyroid disease
- Diabetes
- Hypertension

TERM	WORD PARTS			DEFINITION
iridectomy (ĭr″ ĭ-dĕk′ tō-mē)	irid ectomy	R S	iris excision	Surgical excision of a portion of the iris
iridocyclitis (ĭr″ ĭd-ō-sī-klī′ tĭs)	irido cycl itis	CF R S	iris ciliary body inflammation	Inflammation of the iris and ciliary body
iridodesis (ĭr″ ĭ-dŏd′ ĕ-sĭs)	irido desis	CF S	iris binding	Surgical binding of part of the iris to form an artificial one
iridomalacia (ĭr″ ĭd-ō-mă-lā′ shĭ-ă)	irido malacia	CF S	iris softening	A softening of the iris
iridotasis (ĭr″ ĭ-dŏt′ ă-sĭs)	irido tasis	CF S	iris stretching	A stretching of the iris in treatment of glaucoma
keratitis (kĕr″ ă-tī′ tĭs)	kerat itis	R S	cornea inflammation	Inflammation of the cornea
keratometer (kĕr″ ă-tŏm′ ĕ-tĕr)	kerato meter	CF S	cornea instrument to measure	An instrument used to measure the curve of the cornea
keratoplasty (kĕr′ ă-tō-plăs″ tē)	kerato plasty	CF S	cornea surgical repair	Surgical repair of the cornea
lacrimal (lăk′ rĭm-ăl)	lacrim al	R S	tear pertaining to	Pertaining to tears

continued

Terminology - continued

TERM	WORD PARTS			DEFINITION
myopia (mī-ŏ′ pĭ-ă)	my opia	R S	to shut eye, vision	A defect in vision in which parallel rays come to a focus in front of the retina; *nearsightedness*
nyctalopia (nĭk″tă-lō′ pĭ-ă)	nyctal opia	R S	blind eye, vision	A condition in which the individual has difficulty seeing at night; night blindness
ocular (ŏk′ ū-lar)	ocul ar	R S	eye pertaining to	Pertaining to the eye
ophthalmologist (ŏf″ thăl-mŏl′ ō-jĭst)	ophthalmo log ist	CF R S	eye study of one who specializes	One who specializes in the study of the eye
ophthalmology (ŏf″ thăl-mŏl′ ō-jē)	ophthalmo logy	CF S	eye study of	The study of the eye
ophthalmopathy (of″ thăl-mŏp′ ă-thē)	ophthalmo pathy	CF S	eye disease	Any eye disease
ophthalmoscope (ŏf″ thăl′ mō-skōp)	ophthalmo scope	CF S	eye instrument	An instrument used to examine the interior of the eye
optic (op′ tĭk)	opt ic	R S	eye pertaining to	Pertaining to the eye
optomyometer (ŏp″ tō-mī-ŏm′ ĕt-ĕr)	opto myo meter	CF CF S	eye muscle instrument to measure	An instrument used to measure the strength of the muscles of the eye
phacolysis (făk-ŏl″ ĭ-sĭs)	phaco lysis	CF S	lens destruction, to separate	Surgical destruction and removal of the crystalline lens in the treatment of cataract
phacosclerosis (făk″ ō-sklĕr-ō′ sĭs)	phaco scler osis	CF R S	lens hardening condition of	A condition of hardening of the crystalline lens
photophobia (fō″ tō-fō′ bĭ-ă)	photo phobia	CF S	light fear	Unusual intolerance of light
presbyopia (prĕz″ bĭ-ō′ pĭ-ă)	presby opia	R S	old eye, vision	A defect in vision in which parallel rays come to a focus beyond the retina; occurs normally with aging; *farsightedness*

Terminology - continued

TERM	WORD PARTS			DEFINITION
pupillary (pū′ pĭ-lĕr-ē)	pupill ary	R S	pupil pertaining to	Pertaining to the pupil
retinal (rĕt′ ĭ-năl)	retin al	R S	retina pertaining to	Pertaining to the retina
retinitis (rĕt″ĭ-nī′ tĭs)	retin itis	R S	retina inflammation	Inflammation of the retina
retinoblastoma (rĕt″ ĭ-nō-blăs-tō′ mă)	retino blast oma	CF S S	retina germ cell tumor	A malignant tumor arising from the germ cell of the retina
retinopathy (rĕt″ ĭn-ŏp′ ă-thē)	retino pathy	CF S	retina disease	Any disease of the retina
scleritis (sklē- rī′ tĭs)	scler itis	R S	sclera inflammation	Inflammation of the sclera
tonography (tō-nŏg′ ră-fē)	tono graphy	CF S	tone recording	Recording of intraocular pressure used in detecting glaucoma
tonometer (tŏn-ŏm′ ĕ-tĕr)	tono meter	CF S	tone instrument to measure	An instrument used to measure intraocular pressure
trifocal (trĭ-fō′ căl)	tri foc al	P R S	three focus pertaining to	Pertaining to having three foci
uveal (ū′ vē-ăl)	uve al	R S	uvea pertaining to	Pertaining to the second or vascular coat of the eye
uveitis (ū-vē- ī′ tĭs)	uve itis	R S	uvea inflammation	Inflammation of the uvea
xenophthalmia (zĕn″ŏf-thăl′ mē-ă)	xen ophthalm ia	R R S	foreign material eye condition	Inflamed eye condition caused by foreign material
xerophthalmia (zē-rŏf-thăl′ mĭ-ă)	xer ophthalm ia	R R S	dry eye condition	An eye condition in which there is dryness of the conjunctiva

VOCABULARY WORDS

Vocabulary words are terms that have not been divided into component parts. They are common words or specialized terms associated with the subject of this chapter. These words are provided to enhance your medical vocabulary.

WORD	DEFINITION
accommodation (ă-kŏm″ ō-dā′ shŭn)	The process whereby the eyes make adjustments for seeing objects at various distances
anomaloscope (ă-nŏm′ a-lō-skōp)	Instrument used for detecting color blindness
cataract (kăt″ ə răkt′)	An opacity of the crystalline lens or its capsule; most often occurs in adults past middle age
chalazion (kă-lā′ zĭ-ŏn)	A small, hard, painless cyst of a meibomian gland *(one of the sebaceous follicles of the eyelids)*
conjunctivitis (kŏn-jŭnk″ tĭ-vī′tĭs)	Inflammation of the conjunctiva caused by allergy, trauma, chemical injury, bacterial, viral, or rickettsial infection. The type called "pinkeye" is infectious and contagious.
corneal transplant (kŏr′ nē-ăl trăns′ plănt)	The surgical process of transferring the cornea from a donor to a patient
cryosurgery (krī″ ō-sur′ jur-ē)	A type of surgery that uses extreme cold for destruction of tissue or for production of well-demarcated areas of cell injury; may be used in the removal of cataracts and in the repair of retinal detachment
entropion (ĕn-trō-pē-ŏn)	The turning inward of the margin of the lower eyelid
enucleation (ē- nū″ klē- ā′ shŭn)	A process of removing an entire part or mass without rupture, as the eyeball from its orbit
epiphora (ĕ-pĭf′ō-ră)	The abnormal downpour of tears caused by excessive secretion or obstruction of a lacrimal duct
exotropia (ĕks″ ō-trō′ pē-ă)	The turning outward of one or both eyes
glaucoma (glaw-kō′ mă)	A disease characterized by increased intraocular pressure, which results in atrophy of the optic nerve and blindness
hemianopia (hĕm″ ē-ă-nŏ′ pē-ă)	The inability (blindness) to see half the field of vision

Vocabulary - continued

WORD	DEFINITION
keratoconjunc-tivitis (kĕr″ă-tō-kŏn-jŭnk″ tĭ-vī′ tĭs)	Inflammation of the cornea and the conjunctiva
laser (lā′ zĕr)	An acronym for **l**ight **a**mplification by **s**timulated **e**mission of **r**adiation
laser trabeculo-plasty (tră-bĕk′ ū-lō-plăs″ tē)	The use of a laser to reduce intraocular pressure; may be used to treat glaucoma
microlens (mī′ krō-lĕns)	A small, thin corneal contact lens
miotic (mĭ-ŏt′ ĭk)	Pertaining to an agent that causes the pupil to contract
mydriatic (mĭd″ rĭ-ăt′ ĭk)	Pertaining to an agent that causes the pupil to dilate
nystagmus (nĭs-tăg′ mŭs)	An involuntary, constant, rhythmic movement of the eyeball
optician (ŏp-tĭsh′ ăn)	One who specializes in the making of optical products and accessories. This person is not a physician.
optometrist (ŏp-tŏm′ ĕ-trĭst)	One who specializes in examining the eyes for refractive errors and providing appropriate corrective lenses. This person is not a physician but is trained and licensed as a Doctor of Optometry (OD).
orthoptics (or-thŏp′ tĭks)	The study and treatment of defective binocular vision resulting from defects in ocular musculature; also a technique of eye exercises for correcting defective binocular vision
phacoemulsifi-cation (făk″ ō-ē′ mŭl′sĭ-fĭ-kā″ shŭn)	The process of using ultrasound to disintegrate a cataract. A needle is inserted through a small incision, and the disintegrated cataract is aspirated.
photocoagulation (fō″ tō-kō-ăg″ ū-lā′ shŭn)	The process of altering proteins in tissue by the use of light energy such as the laser beam; used in the treatment of retinal detachment, retinal bleeding, or intraocular tumors
pterygium (tĕr-ĭj′ ĭ-ŭm)	An abnormal triangular fold of membrane that extends from the conjunctiva to the cornea

continued

Vocabulary - continued

WORD	DEFINITION
radial keratotomy (rā′ dē-ăl kĕr-ă′ tŏt′ ō-mē)	A surgical procedure that may be performed to correct nearsightedness *(myopia)*. Delicate spoke-like incisions are made in the cornea to flatten it, thereby shortening the eyeball so that light reaches the retina. Not all patients have their vision improved, and complications could lead to blindness.
retrolental fibroplasia (RLF) (rĕt″ rō-lĕn-tăl fĭ-brō-plā-sē-ă)	A disease of the retinal vessels present in premature infants; may be caused by excessive use of oxygen in the incubator. Retinal detachment and blindness may occur.
Snellen chart (snĕl′ ĕn chart)	A chart for testing visual acuity. It is printed with lines of black letters that are graduated in size from smallest, on the bottom to largest on the top (Fig. 14–3).
strabismus (stră-bĭz′ mŭs)	A disorder of the eye in which the optic axes cannot be directed to the same object; *also called a squint*
sty(e) (stī)	Inflammation of one or more of the sebaceous glands of the eyelid; *also called a hordeolum*
trachoma (trā-kō′ mă)	A chronic contagious disease of the conjunctiva and cornea. The disease affects millions of people, mostly in Asia and Africa, but is also seen in the southwestern part of the United States.
trichiasis (trĭk-ī′ ăs-ĭs)	A condition of ingrowing eyelids that rub against the cornea causing a constant irritation to the eyeball

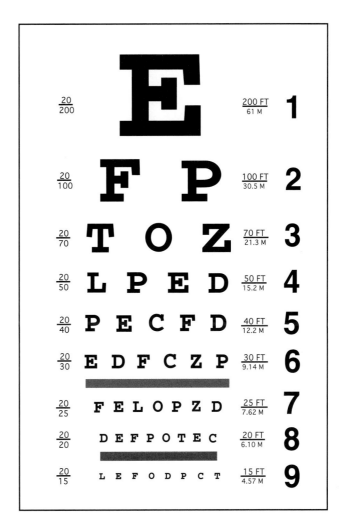

FIGURE 14–3

The Snellen eye chart. Individuals with normal vision can read line 8 of a full-sized chart at 20 feet (6.10 m).

 # ABBREVIATIONS

Acc	accommodation	**IOL**	intraocular lens
ALT	argon laser trabeculoplasty	**IOP**	intraocular pressure
D	diopter	**L & A**	light and accommodation
DVA	distance visual acuity	**LE**	left eye
ECCE	extracapsular cataract extraction	**LTP**	laser trabeculoplasty
EM	emmetropia	**MY**	myopia
EOM	extraocular movement; extraocular muscles	**NVA**	near visual acuity
		OD	oculus dexter (right eye)
HT	hypermetropia (hyperopia)	**OS**	oculus sinister (left eye)
ICCE	intracapsular cataract cryoextraction	**OU**	oculus uterque (each eye)

PERLA	pupils equal, react to light and	VA	visual acuity
	accommodation	VF	visual field
RE	right eye	**XT**	exotropia
REM	rapid eye movement	+	plus or convex
SMD	senile macular degeneration	–	minus or concave
ST	esotropia		

DRUG HIGHLIGHTS

Drugs that are generally used for the eye include those that are used for glaucoma, during diagnostic examination of the eye, and in intraocular surgery. Antibiotics, antifungal, and antiviral drugs are used in the treatment of eye infections.

Drugs Used to Treat Glaucoma   Either increase the outflow of aqueous humor, decrease its production, or produce both of these actions. These drugs may be diuretics, direct-acting miotics, and/or cholinesterase inhibitors.

Diuretics   *Examples: Diamox (acetazolamide), Daranide (dichlorphenamide), Glycerol (glycerin), Osmitrol (mannitol), and Ureaphil (urea).*

Direct-acting miotics   *Examples: Miochol (acetylcholine chloride) and Isopto Carbachol (carbachol).*

Cholinesterase inhibitors   *Examples: Humorsol (demecarium bromide), Phospholine Iodide (echothiophate), Floropryl (isoflurophate), and Eserine Sulfate (physostigmine sulfate).*

Mydriatics   Agents that are used to produce dilation of the pupil (mydriasis) may be anticholinergics or sympathomimetics.

Anticholinergics   Produce dilation of the pupil and interfere with the ability of the eye to focus properly (cycloplegia). They are used primarily as an aid in refraction, during internal examination of the eye, in intraocular surgery, and in the treatment of anterior uveitis and secondary glaucomas.
Examples: Atropisol (atropine sulfate), Cyclogyl (cyclopentolate HCl), Isopto Homatropine (homatropine HBr), Hyoscine (scopolamine HBr), and Mydriacyl (tropicamide).

Sympathomimetics   Produced mydriasis without cycloplegia. Pupil dilation is obtained as the drug causes contraction of the dilator muscle of the iris. They also affect intraocular pressure by decreasing production of aqueous humor while increasing its outflow from the eye.
Examples: Propine (dipivefrin HCl), Paredrine (hydroxyamphetamine HBr), Naphcon (naphazoline HCl), and Murine, Visine (tetrahydrozoline (HCl).

Antibiotics   Used to treat infectious diseases. Those that are used for the eye may be in the form of an ointment, cream, or solution.
Examples: Aureomycin Ophthalmic (chlortetracycline HCl) ointment 1%, erythromycin, bacitracin, tetracycline HCl, chloramphenicol, and polymyxin B sulfate.

Antifungal Agent   *Natacyn (natamycin)* is used in treating fungal infections of the eye, such as blepharitis, conjunctivitis, and keratitis.

Antiviral Agents   *Stoxil, Herplex (idoxuridine)* is a potent antiviral agent used in the treatment of keratitis caused by the herpes simplex virus. *Vira-A (vidarabine) and Viroptic (trifluridine)* are also used to treat viral infections of the eye and are effective in the treatment of herpes simplex infections.

DIAGNOSTIC AND LABORATORY TESTS

Test	Description
color vision tests (kul′ or vĭzh′ ŭn test)	The use of polychromatic plates or an anomaloscope to assess the ability to recognize differences in color.
exophthalmometry (ĕk″ sŏf-thăl-mŏm′ ĕ-trē)	Measurement of the forward protrusion of the eye via an exophthalmometer; used to evaluate an increase or decrease in exophthalmos.
gonioscopy (gō″ nē-ŏs′ kō-pē)	Examination of the anterior chamber of the eye via a gonioscope; used for determining ocular motility and rotation.
keratometry (kĕr″ ă-tŏm′ ĕ-trē)	Measurement of the cornea via a keratometer.
ocular ultrasonography (ŏk′ ū lăr ŭl-tră-sŏn-ŏg′ ră-fē)	The use of high-frequency sound waves (via a small probe placed on the eye) to measure for intraocular lenses and to detect orbital and periorbital lesions; also used to measure the length of the eye and the curvature of the cornea in preparation for surgery.
ophthalmoscopy (ŏf-thăl-mŏs′ kō-pē)	Examination of the interior of the eyes via an ophthalmoscope; used to identify changes in the blood vessels in the eye and to diagnose systemic diseases.
tonometry (tōn-ŏm′ ĕ-trē)	Measurement of the intraocular pressure of the eye via a tonometer; used to screen for and detect glaucoma.
visual acuity (vĭzh′ ū-ăl ă-kū′ ĭ-tē)	Measurement of the acuteness or sharpness of vision. A Snellen eye chart may be used, and the patient reads letters of various sizes from a distance of 20 feet. Normal vision is 20/20.

COMMUNICATION ENRICHMENT

This segment is provided for those who wish to enhance their ability to communicate in either English or Spanish.

▶ Related Terms

English	Spanish	English	Spanish
blind	ciego (sĭ-*ĕ*-gō)	eyelid	párpado (*păr*-pă-do)
blindness	ceguedad (sĕ-gĕ-*dăd*)	eye	ojo (*ō*-hō)
cloudy vision	visión nublada (vĭ-sĭ-*ōn* nū-*blă*-dă)	eyeglasses	anteojos; espejuelos (ăn-tĕ-*ō*-hō; ĕs-pĕ-*hū*-ĕ-lōs)
double vision	visión doble (vĭ-sĭ-*ōn dō*-blĕ)	glaucoma	glaucoma (glă-ū-*cō*-mă)
cataract	catarata (că-tă-*ră*-tă)	pupil	pupila (*pū*-pĭ-lă)
conjunctiva	conjuntiva (cōn-hūn-*tĭ*-vă)	vision	visión (*vĭ*-sĭ-ōn)
contact lens	lente de contacto (*lĕn*-tĕ dĕ *cōn*-tăc-tō)	loss of	pérdida de visión (*pĕr*-dĭ-dă dĕ *vĭ*-sĭ-ōn)
for distance	para distancia (*pă*-ră dĭs-*tăn*-sĭ-ă)	problems	problemas (prō-*blĕ*-măs)
for close-up	para de cerca (*pă*-ră dĕ *sĕr*-kă)	test	examen (ex-*să*-mĕn)
for reading	para leer (*pă*-ră lĕ-*ĕr*)	laser	láser (*lă*-sĕr)
all the time	todo el tiempo (*tō*-dō ĕl tĭ-*ĕm*-pō)	view	paisaje (pă-ĭ-*să*-hĕ)
since when	¿desde cuándo? (dĕs-*dĕ kwan*-dō)	conjunctivitis	conjuntivitis (con-*hūn*-tĭ-vĭ-tĭs)
eyebrow	ceja (*sĕ*-hă)	near	cerca (*sĕr*-kă)
eyelash	pestaña (pĕs-*tan*-yă)	far	lejos (*lĕ*-hōs)

English	Spanish	English	Spanish
see	ver (vĕr)	optic	óptico (ōp-tĭ-kō)
sight	vista (vĭs-tă)	orbit	órbita (ōr-bĭ-tă)
cornea	córnea (cōr-nĕ-ă)	iris	iris (ĭ-rĭs)
lens	lente (lĕn-tĕ)	tear	lágrima (lă-grĭ-ma)

STUDY AND REVIEW SECTION

LEARNING EXERCISES

▶ Anatomy and Physiology

Write your answers to the following questions. Do not refer back to the text.

1. The external structures of the eye are the _____,

   _____, _____, _____,

   and the _____ _____.

2. The orbit is lined with _____ _____, which
   cushions the eyeball.

3. The optic foramen is an opening for the _____ _____

   and _____ _____.

4. State the functions of the muscles of the eye.

   a. _____

   b. _____

5. Each eye has a pair of eyelids that function to protect the eyeball from _____

   _____, _____ _____, and _____.

6. Describe the conjunctiva and state its function. _____

   _____

7. Define lacrimal apparatus. _____

   _____

8. The internal structures of the eye are the _____,

    _____, and the _____ _____.

9. The eyeball is the organ of _____.

10. The point at which nerve fibers from the retina converge to form the optic nerve

    is known as the _____ _____.

11. Define accommodation. _____

    _____

12. Match the following terms and definitions by placing the correct letter on the
    line provided.

    _____   1. Aqueous humor   a. White of the eye

    _____   2. Vitreous humor   b. Colored membrane attached to the ciliary
                                            body
    _____   3. Iris
                                         c. Watery fluid
    _____   4. Sclera
                                         d. Opening in the center of the iris
    _____   5. Uvea
                                         e. Jelly-like material
    _____   6. Pupil
                                         f. Middle layer of the eyeball
    _____   7. Retina
                                         g. Anterior transparent portion of the eyeball
    _____   8. Rods and cones
                                         h. Innermost layer of the eyeball
    _____   9. Lens
                                         i. Photoreceptive cells
    _____ 10. Cornea
                                         j. Colorless crystalline body

► **Word Parts**

1. In the spaces provided, write the definitions for the following prefixes, roots,
    combining forms, and suffixes. Do not refer to the listings of terminology words.
    Leave blank those terms you cannot define.

2. After completing as many as you can, refer back to the terminology word listings to
    check your work. For each word missed or left blank, write the term and its
    definition several times on the margins of these pages or on a separate sheet of
    paper.

3. To maximize the learning process, it is to your advantage to do the following
    exercises as directed. To refer to the terminology listings before completing these
    exercises invalidates the learning process.

Prefixes

Give the definitions of the following prefixes:

1. a- _____
2. bi- _____
3. dipl- _____
4. ec- _____
5. em- _____
6. eso- _____
7. hyper- _____
8. intra- _____
9. tri- _____

Roots and Combining Forms

Give the definitions of the following roots and combining forms:

1. ambly _____
2. ametr _____
3. aniso _____
4. blephar _____
5. blepharo _____
6. choroid _____
7. choroido _____
8. cor _____
9. corne _____
10. cycl _____
11. cyclo _____
12. cyst _____
13. dacry _____
14. dacryo _____
15. electro _____
16. foc _____
17. gonio _____
18. irid _____
19. irido _____
20. kerat _____
21. kerato _____
22. lacrim _____
23. log _____
24. metr _____
25. my _____
26. myo _____
27. nyctal _____
28. ocul _____
29. ophthalm _____
30. ophthalmo _____
31. opt _____
32. opto _____
33. phaco _____
34. phak _____
35. photo _____
36. presby _____
37. pupill _____
38. retin _____
39. retino _____
40. scler _____

41. stigmat _____

42. tono _____

43. trop _____

44. uve _____

45. xen _____

46. xer _____

Suffixes

Give the definitions of the following suffixes:

1. -al _____

2. -ar _____

3. -ary _____

4. -blast _____

5. -desis _____

6. -ectomy _____

7. -gram _____

8. -graphy _____

9. -ia _____

10. -ic _____

11. -ion _____

12. -ism _____

13. -ist _____

14. -itis _____

15. -logy _____

16. -lysis _____

17. -malacia _____

18. -meter _____

19. -oma _____

20. -opia _____

21. -osis _____

22. -pathy _____

23. -phobia _____

24. -plasty _____

25. -plegia _____

26. -ptosis _____

27. -scope _____

28. -tasis _____

▶ Identifying Medical Terms

In the spaces provided, write the medical terms for the following meanings:

1. _____   Dullness of vision

2. _____   Pertaining to having two foci

3. _____   A drooping of the upper eyelid

4. _____   Pertaining to the cornea

5. _____   A tumor-like swelling caused by obstruction of the tear duct

6. _____   Double vision

7. _____ Normal or perfect vision

8. _____ Pertaining to within the eye

9. _____ A softening of the iris

10. _____ Inflammation of the cornea

11. _____ Surgical repair of the cornea

12. _____ Pertaining to tears

13. _____ Pertaining to the eye

14. _____ Any eye disease

15. _____ Unusual intolerance of light

▶ Spelling

In the spaces provided, write the correct spelling of these misspelled terms:

1. atigmatism _____
2. cyloplegia _____
3. irdectomy _____
4. opthalmologist _____
5. pacosclerosis _____
6. pupilary _____
7. retinblastoma _____
8. sleritis _____
9. tonmeter _____
10. ueal _____

WORD PARTS STUDY SHEET

Word Parts	Give the Meaning
a-	_____
bi-	_____
dipl-	_____
ec-	_____
em-	_____
eso-	_____
intra-	_____
tri-	_____
ambly-	_____

ametr- _____

aniso- _____

blephar-, blepharo- _____

choroid-, choroido- _____

cor- _____

corne- _____

cycl-, cyclo- _____

dacry-, dacryo- _____

foc- _____

gonio- _____

irid-, irido- _____

kerat-, kerato- _____

lacrim- _____

nyctal- _____

ocul-, ophthalm-, ophthalmo-, opt-, opto- _____

phaco- _____

phak- _____

photo- _____

presby- _____

pupill- _____

retin-, retino- _____

scler- _____

stigmat- _____

tono- _____

uve- _____

xen- _____

xer- _____

-lysis _____

-opia _____

-ptosis _____

REVIEW QUESTIONS

▶ **Matching**

Select the appropriate lettered meaning for each numbered line.

_____ 1. anomaloscope

_____ 2. entropion

_____ 3. epiphora

_____ 4. hemianopia

_____ 5. phacoemulsification

_____ 6. photocoagulation

_____ 7. radial keratotomy

_____ 8. retrolental fibroplasia

_____ 9. strabismus

_____ 10. sty(e)

a. A squint
b. A disease of the retinal vessels present in premature infants
c. The process of using ultrasound to disintegrate a cataract
d. The use of a laser to treat retinal detachment and/or retinal bleeding
e. An instrument used for detecting color blindness
f. The turning inward of the margin of the lower eyelid
g. A surgical procedure that may be performed to correct myopia
h. The inability to see half the field of vision
i. A hordeolum
j. The abnormal downpour of tears
k. A disease characterized by increased intraocular pressure

▶ **Abbreviations**

Place the correct word, phrase, or abbreviation in the space provided.

1. distance visual acuity _____

2. EM _____

3. HT _____

4. intraocular lens _____

5. light and accommodation _____

6. MY _____

7. OD _____

8. left eye _____

9. each eye _____

10. XT _____

► Diagnostic and Laboratory Tests

Select the best answer to each multiple choice question. Circle the letter of your choice.

1. The measurement of the forward protrusion of the eye.
   a. gonioscopy
   b. keratometry
   c. exophthalmometry
   d. tonometry

2. The measurement of the cornea.
   a. gonioscopy
   b. keratometry
   c. exophthalmometry
   d. tonometry

3. Used to identify changes in the blood vessels in the eye and to diagnose systemic diseases.
   a. exophthalmometry
   b. gonioscopy
   c. ophthalmoscopy
   d. tonometry

4. The measurement of the intraocular pressure of the eye.
   a. exophthalmometry
   b. gonioscopy
   c. ophthalmoscopy
   d. tonometry

5. The measurement of the acuteness or sharpness of vision.
   a. color vision tests
   b. ultrasonography
   c. tonometry
   d. visual acuity

CRITICAL THINKING ACTIVITY

▶ Case Study

Cataracts

Please read the following case study and then answer the questions that follow.

A 67-year-old male was seen by a physician, and the following is a synopsis of the visit.

Present History: The patient states that he has trouble driving at night, bright lights hurt his eyes, his vision seems to blur while watching television, he feels as though his glasses are dirty and there is a film over his eyes, and on occasion he has seen halos around lights. His ophthalmologist previously told him that he was developing cataracts and when the condition began to interfere with his life-style he would be a candidate for surgery. He is back in for his yearly eye examination and to talk to his physician about eye surgery. He would like to have his right eye done first.

Signs and Symptoms: Chief complaint: trouble driving at night, photophobia, blurred vision, feels like there is a film over his eyes, and sees halos around lights.

Diagnosis: Cataracts. The diagnosis was determined by a complete eye examination.

Treatment: Surgical procedure—phacoemulsification. Phacoemulsification is the process of using an ultrasonic device to disintegrate the cataract, which is then aspirated and removed. After surgery, the patient is advised not to lift any heavy objects, run, jog, or ride a horse, The patient should avoid sleeping on the operative side, rubbing the eyes, squeezing the eyelids shut, straining at bowel movement, getting soap in the eyes, sexual relations, driving, coughing, sneezing, vomiting, and bending head down below waist. The patient is advised to report any unusual symptoms such as pain, changes in vision, persistent headache, and discharge from the eye to his physician.

Prevention: Since most cataracts occur as part of the aging process, there are no known preventive measures.

Critical Thinking Questions

1. Signs and symptoms of cataracts include trouble driving at night, _____, blurred vision, film over the eyes, and seeing halos around lights.

2. The diagnosis was determined by a _____ eye examination.

3. Treatment included a surgical procedure known as phacoemulsification where an _____ device is used to disintegrate the cataract.

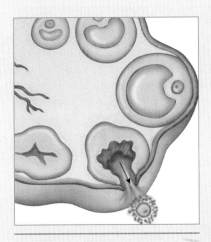

THE FEMALE REPRODUCTIVE SYSTEM

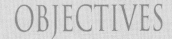

OBJECTIVES

On completion of this chapter, you should be able to:

- Describe the uterus and state its functions.

- Describe the fallopian tubes and state their functions.

- Describe the ovaries and state their functions.

- Describe the vagina and state its functions.

- Describe the breast.

- Describe the menstrual cycle.

- Analyze, build, spell, and pronounce medical words that relate to surgical procedures and pathology.

- Identify and give the meaning of selected vocabulary words.

- Identify and define selected abbreviations.

- Review Drug Highlights presented in this chapter.

- Provide the description of diagnostic and laboratory tests related to the female reproductive system.

- Successfully complete the study and review section.

▶ ANATOMY AND PHYSIOLOGY OVERVIEW

The female reproductive system consists of the left and right *ovaries,* which are the female's primary sex organs, and the following accessory sex organs: two *fallopian tubes,* the *uterus,* the *vagina,* the *vulva,* and two *breasts.* The vital function of the female reproductive system is to perpetuate the species through sexual or germ cell reproduction.

▶ THE UTERUS

The *uterus* is a muscular, hollow, pear-shaped organ having three identifiable areas: the *body* or upper portion, the *isthmus* or central area, and the *cervix,* which is the lower cylindrical portion or neck. The *fundus* is the bulging surface of the body of the uterus extending from the internal os *(mouth)* of the cervix upward above the fallopian tubes. The uterus is suspended in the anterior part of the pelvic cavity, halfway between the sacrum and the symphysis pubis, above the bladder, and in front of the rectum. A number of ligaments support the uterus and hold it in position. These are two broad ligaments, two round ligaments, two uterosacral ligaments, and the ligaments that are attached to the bladder. The normal position of the uterus is with the cervix pointing toward the lower end of the sacrum and the fundus toward the suprapubic region. An average, normal uterus is about 8 cm long, 5 cm wide, and 2.5 cm thick (Figs. 15–1 and 15–2).

THE UTERINE WALL

The wall of the uterus consists of three layers: the *peritoneum* or outer layer, the *myometrium* or muscular middle layer, and the *endometrium,* which is the mucous membrane lining the inner surface of the uterus. The endometrium is composed of columnar ep-

THE FEMALE REPRODUCTIVE SYSTEM

ORGAN/STRUCTURE	PRIMARY FUNCTIONS
The Uterus	Organ of the cyclic discharge of menses; provides place for the nourishment and development of the fetus; contracts during labor to help expel the fetus
The Fallopian Tubes	Serve as a duct for the conveyance of the ovum from the ovary to the uterus; serve as ducts for the conveyance of spermatozoa from the uterus toward the ovary
The Ovaries	Production of ova and hormones
The Vagina	Female organ of copulation; serves as a passageway for the discharge of menstruation; serves as a passageway for the birth of the fetus
The Vulva	External female genitalia
Mons pubis	Provides pad of fatty tissue
Labia majora	Provides two folds of adipose tissue
Labia minora	Lies within the labia majora and encloses the vestibule
Vestibule	Opening for the urethra, the vagina, and two excretory ducts of Bartholin's glands
Clitoris	Erectile tissue that is homologous to the penis of the male; produces pleasurable sensations during the sexual act
The Breast	Following childbirth, mammary glands produce milk

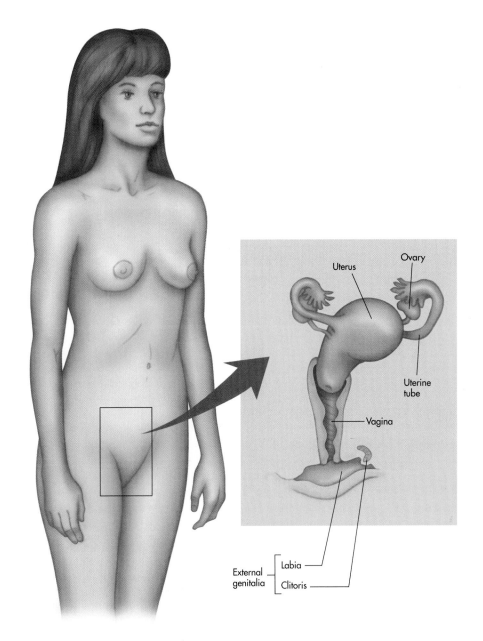

FIGURE 15–1

The female reproductive system.

ithelium and connective tissue and is supplied with blood by both straight and spiral arteries. It undergoes marked changes in response to hormonal stimulation during the menstrual cycle. These changes are discussed in the last section of this overview.

FUNCTIONS OF THE UTERUS

There are three primary functions associated with the uterus:

- It is the organ of the cyclic discharge of a bloody fluid from the uterus and the changes that occur to its endometrium.

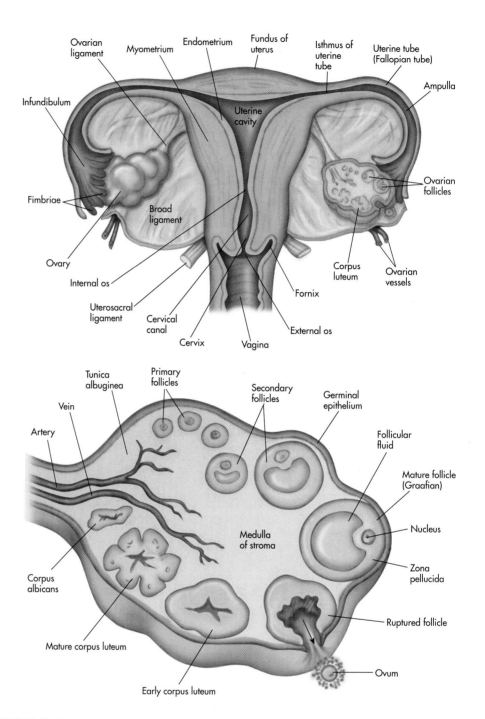

FIGURE 15–2

The uterus, ovaries, and associated structures with an expanded view of a mammalian ovary showing stages of graafian follicle and ovum development.

- It functions as a place for the protection and nourishment of the fetus during pregnancy.
- During labor, the muscular uterine wall contracts rhythmically and powerfully to expel the fetus from the uterus.

ABNORMAL POSITIONS OF THE UTERUS

The uterus may become malpositioned because of weakness of any of its supporting ligaments. Trauma, disease processes of the uterus, or multiple pregnancies may contribute to the weakening of the supporting ligaments. The following terms describe some of the abnormal positions of the uterus:

Anteflexion. The process of bending forward of the uterus at its body and neck

Retroflexion. The process of bending the body of the uterus backward at an angle with the cervix usually unchanged from its normal position

Anteversion. The process of turning the fundus forward toward the pubis, with the cervix tilted up toward the sacrum

Retroversion. The process of turning the uterus backward, with the cervix pointing forward toward the symphysis pubis

▶ THE FALLOPIAN TUBES

Also called the *uterine tubes* or *oviducts,* the *fallopian tubes* extend laterally from either side of the uterus and end near each ovary. An average, normal fallopian tube is about 11.5 cm long and 6 mm wide. Its wall is composed of three layers: the *serosa* or outermost layer, composed of connective tissue; the *muscular layer,* containing inner circular and outer longitudinal layers of smooth muscle; and the *mucosa* or inner layer, consisting of simple columnar epithelium.

ANATOMICAL FEATURES OF THE FALLOPIAN TUBES

The *isthmus* is the constricted portion of the tube nearest the uterus (see Fig. 15–2). From the isthmus, the tube continues laterally and widens to form a section called the *ampulla.* Beyond the ampulla, the tube continues to expand and ends as a funnel-shaped opening. This end of the tube is called the *infundibulum,* and its opening is the *ostium.* Surrounding each ostium are *fimbriae* or *finger-like processes* that work to propel the discharged ovum into the tube, where ciliary action aids in moving it toward the uterus. Should the ovum become impregnated by a spermatozoon while in the tube, the process of *fertilization* occurs.

FUNCTIONS OF THE FALLOPIAN TUBES

The two basic functions of the fallopian tubes are as follows:

- Each tube serves as a duct for the conveyance of the ovum from the ovary to the uterus.
- The tubes serve as ducts for the conveyance of spermatozoa from the uterus toward each ovary.

▶ THE OVARIES

Located on either side of the uterus, the *ovaries* are almond-shaped organs attached to the uterus by the ovarian ligament and lie close to the fimbriae of the fallopian tubes. The anterior border of each ovary is connected to the posterior layer of the broad ligament by the *mesovarium.* Each ovary is attached to the side of the pelvis by the *suspensory ligaments.* An average, normal ovary is about 4 cm long, 2 cm wide, and 1.5 cm thick.

MICROSCOPIC ANATOMY

Each ovary consists of two distinct areas: the *cortex* or outer layer and the *medulla* or inner portion. The cortex contains small secretory sacs or follicles in three stages of development. These stages are known as *primary, growing,* and *graafian,* which is the follicles' mature stage (see Fig. 15–2). The ovarian medulla contains connective tissue, nerves, blood and lymphatic vessels, and some smooth muscle tissue in the region of the hilus.

FUNCTION OF THE OVARIES

The functional activity of the ovary is primarily controlled by the anterior lobe of the pituitary gland, which produces the *gonadotropic hormones* FSH and LH. These abbreviations are for follicle-stimulating hormone, instrumental in the development of the ovarian follicles, and luteinizing horome, which stimulates the development of the *corpus luteum,* a small yellow mass of cells that develops within a ruptured ovarian follicle.

Two functions have been identified for the ovary: the production of ova or female reproductive cells and the production of hormones.

The Production of Ova

Each month a *graafian follicle* ruptures on the ovarian cortex, and an *ovum* (singular of ova) discharges into the pelvic cavity, where it enters the fallopian tube. This process is known as *ovulation.* In an average, normal woman more than 400 ova may be produced during her reproductive years (see Fig. 15–2).

The Production of Hormones

The ovary is also an endocrine gland, producing *estrogen* and *progesterone.* Estrogen is the female sex hormone secreted by the follicles. Progesterone is a steroid hormone secreted by the corpus luteum. These hormones are essential in promoting growth, development, and maintenance of the female secondary sex organs and characteristics. They also prepare the uterus for pregnancy, promote development of the mammary glands, and play a vital role in a woman's emotional well-being and sexual drive.

▶ THE VAGINA

The *vagina* is a musculomembranous tube extending from the vestibule to the uterus (Fig. 15–2). It is 10 to 15 cm in length and is situated between the bladder and the rectum. It is lined by mucous membrane made up of *squamous epithelium.* A fold of mucous membrane, the *hymen,* partially covers the external opening of the vagina.

FUNCTIONS OF THE VAGINA

The vagina has three basic functions:

- It is the female organ of copulation. The vagina receives the seminal fluid from the male penis.

- It serves as a passageway for the discharge of menstruation.
- It serves as a passageway for the birth of the fetus.

▶ THE VULVA

The *vulva* consists of the following five organs that comprise the external female genitalia (Fig. 15–3):

Mons pubis. A pad of fatty tissue of triangular shape and, after puberty, covered with pubic hair. It may be referred to as the mons veneris or "mound of Venus," and is the rounded area over the symphysis pubis.

Labia majora. The two folds of adipose tissue, which are large lip-like structures, lying on either side of the vaginal opening.

Labia minora. Two thin folds of skin that lie within the labia majora and enclose the vestibule.

Vestibule. The cleft between the labia minora. It is approximately 4 to 5 cm long and 2 cm wide. Four major structures open into it: the urethra, the vagina, and two excretory ducts of the Bartholin glands.

Clitoris. A small organ consisting of sensitive erectile tissue that is homologous to the penis of the male.

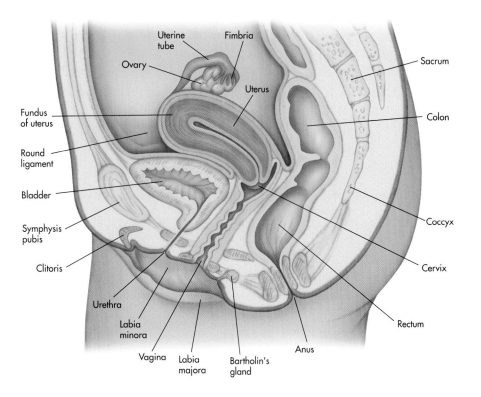

FIGURE 15–3

Sagittal section of the female pelvis, showing organs of the reproductive system.

Between the vulva and the anus is an external region known as the *perineum.* It is composed of muscle covered with skin. During the second stage of labor, a decision is made by the attending physician as to the need to perform an *episiotomy,* a surgical procedure to prevent tearing of the perineum and to facilitate delivery of the fetus.

▶ THE BREAST

The *breasts* or mammary glands are compound *alveolar structures* consisting of 15 to 20 glandular tissue lobes separated by septa of connective tissue. Most women have two breasts that lie anterior to the pectoral muscles and curve outward from the lateral margins of the sternum to the anterior border of the axilla. The size of the breast may greatly vary according to age, heredity, and adipose *(fatty)* tissue present. The *areola* is the dark, pigmented area found in the skin over each breast, and the nipple is the elevated area in the center of the areola. During pregnancy, the areola changes from its pinkish color to a dark brown or reddish color. The areola is supplied with a row of small sebaceous glands that secrete an oily substance to keep it resilient. The *lactiferous glands* consist of 20 to 24 glands in the areola of the nipple and, during lactation, secrete and convey milk to a suckling infant (Fig. 15–4). The hormone *prolactin,* which is pro-

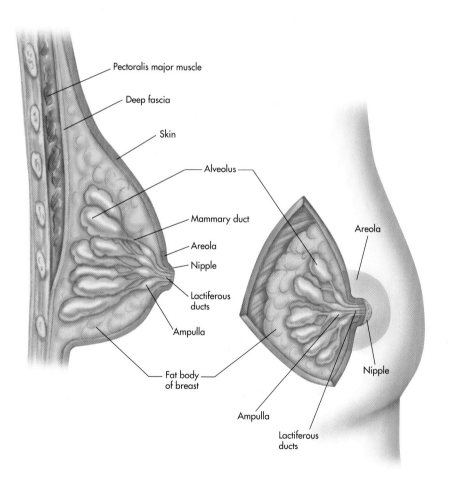

FIGURE 15–4

The breast.

duced by the anterior lobe of the pituitary, stimulates the mammary glands to produce milk after childbirth. Other hormones playing a role in milk production are insulin and glucocorticoids. *Colostrum*, a thin yellowish secretion, is the "first milk" and contains mainly serum and white blood cells. Suckling stimulates the production of oxytocin by the posterior lobe of the pituitary gland. It acts on the mammary glands to stimulate the release of milk and stimulates the uterus to contract during parturition.

BREAST-FEEDING

Among the natural advantages of breast-feeding are the following:

- It provides an ideal food for most newborn babies.
- The milk provides essential nutrients for growth and development.
- The milk is virtually free from harmful bacteria.

After the first 2 weeks, the nursing mother may produce 1 or more pints of milk per day. Milk production may be affected by emotions, food, fluids, physical health, and medications. The nursing mother will usually have a supply of milk for her suckling infant for a period of 6 to 9 months. The nursing process is usually a satisfying experience for both mother and infant. For the mother, the nursing causes contractions of the muscles of the uterus, which aid in its rapid return to normal size. For the infant, breast milk is a natural substance that provides almost everything needed for the first months of life.

▶ THE MENSTRUAL CYCLE

The onset of the *menstrual cycle* occurs at the age of *puberty* and its cessation is at *menopause.* It is a periodic recurrent series of changes occurring in the uterus, ovaries, vagina, and breasts approximately every 28 days. The menstrual cycle is divided into four phases, each of which is described for you.

MENSTRUATION PHASE

The *menstruation phase* is characterized by the discharge of a bloody fluid from the uterus accompanied by a shedding of the endometrium. This phase averages 4 to 5 days and is considered to be the first to the fifth days of the cycle.

PROLIFERATION PHASE

The *proliferation phase* is characterized by the stimulation of estrogen, the thickening and vascularization of the endometrium, along with the maturing of the ovarian follicle. This phase begins about the fifth day and ends at the time of rupture of the graafian follicle—about 14 days before the onset of menstruation.

LUTEAL OR SECRETORY PHASE

The *luteal phase is* characterized by continued thickening of the endometrium, by the glands within the endometrium becoming tortuous, and by the appearance of coiled arteries in its tissues. The endometrium becomes edematous, and the stroma becomes compact. During this phase, the corpus luteum in the ovary is developing and secreting progesterone. The progesterone level is highest during this phase as the estrogen level decreases. This phase lasts about 10 to 14 days.

PREMENSTRUAL OR ISCHEMIC PHASE

During the *premenstrual phase,* the coiled arteries become constricted, the endometrium becomes anemic and begins to shrink, and the corpus luteum decreases in functional activity. This phase lasts about 2 days and ends with the occurrence of menstruation.

Premenstrual syndrome is a condition that affects certain women and may cause distressful symptoms such as constipation, diarrhea, nausea, anorexia, appetite cravings, headache, backache, muscular aches, edema, insomnia, clumsiness, malaise, irritability, indecisiveness, mental confusion, and depression. These symptoms may begin 2 weeks before the onset of *menstruation.* Although the exact cause of this syndrome has not been determined, it may be due to the amount of prostaglandin produced, a deficient or excessive amount of estrogen or progesterone, or an interrelationship between these factors.

▶ THE CHILD

The sex of the child is determined at the time of **fertilization.** When a spermatozoon carrying the X sex chromosome fertilizes the X-bearing ovum, the result is a female child (X + X = female). When the X-bearing ovum is fertilized by the Y-bearing spermatozoon, a male child is produced (X + Y = male). Sex differentiation occurs early in the embryo. At 16 weeks the external **genitals** of the fetus are recognizably male or female. This difference may be seen during ultrasonography. See Figure 15–5.

The genitals of the newborn are not fully developed at birth. They may be slightly swollen, and in the female infant, blood-tinged mucus may be discharged from the vagina. This is due to hormones transmitted from the mother to the infant. The labia minora may protrude beyond the labia majora.

The sex organs do not mature until the onset of **puberty.** At puberty the female experiences breast development, vaginal secretions, and menarche. A study published in the *Journal of Pediatrics,* April 1997, revealed that many girls begin to develop sexually by age 8. This study involved 17,000 American girls ages 3 to 12, who were seen in 65 pediatric practices nationwide. At age 8, 48.3% of African-American girls and 14.7% of white girls had begun developing breasts, pubic hair, or both. Among African-American girls, menstruation began on average at 12.16 years; among white girls, the average was 12.88 years. The study raised questions about whether environmental estrogens, chemicals that mimic the female hormone estrogen, are bringing on puberty at an earlier age. The study also suggested that sex education should begin sooner than it often does.

▶ THE OLDER ADULT

At about 50 years of age, men and women begin experiencing bodily changes that are directly related to **hormonal** production. In women, the ovaries cease to produce estrogen and progesterone. With decreased production of the female hormones, estrogen and progesterone, women enter the phase of life known as **menopause.** Natural menopause will occur in 25% of women by age 47, in 50% by age 50, 75% by age 52, and in 95% by age 55.

The symptoms of menopause vary from being hardly noticeable to being severe. Symptoms may include irregular periods, hot flashes, vaginal dryness, insomnia, joint pain, headache, emotional instability, irritability, and depression. Breast tissue may lose its firmness, and pubic and axillary hair becomes sparse. Without estrogen, the uterus becomes smaller, the vagina shortens and vaginal tissues become drier. There may be loss of bone mass leading to **osteoporosis.**

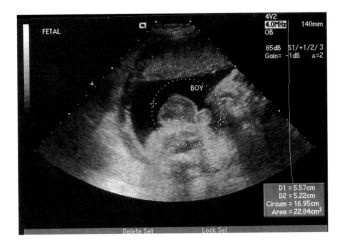

FIGURE 15–5

Ultrasonogram showing a male fetus. *(Courtesy of Nancy West.)*

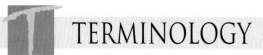 TERMINOLOGY

WITH SURGICAL PROCEDURES & PATHOLOGY

TERM	WORD PARTS			DEFINITION
abortion (ă-bōr′ shŭn)	abort ion	R S	to miscarry process	The process of miscarrying
amenorrhea (ă-měn″ ō-rē′ ă)	a meno rrhea	P CF S	lack of month flow	A lack of the monthly flow or menstruation
amniocentesis (ăm″ nĭ-ō-sĕn-tē′ sĭs)	amnio centesis	CF S	lamb surgical puncture	Surgical puncture of the amniotic sac to obtain a sample of amniotic fluid
amniotome (ăm′ nĭ-ō-tōm)	amnio tome	CF S	lamb instrument to cut	An instrument used to cut fetal membranes
anovular (ăn-ŏv′ ū-lăr)	an ovul ar	P R S	lack of ovary pertaining to	Pertaining to the lack of production and discharge of an ovum
antenatal (ăn″ tē- nā′ tal)	ante nat al	P R S	before birth pertaining to	Pertaining to before birth
ante partum (ăn′ tē păr′ tŭm)	ante partum	P R	before labor	The time before the onset of labor
bartholinitis (bar″ tō-lĭn-ī′ tĭs)	bartholin itis	R S	Bartholin's glands inflammation	Inflammation of Bartholin's glands
catamenia (kăt ă-mē′ nĭ-ă)	cata men ia	P R S	down month condition	The condition of monthly discharge of blood from the uterus
cervicitis (sĕr-vĭ-sī′ tĭs)	cervic itis	R S	cervix inflammation	Inflammation of the uterine cervix
colpoperineo- **plasty** (kŏl″ pō-pĕr″ĭn-ē′ ō-plăs″ tē)	colpo perineo plasty	CF CF S	vagina perineum surgical repair	Surgical repair of the vagina and perineum
colporrhaphy (kŏl-pōr′ ă-fē)	colpo rrhaphy	CF S	vagina suture	Suture of the vagina

Terminology - continued

TERM	WORD PARTS			DEFINITION
colposcope (kŏl′ pō-skōp)	colpo scope	CF S	vagina instrument	An instrument used to examine the vagina and cervix by means of a magnifying lens
conception (kŏn-sĕp′ shŭn)	con cept ion	P R S	together receive process	Process of the union of the male's sperm and the female's ovum; *fertilization*
contraception (kŏn″ tră-sĕp′ shŭn)	contra cept ion	P R S	against receive process	Process of preventing conception

TERMINOLOGY SPOTLIGHT

Contraception is the process of preventing conception. According to the Association of Reproductive Health Professional's survey, 4 out of 5 American women ages 18 to 50 are sexually active. Of these, 9 out of 10, were interested in becoming more educated about various methods of birth control.

In the United States, there are numerous methods that may be used for contraception; some of these are birth control pills, condoms, a diaphragm, foams, jellies, suppositories, natural planning (rhythm method), an intrauterine device (IUD), a cervical cap, a contraceptive sponge, a vasectomy, female sterilization, the Norplant system, Depo-Provera contraceptive injection, and the female condom (Reality).

The most frequently used contraceptives cited by 4000 women ages 18 to 50 were:

Pill	86%
Barrier method (condom, diaphragm, etc.)	76%
Sterilization	34%
Natural planning	25%
IUD	14%
Depo-Provera	2%
Norplant system	1%
None	5%

TERM	WORD PARTS			DEFINITION
culdocentesis (kŭl″ dō-sĕn-tē′ sĭs)	culdo centesis	CF S	cul-de-sac surgical puncture	Surgical puncture of the cul-de-sac for removal of fluid
cystocele (sĭs′ tō-sēl)	cysto cele	CF S	bladder hernia	A hernia of the bladder that protrudes into the vagina
dysmenorrhea (dĭs″ mĕn-ō-rē′ ă)	dys meno rrhea	P CF S	difficult, painful month flow	Difficult or painful monthly flow

continued

Terminology - continued

TERM	WORD PARTS			DEFINITION
dyspareunia (dĭs′ pă-rū′ nĭ-ă)	dys	P	difficult, painful	Difficult or painful sexual intercourse
	par	P	beside	
	eunia	R	a bed	
dystocia (dĭs-tō′ sĭ-ă)	dys	P	difficult, painful	The condition of a difficult and painful childbirth
	toc	R	birth	
	ia	S	condition	
endometriosis (ĕn″ dō-mē″ trĭ-ō′ sĭs)	endo	P	within	A condition in which endometrial tissue occurs in various sites in the abdominal or pelvic cavity
	metri	CF	uterus	
	osis	S	condition of	
episiotomy (ĕ-pĭs″ ĭ-ŏt′ ō-mē)	episio	CF	vulva, pudenda	Incision of the perineum to prevent tearing of the perineum and to facilitate delivery
	tomy	S	incision	
eutocia (ū-tō′ sĭ-ă)	eu	P	good, normal	The condition of a good, normal childbirth
	toc	R	birth	
	ia	S	condition	
fibroma (fī-brō′ mă)	fibr	R	fibrous tissue	A fibrous tissue tumor
	oma	S	tumor	
genitalia (jĕn-ĭ-tăl′ ĭ-ă)	genital	R	belonging to birth	The male or female reproductive organs
	ia	S	condition	
gynecologist (gī″ nĕ-kōl′ ō-jĭst)	gyneco	CF	female	One who specializes in the study of the female
	log	R	study of	
	ist	S	one who specializes	
gynecology (gī″ nĕ-kōl′ ō-jē)	gyneco	CF	female	The study of the female
	logy	S	study of	
hematosalpinx (hē″ mă-tō-săl′ pĭnks)	hemato	CF	blood	A collection of blood in the fallopian tube that may be associated with tubal pregnancy
	salpinx	R	tube	
hymenectomy (hī″ mĕn-ĕk′ tō-mē)	hymen	R	hymen	Surgical excision of the hymen
	ectomy	S	excision	
hysterectomy (hĭs″ tĕr-ĕk′ tō-mē)	hyster	R	womb, uterus	Surgical excision of the uterus
	ectomy	S	excision	

Terminology - continued

TERM	WORD PARTS			DEFINITION
hysterotomy (hĭs″ tĕr-ŏt′ ō-mē)	hystero tomy	CF S	womb, uterus incision	Incision into the uterus; also called a cesarean section
intrauterine (ĭn′ tră-ū′ tĕr-ĭn)	intra uter ine	P R S	within uterus pertaining to	Pertaining to within the uterus
mammography (măm-ŏg′ ră-fē)	mammo graphy	CF S	breast recording	Process of obtaining pictures of the breast by the use of x-rays
mammoplasty (măm′ ō-plăs″ tē)	mammo plasty	CF S	breast surgical repair	Surgical repair of the breast
mastectomy (măs-tĕk′ tō-mē)	mast ectomy	R S	breast excision	Surgical excision of the breast
mastitis (măs-tī′ tĭs)	mast itis	R S	breast inflammation	Inflammation of the breast
menopause (mĕn′ ō-pawz)	meno pause	CF R	month cessation	Cessation of the monthly flow; *also called climacteric*
menorrhagia (mĕn″ ō-rā′ jĭ-ă)	meno rrhagia	CF S	month to burst forth	Excessive bursting forth of blood at the time of the monthly flow
menorrhea (mĕn″ ō-rē′ ă)	meno rrhea	CF S	month flow	A normal monthly flow
multipara (mŭl-tĭp′ ă-ră)	multi para	P R	many to bear	A woman who has borne more than one child
myometritis (mī″ ō-mē-trī′ tĭs)	myo metr itis	CF R S	muscle womb, uterus inflammation	Inflammation of the muscular wall of the uterus
neonatal (nē″ ō-nā′ tăl)	neo nat al	P R S	new birth pertaining to	Pertaining to the first 4 weeks after birth
nullipara (nŭl-ĭp′ ă-ră)	nulli para	P R	none to bear	A woman who has borne no offspring
oligomenorrhea (ŏl″ ī-gō-mĕn″ ō-rē′ ă)	oligo meno rrhea	P CF S	scanty month flow	A scanty monthly flow

continued

Terminology - continued

TERM	WORD PARTS			DEFINITION
oogenesis (ō″ ō-jĕn′ ĕ-sĭs)	oo genesis	CF S	ovum, egg formation, produce	Formation of the ovum
oophorectomy (ō″ŏf-ō-rĕk′ tō-mē)	oophor ectomy	R S	ovary excision	Surgical excision of an ovary
oophoritis (ō″ŏf-ō-rī′ tĭs)	oophor itis	R S	ovary inflammation	Inflammation of an ovary
panhysterectomy (păn″ hĭs-tĕr-ĕk′ tō-mē)	pan hyster ectomy	P R S	all womb, uterus excision	Surgical excision of the entire uterus
pelvimetry (pĕl-vĭm′ ĕt-rē)	pelvi metry	CF S	pelvis measurement	Measurement of the pelvis to determine its capacity and diameter
perinatalogy (pĕr″ ĭ-nă-tŏl′ ō-jē)	peri nata logy	P CF S	around birth study of	Study of the fetus and infant from 20 to 29 weeks of gestation to 1 to 4 weeks after birth
postcoital (pōst-kō′ ĭt-ăl)	post coit al	P R S	after a coming together pertaining to	Pertaining to after sexual intercourse
postpartum (pōst păr′ tŭm)	post partum	P R	after labor	Pertaining to after childbirth
prenatal (prē- nā′ tl)	pre nat al	P R S	before birth pertaining to	Pertaining to before birth
primipara (prī-mĭp′ ă-ră)	primi para	P R	first to bear	A woman who is bearing her first child
pseudocyesis (sū″ dō-sī-ē′ sĭs)	pseudo cyesis	P S	false pregnancy	A false pregnancy
pyometritis (pī″ ō-mē- trī′ tĭs)	pyo metr itis	CF R S	pus womb, uterus inflammation	Purulent (pus) inflammation of the uterus
pyosalpinx (pī″ ō-săl′ pĭnks)	pyo salpinx	CF R	pus tube	Accumulation of pus in the fallopian tube

Terminology - continued

TERM	WORD PARTS			DEFINITION
rectovaginal (rĕk″ tō-văj′ ĭ-năl)	recto vagin al	CF R S	rectum vagina pertaining to	Pertaining to the rectum and vagina
retroversion (rĕt″ rō-vur′ shŭn)	retro vers ion	P R S	backward turning process	The process of being turned backward, such as the displacement of the uterus with the cervix pointed forward
salpingectomy (săl″ pĭn-jĕk′ tō-mē)	salping ectomy	R S	tube excision	Surgical excision of a fallopian tube
salpingitis (săl″ pĭn-jī′ tĭs)	salping itis	R S	tube inflammation	Inflammation of a fallopian tube
salpingo-oophor-ectomy (săl′ pĭng″ gō-ō″ ŏf-ō-rĕk′ tō-mē)	salpingo oophor ectomy	CF R S	tube ovary excision	Surgical excision of an ovary and a fallopian tube
trimester (trī-mĕs′ tĕr)	tri mester	P R	three month	A period of 3 months
vaginitis (văj″ ĭn-ī′ tĭs)	vagin itis	R S	vagina inflammation	Inflammation of the vagina
venereal (vē-nē′ rē-ăl)	venere al	R S	sexual intercourse pertaining to	Pertaining to or resulting from sexual intercourse

VOCABULARY WORDS

Vocabulary words are terms that have not been divided into component parts. They are common words or specialized terms associated with the subject of this chapter. These words are provided to enhance your medical vocabulary.

WORD	DEFINITION
amniocentesis (ăm″ nĭ-ō-sĕn-tē′ sĭs)	A surgical puncture of the amniotic sac to obtain amniotic fluid from which it can be determined if the fetus has Down syndrome, neural tube defects, Tay-Sachs disease, or other genetic defects
biotics (bī-ŏt′ ĭks)	The science of living organisms and the sum of knowledge regarding the life process
blastocyst (blăs′ tō-sĭst)	An embryonic cell mass that attaches to the uterus wall and is a stage in the development of a mammalian embryo
decidua (dē- sĭd′ ū-ă)	The endometrium or mucous membrane of the pregnant uterus that envelops the impregnated ovum
diagnostic ultrasound (dī″ ăg-nŏs′ tĭk ŭl′ tră-sŏund)	The use of extremely high-frequency sound waves for the purpose of diagnosing genetic defects and hydrocephalic conditions in the unborn fetus
Doppler ultrasound (dăp′ lər ŭl′ trăh-sŏund)	A procedure using an audio transformation of high-frequency sounds to monitor the fetal heartbeat
fetus (fē′ tŭs)	The developing young in the uterus from the third month to birth
gamete intrafallopian transfer (GIFT) (găm′ ēt ĭn″ tră-fă-lō′ pē-ăn)	A procedure that places the sperm *(spermatozoa)* and eggs *(oocytes)* directly in the fimbriated end of the fallopian tube via a laparoscope
genetics (jĕn-ĕt′ ĭks)	The science of biology that studies the phenomenon of heredity and the laws governing it
hysteroscope (hĭs′ tĕr-ō-skōp)	An instrument used in the biopsy of uterine tissue before 12 weeks of gestation. This tissue is then analyzed for chromosome arrangement, DNA sequence, and genetic defects.

Vocabulary - continued

WORD	DEFINITION
laser ablation (lā′ zĕr ăb-lā′ shŭn)	A procedure that uses a laser to destroy the uterine lining. A biopsy is performed before the procedure to make sure no cancer is present. This procedure may be used for disabling menstrual bleeding. *It does cause sterility.*
laser laparoscopy (lā′ zĕr lăp-ăr-ŏs′ kō-pē)	A procedure that uses a long, telescope-like instrument equipped with a laser, lights, and a tiny video camera. It may be used to explore the abdominal area and to treat ectopic pregnancy.
laser lumpectomy (lā-zĕr lŭm-pĕk′ tō-mē)	The use of a contact Yag laser to remove a tumor from the breast. It appears to cause less pain for the patient and discharge time from the hospital is sooner.
lumpectomy (lŭm-pĕk′ tō-mē)	The surgical removal of a tumor from the breast. In this procedure, no other tissue or lymph nodes are removed, only the tumor; usually not considered for large tumors, although the latest strategy involves shrinking large tumors with chemotherapy so that they become small enough to be removed by this method
menarche (mĕn-ar′ kē)	The beginning of the monthly flow; *menses*
mittelschmerz (mĭt′ ĕl-shmārts)	Abdominal pain that occurs midway between the menstrual periods at ovulation
morula (mor′ ū-lă)	A solid mass of cells resulting from cell division after fertilization of an ovum
nonstress test (nŏn′ strĕs tĕst)	A diagnostic procedure, often done in a physician's office, wherein a monitor is placed on the mother's abdomen and fetal heartbeats are recorded. The fetal heartbeats should accelerate if the fetus moves.
ovulation (ŏv″ ū-lā′ shăn)	The process in which an ovum is discharged from the cortex of the ovary
ovum transfer (ō′ vum trăns′ fer)	A method of fertilization for women who cannot conceive children. A donor ovum is impregnated within the donor's body by artificial insemination and later transferred to the recipient female.
"parking" (părk′ ĭng)	A surgical procedure in which the fallopian tube is detached from the ovary. An incision is made into the peritoneum and the tube is sewn into it. This is a reversible sterilization procedure.
parturition (par″ tū-rĭsh′ ŭn)	The act of giving birth; *also known as childbirth or delivery*
pudendal (pū-dĕn′ dăl)	Pertaining to the external female genitalia

continued

Vocabulary - continued

WORD	DEFINITION
puerperium (pū″ ĕr-pē′ rĭ-ŭm)	The 4 to 6 weeks after childbirth when the female generative organs usually return to a normal state
quickening (kwĭk′ ĕn-ĭng)	The first movement of the fetus felt in the uterus, occurring during the 16th to 20th week of pregnancy
secundines (sĕk′ ŭn-dīnz)	The afterbirth consisting of the placenta, umbilical cord, and fetal membranes
sonogram (sō′ nŏ-grăm)	A procedure using high-frequency sound waves to display a visual echo image of the fetus; used to determine size of the fetus and to diagnose genetic defects
surrogate mother (sur′ ō-gāt mŭth′ ēr)	A female who contracts to bear a child for another. Pregnancy may occur as a result of artificial insemination
"test-tube baby" (tĕs′ tūb bā′ bē)	An in vitro fertilization technique whereby the ovum is fertilized outside the body and later implanted in the host female
toxic shock syndrome (tŏk′ sĭk shŏk sĭn′ drōm)	A poisonous *Staphylococcus aureus* infection that may strike young, menstruating women
uterine adnexa (ū′ tĕr-ĭn ăd-nĕk′ sah)	The ovaries and fallopian tubes
zygote (zī′ gōt)	The fertilized ovum. The zygote is produced by the union of two gametes.

 ABBREVIATIONS

AB	abortion		**CS**	cesarean section
AFP	alpha-fetoprotein		**CVS**	chorionic villus sampling
AH	abdominal hysterectomy		**D&C**	dilation (dilatation) and curettage
Ascus	atypical squamous cells of undetermined significance		**DES**	diethylstilbestrol
			DUB	dysfunctional uterine bleeding
BBT	basal body temperature		**EDC**	expected date of confinement
C-section	cesarean section		**FSH**	follicle-stimulating hormone
CIN	cervical intraepithelial neoplasia		**GIFT**	gamete intrafallopian transfer
CIS	carcinoma-in-situ		**grav I**	pregnancy one

Gyn	gynecology	**OB**	obstetrics
HCG	human chorionic gonadotropin	**Pap**	Papanicolaou (smear)
HPV	human papillomavirus	**PID**	pelvic inflammatory disease
HRT	hormone replacement therapy	**PMP**	previous menstrual period
HSG	hysterosalpingography	**PMS**	premenstrual syndrome
IUD	intrauterine device	**TSS**	toxic shock syndrome
LH	luteinizing hormone	**UC**	uterine contractions
LMP	last menstrual period	**WNL**	within normal limits
MH	marital history		

 ## DRUG HIGHLIGHTS

Drugs that are generally used for the female reproductive system include hormones, contraceptives, and those used during labor and delivery.

Female Hormones

Estrogens

Are used for a variety of conditions. They may be used in the treatment of amenorrhea, dysfunctional bleeding, and hirsutism and in palliative therapy for breast cancer in women and prostatic cancer in men. They are also used as replacement therapy in the treatment of uncomfortable symptoms that are related to menopause. In this instance, it is believed that estrogen replacement therapy is useful in preventing osteoporosis and possibly heart disease.

Examples: TACE (chlorotrianisene), Premarin (conjugated estrogens, USP), DES (diethylstilbestrol), Estrace (estradiol), Theelin (estrone), and Estraderm (estradiol) transdermal system.

Progestogens/ progestins

Synthetic preparations of progesterone. They are used to prevent uterine bleeding and are combined with estrogen for treatment of amenorrhea. They may be used in cases of infertility and threatened or habitual miscarriage. Progesterone is responsible for changes in the uterine endometrium during the second half of the menstrual cycle, development of maternal placenta after implantation, and development of mammary glands.

Examples: Provera (medroxyprogesterone acetate), Norlutin (norethindrone), Norlutate (norethindrone acetate), and Gesterol (progesterone).

Contraceptives

Oral

Nearly 100% effective when used as directed. These pills contain mixtures of estrogen and progestin in various levels of strength. The estrogen in the pill inhibits ovulation and the progestin inhibits pituitary secretion of luteinizing hormone (LH), causes changes in the cervical mucus that renders it unfavorable to penetration by sperm, and alters the nature of the endometrium.

Examples: Ortho-Novum 10/11-21, Triphasil-21, Micronor, Enovid-E 21, Ovulen-28, Brevicon 21-day, Demulen 1/50-21, and Lo/Ovral-21.

The Norplant system

Consists of six thin capsules that contain levonorgestrel (a progestin). The capsules are made of a soft flexible material and are placed in a fan-like pattern just under the skin on the inside surface of the upper arm. They have a 99% effective contraceptive action that begins within hours after placement and lasts up to 5 years.

Uterine Stimulants   Oxytocic agents (uterine stimulants) may be used in obstetrics to induce labor at term. They are also used to control postpartum hemorrhage and to induce therapeutic abortion.
Examples: Ergotate Maleate (ergonovine maleate) and Pitocin (oxytocin).

Uterine Relaxants   May be administered to delay labor until the fetus has gained sufficient maturity as to be likely to survive outside the uterus.
Examples: Ethanol (ethyl alcohol) and Yutopar (ritodrine HCl).

 # DIAGNOSTIC AND LABORATORY TESTS

Test	Description
amniotic fluid analysis (ăm-nē-ŏt′ ĭk floo′ ĭd ă-năl′ ĭ-sĭs)	A procedure that involves the removal of amniotic fluid via a large needle. Ultrasound is used to give the location of the fetus, and then the needle is inserted into a suprapubic site of the mother. Abnormal results can indicate spina bifida, Down syndrome, hemophilia, hemolytic disease, and/or poor fetal maturity.
breast examination (brest ĕks-ăm″ ĭ-nā′ shŭn)	Visual inspection and manual examination of the breast for changes in contour, symmetry, "dimpling" of skin, retraction of the nipple(s), and for the presence of lumps.
chorionic villus sampling (CVS) (kō-rē-ŏn′ ĭk vĭl′ ŭs sam′ plĭng)	A procedure that involves the insertion of a catheter into the cervix and into the outer portion of the membranes surrounding the fetus. A sample of the chorionic villi can be examined for the chromosomal abnormalities and biochemical disorders. This procedure can be done 8 weeks into pregnancy.
colposcopy (kŏl-pŏs′ kō-pē)	Visual examination of the vagina and cervix via a colposcope. Abnormal results may indicate cervical or vaginal erosion, tumors, and dysplasia.
culdoscopy (kŭl-dŏs′ kō-pē)	Visual examination of the viscera of the female pelvis via a culdoscope. May be used in suspected ectopic pregnancy and unexplained pelvic pain, and to check for pelvic masses.
estrogens (es′ trō-jĕns)	A urine test or blood serum test to determine the level of estrone, estradiol, and estriol.

human chorionic gonadotropin (HCG)
(hū′ măn kō-rē-ŏn′ ĭk gŏn″ ă-dō- trō′ pĭn)

A urine test or blood serum test to determine the presence of HCG. A positive result may indicate pregnancy.

hysterosalpingography
(hĭs″ tĕr-ō-săl″ pĭn-gŏg′ ră-fē)

X-ray of the uterus and fallopian tubes after the injection of a radiopaque substance. Size and structure of the uterus and fallopian tubes can be evaluated. Uterine tumors, fibroids, tubal pregnancy, and tubal occlusion may be observed. Also used for treatment of an occluded fallopian tube.

laparoscopy
(lăp-ăr-ŏs′ kō-pē)

Visual examination of the abdominal cavity via a laparoscope. Used to examine the ovaries and fallopian tubes.

mammography
(măm-ŏg′ ră-fē)

The process of obtaining pictures of the breast by use of x-rays. This procedure is able to locate breast tumors before they grow to 1 cm. It is the most effective means of detecting early breast cancers.

Papanicolaou (Pap smear)
(păp′ ăh-nĭk″ ō-lă′ oo)

A screening technique to aid in the detection of cervical/uterine cancer and cancer precursors. It is not a diagnostic procedure. Both false-positive and false-negative results have been experienced with Pap smears. Any lesion should be biopsied unless not indicated clinically. The Pap smear should not be used as a sole means to diagnose or exclude malignant and premalignant lesions. It is a screening procedure only.

Pap smear results are generally reported as: within normal limits (WNL); abnormal squamous cells of undetermined significance (Ascus); mild dysplasia (CIN I); moderate dysplasia (CIN II); and severe dysplasia and/or carcinoma-in-situ (CIN III).

pregnanediol
(prĕg″ nān-dī-ŏl)

A urine test that determines menstrual disorders or possible abortion.

wet mat or wet-prep
(wĕt măt or wĕt-prĕp)

Examination of vaginal discharge for the presence of bacteria and yeast. A vaginal smear is placed on a microscopic slide, wet with normal saline, and then viewed under a microscope by the physician.

COMMUNICATION ENRICHMENT

This segment is provided for those who wish to enhance their ability to communicate in either English or Spanish.

▶ **Related Terms**

English	Spanish
abortion	aborto (ă-bō̄r-tō)
breast examination	examen de pecho (ex-să-mĕn dĕ pĕ̄-chō)
breasts	pechos; senos (pe-chō̄s; sĕ̄-nō̄s)
cesarean	cesarea (sĕ-să-rĕ-ă)
contraception	contracepción (cō̄n-tră-cĕp-sĭ-ō̄n)
Do you use?	¿usa? (¿ū-să?)
the pill	la píldora (lă pĭl-dō̄-ră)
the diaphragm	el diafragma (ĕl dĭ-ă-frăg-mă)
an IUD	un dispositivo ultra intrauterino (ūn dĭs-pō̄-sĭ-tĭ-vō̄ ūl-tră ū-tĕ-rĭ-nō̄)
foam	espuma (ĕs-pū̄-mă)
condoms	preservativos (condones) (prĕ̄-sĕr-vă-tĭ-vō̄s; cō̄n-dō̄-nĕs)
the rhythm method	el método de ritmo (ĕl mĕ̄-tō̄-dō̄ dĕ rĭt-mō̄)
the method of withdrawal	el método de retirar (ĕl mĕ̄-tō̄-dō̄ dĕ rĕ̄-tĭ-răr)
abstinence	abstinencia (ăbs-tĭ-nĕ̄n-sĭ-ă)
injection	inyección (ĭn-jĕc-sĭ-ō̄n)

English	Spanish
cramps	calambres (că-*lăm*-brĕs)
delivery	parto (*păr*-tō)
episiotomy	episiotomia (ĕ-*pĭ*-sĭ-ō-tō-mĭ-ă)
intercourse	acto sexual; cópula (ăk-*tō sĕx*-sū-ăl; *cō*-pū-lă)
lump	protuberancia (prō-tū-bĕ-*răn*-sĭ-ă)
marital status	estado civil (ĕs-*tă*-dō *sĭ*-vĭl)
menopause	menopausia (mĕ-nō-*pă*-ū-sĭ-ă)
menstrual history	historia menstrual (ĭs-*tō*-rĭ-ă *mĕns*-trū-ăl)
multiple births	nacimientos múltiples (*nă*-sĭ-mĭ-ĕn-tōs *mūl*-tĭ-plĕs)
nipple	pezón (pĕ-*zōn*)
ovary	ovario (ō-*vă*-rĭ-ō)
Pap smear	papanicolao (*pă*-pă-nĭ-kō-lă-ō)
pelvic examination	examen de la pelvis (ĕx-*să*-mĕn dĕ lă pĕlvĭs)
period	periódo (pĕ-rĭ-*ō*-dō)
placenta	placenta (plă-*cĕn*-tă)
pregnancy	embarazo; preñez (ĕm-bă-*ră*-zō; prĕn-*yĕz*)
pregnant	embarazada (ĕm-bă-ră-*să*-dă)
premature	prematuro (prĕ-mă-*tū*-rō)

English	Spanish
sanitary napkin	toalla sanitaria (tō-ă-jă săn-nĭ-tă-rĭ-ă)
uterus	útero (ū-tĕ-rō)
vagina	vagina (vă-hĭ-nă)
womb	matriz (mă-trĭz)

STUDY AND REVIEW SECTION

LEARNING EXERCISES

▶ Anatomy and Physiology

Write your answers to the following questions. Do not refer back to the text

1. List the primary and accessory sex organs of the female reproductive system.

    a. _____   b. _____

    c. _____   d. _____

    e. _____   f. _____

2. State the vital function of the female reproductive system. _____

    _____

3. Name the three identifiable areas of the uterus.

    a. _____   b. _____

    c. _____

4. Define fundus. _____

    _____

5. Name the ligaments that support the uterus and hold it in position.

    a. _____   b. _____

    c. _____   d. _____

6. Name the three layers of the uterine wall.

   a. _____   b. _____

   c. _____

7. State the three primary functions associated with the uterus.

   a. _____

   b. _____

   c. _____

8. Define the following terms:

   a. Anteflexion_____

   _____

   b. Retroflexion _____

   _____

   c. Anteversion _____

   _____

   d. Retroversion _____

   _____

9. The fallopian tubes are also called the _____ _____

   or _____.

10. Name the three layers of the fallopian tubes.

   a. _____   b. _____

   c. _____

11. Define fimbriae. _____

   _____

12. Should the ovum become impregnated by a spermatozoon while in the fallopian

   tube, the process of _____ occurs.

13. State two functions of the fallopian tubes.

   a. _____   b. _____

   c. _____

14. Describe the ovaries. _____

   _____

15. Name the three stages of an ovarian follicle.

a. _____   b. _____

c. _____

16. The functional activity of the ovary is controlled by the _____ .

17. State the two functions of the ovary.

a. _____   b. _____

18. The vagina is a _____ tube extending from the _____ to the uterus.

19. State the three functions of the vagina.

a. _____   b. _____

c. _____

20. Name the organs that comprise the external female genitalia.

a. _____   b. _____

c. _____   d. _____

e. _____

21. Between the vulva and the anus is an external region known as the _____

_____ .

22. Define episiotomy. _____

_____

23. The breasts or _____ _____ are compound alve-olar structures.

24. The _____ is the dark pigmented area found in the skin over each

breast and the _____ is the elevated area in its center.

25. Name the three hormones that play a role in milk production.

a. _____   b. _____

c. _____

26. Define colostrum. _____

_____

27. Name the four phases of the menstrual cycle.

a. _____   b. _____

c. _____   d. _____

28. Define premenstrual syndrome. _____

_____

_____

▶ ## Word Parts

1. In the spaces provided, write the definitions of these prefixes, roots, combining forms, and suffixes. Do not refer to the listings of terminology words. Leave blank those terms you cannot define.

2. After completing as many as you can, refer back to the terminology word listings to check your work. For each word missed or left blank, write the term and its definition several times on the margins of these pages or on a separate sheet of paper.

3. To maximize the learning process, it is to your advantage to do the following exercises as directed. To refer to the terminology listings before completing these exercises invalidates the learning process.

Prefixes

Give the definitions of the following prefixes:

1. a- _____ 2. an- _____

3. ante- _____ 4. cata- _____

5. con- _____ 6. contra- _____

7. dys- _____ 8. endo- _____

9. eu- _____ 10. intra- _____

11. multi- _____ 12. neo- _____

13. nulli- _____ 14. oligo- _____

15. pan- _____ 16. par- _____

17. peri- _____ 18. post- _____

19. pre- _____ 20. primi- _____

21. pseudo- _____ 22. retro- _____

23. tri- _____

Roots and Combining Forms

Give the definition of the following roots and combining forms:

1. abort _____
2. amnio _____
3. bartholin _____
4. cept _____
5. cervic _____
6. coit _____
7. colpo _____
8. culdo _____
9. cysto _____
10. episio _____
11. eunia _____
12. fibr _____
13. genital _____
14. gyneco _____
15. hemato _____
16. hymen _____
17. hyster _____
18. hystero _____
19. log _____
20. mammo _____
21. mast _____
22. men _____
23. meno _____
24. mester _____
25. metr _____
26. metri _____
27. myo _____
28. nat _____
29. nata _____
30. oo _____
31. oophor _____
32. ovul _____
33. para _____
34. partum _____
35. pause _____
36. pelvi _____
37. perineo _____
38. pyo _____
39. recto _____
40. salping _____
41. salpingo _____
42. salpinx _____
43. toc _____
44. uter _____
45. vagin _____
46. venere _____
47. vers _____

Suffixes

Give the definitions of the following suffixes:

1. -al _____
2. -ar _____

3. -cele _____   4. -centesis _____

5. -cyesis _____   6. -ectomy _____

7. -genesis _____   8. -graphy _____

9. -ia _____   10. -ine _____

11. -ion _____   12. -ist _____

13. -itis _____   14. -logy _____

15. -metry _____   16. -oma _____

17. -osis _____   18. -plasty _____

19. -rrhagia _____   20. -rrhaphy _____

21. -rrhea _____   22. -scope _____

23. -tome _____   24. -tomy _____

▶ Identifying Medical Terms

In the spaces provided, write the medical terms for the following meanings:

1. _____   The process of miscarrying

2. _____   An instrument used to cut fetal membranes

3. _____   The time before the onset of labor

4. _____   Inflammation of the uterine cervix

5. _____   Suture of the vagina

6. _____   A difficult or painful monthly flow

7. _____   A good, normal childbirth

8. _____   A fibrous tissue tumor

9. _____   The study of the female

10. _____   Surgical excision of the hymen

11. _____   Surgical repair of the breast

12. _____   A normal monthly flow

13. _____   Pertaining to the first 4 weeks after birth

14. _____   Formation of the ovum

15. _____   Pertaining to after childbirth

▶ Spelling

In the spaces provided, write the correct spelling of these misspelled terms:

1. amiocentesis _____

2. bartolinitis _____

3. dytocia _____

4. epsiotomy _____

5. hystrotomy _____

6. menorhagia _____

7. oophritis _____

8. salpinitis _____

9. vajinitis _____

10. veneral _____

WORD PARTS STUDY SHEET

Word Parts	Give the Meaning
ante-	_____
contra-	_____
dys-	_____
multi-	_____
nulli-	_____
primi-	_____
tri-	_____
abort-	_____
amnio-	_____
bartholin-	_____
cervic-	_____
coit-	_____
colpo-	_____
genital-	_____
gyneco-	_____
hymen-	_____
hyster-, hystero-	_____
mammo-, mast-	_____

men-, meno- _____

metr-, metri-, metro- _____

oo- _____

oophor- _____

partum- _____

perineo- _____

salping-, salpingo- _____

uter- _____

vagin- _____

venere- _____

-cele _____

-centesis _____

-cyesis _____

-genesis _____

-ia, -osis _____

-oma _____

-plasty _____

-rrhagia _____

-rrhaphy _____

-rrhea _____

-scope _____

-tome _____

-tomy _____

REVIEW QUESTIONS

▶ **Matching**

Select the appropriate lettered meaning for each numbered line.

_____	1. gamete intrafallopian transfer	a. A solid mass of cells resulting from cell division after fertilization of an ovum
_____	2. laser ablation	b. Pertaining to the external female genitalia
_____	3. lumpectomy	c. The beginning of the monthly flow; menses
_____	4. menarche	d. Surgical removal of a tumor from the breast
_____	5. mittelschmerz	e. Abdominal pain that occurs midway between the menstrual periods at ovulation
_____	6. morula	f. A procedure that places the sperm and eggs directly in the fimbriated end of the fallopian tube
_____	7. ovulation	g. The process in which an ovum is discharged from the cortex of the ovary
_____	8. parturition	h. The act of giving birth
_____	9. pudendal	i. The first movement of the fetus felt in the uterus, occurring during the 16th to 20th week of pregnancy
_____	10. quickening	j. A procedure that uses a laser to destroy the uterine lining
		k. The fertilized ovum

▶ **Abbreviations**

Place the correct word, phrase, or abbreviation in the space provided.

1. AB _____

2. alpha-fetoprotein _____

3. AH _____

4. cesarean section _____

5. DES _____

6. expected date of confinement _____

7. grav I _____

8. Gyn _____

9. intrauterine device _____

10. pelvic inflammatory disease _____

▶ Diagnostic and Laboratory Tests

Select the best answer to each multiple choice question. Circle the letter of your choice.

1. A procedure that involves the insertion of a catheter into the cervix and into the outer portion of the membranes surrounding the fetus.
    a. amniotic fluid analysis
    b. chorionic villus sampling
    c. colposcopy
    d. culdoscopy

2. A positive result may indicate pregnancy.
    a. colposcopy
    b. culdoscopy
    c. HCG
    d. laparoscopy

3. X-ray of the uterus and fallopian tubes after the injection of a radiopaque substance.
    a. hysterosalpingography
    b. laparoscopy
    c. culdoscopy
    d. mammography

4. Used to examine the ovaries and fallopian tubes.
    a. colposcopy
    b. culdoscopy
    c. laparoscopy
    d. mammography

5. The process of obtaining pictures of the breast by use of x-rays.
    a. colposcopy
    b. culdoscopy
    c. laparoscopy
    d. mammography

CRITICAL THINKING ACTIVITY

▶ **Case Study**

Menopause

Please read the following case study and then answer the questions that follow.

A 52-year-old female was seen by a physician and the following is a synopsis of the visit.

Present History: The patient states that her periods have become very irregular, that she has hot flashes and trouble sleeping, that sex with her husband has become uncomfortable, and that she is very moody.

Signs and Symptoms: Chief complaint: irregular periods, hot flashes, insomnia, dyspareunia, and emotional instability.

Diagnosis: Menopause. The diagnosis was determined by a complete gynecologic examination.

Treatment: Hormone replacement therapy (HRT) consisting of estrogens combined with progestin. The patient was placed on Prempro (conjugated estrogens/medroxyprogesterone acetate tablets) one tablet daily. Prempro is packaged in a special calendar blister pack that shows one instantly whether she has taken the pill for that day. The package is designed for 2 weeks, with directions for use: Begin either card with the tablet that is labeled for the day of the week on which your first day of therapy falls. Complete one card, then begin the second card the very next day. Complete second card.

Prevention: There are no known preventive measures.

Critical Thinking Questions

1. Symptoms of menopause include irregular periods, hot flashes, insomnia, _____, and emotional instability.

2. The diagnosis was determined by a complete _____ examination.

3. Treatment included hormone replacement therapy _____, a combination of estrogens and progestin.

4. The abbreviation for hormone replacement therapy is _____.

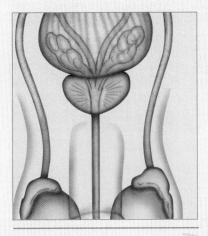

THE MALE REPRODUCTIVE SYSTEM

OBJECTIVES

On completion of this chapter, you should be able to:

- Describe the male's external organs of reproduction.

- Describe and state the functions of the testes, epididymis, ductus deferens, seminal vesicles, prostate gland, bulbourethral glands, and urethra.

- Analyze, build, spell, and pronounce medical words that relate to surgical procedures and pathology.

- Identify and give the meaning of selected vocabulary words.

- Identify and define selected abbreviations.

- Review Drug Highlights presented in this chapter.

- Provide the description of diagnostic and laboratory tests related to the male reproductive system.

- Successfully complete the study and review section.

▶ ANATOMY AND PHYSIOLOGY OVERVIEW

The male reproductive system consists of the *testes, various ducts,* the *urethra,* and the following accessory glands: *bulbourethral, prostate,* and the *seminal vesicles.* The supporting structures and accessory sex organs are the *scrotum* and the *penis* (Fig. 16–1). The vital function of the male reproductive system is to provide the sperm cells necessary to fertilize the ovum thereby perpetuating the species. The following is a general overview of the organs and functions of this system.

▶ EXTERNAL ORGANS

In the male, the scrotum and the penis are the external organs of reproduction.

THE SCROTUM

The *scrotum* is a pouch-like structure located behind the penis. It is suspended from the perineal region and is divided by a septum into two sacs, each containing one of the testes along with its connecting tube called the *epididymis.* Within the tissues of the scrotum are fibers of smooth muscle that contract in the absence of sufficient heat, giving the scrotum a wrinkled appearance. This contractile action brings the testes closer to the perineum where they can absorb sufficient body heat to maintain the viability of the *spermatozoa.* Under normal conditions, the walls of the scrotum are generally free of wrinkles, and it hangs loosely between the thighs (Fig. 16–1).

THE PENIS

The *penis* is the external male sex organ and is composed of erectile tissue covered with skin. The size and shape of the penis varies, with an average erect penis being 15 to 20 cm in length. The penis has three longitudinal columns of erectile tissue that are capa-

THE MALE REPRODUCTIVE SYSTEM

ORGAN/STRUCTURE	PRIMARY FUNCTIONS
The Scrotum	Contains testes and connecting tubes; contractile action brings the testes closer to the perineum, where they can absorb sufficient body heat to maintain the viability of the spermatozoa
The Penis	Male organ of copulation; site of the orifice for the elimination of urine and semen from the body
The Testes	Contains seminiferous tubules that are the site of the development of spermatozoa; cells within the testes also produce the male sex hormone, testosterone
The Epididymis	Storage site for the maturation of sperm
The Ductus Deferens or Vas Deferens	Excretory duct of the testis
The Seminal Vesicles	Produce a slightly alkaline fluid that becomes a part of the seminal fluid or semen
The Prostate Gland	Secretes an alkaline fluid that aids in maintaining the viability of spermatozoa
The Bulbourethral or Cowper's Glands	Produce a mucous secretion before ejaculation, which becomes a part of the semen
The Urethra	Transmits urine and semen out of the body

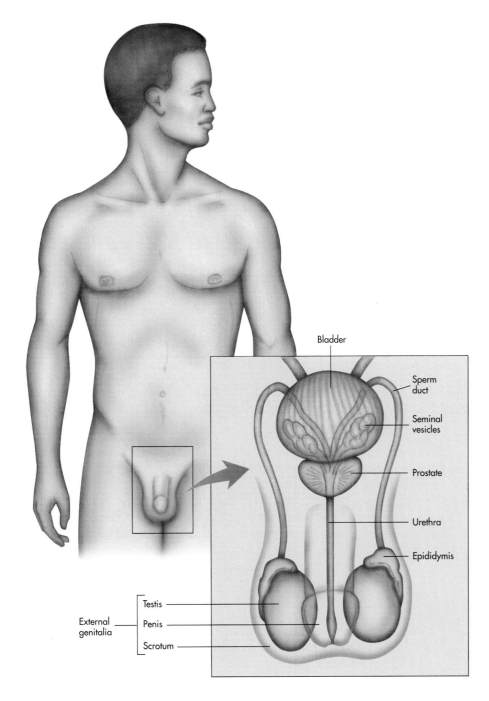

FIGURE 16-1

The male reproductive system: seminal vesicles, prostate, urethra, sperm duct, epididymis, and external genitalia.

ble of significant enlargement when engorged with blood, as is the case during sexual stimulation. Two of these columns, located side by side, form the greater part of the penis. These columns are known as the *corpora cavernosa penis*. The third longitudinal column, the *corpus spongiosum*, has the same function as the first two columns but is transversed by the penile portion of the urethra and tends to be more elastic when in an erectile state. The *corpus spongiosum*, at its distal end, expands to form the *glans penis*.

The glans penis is the cone-shaped head of the penis and is the site of the urethral orifice. It is covered with loose skin folds called the *foreskin* or prepuce. See Figure 16–2. The foreskin contains glands that secrete a lubricating fluid called *smegma.* The foreskin may be removed by a surgical procedure known as *circumcision.*

The erectile state in the penis results when sexual stimulation causes large quantities of blood from dilated arteries supplying the penis to fill the cavernous spaces in the erectile tissue. When the arteries constrict, the pressure on the veins in the area is reduced, thus allowing more blood to leave the penis than enters, and the penis returns to its normal state. The functions of the penis are to serve as the male organ of *copulation* and as the site of the orifice for the elimination of urine and semen from the body.

▶ THE TESTES

The male has two ovoid-shaped organs, the *testes,* located in the scrotum. Each testis is about 4 cm long and 2.5 cm wide. The interior of each testis is divided into about 250 wedge-shaped lobes by fibrous tissues. Coiled within each lobe are one to three small tubes called the *seminiferous tubules.* These tubules are the site of the development of male reproductive cells, the *spermatozoa.* Cells within the testes also produce the male sex hormone, *testosterone,* which is responsible for the development of secondary male characteristics during puberty. Testosterone is essential for normal growth and development of the male accessory sex organs. It plays a vital role in the erection process of the penis, and thus, is necessary for the reproductive act, copulation. Additionally, it affects the growth of hair on the face, muscular development, and vocal timbre. The *seminiferous tubules* form a plexus or network called the rete testis from which 15 to 20 small ducts, the efferent ductules, leave the testis and open into the epididymis (Figs. 16–1 and 16–2).

▶ THE EPIDIDYMIS

Each testis is connected by efferent ductules to an *epididymis,* which is a coiled tube lying on the posterior aspect of the testis. The epididymis is between 13 and 20 feet in length but is coiled into a space less than 2 inches (5 cm) long and ends in the ductus deferens. Each epididymis functions as a storage site for the maturation of *sperm* (Fig. 16–3) and as the first part of the duct system through which sperm pass on their journey to the urethra (see Figs. 16–1 and 16–2).

▶ THE DUCTUS DEFERENS OR VAS DEFERENS

The *ductus deferens* is a slim muscular tube, about 45 cm in length, and is a continuation of the epididymis. It has been described as the *excretory duct* of the testis and extends from a point adjacent to the testis to enter the abdomen through the inguinal canal. It is later joined by the duct from the seminal vesicle. Between the testis and the part of the abdomen known as the internal inguinal ring, the ductus deferens is contained within a structure known as the *spermatic cord.* The spermatic cord also contains arteries, veins, lymphatic vessels, and nerves (see Fig. 16–4).

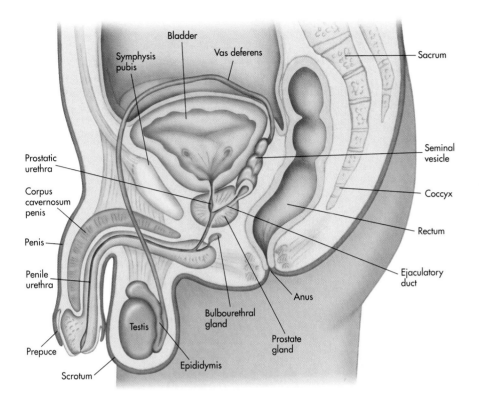

FIGURE 16–2

Sagittal section of the male pelvis, showing the organs of the reproductive system.

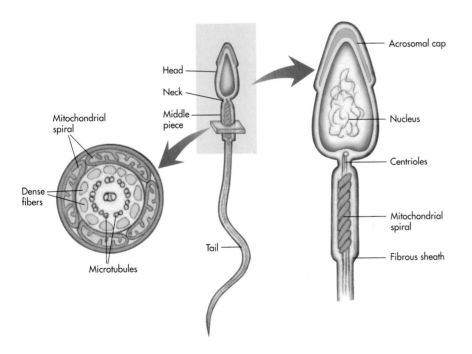

FIGURE 16–3

The basic structure of a spermatozoon (sperm).

▶ THE SEMINAL VESICLES

There are *two seminal vesicles,* each connected by a narrow duct to a ductus deferens, which then forms a short tube, the *ejaculatory duct,* that penetrates the base of the prostate gland and opens into the prostatic portion of the urethra. The seminal vesicles produce a slightly alkaline fluid that becomes a part of the seminal fluid or semen (see Fig. 16–4).

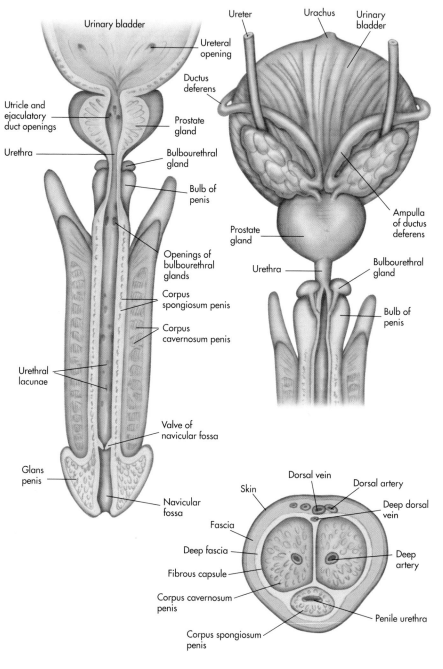

FIGURE 16–4

The structures of the bladder, prostate gland, and penis.

▶ THE PROSTATE GLAND

The *prostate gland* is about 4 cm wide and weighs about 20 g. It is composed of glandular, connective, and muscular tissue and lies behind the urinary bladder. It surrounds the first 2.5 cm of the urethra and secretes an alkaline fluid that aids in maintaining the viability of spermatozoa. Enlargement of the prostate *(benign prostatic hyperplasia)* is a condition that sometimes occurs in older men. In this condition, the prostate obstructs the urethra and causes interference with the normal passage of urine. When this occurs, a *prostatectomy* may be performed to remove a part of the gland. The prostate gland may also be a site for cancer in older men (see Fig. 16–4).

▶ THE BULBOURETHRAL OR COWPER'S GLANDS

The *bulbourethral glands* are two small pea-sized glands located below the prostate and on either side of the urethra. A duct about 2.5 cm long connects them with the wall of the urethra. The bulbourethral glands produce a mucous secretion before ejaculation, which becomes a part of the semen (see Fig. 16–4).

▶ THE URETHRA

The male *urethra* is approximately 20 cm long and is divided into three sections: prostatic, membranous, and penile. It extends from the urinary bladder to the external urethral orifice at the head of the penis. It serves the function of transmitting urine and semen out of the body (see Fig. 16–4).

LIFE SPAN CONSIDERATIONS

▶ THE CHILD

In the newborn, the **testicles** may appear large at birth. They may fail to descend into the scrotum, causing a condition, **cryptorchism.** The foreskin of the penis may be tight at birth, causing **phimosis,** a condition of narrowing of the opening of the prepuce wherein the foreskin cannot be drawn back over the glans penis.

Puberty is defined as a period of rapid change in the lives of boys and girls during which time the reproductive systems mature and become functionally capable of reproduction. In the male, puberty begins around 12 years of age, when the genitals start to increase in size and the shoulders broaden and become muscular. As testosterone is released, secondary sexual characteristics develop, such as pubic and axillary hair, increase in size of the penis and testes, voice changes, facial hair, erections, and noctural emissions.

▶ THE OLDER ADULT

With aging, the **prostate gland** enlarges and its glandular secretions decrease, the **testes** become smaller and more firm, there is a gradual decrease in the production of **testosterone,** and pubic hair becomes sparser and stiffer. This period of change in the male has been referred to as the "male climacteric" and may be associated with symptoms such as hot flashes, feelings of suffocation, insomnia, irritability, and emotional instability. Testosterone replacement therapy may be recommended for the "male climacteric."

In a healthy, normal male **spermatogenesis** and the ability to have erections lasts a lifetime. However, sexual arousal may be slowed with a longer refractory period between erections. In men, a "refractory period" is a time after one orgasm during which they are not physically able to have another one.

According to the National Institutes of Health (NIH) **erectile dysfunction** (*impotence*) affects as many as 20 million men in the United States. It was once thought to be an unavoidable result of aging, but now, erectile dysfunction is understood to be caused by a variety of factors. Erectile dysfunction is defined as the inability to achieve or maintain an erection sufficient for sexual intercourse. It occurs when not enough blood is supplied to the penis, when the smooth muscle in the penis fails to relax, or when the penis does not retain the blood that flows into it. According to studies by the NIH, 5% of men have some degree of erectile dysfunction at age 40 and approximately 15 to 25% at age 65 or older. Although the likelihood of erectile dysfunction increases with age, it is not an inevitable part of aging. About 80% of erectile dysfunction has a physical cause. See Table 16–1 for physical causes of erectile dysfunction.

TABLE 16–1   Some Physical Causes of Erectile Dysfunction

Vascular Diseases	Arteriosclerosis, hypertension, high cholesterol, and other medical conditions can obstruct blood flow and cause erectile dysfunction
Diabetes	Can alter nerve function and blood flow to the penis and cause erectile dysfunction
Prescription Drugs	Certain antihypertensive and cardiac medications, antihistamines, psychiatric medications, and other prescription drugs can cause erectile dysfunction
Substance Abuse	Excessive smoking, alcohol, and illegal drugs constrict blood vessels and can cause erectile dysfunction
Neurologic Diseases	Multiple sclerosis, Parkinson's disease, and other diseases can interrupt nerve impulses to the penis and cause erectile dysfunction
Surgery	Prostate, colon, bladder, and other types of pelvic surgery may damage nerves and blood vessels and cause erectile dysfunction
Spinal Injury	Interruptions of nerve impulses from the spinal cord to the penis can cause erectile dysfunction
Other	Hormonal imbalance, kidney failure, dialysis, and reduced testosterone levels can cause erectile dysfunction

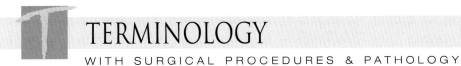

TERMINOLOGY

WITH SURGICAL PROCEDURES & PATHOLOGY

TERM	WORD PARTS			DEFINITION
anorchism (ăn-ōrʹ kĭzm)	an orch ism	P R S	lack of testicle condition of	A condition in which there is a lack of one or both testes
aspermatism (ă-spĕrʹ mă-tĭzm)	a spermat ism	P R S	lack of seed condition of	A condition in which there is a lack of secretion of the male seed
azoospermia (ă-zōʺ ō-spĕrʹ mē-ă)	a zoo sperm ia	P CF R S	lack of animal seed condition	A condition in which there is a lack of spermatozoa in the semen
balanitis (bălʺ ă-nīʹ tĭs)	balan itis	R S	glans inflammation	Inflammation of the glans penis
circumcision (sĕrʺ kŭm-sĭʹ shŭn)	circum cis ion	P R S	around to cut process	The surgical process of removing the foreskin of the penis
cryptorchism (krĭpt-ōrʹ kĭzm)	crypt orch ism	R R S	hidden testicle condition of	A condition in which the testes fail to descend into the scrotum
epididymectomy (ĕpʺ ĭ-dĭdʺ ĭ-mĕkʹ tō-mē)	epi didym ectomy	P R S	upon testis excision	Surgical excision of the epididymis
epididymitis (ĕpʺ ĭ-dĭdʺ ĭ-mīʹ tĭs)	epi didym itis	P R S	upon testis inflammation	Inflammation of the epididymis
epispadias (ĕpʺ ĭ-spāʹ dĭ-ăs)	epi spadias	P R	upon a rent, an opening	A congenital defect in which the urethra opens on the dorsum of the penis
hydrocele (hīʹ drō-sēl)	hydro cele	P S	water hernia	A collection of serous fluid in a sac-like cavity; specifically the tunica vaginalis testis
hypospadias (hīʺ pō-spāʹ dĭ-ăs)	hypo spadias	P R	under a rent, an opening	A congenital defect in which the urethra opens on the underside of the penis

continued

Terminology - continued

TERM	WORD PARTS			DEFINITION
oligospermia (ŏl″ ĭ-gō-spĕr′ -mĭ-ă)	oligo sperm ia	P R S	scanty seed condition	A condition in which there is a scanty amount of spermatozoa in the semen
orchidectomy (or″ kĭ-dĕk′ tō-mē)	orchid ectomy	R S	testicle excision	Surgical excision of a testicle
orchidopexy (or′ kĭd-ō-pēk ″ sē)	orchido pexy	CF S	testicle fixation	Surgical fixation of a testicle
orchidoplasty (or′ kĭd-ō-plăs″ tē)	orchido plasty	CF S	testicle surgical repair	Surgical repair of a testicle
orchidotomy (or″ kĭd-ŏt′ ō-mē)	orchido tomy	CF S	testicle incision	Incision into a testicle
orchitis (or-kī′ tĭs)	orch itis	R S	testicle inflammation	Inflammation of a testicle
parenchyma (păr-ĕn′ kĭ-mă)	par enchyma	P R	beside to pour	The essential cells of a gland or organ that are concerned with its function
penitis (pē-nī′ tĭs)	pen itis	R S	penis inflammation	Inflammation of the penis
phimosis (fī-mō′ sĭs)	phim osis	R S	a muzzle condition of	A condition of narrowing of the opening of the prepuce wherein the foreskin cannot be drawn back over the glans penis
prostatalgia (prŏs″ tă-tăl′ jĭ-ă)	prostat algia	R S	prostate pain	Pain in the prostate
prostatectomy (prŏs″ tă-tĕk′ tō-mē)	prostat ectomy	R S	prostate excision	Surgical excision of the prostate
prostatitis (prŏs″ tă-tī′ tĭs)	prostat itis	R S	prostate inflammation	Inflammation of the prostate
prostatocystitis (prŏs″ tă-tō-sĭs-tĭ′ tĭs)	prostato cyst itis	CF R S	prostate bladder inflammation	Inflammation of the prostate and bladder
prostatomegaly (prŏs″ tă-tō-mĕg′ ă-lē)	prostato megaly	CF S	prostate enlargement	Enlargement of the prostate

Terminology - continued

TERM	WORD PARTS			DEFINITION

TERMINOLOGY SPOTLIGHT

Prostatomegaly is defined as enlargement of the prostate. Enlargement of the prostate gland may occur in men who are 50 years of age and older and is referred to as **benign prostatic hyperplasia** (BPH). By age 60, four out of five men may have an enlarged prostate. As the prostate enlarges, it compresses the **urethra,** thereby restricting the normal flow of urine. This restriction generally causes a number of symptoms and can be referred to as **prostatism.** Prostatism is any condition of the prostate gland that interferes with the flow of urine from the bladder. Symptoms usually include:

- A weak or hard-to-start urine stream
- A feeling that the bladder is not empty
- A need to urinate often, especially at night
- A feeling of urgency (a sudden need to urinate)
- Abdominal straining; a decrease in size and force of the urinary stream
- Interruption of the stream
- Acute urinary retention
- Recurrent urinary infections

Treatment for benign prostatic hyperplasia may include surgery, medication, and/or balloon dilation of the urethra.
Surgery. Transurethral resection of the prostate (TURP or TUR). During this procedure, an endoscopic instrument that has ocular and surgical capabilities is introduced directly through the urethra to the prostate and small pieces of the prostate gland are removed by using an electrical cutting loop.
Medication. Proscar (finasteride), an oral medication, may be prescribed by a physician to help relieve the symptoms of BPH. It lowers the levels of dihydrotestosterone (DHT), which is a major factor in enlargement of the prostate. Lowering of DHT leads to shrinkage of the enlarged prostate gland in most men. Although this can lead to gradual improvement in urine flow and symptoms, it does not work for all cases. Side effects may include impotence and less desire for sex. Proscar can alter the prostate-specific antigen test (PSA) that is used to screen for prostate cancer.
Balloon dilation. During this procedure, a balloon catheter is placed in the distal urethra and inflated by injecting a dilute contrast media at high pressure. The balloon is left in place for approximately 10 minutes and then the pressure is released.

TERM	WORD PARTS			DEFINITION
spermatoblast (spĕr-măt′ ō-blăst)	spermato blast	CF S	seed, sperm immature cell, germ cell	The sperm germ cell
spermatocyst (spĕr-măt′ ō-sĭst)	spermato cyst	CF R	seed, sperm sac, bladder	A cyst of the epididymis that contains spermatozoa
spermatogenesis (spĕr″ măt-ō-jĕn′ ĕ-sĭs)	spermato genesis	CF S	seed, sperm formation, produce	Formation of spermatozoa
spermatozoon (spĕr″ măt-ō-zō′ ŏn)	spermato zoon	CF R	seed, sperm life	The male sex cell. *The plural form is spermatozoa*

continued

Terminology - continued

TERM	WORD PARTS			DEFINITION
spermaturia (spĕr″ mă-tū′ rĭ-ă)	spermat uria	R S	seed, sperm urine	Discharge of semen with the urine
spermicide (spĕr′ mĭ-sīd)	spermi cide	CF S	sperm to kill	An agent that kills sperm
testicular (tĕs-tĭk′ ū-lar)	testicul ar	R S	testicle pertaining to	Pertaining to a testicle
varicocele (văr′ ĭ-kō-sēl)	varico cele	CF S	twisted vein hernia	An enlargement and twisting of the veins of the spermatic cord
vasectomy (văs-ĕk′ tō-mē)	vas ectomy	R S	vessel excision	Surgical excision of the vas deferens
vesiculitis (vĕ-sĭk″ ū-lī′ tĭs)	vesicul itis	R S	vesicle inflammation	Inflammation of a vesicle; in particular, the seminal vesicle

VOCABULARY WORDS

Vocabulary words are terms that have not been divided into component parts. They are common words or specialized terms associated with the subject of this chapter. These words are provided to enhance your medical vocabulary.

WORD	DEFINITION
artificial insemination (ăr″ tĭ-fĭsh′ ăl ĭn-sĕm″ ĭn-ā′ shŭn)	The process of artificial placement of semen into the vagina so that conception may take place
capacitation (kăh-păs″ ĭ-tā′ shŭn)	The process by which spermatozoa are conditioned to fertilize an ovum in the female genital tract
castrate (kăs′ trāt)	To remove the testicles or ovaries; *to geld, to spay*
cloning (klōn′ ing)	The process of creating a genetic duplicate of an individual organism through asexual reproduction

Vocabulary - continued

WORD	DEFINITION
coitus (kō′ ĭ-tŭs)	Sexual intercourse between a man and a woman
condom (kŏn′ dŭm)	A thin, flexible protective sheath, usually rubber, worn over the penis during copulation to help prevent impregnation or venereal disease
condyloma (kŏn″ dĭ-lō′ mă)	A wart-like growth of the skin, most often seen on the external genitalia; is either viral or syphilitic in origin
ejaculation (ē-jăk″ ū-lā′ shŭn)	The process of expulsion of seminal fluid from the male urethra
Ericsson sperm separation method (er′ ik-son sperm sĕp″ ă-rā′ shŭn mĕth′ od	A process of separating the Y-chromosome sperm from the X-chromosome sperm. A sperm sample is taken and placed in a tube of albumin. Those that survive are Y-chromosome sperm, which make male babies. Women inseminated with these sperm have a 75 to 80% chance of producing a male child.
eugenics (ū-jĕn′ ĭks)	The study and control of the bringing forth of offspring as a means of improving genetic characteristics of future generations
eunuch (ū′ nŭk)	A male who has been castrated, ie, had his testicles removed
gamete (găm′ ēt)	A mature reproductive cell of the male or female; *a spermatozoon or ovum*
gonorrhea (gŏn″ŏ-rē′ ă)	A highly contagious venereal disease of the genital mucous membrane of either sex; the infection transmitted by the gonococcus *Neisseria gonorrhoeae*
gossypol (gŏs′ sĕ-pŏl)	An extract of cottonseed oil that acts as a spermicide and may inhibit or prevent herpes simplex virus infection
gynecomastia (jĭ″ nĕ-kō-măs′ tĭ-ă)	A condition of excessive development of the mammary glands in the male
herpes genitalis (hĕr′ pēz jĕn-ĭ-tăl′ ĭs)	A highly contagious venereal disease of the genitalia of either sex; caused by herpes simplex virus-2 (HSV-2)
heterosexual (hĕt″ ĕr-ō-sĕk′ shū-ăl)	Pertaining to the opposite sex; refers to an individual who has a sexual preference for the opposite sex
homosexual (hō″ mō-sĕks′ ū-ăl)	Pertaining to the same sex; refers to an individual who has a sexual preference for the same sex

continued

Vocabulary - continued

WORD	DEFINITION
infertility (ĭn″ fĕr-tĭl′ ĭ-tē)	The inability to produce a viable offspring
mitosis (mī-tō′ sĭs)	The ordinary condition of cell division
prepuce (prē′ pūs)	The foreskin over the glans penis in the male
puberty (pū′ ber-tē)	The stage of development in the male and female when secondary sex characteristics begin to develop and become functionally capable of reproduction
semen (sē′ mĕn)	The fluid-transporting medium for spermatozoa discharged during ejaculation
syphilis (sĭf′ ĭ-lĭs)	A chronic infectious venereal disease caused by *Treponema pallidum,* which is transmitted sexually
trisomy (trī′ sōm-ē)	A genetic condition of having three chromosomes instead of two. The condition causes various birth defects.

ABBREVIATIONS

AIH	artificial insemination homologous	**SPP**	suprapubic prostatectomy
BPH	benign prostatic hyperplasia	**STDs**	sexually transmitted diseases
FTA-ABS	fluorescent treponemal antibody absorption	**STS**	serologic test for syphilis
		TPA	*Treponema pallidum* agglutination
Gc	gonorrhea	**TUR**	transurethral resection
HLA	human leukocyte antigen	**UG**	urogenital
HPV	human papilloma virus	**VD**	venereal disease
HSV-2	herpes simplex virus-2	**VDRL**	venereal disease research laboratory
NPT	nocturnal penile tumescence	**WR**	Wassermann reaction
PSA	prostate-specific antigen		

DRUG HIGHLIGHTS

Drugs that are generally used for the male reproductive system include androgenic hormones. Testosterone is the most important androgen and adequate secretions of this hormone are necessary to maintain normal male sex characteristics, the male libido, and sexual potency.

Testosterone	Is responsible for growth, development, and maintenance of the male reproductive system, and secondary sex characteristics.
Therapeutic use	As replacement therapy in primary hypogonadism, and to stimulate puberty in carefully selected males. It may be used to relieve male menopause symptoms due to androgen deficiency. It may also be used to help stimulate sperm production in oligospermia and in impotence due to androgen deficiency. It may be used when there is advanced inoperable metastatic breast cancer in women who are 1 to 5 years postmenopausal and to prevent postpartum breast pain and engorgement in the non-nursing mother. *Examples: Halotestin (fluoxymesterone), Metandren (methyltestosterone), Andro (testosterone enanthate in oil), and Testex (testosterone propionate in oil).*
Patient teaching	Educate the patient to be aware of possible adverse reactions and report any of the following to the physician. *All patients:* nausea, vomiting, jaundice, edema. *Males:* frequent or persistent erection of the penis. Adolescent males: signs of premature epiphyseal closure. Should have bone development checked every 6 months. *Females:* hoarseness, acne, changes in menstrual periods, growth of hair on face and/or body.
Special Considerations	In diabetic patients, the effects of testosterone may decrease blood glucose and insulin requirements. Testosterone may decrease the anticoagulant requirements of patients receiving oral anticoagulants. These patients require close monitoring when testosterone therapy is begun and then when it is stopped. Anabolic steroids (testosterone) may be abused by individuals who seek to increase muscle mass, strength, and overall athletic ability. This form of use is illegal and signs of abuse may include flu-like symptoms, headaches, muscle aches, dizziness, bruises, needle marks, increased bleeding (nosebleeds, petechiae, gums, conjunctiva), enlarged spleen, liver, and/or prostate, edema, and in the female increased facial hair, menstrual irregularities, and enlarged clitoris.

DIAGNOSTIC AND LABORATORY TESTS

Test	Description
fluorescent treponemal antibody absorption (floo-ō-rĕs′ ĕnt trĕp″ ō-nē′ măl ăn′ tĭ-bŏd″ ē ab-sorp′ shŭn)	A test performed on blood serum to determine the presence of *Treponema pallidum*. Used to detect syphilis.
paternity (pă-tĕr′ nĭ-tē)	A test to determine whether a certain man could be the father of a specific child. The test can indicate only who is not the father. Types of tests that may be used are blood type, human leukocyte antigen (HLA), white blood cell, enzyme and protein, and genetic. The blood type of the child and accused father are analyzed for compatibility. For example, a parent with type O blood cannot be the parent of a child with type AB blood. The HLA looks at the body's tissue compatibility system, and the white blood cell test looks at chemical markers (antigens) on the surface of the white blood cells. Enzyme and protein looks at red blood cell enzymes, and a new genetic test is being developed that uses molecular and protein biology to look at family-related patterns among genes.
prostate-specific antigen (PSA) immunoassay (prŏs′ tāt-spĕ-sĭf′ ĭk ăn′ tĭ-jĕn ĭm″ ū-nō-ăs′ sā)	A blood test that measures concentrations of a special type of protein known as prostate-specific antigen. Increased level indicates prostate disease or possibly prostate cancer.
semen (sē′ mĕn)	A test performed on semen that looks at the volume, pH, sperm count, sperm motility, and morphology. Used to evaluate infertility in men.
testosterone toxicology (tĕs-tŏs′ tĕr-ōn tŏks″ ĭ-kŏl′ ō-jē)	A test performed on blood serum to identify the level of testosterone. Increased level may indicate benign prostatic hyperplasia. Decreased level may indicate hypogonadism, testicular hypofunction, hypopituitarism, and/or orchidectomy.
venereal disease research laboratory (vē- nē′ rē-ăl dĭ-zēz rē′ sĕrch lăb′ ră-tor″ ē)	A test performed on blood serum to determine the presence of *Treponema pallidum*. Used to detect syphilis.

SEXUALLY TRANSMITTED DISEASES (STDS)

Sexually transmitted diseases can occur in men, women, and children. They are passed from person to person through sexual contact or from mother to child. The following is a summary of the most common sexually transmitted diseases:

Disease	Cause	Symptoms	Treatment
Chlamydia (klă-mĭd′ ē-ă)	*Chlamydia trachomatis* (bacterium)	**MAY BE ASYMPTOMATIC OR** **MALE:** Mucopurulent discharge from penis, burning, itching in genital area, dysuria, swollen testes. Can lead to sterility **FEMALE:** Mucopurulent discharge from vagina, cystitis, pelvic pain, cervicitis. Can lead to pelvic inflammatory disease (PID) and sterility **NEWBORN:** Eye infection, pneumonia. Can cause death	Antibiotics—tetracycline or erythromycin
Genital warts (jĕn′ ĭ-tăl wŏrts)	Human papilloma virus (HPV)	**MALE:** Cauliflower-like growths on the penis and perianal area **FEMALE:** Cauliflower-like growths around vagina and perianal area	Laser surgery, chemotherapy, cryosurgery, cauterization
Gonorrhea (gŏn″ ŏ-rē′ ă)	*Neisseria gonorrhoeae* (bacterium)	**MALE:** Purulent urethral discharge, dysuria, urinary frequency **FEMALE:** Purulent vaginal discharge, dysuria, urinary frequency, abnormal menstrual bleeding, abdominal tenderness. Can lead to PID and sterility **NEWBORN:** Gonorrheal ophthalmia neonatorum, purulent eye discharge. Can cause blindness	Antibiotics—penicillin or tetracycline
Herpes genitalis (hĕr′ pēz jĕn-ĭ-tāl′ ĭs)	Herpes simplex virus-2 (HSV-2)	**ACTIVE PHASE MALE:** Fluid-filled vesicles (blisters) on penis. Rupture causes acute pain and itching **FEMALE:** Blisters in and around vagina **NEWBORN:** Can be infected during vaginal delivery. Severe infection, physical and mental damage **GENERALIZED:** "Flu-like" symptoms, fever, headache, malaise, anorexia, muscle pain	**NO CURE:** Antiviral drug acyclovir (Zovirax) may be used to relieve symptoms during acute phase
Syphilis (sĭf′ ĭ-lĭs)	*Treponema pallidum* (bacterium)	**PRIMARY**—1st stage Chancre at point of infection. See Figures 16–5 and 16–6. **Male**—penis, anus, rectum. **Female**—vagina, cervix. **Both**—lips, tongue, fingers, or nipples **SECONDARY**—2nd stage "Flu-like" symptoms with a skin rash over moist, fatty areas of the body. See Figure 16–7. Alopecia	Antibiotics—penicillin, tetracycline, or erythromycin

Disease	Cause	Symptoms	Treatment
		TERTIARY—latent-3rd stage No symptoms —damage to internal organs **NEWBORN:** Congenital syphilis—may have a heart defect, bone deformity, or other deformities	
Trichomoniasis (trĭk″ ō-mō-nī′ ă-sĭs)	*Trichomonas* (parasitic protozoa)	**MALE:** Usually asymptomatic. Can lead to cystitis, urethritis, prostatitis **FEMALE:** White frothy vaginal discharge, burning and itching of vulva. Can lead to cystitis, urethritis, vaginitis	Metronidazole (Flagyl)

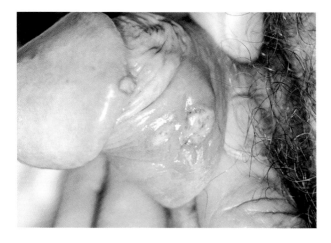

FIGURE 16–5

Chancre. *(Courtesy of Jason L. Smith, MD.)*

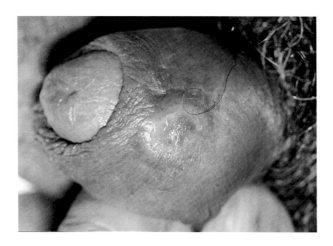

FIGURE 16–6

Chancre. *(Courtesy of Jason L. Smith, MD.)*

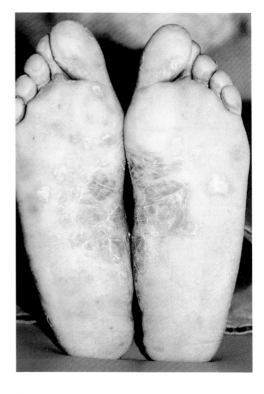

FIGURE 16–7

Secondary syphilis. *(Courtesy of Jason L. Smith, MD.)*

COMMUNICATION ENRICHMENT

This segment is provided for those who wish to enhance their ability to communicate in either English or Spanish.

▶ **Related Terms**

English	Spanish	English	Spanish
AIDS (Acquired Immune Deficiency Syndrome)	SIDA (Síndrome de Immune Deficiencia Adquirida) (sĭ-*dă* [sĭn-*drō*-mĕ dĕ ĭmm-*mū*-n-dĕ-fĭ-cĭ-ĕn-cĭ-ă *ăd*-kĭ-rĭ-dă])	homosexual	homosexual (*ō*-mō-sĕx-sū-ăl)
		impotence	impotencia (ĭm-pō-*tĕn*-sĭ-ă)
		masturbate	masturbarse (*măs*-tūr-băr-sĕ)
bisexual	bisexual (bĭ-*sĕx*-sū-ăl)	masturbation	masturbación (*măs*-tūr-bă-sĭ-ōn)
chlamydia	chlamydia (klă-*mĭ*-dĭ-ă)	penis	pene (*pĕ*-nĕ)
circumcision	circuncisión (sĭr-*cūn*-sĭ-ōn)	prostate	prostático; prostata (prōs-*ta*-tĭ-kō; prōs-*tă*-tă)
condom	condon (*cōn*-dōn)	prostatectomy	prostatectomia (prōs-*tă*-tĕk-tō-mĭ-ă)
ejaculation	eyaculación (ĕ-yă-kū-lă-sĭ-*ōn*)		
ejaculate	eyacular (ĕ-yă-kū-*lăr*)	prostate gland	glándula prostática (*glăn*-dū-lă prōs-*tă*-tĭ-ka)
erection	erección (ĕ-rĕk-sĭ-*ōn*)	reproduction	reproducción (rĕ-prō-dūk-sĭ-*ōn*)
genitals	genitales (hĕ-nĭ-*tă*-lĕs)	reproductive system	sistema reproductivo (sĭs-*tĕ*-mă rĕ-prō-*dūk*-tĭ-vō)
gonorrhea	gonorrea (gō-*nō*-rĕ-ă)		
herpes	herpe (*ĕr*-pĕ)	semen	semen (*sĕ*-mĕn)
heterosexual	heterosexual (ĕ-tĕ-rō-sĕx-sū-ăl)	sexual desires	deseos sexual (dĕ-*sĕ*-ōs *sĕx*-sū-ăl)

English	Spanish	English	Spanish
sexual relations	relaciones sexual (re-*lă*-sĭ-ō-nĕs *sĕx*-sū-ăl)	underwear	ropa interior (*rŏ*-pă ĭn-*tĕ*-rĭ-ōr)
sterile	estéril (ĕs-*tĕ*-rĭl)	venereal	venéreo (vĕ-*nĕ*-rĕ-ō)
syphilis	sífilis (*sĭ*-fĭ-lĭs)	veneral infection	enfermedad venérea (ĕn-*fĕr*-mĕ-dăd vĕ-*nĕ*-rĕ-ă)
testicle	testículo (tĕs-*tĭ*-kū-lō)		

STUDY AND REVIEW SECTION

LEARNING EXERCISES

▶ Anatomy and Physiology

Write your answers to the following questions. Do not refer back to the text.

1. List the primary and accessory glands of the male reproductive system.

   a. _____   b. _____

   c. _____   d. _____

   e. _____   f. _____

2. Name the supporting structure and accessory sex organs of the male reproductive system.

   a. _____   b. _____

3. State the vital function of the male reproductive system. _____

   _____

4. Describe the scrotum. _____

   _____

5. The _____ _____ _____ and the

   _____ _____ are names of the three longitudinal columns of erectile tissue in the penis.

6. The average erect penis measures _____ to _____ cm in length.

7. The _____ _____ is the cone-shaped head of the penis.

8. Define prepuce. _____

   _____

9. Define smegma. _____

10. State two functions of the penis.

    a. _____   b. _____

11. Describe the testes. _____

    _____

    _____

12. _____ _____ are the site of the development of spermatozoa.

13. List five effects of testosterone regarding male development.

    a. _____   b. _____

    c. _____   d. _____

    e. _____

14. Name the plexus that the seminiferous tubules form. _____

15. Describe the epididymis. _____

    _____

16. State two functions of the epididymis.

    a. _____   b. _____

17. The excretory duct of the testes is known by two names, _____

    _____ or _____ _____.

18. The spermatic cord contains five types of structures and connects the testes with organs in the abdomen. Name these five structures.

    a. _____   b. _____

    c. _____   d. _____

    e. _____

19. State the function of the seminal vesicles. _____

    _____

20.   Describe the prostate gland. _____

_____

21.   Define the condition known as benign prostatic hyperplasia. _____

_____

22.   The two small pea-sized glands located below the prostate and on either side of the urethra are known as the _____ glands or as _____ glands.

23.   Name the three sections of the male urethra.

a. _____   b. _____

c. _____

24.   State a function of the male urethra. _____

25.   The male urethra is approximately _____ cm long.

▶   Word Parts

1.   In the spaces provided, write the definitions of these prefixes, roots, combining forms, and suffixes. Do not refer to the listings of terminology words. Leave blank those terms you cannot define.

2.   After completing as many as you can, refer back to the terminology word listings to check your work. For each word missed or left blank, write the term and its definition several times on the margins of these pages or on a separate sheet of paper.

3.   To maximize the learning process, it is to your advantage to do the following exercises as directed. To refer to the terminology listings before completing these exercises invalidates the learning process.

Prefixes

Give the definitions of the following prefixes:

1.   a- _____   2.   an- _____

3.   circum- _____   4.   epi- _____

5.   hydro- _____   6.   hypo- _____

7.   oligo- _____   8.   par- _____

Roots and Combining Forms

Give the definitions of the following roots and combining forms:

1.   balan _____   2.   cis _____

3. crypt _____

4. cyst _____

5. didym _____

6. enchyma _____

7. orch _____

8. orchid _____

9. orchido _____

10. pen _____

11. phim _____

12. prostat _____

13. prostato _____

14. spadias _____

15. sperm _____

16. spermat _____

17. spermato _____

18. spermi _____

19. testicul _____

20. varico _____

21. vas _____

22. vesicul _____

23. zoo _____

24. zoon _____

Suffixes

Give the definitions of the following suffixes:

1. -algia _____

2. -ar _____

3. -blast _____

4. -cele _____

5. -cide _____

6. -ectomy _____

7. -genesis _____

8. -ia _____

9. -ion _____

10. -ism _____

11. -itis _____

12. -megaly _____

13. -osis _____

14. -pexy _____

15. -plasty _____

16. -tomy _____

17. -uria _____

▶ Identifying Medical Terms

In the spaces provided, write the medical terms for the following meanings:

1. _____   Inflammation of the glans penis

2. _____   Surgical excision of the epididymis

3. _____   Surgical excision of a testicle

4. _____   Surgical repair of a testicle

5. _____ Pain in the prostate

6. _____ Inflammation of the prostate and bladder

7. _____ The sperm germ cell

8. _____ The male sex cell

9. _____ An agent that kills sperm

10. _____ Pertaining to a testicle

▶ **Spelling**

In the spaces provided, write the correct spelling of these misspelled terms:

1. crptorchism _____   2. hyospadias _____

3. orchdotomy _____   4. prostatmegaly _____

5. spermauria _____

WORD PARTS STUDY SHEET

Word Parts	Give the Meaning
circum-	_____
epi-	_____
hydro-	_____
hypo-	_____
oligo-	_____
balan-	_____
cis-	_____
crypt-	_____
cyst-	_____
didym-	_____
orch-, orchid-, orchido-	_____
pen-	_____
phim-	_____
prostat-, prostato-	_____

spadias-   _____

sperm-, spermat-, spermi-, spermato-   _____

testicul-   _____

varico-   _____

vas-   _____

vesicul-   _____

zoo-   _____

zoon-   _____

-algia   _____

-blast   _____

-cele   _____

-cide   _____

-ectomy   _____

-genesis   _____

-ia, -ism, -osis   _____

-ion   _____

-itis   _____

-megaly   _____

-pexy   _____

-plasty   _____

-tomy   _____

-uria   _____

REVIEW QUESTIONS

▶ Matching

Select the appropriate lettered meaning for each numbered line.

_____ 1. circumcision

_____ 2. coitus

_____ 3. condom

a. Caused by the bacterium *Treponema pallidum*
b. A mature reproductive cell of the male or female
c. Sexual intercourse between a man and a woman

_____ 4. gamete

_____ 5. genital warts

_____ 6. gonorrhea

_____ 7. infertility

_____ 8. prepuce

_____ 9. syphilis

_____ 10. trichomoniasis

d. Caused by a parasitic protozoa

e. The surgical process of removing the foreskin of the penis

f. A thin, flexible protective sheath worn over the penis during copulation to help prevent impregnation or venereal disease

g. Caused by the human papilloma virus

h. The inability to produce a viable offspring

i. Causes purulent urethral discharge in the male and purulent vaginal discharge in the female

j. Caused by the bacterium *Chlamydia trachomatis*

k. The foreskin over the glans penis in the male

▶ Abbreviations

Place the correct word, phrase, or abbreviation in the space provided.

1. benign prostatic hyperplasia _____

2. Gc _____

3. human papilloma virus _____

4. HSV-2 _____

5. STDs _____

6. *Treponema pallidum* agglutination _____

7. TUR _____

8. UG _____

9. venereal disease _____

10. Wassermann reaction _____

▶ Diagnostic and Laboratory Tests

Select the best answer to each multiple choice question. Circle the letter of your choice.

1. A test performed on blood serum to detect syphilis.
    a. paternity
    b. semen
    c. FTA-ABS
    d. HSV-2

2. A test to determine whether a certain man could be the father of a specific child.
    a. paternity
    b. semen
    c. FTA-ABS
    d. HSV-2

3. An increased level indicates prostate disease or possibly prostate cancer.
    a. fluorescent treponemal antibody
    b. prostate-specific antigen
    c. semen
    d. testosterone toxicology

4. Used to determine infertility in men.
    a. paternity
    b. prostate-specific antigen
    c. semen
    d. testosterone toxicology

5. An increased level may indicate benign prostatic hyperplasia.
    a. fluorescent treponemal antibody
    b. prostate-specific antigen
    c. testosterone toxicology
    d. venereal disease research

CRITICAL THINKING ACTIVITY

▶ Case Study

Benign Prostatic Hyperplasia

Please read the following case study and then answer the questions that follow.

A 58-year-old male was seen by a physician, and the following is a synopsis of the visit.

Present History: The patient states that he is having difficulty with urination. He is having a need to urinate often, especially at night, urgency, and a decrease in size and force of the urinary stream.

Signs and Symptoms: Chief complaint: frequency, urgency, and decrease in size and force of the urinary stream.

Diagnosis: Benign prostatic hyperplasia

Treatment: Proscar (finasteride) was ordered by the physician to help relieve the symptoms of benign prostatic hyperplasia. It lowers the levels of dihydrotestosterone (DHT), which is a major factor in enlargement of the prostate. Lowering of DHT leads to shrinkage of the enlarged prostate gland in most men. It may take 6 months or more to determine if it is working for an individual. The patient was scheduled for a follow-up visit in 6 months and informed that side effects of Proscar may include impotence and less desire for sex, and that this medication can alter the prostate-specific antigen test (PSA) that is used to screen for prostate cancer.

Critical Thinking Questions

1. Signs and symptoms of benign prostatic hyperplasia include frequency, _____, and decrease in size and force of the urinary stream.

2. Treatment included _____ (finasteride).

3. Side effects of this medication may include _____ and less desire for sex.

4. This medication can alter the _____-specific antigen test that is used to screen for prostate cancer.

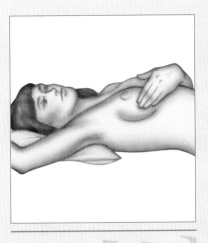

17

ONCOLOGY

OBJECTIVES

On completion of this chapter, you should be able to:

- Describe cancer.
- Describe the three main classifications of cancer.
- Describe cell differentiation.
- Describe the invasive process.
- Identify the staging system that evaluates the spread of a tumor.
- Describe various methods that may be used in diagnosing cancer.
- Describe the various forms of treatment for cancer.
- List several recommended cancer preventive methods.
- Analyze, build, spell, and pronounce medical words that relate to surgical procedures and pathology.
- Identify and give the meaning of selected vocabulary words.
- Identify and define selected abbreviations.
- Successfully complete the study and review section.

► AN OVERVIEW OF CANCER

Cancer was first identified around 400 BC during the time of Hippocrates and is a Latin term meaning *a crab*. Early reports on cancer compared the disease to a crab because of its tendency to stretch out and spread like the crab's four pairs of legs. Today, cancer refers to any malignant tumor (neoplasm, oncoma). More than 200 different types of cancer have been identified; however, the majority of tumors can be classified into three main groups: *carcinomas*, which account for about 80% of cancers; *sarcomas*, which are the next largest group; and *mixed cancers*, which have characteristics of both carcinomas and sarcomas (see Classification of Cancer).

The incidence of cancer is now five times greater than it was 100 years ago. Cancer will strike one of every three Americans, according to recent statistics from the American Cancer Society. However, there is hope for those afflicted. Cancer has become one of the most curable of the major diseases in the United States, and those tumors that cannot be cured can be controlled through treatment, thereby giving the patient an extended life span. With early detection followed by immediate treatment, the cure rate for cancer is now one in every two. Highly advanced surgical techniques are being used to remove cancerous tissue, and it is usually possible to excise all the cancer cells when the malignancy is discovered in its earliest stages. *Chemotherapy* and *radiation therapy* are the other two principal means of treatment for patients with cancer. These treatments employ agents to kill cancerous cells that remain after surgery or in malignancies deemed inoperable. Other forms of treatment are under investigation as scientists continue their research into the causes of cancer. Although the exact cause or causes remain unknown, research has shown that some cancers can be prevented, especially those associated with environmental factors. Oncologists searching for the causes of cancer have identified numerous factors that play a role in the development of cancer. These factors are generally grouped under three main classifications: environmental, hereditary, and biological. Viruses have long been suspected of playing a role in the development of cancer; however, the human T-cell leukemia-lymphoma virus (HTLV) is the first known to cause cancer in humans. It has been found to be present in the cells of individuals with certain types of leukemia and lymphoma. Fortunately, not everyone affected by HTLV develops cancer. Scientists are studying the complex biological relation among viruses, genes, and the development of cancer with the hope of uncovering information leading to the prevention, control, and possible cure of cancer. The American Cancer Society has published the following list of safeguards against cancer, which encourages individuals to take specific steps to safeguard their health and aids in the early detection of cancer.

SITE	ACTION
Breast	Monthly self-examination
Uterus	Pap test once a year
Lung	Don't smoke cigarettes
Skin	Avoid excess sun
Colon-rectum	Procto annually, especially after 40
Mouth	Exams regularly
Whole body	Annual health checkup

► CLASSIFICATION OF CANCER

The more than 200 types of cancer have been grouped into three main classifications: *carcinomas, sarcomas,* and *mixed cancers.*

CARCINOMAS

As mentioned earlier, *carcinomas* make up the great majority of all cancers and are malignant tumors of epithelial tissues. They are named according to the type of epithelial cell in which the malignancy occurs or the primary site of the tumor. For example, a cancer of squamous epithelium is a *squamous carcinoma.* See Figures 17–1 and 17–2. Likewise a cancer originating in the bronchus of the respiratory tract is a *bronchogenic carcinoma.* Epithelial tissue lines body surfaces including those of glands and organs; therefore, carcinomas make up the majority of the glandular cancers and are generally found in the breast, stomach, uterus, tongue, and skin.

SARCOMAS

Sarcomas are a less prevalent type of cancer that develops from embryonic cells of connective tissue such as muscle, fat, bone, and blood vessels. They are named by adding the suffix-oma (tumor) with the root sarc (flesh), to the word part that identifies the tissue of origin. A cancer of the bone, for examples, is an *osteosarcoma:* osteo (CF), bone; sarc (R), flesh; and -oma (S), tumor.

MIXED CANCERS

Mixed cancers originate in cells capable of differentiating into epithelial or connective tissue or when malignancies occur concurrently in adjacent tissue types. For example, stomach cancer may be a mixed cancer when carcinoma originates in the epithelial lining of the stomach wall and a *sarcoma* arises in the adjacent muscular layer underlying the epithelium.

OTHER TYPES

Other types of cancer may be classified as *leukemias, lymphomas,* or *melanomas.* Leukemias are cancers of the blood-forming tissues. Lymphomas are cancers of lymphoid tissue, and melanomas are cancers of black moles.

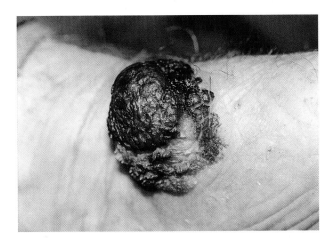

FIGURE 17–1

Squamous cell carcinoma. *(Courtesy of Jason L. Smith, MD.)*

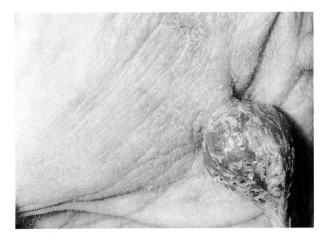

FIGURE 17–2

Squamous cell carcinoma. *(Courtesy of Jason L. Smith, MD.)*

▶ CELL DIFFERENTIATION

Normal cells reproduce themselves through an orderly process that assures growth, tissue repair, and cell reproduction or *mitosis*. Normal cells have a distinct appearance and a specialized function. In normal cell development, immature cells undergo normal changes as they mature and assume their specialized functions. This process is called *differentiation*. Knowledge of cell differentiation allows a pathologist or histologist, looking at a sample of tissue through a microscope, to identify the body area from which the tissue was removed. In cancer, there is an abnormal process wherein a cell or group of cells undergoes changes and no longer carries on normal cell functions. This failure of immature cells to develop specialized functions is called dedifferentiation. It is believed that this process involves a disturbance in the DNA of the affected cells. *Malignant cells* usually multiply rapidly, forming a mass of abnormal cells that enlarges, ulcerates, and sheds malignant cells to surrounding tissues. This process destroys the normal cells, with malignant cells taking their places. Microscopic analysis of a malignant cell reveals a loss of differentiation, anaplasia, nuclei of various sizes that are hyperchromatic, and cells in the process of rapid and disorderly division. Based on microscopic analysis, malignant tumors are further classified as grades I, II, III, or IV. The following describes each of the four grades of tumors in this system:

- **Grade I.** The most differentiated and the least malignant tumors. Only a few cells are undergoing mitosis; however, some abnormality does exist.
- **Grade II.** Moderately undifferentiated. More cells are undergoing mitosis, and the pattern is fairly irregular.
- **Grade III.** Many cells are undifferentiated, and tissue origin may be difficult to recognize. Many cells are undergoing mitosis.
- **Grade IV.** The least differentiated and a high degree of malignancy.

This system of grading tumors is used to report the prognosis of the disease and also to determine whether the tumor is likely to respond to radiation therapy.

▶ THE INVASIVE PROCESS

Two ways in which malignant cells spread to body parts are by *invasive growth (by active migration or direct extension)* and *metastasis*.

INVASIVE GROWTH

Invasive growth is the spreading process of a malignant tumor into adjacent normal tissue. Young malignant cells divide at the periphery of the tumor and spread by active migration or direct extension. In *active migration,* the malignant cells break away from the neoplasm, invade surrounding tissue, divide, form secondary neoplasms, and then reunite with the primary tumor as growth continues. In *direct extension,* multiplication of malignant cells is rapid, and there is subsequent spreading into surrounding tissues via the interstitial spaces accompanied by engulfment and destruction of normal cells. As a tumor's mass enlarges, its weight is supported by connective fibers that attach to surrounding structures. Adjacent veins and lymph vessels are invaded by these fibers and become pathways for the spread of malignant cells.

METASTASIS

Metastasis is the process whereby cancer cells are spread from a primary site to distant secondary sites elsewhere in the body. This process usually occurs when malignant cells invade the bloodstream or lymph system and are transported to a secondary site where they become lodged and form a neoplasm. Malignant cells carried in the bloodstream may lodge in highly vascular organs such as the lungs or liver, and the development of a secondary neoplasm depends on the viability and the reception of the organ.

▶ STAGING

Further reporting of the development and spread of cancer cells may be made through the use of a system that evaluates the spread of the tumor. The staging system uses the letters **T** (tumor), **N** (node), and **M** (metastasis) to indicate spread and uses numerical subscripts to indicate degree of tumor involvement. For example, $T_2N_1M_0$ indicates a primary tumor at stage 2, abnormality of regional lymph nodes at stage 1, and no evidence of distant metastasis.

▶ CHARACTERISTICS OF NEOPLASMS

Neoplasms or tumors, as they are commonly called, may be *benign* or *malignant.* The following characteristics will distinguish the differences between benign and malignant neoplasms:

BENIGN TUMORS	MALIGNANT TUMORS
1. Grow slowly	1. Grow rapidly
2. Encapsulated	2. Not encapsulated
3. Cells resemble the normal cells from which they arose	3. Cells undergo permanent change, abnormal rapid proliferation
4. Grow by expansion and cause pressure on surrounding tissue	4. Invasive growth and metastasis
5. Remain localized	5. Spread via the bloodstream
6. Do not recur when surgically removed	6. May recur when surgically removed if invasive growth has occurred
7. Tissue destruction is minimal	7. Tissue destruction is extensive if invasive growth has occurred
8. No cachexia	8. Cancer cachexia (extreme weakness, fatigue, wasting, and malnutrition)
9. Usually not a threat to life	9. Threat to life unless detected early and properly treated

As malignant cells proliferate and begin the invasive process, the patient is unaware of the development of the cancer. In its early stages, cancer is said to be silent; however, cytologic changes are occurring that could be detected if a tissue sample were taken and analyzed by a pathologist. With the proliferation of malignant cells and the continuation of the invasive process, tissues, organs, and surrounding structures become compressed, and ischemia may occur, causing necrosis, inflammation, ulceration, and bleeding. This bleeding is usually *occult (hidden)* and is not noted by the patient. The enlarging tumor eventually causes sufficient pressure on surrounding tissues and organs to create a feeling of numbness, tingling, and pain. Because the tumor itself does not have nerve endings, pain is not an early symptom of its development. Because of the "silent" development of cancer, the patient does not usually become aware of its symptoms until its systemic effects are evident. These systemic effects depend on the site and type of cancer but usually result in an imbalance in the patient's physiology, leading to subtle but noticeable changes that may warn of the disease.

The American Cancer Society lists seven warning signals of cancer. The first letters of each warning signal combine to spell the word CAUTION, and persons who develop any of the following symptoms should bring it to the attention of a physician immediately:

- **C**hange in bowel or bladder habits
- **A** sore that does not heal
- **U**nusual bleeding or discharge
- **T**hickening or lump in breast or elsewhere
- **I**ndigestion or difficulty in swallowing
- **O**bvious change in a wart or mole
- **N**agging cough or hoarseness

▶ DIAGNOSIS

A variety of *diagnostic tools* and *procedures* is used to detect the possible presence of cancer. Principal among these are examination, visualization by endoscopy, laboratory analysis, biopsy, and diagnostic radiology.

EXAMINATION

An *annual physical examination* may be the best means of protecting one's state of health. The American Cancer Society publishes a cancer detection examination that recommends certain tests be included in an annual physical examination in addition to the medical history and usual tests.* These tests are listed below:

Skin. Entire skin

Head and neck. Eyes; nose; mouth, under all dentures; vocal cords with mirror, if hoarseness

Chest. Listen to heart and lungs; x-ray record of chest when indicated

Breast. Palpation of breasts and under arms for any abnormalities; biopsy of lump in breast when indicated; instruct and encourage breast self-examination; ages 40 to 49 get a mammogram every 1 to 2 years, after age 49 every year

Abdomen. Palpation for any abnormalities

Pelvis. Pelvic examination, including a Pap test for all women

Colon and rectum. Digital examination of rectum; proctosigmoidoscopic examination; x-ray record of colon or intestinal tract when indicated

Prostate. Digital examination of prostate; palpation of male testes; palpation of groin for enlarged lymph nodes; age 50 and over should have a prostate-specific antigen (PSA) blood test each year

Blood. For leukemia or anemia

Urinalysis. For indication of bladder or kidney cancer

---

*This information was taken from American Cancer Society Professional Education publications.

VISUALIZATION BY ENDOSCOPY

Endoscopy provides the physician with a direct view of certain portions of the body. The following is a list of endoscopic procedures used to assess specific locations within the body:

Sigmoidoscopy. The process of using a sigmoidoscope to examine the lower 10 inches of the large intestines

Laryngoscopy. The process of using a laryngoscope to examine the interior of the larynx

Bronchoscopy. The process of using a bronchoscope to examine the bronchi

Gastroscopy. The process of using a gastroscope to examine the interior of the stomach

Cystoscopy. The process of using a cystoscope to examine the bladder

Colposcopy. The process of using a colposcope to examine the cervix and vagina

Proctoscopy. The process of using a proctoscope to examine the anus and rectum

Colonoscopy. The process of using a colonoscope to examine the colon

Laparoscopy. The process of using a laparoscope to examine the abdomen

LABORATORY ANALYSIS

Laboratory analysis plays a key role in detecting specific types of cancer. The following are some of the laboratory tests used to diagnose cancer:

Pap smear/test. A cytologic screening test developed by Dr. George Papanicolaou and used to detect the presence of abnormal or cancerous cells from the cervix and vagina

Fecal occult blood test. A test used to detect occult (hidden) blood. This test may be used to check for cancer of the colon

Sputum cytology test. Microscopic examination of sputum to detect abnormal or cancerous cells of the bronchi and lungs

Blood serum test. Analysis of blood serum provides useful information about certain proteins synthesized by cancer

Abbot Lab's AFP-EIA test. An immunoassay test that uses alpha-fetoprotein to mark tumor cells when testing for cancer of the testicles

Bone marrow study. A test used to detect abnormal bone marrow cells, which may indicate leukemia

Urine assay tests. Tests providing useful information about catecholamines, which may indicate pheochromocytoma of the adrenal medulla

Gravlee jet washer. A device developed by Dr. Clark Gravlee to check for endometrial abnormalities as surface cells of the uterine cavity are studied under a microscope

BIOPSY

The surgical removal of a small piece of tissue for microscopic examination is known as *biopsy*. It is the method of providing the proof of cancer in the diagnosis of the disease. The following different types of biopsy may be used for tissue removal:

Excisional biopsy. Surgical removal of a piece of tissue from the suspected body site

Incisional biopsy. A surgical incision to remove a section or wedge of tissue from the suspected body site

Needle biopsy. Puncture of a tumor for the removal of a core of tissue through the lumen of a needle

Cone biopsy. Removal of a cone of tissue from the uterine cervix

Sternal biopsy. Removal of a piece of bone marrow from the sternum

Endoscopic biopsy. Removal of a piece of tissue through an endoscope

Punch biopsy. Removal of a plug of tissue (epidermis, dermis, and subcutaneous tissue) from the skin

DIAGNOSTIC RADIOLOGY

Encompassing a wide range of tests and procedures, *diagnostic radiology* can reveal tumors that may not have been detected by other diagnostic procedures (see Chapter 18, Radiology and Nuclear Medicine).

▶ TREATMENT

The treatment of cancer may be any one or a combination of the following methods: *surgery, chemotherapy, radiation therapy,* or *immunotherapy*. The treatment of choice will depend on the type of cancer, its location, its invasive process, and the state of health of the patient.

SURGERY

Surgery may be the treatment of choice when the tumor is small and localized and the surrounding tissue is accessible for removal. The aim of surgery is the removal of all cancerous tissue plus some of the surrounding normal tissue. Surgery may also be used to alleviate some of the complications of cancer, such as the obstruction of an area caused by the enlargement of a tumor.

CHEMOTHERAPY

Chemotherapy may be the treatment of choice when the cancer is disseminated and cannot be surgically removed. It is also used when a tumor fails to respond to radiation therapy. Antineoplastic, anticancer drugs do injury to individual cells, interfere with their vital functions, and kill or destroy malignant cells. In rendering cancerous cells harmless, certain normal cells may also be destroyed. The normal cells with the greatest sensitivity to destruction are the hematopoietic cells, epithelial cells, and the hair follicles. The plan of treatment for patients undergoing chemotherapy is individualized. The aim of chemotherapy is to put the patient in remission so that life may continue without *exacerbation* of symptoms. The following are classifications of chemotherapeutic drugs used in the treatment of cancer.

Alkylating Agents
Alkylating agents are chemical compounds that cause chromosome breakage and prevent the formation of new DNA, thereby interfering with cell division. These agents are used in the treatment of leukemia, lymphoma, or disseminated malignancies. *Nitrogen mustard, cyclophosphamide, melphalan, chlorambucil, busulfan,* and *thiotepa* are some of the alkylating agents available.

Antimetabolites

Antimetabolites are substances that interfere with the metabolic process of the cell, thus preventing cell reproduction. They are used in the treatment of leukemia, disseminated solid tumors, and choriocarcinoma. Some of the antimetabolites used are *methotrexate, 6-mercaptopurine, 5-fluorouracil, cytosine arabinoside,* and *thioguanine.*

Vinca Alkaloids

The *vinca alkaloids* are compounds that interfere with cell division by interacting with the cell's miotic process. Alkaloids are used in the treatment of leukemia, lymphoma, Wilm's tumor, and neuroblastoma. *Vincristine* and *vinblastine* are alkaloids.

Antibiotics

Certain *antibiotics* have an antineoplastic effect and are used in the treatment of leukemia, Wilm's tumor, choriocarcinoma, and cancer of the testes. *Actinomycin-D* and *mithramycin* are such antibiotics.

Steroid Hormones

Steroid hormones are substances that alter the hormonal environment. Commonly used steroids and the cancers they treat include the following:

- **Androgen**—breast cancer
- **Estrogen**—prostate cancer
- **Progesterone**—endometrial cancer
- **Adrenocortical hormones**—leukemia

IMMUNOTHERAPY

Immunotherapy is the treatment of disease by stimulation of the body's immune system. It may be used as an adjuvant to other types of treatment. There are three types of immunotherapy: *active specific, passive,* and *adoptive.*

Active Immunotherapy

Active specific immunotherapy is the use of various agents to produce a specific host–immune response. The patient's own tumor cells, tumor antigens, oncogenic viruses, and bacterial products are a few of the agents that are being used to create an immune response of a specific nature.

Passive Immunotherapy

Passive immunotherapy is the use of serum or other products from an immunocompetent individual that are given to an immunodeficient individual to produce an immune response.

Adoptive Immunotherapy

Adoptive immunotherapy is the process of transferring a form of specific immune response from a donor to a recipient.

OTHER FORMS OF TREATMENT

Differentiation Agents/Maturation Agents

This is a new classification of drugs that invade cancer cells and somehow cause them to mature into cells that are almost normal. They are being tested on humans and have demonstrated good activity against colon cancer.

Interleukin-2 (IL-2)

This is a genetically engineered immune-boosting drug that stimulates the patient's immune system to produce *lymphokine-activated killer* (LAK) cells that destroy some forms of tumor cells. It is used in the treatment of certain types of cancer.

Intraoperative Radiation Therapy

This is the delivery of *tumoricidal* doses of radiation directly onto a tumor bed while the surgical wound is still open. The surgeon and radiotherapist decide on the target area, and then the radiotherapist positions the sterile treatment cone in the incision. The treatment is usually for 15 to 30 minutes, and the incision is closed after the treatment is completed.

Photodynamic Therapy

This is the use of a *red laser* to kill cancerous cells. *Hematoporphyrin derivative* (Hpd), a light-sensitizing agent, is intravenously injected, and 3 days after the injection the physician uses the red laser. Normal cells eliminate Hpd and are not harmed during the treatment. Cancerous cells retain Hpd, and the red light kills them.

Recombinant Interferon Therapy

This is a genetically engineered *immune system activator.* It strengthens the body's immune system and helps it fight cancer cells. It is indicated for use in the treatment of hairy cell leukemia in people 18 years of age or older.

Tumor Necrosis Factor (TNF)

This is a lymphokine produced by *macrophages (white blood cells).* It triggers the macrophages to destroy malignant tumors. It is being tested in the treatment of low-grade lymphoma.

Whole Body Hyperthermia

This is the process of elevating the patient's body temperature to 108°F (42.2°C) to enhance the effect of radiation or chemotherapy. Cancer cells are sensitive to heat, so after radiation therapy, *hyperthermia* is employed to inhibit the cancer cells from repairing themselves. It is used before chemotherapy to increase the vulnerability of the cancer cells to the drug being used in the treatment process.

▶ PREVENTION OF CANCER

STOP SMOKING OR DON'T EVER START

Smoking is the most preventable cause of death in man. In the United States, tobacco use is responsible for more than one in six deaths. Cigarette smoking is responsible for 90% of lung cancer among men and 79% among women. Smoking accounts for about 30% of all cancer deaths. Those who smoke two or more packs of cigarettes a day have lung cancer mortality rates 15 to 25 times greater than nonsmokers. According to the World Health Organization, approximately 2.5 million people each year worldwide die as a result of smoking.

STOP USING SMOKELESS TOBACCO OR DON'T EVER START

There has been a resurgence in the use of all forms of smokeless tobacco. The greatest cause of concern centers on the increased use of "dipping snuff." In this practice, tobacco that has been processed into a coarse, moist powder is placed between the cheek and gum, and nicotine, along with a number of carcinogens, is absorbed through the oral mucosa. Use of chewing tobacco or snuff increases the risk of cancer of the mouth, larynx (voice box), pharynx (throat), and esophagus (food tube).

AVOID DIRECT SUNLIGHT AND/OR USE PROTECTIVE SUNSCREEN

Epidemiologic evidence shows that sun exposure is a major factor in the development of melanoma and that incidence increases for those living near the equator. Almost all of the more than 700,000 cases of basal and squamous cell skin cancer diagnosed each year in the United States are sun related (ultraviolet radiation).

AVOID IONIZING RADIATION AND/OR LIMIT EXPOSURE

Excessive exposure to ionizing radiation can increase cancer risk. Excessive radon exposure in homes, schools, and one's workplace may increase the risk of lung cancer, especially in cigarette smokers.

"EAT-RIGHT" NUTRITION AND DIET

More and more evidence shows that *proper nutrition* and *diet* can help prevent disease. One may reduce his or her cancer risk by:

- Maintaining desirable weight. Individuals 40% or more overweight increase their risk of colon, breast, prostate, gallbladder, ovary, and uterus cancer.
- Eat a variety of food.
- Eat a variety of vegetables and fruits each day. The National Institute (NCI) suggest eating at least 5 servings of fruits and vegetables each day: "5 a Day for Better Health." Studies have shown that a daily consumption of vegetables and fruits may decrease the risk of lung, prostate, esophagus, colorectal, and stomach cancers.
- Eat more foods that are high in fiber, such as whole grains, breads, pasta, vegetables, and fruits. High-fiber diets may reduce the risk of colon cancer.
- Cut down on total fat intake. It is recommended that only 30% or less of one's daily intake be from fat. A high-fat diet may contribute to breast, colon, and prostate cancer.
- If you drink, limit the consumption of alcohol to a minimum. The heavy use of alcohol, especially when accompanied by cigarette smoking or smokeless tobacco use, increases the risk of cancers of the mouth, larynx, pharynx, esophagus, and liver.
- Limit the consumption of salt-cured, smoked, and nitrite-cured foods. In areas of the world where salt-cured and smoked foods are eaten frequently, there is higher incidence of cancer of the esophagus and stomach.

AVOID OCCUPATIONAL HAZARDS

Exposure to several different *industrial agents* (nickel, chromate, asbestos, vinyl chloride, etc.) increases risk of various cancers. Risk of lung cancer from *asbestos* is greatly increased when combined with cigarette smoking.

FYI: THE NATIONAL CANCER INSTITUTE (NCI) AND THE AMERICAN CANCER SOCIETY

The National Cancer Institute has designated several medical centers throughout the United States as Comprehensive Cancer Centers (CCCs). These centers develop comprehensive cancer programs and provide up-to-date regimens. For information on oncology you may call 1–800–4–CANCER or 800–422–6237.

The American Cancer Society is a voluntary organization dedicated to the control and eradication of cancer. National headquarters are in Atlanta, and there are 58 incorporated chartered Divisions: one in each state, in Puerto Rico, the District of Columbia, and six metropolitan areas. For information you may call 800–ACS–2345 or write: American Cancer Society, Inc., 1599 Clifton Road, N. E., Atlanta, GA 30329–4251.

The American Cancer Society Society is the nationwide, community-based, voluntary health organization dedicated to eliminating cancer as a major health problem by preventing cancer, saving lives from cancer, and diminishing suffering from cancer through research, education, and service.

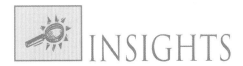INSIGHTS

BREAST CANCER

This year approximately 182,000 women and approximately 1000 men will be diagnosed with breast cancer. It kills about 46,000 women a year, and is the leading cause of death in women between the ages of 32 and 52.

In cancer, there is an abnormal process wherein a cell or group of cells undergoes changes and no longer carries on normal cell functions. This failure of immature cells to develop specialized functions is called dedifferentiation. It is believed that this process involves a disturbance in the DNA of the affected cells. Malignant cells usually multiply rapidly, forming a mass of abnormal cells that enlarges, ulcerates, and sheds malignant cells to surrounding tissues. This process destroys the normal cells, with malignant cells taking their places, and often results in the formation of a tumor.

If cancer is not detected and treated early, it will continue to grow, invade, and destroy adjacent tissue, and spread into surrounding lymph nodes. See Figure 17–4. It can be carried by the lymph and/or blood to other areas of the body and once this process, known as **metastasis,** has occurred, the cancer is usually advanced and/or disseminated and the 5-year survival rate is low. Early detection of breast cancer is extremely important. The 5-year survival rate for women with localized, and properly treated breast cancer is 92%.

Approximately 50% of malignant tumors of the breast appear in the upper, outer quadrant and extend into the armpit. Eighteen percent of breast cancers occur in the nipple area, 11% in the lower outer quadrant, and 6% in the inner quadrant.

Signs and symptoms of breast cancer are generally insidious and may include:

- Unusual secretions from the nipple
- Changes in the nipple's appearance
- Nontender, movable lump
- Well-localized discomfort that may be described as a burning, stinging, or aching sensation

- Dimpling or peau d'orange (orange-peel appearance) may be present over the area of cancer of the breast
- Asymmetry and an elevation of the affected breast
- Nipple retraction
- Pain in the later stages

Know Your Breast and Your Risk Factors

More than 90% of all breast lumps are discovered by women themselves. The majority of these lumps are benign (noncancerous) but of those that are not, early detection and treatment are essential.

Your Breast:

Being Informed Could Save Your Life
Risk Factors in Order of Importance:

1. Family history—Increased risk when breast cancer occurs before menopause in mother, sister, or daughter especially if cancer occurs in both breasts.

2. Over age 50 and nullipara.

3. Having a first baby after age 30.

4. History of chronic breast disease, especially epithelial hyperplasia.

5. Exposure to ionizing radiation of more than 50 rad during adolescence.

6. Obesity.

7. Early menarche, late menopause.

Examine your breast every month
(BSE, Breast Self-Examination—see Fig. 17–3)
Appearance
Size, shape, symmetry
Tenderness, thickening, texture changes

WHY DO THE BREAST SELF-EXAM?

There are many good reasons for doing a breast self-exam each month. One reason is that it is easy to do and the more you do it, the better you will get at it. When you get to know how your breasts normally feel, you will quickly be able to feel any change, and early detection is the key to successful treatment and cure.

REMEMBER: A breast self-exam could save your breast – and save your life. Most breast lumps are found by women themselves, but in fact, most lumps in the breast are not cancer. Be safe, be sure.

WHEN TO DO BREAST SELF-EXAM

The best time to do breast self-exam is right after your period, when breasts are not tender or swollen. If you do not have regular periods or sometimes skip a month, do it on the same day every month.

NOW, HOW TO DO BREAST SELF-EXAM

1. Lie down and put a pillow under your right shoulder. Place your right arm behind your head.

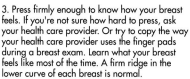

2. Use the finger pads of your three middle fingers on your left hand to feel for lumps or thickening. Your finger pads are the top third of each finger.

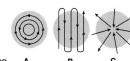

3. Press firmly enough to know how your breast feels. If you're not sure how hard to press, ask your health care provider. Or try to copy the way your health care provider uses the finger pads during a breast exam. Learn what your breast feels like most of the time. A firm ridge in the lower curve of each breast is normal.

4. Move around the breast in a set way. You can choose either the circle (A), the up and down line (B), or the wedge (C). Do it the same way every time. It will help you to make sure that you've gone over the entire breast area, and to remember how your breast feels.

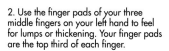

A   B   C

5. Now examine your left breast using your right hand finger pads.

6. If you find any changes, see your doctor right away.

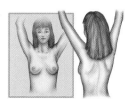

FOR ADDED SAFETY:

You should also check your breasts while standing in front of a mirror right after you do your breast self-exam each month. See if there are any changes in the way your breasts look: dimpling of the skin, changes in the nipple, or redness or swelling.

You might also want to do a breast self-exam while you're in the shower. Your soapy hands will glide over the wet skin, making it easy to check how your breasts feel.

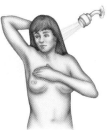

FIGURE 17–3

Breast self-examination.

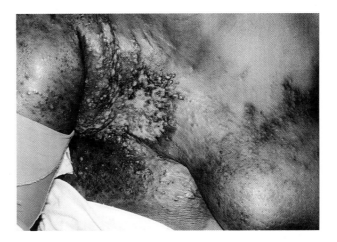

FIGURE 17–4

Metastatic breast cancer. *(Courtesy of Jason L. Smith, MD.)*

TERMINOLOGY
WITH SURGICAL PROCEDURES & PATHOLOGY

TERM	WORD PARTS			DEFINITION
adenocarcinoma (ăd″ ĕ-nō-kăr″ sĭn-ō′ maă)	adeno carcin oma	CF R S	gland cancer tumor	A cancerous tumor of a gland
anaplasia (ăn″ ă-plā′ zĭ-ă)	ana plasia	P S	up formation	A characteristic of most cancerous cells in which there is a loss of differentiation
astrocytoma (ăs″ trō-sī-tō′ mă)	astro cyt oma	P R S	star-shaped cell tumor	A tumor composed of star-shaped neuroglial cells
carcinogen (kăr″ sĭn′ ō-jĕn)	carcino gen	CF S	cancer formation	Any agent or substance that incites or produces cancer
carcinoma (kăr″ sĭ-nō′ mă)	carcin oma	R S	cancer tumor	A cancerous tumor. See Figure 17–5.
chondrosarcoma (kŏn″ drō-săr-kō′ mă)	chondro sarc oma	CF R S	cartilage flesh tumor	A cancerous tumor derived from cartilage cells
choriocarcinoma (kō″ rĭ-ō-kăr″ sĭ-nō′ mă)	chorio carcin oma	CF R S	chorion cancer tumor	A cancerous tumor of the uterus or at the site of an ectopic pregnancy
fibrosarcoma (fī″ brō-săr-kō′ mă)	fibro sarc oma	CF R S	fiber flesh tumor	A cancerous tumor arising from collagen-producing fibroblasts
glioblastoma (glī′ ō-blăs-tō′ mă)	glio blast oma	CF S S	glue immature cell tumor	A cancerous tumor of the brain, usually of the cerebral hemispheres
glioma (gli-ō′ mă)	gli oma	R S	glue tumor	A cancerous tumor of the brain
hemangiosarcoma (hē- măn″ jĭ-ō-săr-kō′ mă)	hem angio sarc oma	R CF R S	blood vessel flesh tumor	A cancerous tumor originating from blood vessels

Terminology - continued

TERM	WORD PARTS			DEFINITION
hypernephroma (hī″ pĕr-nĕ-frō′ mă)	hyper nephr oma	P R S	excessive kidney tumor	A cancerous tumor of the kidney
hyperplasia (hī″ pĕr-plā′ zĭ-ă)	hyper plasia	P S	excessive formation	Excessive formation and growth of normal cells
immunotherapy (ĭm″ mū-nō-thĕr′ ă pē)	immuno therapy	CF S	safe treatment	Treatment of disease by active, passive, or adoptive immunity
leiomyosarcoma (lī″ ō-mī″ ō-săr-kō′ mă)	leio myo sarc oma	CF CF R S	smooth muscle flesh tumor	A cancerous tumor of smooth muscle tissue
leukemia (lū-kē′ mĭ-ă)	leuk emia	R S	white blood condition	A disease of the blood characterized by overproduction of leukocytes; *cancer of the blood-forming tissues*
leukoplakia (lū″ kō-plā′ kĭ-ă)	leuko plakia	CF S	white plate	White, thickened patches formed on the mucous membranes of the cheeks, gums, or tongue. These patches tend to become cancerous
liposarcoma (lĭp″ ō-săr-kō′ mă)	lipo sarc oma	CF R S	fat flesh tumor	A cancerous tumor of fat cells
lymphan-giosarcoma (lĭm-făn″ jē-ō-săr-kō′ mă)	lymph angio sarc oma	R CF R S	lymph vessel flesh tumor	A cancerous tumor of lymphatic vessels
lymphoma (lĭm-fō′ mă)	lymph oma	R S	lymph tumor	A cancerous tumor of the lymph nodes
lymphosarcoma (lĭm″ fō-săr-kō′ mă)	lympho sarc oma	CF R S	lymph flesh tumor	A cancerous disease of lymphatic tissue
medulloblastoma (mĕ-dŭl″ ō-blăs-tō′ mă)	medullo blast oma	CF S S	marrow immature cell tumor	A cancerous tumor of the brain, the fourth ventricle, and the cerebellum

continued

Terminology - continued

TERM	WORD PARTS			DEFINITION
melanoma (mĕl″ ă-nō′ mă)	melan oma	R S	black tumor	A cancerous black mole or tumor. See Figure 17–6.
meningioma (mĕn-ĭn″ jĭ-ō′ mă)	meningi oma	CF S	membrane tumor	A cancerous tumor arising in the arachnoidal tissue of the brain
mucositis (mū″ kō-sī′ tĭs)	mucos itis	R S	mucus inflammation	Inflammation of the oral mucosa caused by exposure to high-energy beams delivered by radiation therapy
mycotoxin (mī″ kō-tŏk′ sĭn)	myco tox in	CF R S	fungus poison pertaining to	Pertaining to a fungus growing in food or animal feed that, if ingested, may cause cancer
myeloma (mī″ ĕ-lō′ mă)	myel oma	R S	marrow tumor	A tumor arising in the hemopoietic portion of the bone marrow
myosarcoma (mī″ ō-săr-kō′ mă)	myo sarc oma	CF R S	muscle flesh tumor	A cancerous tumor of muscle tissue
neoplasm (nē′ ō-plăzm)	neo plasm	P S	new a thing formed	A new thing formed, such as an abnormal growth or tumor
nephroblastoma (nĕf″ rō-blăs-tō′ mă)	nephro blast oma	CF S S	kidney immature cell tumor	A cancerous tumor of the kidney; *also called Wilm's tumor*
neuroblastoma (nū″ rō-blăs-tō′ mă)	neuro blast oma	CF S S	nerve immature cell tumor	A cancerous tumor composed chiefly of neuroblasts; usually found in infants or young children
oligodendro-glioma (ŏl″ ĭ-gō-dĕn″ drō-glī-ō′ mă)	oligo dendro gli oma	P CF R S	little tree glue tumor	A cancerous tumor composed chiefly of neuroglial cells and located in the cerebrum
oncogenes (ŏng″ kō-jēn z′)	onco genes	CF S	tumor produce	Cancer-causing genes
oncogenic (ŏng″ kō-jēn′ ĭk)	onco genic	CF S	tumor formation, produce	The formation of tumors, especially cancerous tumors

Terminology - continued

TERM	WORD PARTS			DEFINITION
osteogenic sarcoma (ŏs″ tē- ō-jĕn′ ĭk săr-kō′ mă)	osteo genic sarc oma	CF S R S	bone formation, produce flesh tumor	A cancerous tumor composed of osseous tissue
precancerous (prē- kăn′ sĕr-ŭs)	pre cancer ous	P R S	before crab pertaining to	Pertaining to the state of a growth or condition before the onset of cancer
reticulosarcoma (rĕ-tĭk″ ū-lō-săr-kō′ mă)	reticulo sarc oma	CF R S	net flesh tumor	A cancerous tumor of the lymphatic system
retinoblastoma (rĕt″ ĭ-nō-blăs-tō′ mă)	retino blast oma	CF S S	retina immature cell tumor	A cancerous tumor of the retina
rhabdomyo-sarcoma (răb″ dō-mī″ ō-săr-kō′ mă)	rhabdo myo sarc oma	CF CF R S	rod muscle flesh tumor	A cancerous tumor arising in striated muscle tissue
sarcoma (săr-kō′ mă)	sarc oma	R S	flesh tumor	A cancerous tumor arising from connective tissue
sarcopoietic (săr″ kō-poy-ĕt′ ĭk)	sarco poietic	CF S	flesh formation	The formation of flesh or muscle
seminoma (sĕm″ ĭ-nō′ mă)	semin oma	R S	seed tumor	A cancerous tumor of the testis
teratoma (tĕr″ ă-tō′ mă)	terat oma	R S	monster tumor	A cancerous tumor of the ovary or testis; may contain embryonic tissues of hair, teeth, bone, or muscle
thymoma (thī-mō′ mă)	thym oma	R S	thymus tumor	A tumor of the thymus gland
trismus (trĭz′ mŭs)	trism us	R S	grating pertaining to	Pertaining to the inability to open the mouth fully; occurs in patients with oral cancer who undergo a combination of surgery and radiation therapy
xerostomia (zē″ rō-stō′ mē-ă)	xero stom ia	CF R S	dry mouth condition	A condition of dryness of the mouth; an oral change caused by radiation therapy or chemotherapy

continued

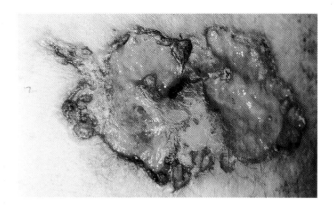

FIGURE 17–5

Basal cell carcinoma. *(Courtesy of Jason L. Smith, MD.)*

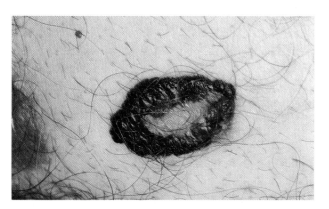

FIGURE 17–6

Melanoma. *(Courtesy of Jason L. Smith, MD.)*

 VOCABULARY WORDS

Vocabulary words are terms that have not been divided into component parts. They are common words or specialized terms associated with the subject of this chapter. These words are provided to enhance your medical vocabulary.

WORD	DEFINITION
Burkitt's lymphoma (bŭrk′ ĭtz lĭm-fō′ mă)	A malignant tumor, most commonly found in Africa, that affects children. The characteristic symptom is a massive, swollen jaw.
dedifferentiation (dē-dĭf″ ĕr-ĕn″ shē-ā′ shŭn)	The process whereby normal cells lose their specialization *(differentiation)* and become malignant
deoxyribonucleic acid (dē-ŏk″ sĭ-rī″ bō-nū-klē′ ĭk ăs′ ĭd)	A complex protein of high molecular weight that is found in the nucleus of every cell. DNA controls all the cell's activities and contains the genetic material necessary for the organism's heredity.
differentiation (dĭf″ ĕr-ĕn″ shē-ā″ shŭn)	The process whereby normal cells have a distinct appearance and specialized function
encapsulated (ĕn-kăp″ sū-lā′ tĕd)	Enclosed within a sheath or capsule

Vocabulary - continued

WORD	DEFINITION
Ewing's sarcoma (ū′ ingz săr-kō′ mă)	A primary bone cancer occurring in the pelvic area or in one of the long bones
exacerbation (ĕks-ăs″ ĕr-bā′ shŭn)	The process of increasing the severity of symptoms. A time when the symptoms of a disease are most prevalent
fungating (fŭn′ gāt-ĭng)	The process of growing rapidly, like a fungus
Hodgkin's disease (hŏj′ kĭns dĭ-zēz″)	A form of lymphoma that occurs in young adults. See Figure 17–7.
human T-cell leukemia-lymphoma virus (HTLV) (hū′ măn tē′ sĕl lū-kē′ mĭ-ă lĭm-fō′ mă vī′ rŭs)	The first virus known to cause cancer in humans
immuno-suppression (ĭm″ ū-nō-sŭ-prĕsh′ ŭn)	The process of preventing formation of the immune response
infiltrative (ĭn′ fĭl-trā″ tĭve)	Pertaining to the process of extending or growing into normal tissue; invasive
in situ (ĭn sī′ too)	To stay within a site; refers to tumor cells that remain at a site and have not invaded adjacent tissue
interstitial (ĭn″ tĕr-stĭsh′ ăl)	Pertaining to between spaces
invasive (ĭn-vā′ sĭv)	The spreading process of a malignant tumor into normal tissue
Kaposi's sarcoma (kăp′ ō-sēz săr-kō′ mă)	A malignant neoplasm that causes violaceous vascular lesions and general lymphadenopathy
lesion (lē′ zhŭn)	A wound; an injury, altered tissue, or a single infected patch of skin
macrofollicular (măk″ rō-fō-lĭk′ ū-lăr)	A giant follicle lymphoma; occurs as a painless swelling of a lymph node but may be found in the spleen

continued

Vocabulary - continued

WORD	DEFINITION
malignant (mă-lĭg′ nănt)	Pertaining to a bad wandering; refers to the spreading process of cancer from one area of the body to another
metastasis (mĕ-tăs′ tă-sis)	The spreading process of cancer from a primary site to a secondary site
mutagen (mū′ tă-jĕn)	Any agent that causes a change in the genetic structure of an organism
mutation (mū-tā′ shŭn)	The process whereby the genetic structure is changed
Paget's disease (păj′ ĕts dĭ-zēz ′)	An inflammatory bone disease that may precede the development of bone cancer. See Figure 17–8.
palliative (păl′ ĭ-ā-tĭv)	Pertaining to a form of treatment that will relieve or alleviate symptoms without curing
primary site (prī′ mă-rē sīt)	The original, initial, or principal site
proliferation (prō-lĭf″ ĕr-ā′ shŭn)	The process of rapid production; to grow by multiplying
remission (rē- mĭsh′ ŭn)	The process of lessening the severity of symptoms. A time when symptoms of a disease are at rest
ribonucleic acid (RNA) (rī″ bō-nū′ klē′ ĭk ăs′ ĭd)	A nucleic acid found in all living cells that is responsible for protein synthesis. The three types are mRNA—messenger RNA; tRNA—transfer RNA; and rRNA—ribosomal RNA.
scirrhus (skĭr′ ŭs)	A hard, cancerous tumor composed of connective tissue
secondary site (sĕk′ ăn-dĕr″ē sīt)	The second site usually derived from the primary site
tamponade (cardiac) (tam′ pŏn-ād [kăr′ dē-ăk])	A pathologic condition of the heart in which there is accumulation of excess fluid in the pericardium. It may be caused by advanced cancer of the lung or a tumor that has metastasized to the pericardium.
tumor (tū′ mor)	An abnormal growth, swelling, or enlargement
violaceous (vĭ″-ō-lā′ shăs)	Pertaining to having a violet color

Vocabulary - continued

WORD	DEFINITION
viral (vī′ răl)	Pertaining to a virus, which means poison in Latin. A virus is a minute organism that may be responsible for 50% of all diseases.
Wilms' tumor (vĭlmz tū′ mor)	A cancerous tumor of the kidney occurring mainly in children

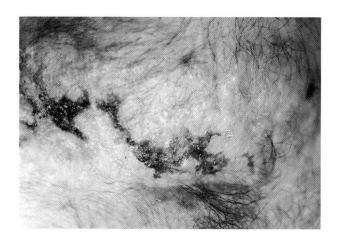

FIGURE 17–7

Cutaneous Hodgkin's disease. *(Courtesy of Jason L. Smith, MD.)*

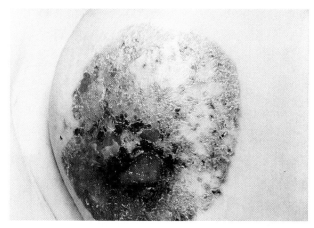

FIGURE 17–8

Paget's disease of the breast. *(Courtesy of Jason L. Smith, MD.)*

 # ABBREVIATIONS

Adeno-Ca	adenocarcinoma	**HTLV**	human T-cell leukemia-lymphoma virus
AFP	alpha-fetoprotein	**IL-2**	interleukin-2
Bx	biopsy	**LAK**	lymphokine-activated killer (cells)
CA	cancer	**Mets**	metastases
chem	chemotherapy	**RNA**	ribonucleic acid
DNA	deoxyribonucleic acid	**St**	stage (of disease)
HD	Hodgkin's disease	**TNF**	tumor necrosis factor
Hpd	hematoporphyrin derivative	**TNM**	tumor, node, metastasis

COMMUNICATION ENRICHMENT

This segment is provided for those who wish to enhance their ability to communicate in either English or Spanish.

▶ **Seven Warning Signals of Cancer**

Siete Señales Canserosas
(sĭ-ĕ́-tĕ sĕ-ñắ-lĕs kăn-sĕ-rō-săs)

English	Spanish
CAUTION	CAUTELA (kă-ū-tĕ-lă)
Change in bowel or bladder habits	Cambio en movimentos fecales (kăm-bĭ-ō ĕn mō-vĭ-mĭ-ĕn-tōs fĕ-kă-lĕs)
A sore that does not heal	Ulcera que no se cura ūl-sĕ-ră kĕ nō sĕ cū-ră)
Unusual bleeding or discharge	Sangramiento inhabitual (săn-gră-mĭ-ĕn-tō ĭn-ă-bĭ-tū-ăl)
Thickening or lump in breast or elsewhere	Espesor o protuberancia en el seno o peson (ĕs-pe-sōr ō prō-tū-bĕ-răn-sĭ-ă ĕn ĕl sĕ-nō ō pĕ-zōn)
Indigestion or difficulty in swallowing	Indigestion o dificultad al tragar (ĭn-dĭ-hĕs-tĭ-ōn ō dĭ-fĭ-kŭl-tăd ăl tră-găr)
Obvious change in wart or mole	Cambio en una verruga (kăm-bĭ-ō ĕn ū-nă vĕ-rū-gă)
Nagging cough or hoarseness	Tos o ronquera persistente (tōs ō rōn-kĕ-ră pĕr-sĭs-tĕn-tĕ)

▶ **Related Terms**

English	Spanish	English	Spanish
cancer	cancer (kăn-cĕr)	malignant	maligno (mă-lĭg-nō)
gland	glandula (glăn-dū-lă)	spread	extensión (ex-tĕn-sĭ-ōn)
treatment	tratamiento (tră-tă-mĭ-ĕn-tō)	remission	remiso; remision (rĕ-mĭ-sō; rĕ-mĭ-sĭ-ōn)

STUDY AND REVIEW SECTION

LEARNING EXERCISES

▶ An Overview of Oncology

Write your answers to the following questions. Do not refer back to the text.

1. Name the three main classifications of cancer.

    a. _____ b. _____ c. _____

2. Define cell differentiation. _____

    _____

3. Define dedifferentiation. _____

    _____

4. Name three ways that malignant cells spread to body parts.

    a. _____ b. _____ c. _____

5. List the seven warning signals for cancer.

    a. _____ b. _____

    c. _____ d. _____

    e. _____ f. _____

    g. _____

6. Name four methods that may be used in the treatment of cancer.

    a. _____ b. _____

    c. _____ d. _____

▶ Word Parts

1. In the spaces provided, write the definitions of these prefixes, roots, combining forms, and suffixes. Do not refer to the listings of terminology words. Leave blank those terms you cannot define.

2. After completing as many as you can, refer back to the terminology word listings to check your work. For each word missed or left blank, write the term and its definition several times on the margins of these pages or on a separate sheet of paper.

3. To maximize the learning process, it is to your advantage to do the following exercises as directed. To refer to the terminology listings before completing these exercises invalidates the learning process.

Prefixes

Give the definitions of the following prefixes:

1. ana- _____
2. astro- _____
3. hyper- _____
4. neo- _____
5. oligo- _____
6. pre- _____

Roots and Combining Forms

Give the definitions of the following roots and combining forms:

1. adeno _____
2. angio _____
3. cancer _____
4. carcin _____
5. carcino _____
6. chondro _____
7. chorio _____
8. cyt _____
9. dendro _____
10. fibro _____
11. gli _____
12. glio _____
13. hem _____
14. immuno _____
15. leio _____
16. leuk _____
17. leuko _____
18. lipo _____
19. lymph _____
20. lympho _____
21. medullo _____
22. melan _____
23. meningi _____
24. mucos _____
25. myco _____
26. myel _____
27. myo _____
28. nephr _____
29. nephro _____
30. neuro _____
31. onco _____
32. osteo _____
33. reticulo _____
34. retino _____
35. rhabdo _____
36. sarc _____
37. sarco _____
38. semin _____

39. stom _____   40. terat _____

41. thym _____   42. tox _____

43. trism _____   44. xero _____

Suffixes

Give the definitions of the following suffixes:

1. -blast _____   2. -emia _____

3. -gen _____   4. -genes _____

5. -genic _____   6. -ia _____

7. -in _____   8. -itis _____

9. -oma _____   10. -ous _____

11. -plakia _____   12. -plasia _____

13. -plasm _____   14. -poietic _____

15. -therapy _____   16. -us _____

▶ Identifying Medical Terms

In the spaces provided, write the medical terms for the following meanings:

1. _____   Any agent or substance that incites or produces cancer

2. _____   A cancerous tumor derived from cartilage cells

3. _____   A cancerous tumor of the brain

4. _____   A cancerous tumor of the kidney

5. _____   Cancer of the blood-forming tissues

6. _____   A cancerous tumor of lymphoid tissue

7. _____   A cancerous black mole or tumor

8. _____   A cancerous tumor of muscle tissue

9. _____   A cancerous tumor composed of osseous tissue

10. _____   A cancerous tumor arising from connective tissue

▶ **Spelling**

In the spaces provided, write the correct spelling of these misspelled terms:

1. anplasia _____
2. fibrsarcoma _____
3. lymphsarcoma _____
4. myloma _____
5. oncgenic _____
6. semioma _____

WORD PARTS STUDY SHEET

Word Parts	Give the Meaning
ana-	_____
astro-	_____
hyper-	_____
neo-	_____
oligo-	_____
pre-	_____
adeno-	_____
carcin-, carcino-	_____
chorio-	_____
dendro-	_____
fibro-	_____
gli-, glio-	_____
immuno-	_____
leio-	_____
leuk-, leuko-	_____
lipo-	_____
lymph-, lympho-	_____
medullo-	_____
melan-	_____
mucos-	_____
onco-	_____

reticulo-   _____

rhabdo-   _____

sarc-, sarco-   _____

stom-   _____

terat-   _____

tox-   _____

trism-   _____

xero-   _____

-blast   _____

-gen, -genes, -genic   _____

-in   _____

-oma   _____

-plakia   _____

-plasia   _____

-plasm   _____

-poietic   _____

-therapy   _____

-us   _____

REVIEW QUESTIONS

▶ Matching

Select the appropriate lettered meaning for each numbered line.

_____ 1. Hodgkin's disease

_____ 2. exacerbation

_____ 3. differentiation

_____ 4. in situ

_____ 5. interleukin-2

_____ 6. photodynamic therapy

_____ 7. recombinant interferon

a. The spreading process of cancer from one area of the body to another
b. A lymphokine produced by macrophages
c. A genetically engineered immune-boosting drug that stimulates the patient's immune system
d. The process whereby normal cells have a distinct appearance and specialized function
e. A form of lymphoma that occurs in young adults

_____ 8.   tumor necrosis factor

_____ 9.   Kaposi's sarcoma

_____ 10. malignant

f. The use of a red laser to kill cancerous cells

g. To stay within a site

h. A malignant neoplasm that causes violaceous vascular lesions and general lymphadenopathy

i. The process of increasing the severity of symptoms

j. A genetically engineered immune system activator

k. Any agent that causes a change in the genetic structure of an organism

▶ **Abbreviations**

Place the correct word, phrase, or abbreviation in the space provided.

1. adenocarcinoma _____

2. biopsy _____

3. CA _____

4. chem _____

5. deoxyribonucleic acid _____

6. IL-2 _____

7. lymphokine-activated killer _____

8. Mets _____

9. TNF _____

10. tumor, node, metastases _____

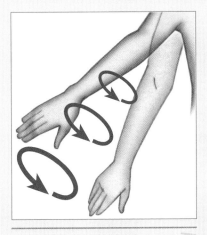

18

RADIOLOGY AND NUCLEAR MEDICINE

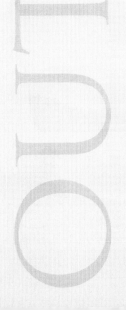
OBJECTIVES

On completion of this chapter, you should be able to:

- Define radiology.

- Describe dangers and safety precautions associated with x-rays.

- Describe the positions used in radiography.

- Describe diagnostic radiology.

- Describe interventional radiology.

- Describe nuclear medicine.

- Define radiation therapy.

- Describe important factors that must be considered when determining the use of radiotherapy for the cancer patient.

- Define the techniques of radiotherapy: external and internal.

- List 13 side effects of radiation.

- Analyze, build, spell, and pronounce medical words that relate to surgical procedures and pathology.

- Identify and give the meaning of selected vocabulary words.

- Identify and define selected abbreviations.

- Successfully complete the study and review section.

▶ AN OVERVIEW OF RADIOLOGY AND NUCLEAR MEDICINE

▶ RADIOLOGY

Radiology is the study of x-rays, radioactive substances, radioactive isotopes, and ionizing radiation. Sometimes called *roentgenology,* this medical specialty was developed after the discovery of an unknown ray in 1895 by Wilhelm Konrad Roentgen, a German physicist, who called his discovery an x-ray. An x-ray is produced by the collision of a stream of electrons against a target (usually an anode of one of the heavy metals) contained within a vacuum tube. This collision produces electromagnetic rays of short wavelengths and high energy. The physician who specializes in radiology, roentgen diagnosis, and roentgen therapy is called a *radiologist.* A *roentgenologist* is a physician who has specialized only in the use of x-rays for diagnosis and the treatment of disease.

CHARACTERISTICS OF X-RAYS

1. X-rays are an invisible form of radiant energy with short wavelengths traveling at 186,000 miles per second. They are able to penetrate different substances to varying degrees.
2. X-rays cause *ionization* of the substances through which they pass. Ionization is a process resulting in the gain or loss of one or more electrons in neutral atoms. The gain of an electron creates a negative electrical charge, whereas the loss of an electron results in a positively charged particle. These negatively or positively charged particles are called ions.
3. X-rays cause fluorescence of certain substances, thus allowing for the process known as *fluoroscopy* (Fig. 18–1). With this technique, internal structures show up as dark images on a glowing screen as x-rays pass through the area being

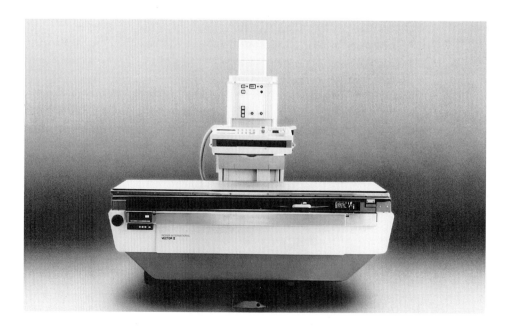

FIGURE 18–1

Vector II R/F table used for fluoroscopic examination of internal structures of the body. *(Courtesy of Picker International. Cleveland, OH.)*

examined. Fluoroscopy also allows the physician an opportunity to visualize internal structures that are in motion. It is also possible to make permanent records of the fluoroscopic examination for future study.

4. X-rays travel in a straight line, thus allowing the x-ray beam to be directed at a specific site during radiotherapy or to produce high-quality shadow images on film (radiographs).

5. X-rays are able to penetrate substances of different densities. In the body, x-rays pass through air in the lungs, fluids such as blood and lymph, and fat around muscles. Such substances are said to be *radiolucent*. Substances that obstruct the passage of radiant energy, in other words absorb radiant energy, such as calcium in bones, lead, or barium, are *radiopaque*. Control of the voltage and amperage applied to the x-ray tube, plus the duration of the exposure, allow images of body structures of varying densities. A contrast medium can be introduced into the body to enhance certain x-ray images. This characteristic allows x-rays to be used as a diagnostic tool.

6. X-rays can destroy body cells. Radiation can be used in the treatment of malignant tumors. In these cases, the x-ray voltage is administered by a radiotherapist using radiotherapy machines such as a linear accelerator or the betatron. Care must be exercised in the administration of radiotherapy, as x-rays can destroy healthy as well as abnormal tissue.

DANGERS AND SAFETY PRECAUTIONS

Because *x-rays* are invisible and produce no sound or smell, those working around and with them need to take certain precautions to avoid unnecessary exposure. Listed are some of the dangers known to be associated with x-rays and the safety precautions designed to prevent unnecessary exposure.

Prolonged Exposure

Prolonged and continued exposure to x-rays can cause damage to the gonads and/or depress the hematopoietic system, which can cause leukopenia and/or leukemia. Personnel involved with radiation therapy should spend the minimal amount of time necessary when caring for patients receiving internal radiation therapy. The farther away one is from the source of radiation, the less the degree of exposure.

Secondary Radiation

X-rays can scatter or be diverted from their normal straight paths when they strike radiopaque objects. This scatter or secondary radiation tends to add unwanted density to the image; therefore, a device known as a *grid* is positioned between the x-ray machine and the patient to absorb scatter before it reaches the x-ray film. The *Potter-Bucky diaphragm*, commonly known as the Bucky, is the most frequently used grid. It consists of alternating strips of lead and radiolucent material. The lead strips are arranged parallel to the stream of x-rays and are kept in motion by a mechanism to prevent them from becoming superimposed on the exposed film.

Safety Precautions

Not all scatter or secondary radiation is absorbed by a grid; therefore, those working in areas adjacent to x-ray equipment risk unintentional exposure from this source unless proper safety precautions are observed. Generally, these safety precautions include the five described below.

Film Badge.   A *film badge* is a device, usually pinned to the clothing, that is sensitive to ionizing radiation and monitors exposure to beta and gamma rays. A periodic analysis of the film badge reveals the amount of radiation the individual has received.

Lead Barrier.   Persons who operate x-ray machines do so from behind barriers equipped with a lead-treated window for viewing the patient.

Lead-lined Room.   X-ray equipment should be housed in an area featuring lead-lined walls, floors, and doors to prevent the escape of radiation from the room.

Protective Clothing.   Lead-lined gloves and aprons are worn by people who hold or position patients for x-ray examination, especially if they hold a patient, such as a child, while an x-ray is being taken.

Gonad Shield.   The reproductive organs are radiosensitive and must be protected by a lead shield while x-rays are being taken. X-rays can cause damage to the genetic material within the reproductive organs, which could lead to birth defects or cancer.

POSITIONS USED IN RADIOGRAPHY

Anteroposterior (AP) Position

In the *anteroposterior position,* the patient is placed with the anterior (front) part of the body facing the x-ray tube and the posterior (back) of the body facing the film. X-rays will pass through the body from the front to the back in reaching the film.

Posteroanterior (PA) Position

In the *posteroanterior position,* the patient is placed with the posterior (back) portion of the body facing the x-ray tube and the anterior (front) of the body facing the film. The x-rays will pass through the body from the back to the front to reach the film.

Lateral Position

In the *lateral position,* the x-ray beam passes from one side of the patient's body to the opposite side to reach the film. Placing the patient's right side next to the film and passing x-rays through the body from left to right is known as the right lateral position. Placing the patient's left side next to the film and passing x-rays through the body from right to left is known as the left lateral position.

Supine Position

In the *supine position,* the patient rests on the back, face upward, allowing the x-rays to pass through the body from the front to the back.

Prone Position

In the *prone position,* the patient is placed lying face down with the head turned to one side. The x-rays will pass from the back to the front side of the body.

Oblique Position

In the *oblique position,* the patient is placed so that the body or body part to be imaged is at an angle to the x-ray beam.

DIAGNOSTIC IMAGING

Diagnostic imaging involves the use of x-rays, ultrasound, radiopharmaceuticals, radiopaque media, and computers to provide the radiologist with images of internal body organs and processes. These images are used in identifying and locating tumors, fractures, hematomas, disease processes, and other abnormalities within the body. In recent years, advances in the field of electronics have produced a variety of computer-assisted x-ray machines to enhance the images obtained by the radiologist. These sophisticated machines now make possible noninvasive procedures for the visualization of organs and processes that were previously not accessible or that required exploratory surgical procedures for examination. Of the computer-assisted radiology equipment now in general use, the computed tomography (CT) scanner and the magnetic resonance imaging (MRI) machine offer the greatest range of diagnostic potential. A brief description of each of these diagnostic tools is given below.

Computed Tomography

When first introduced, *computed tomography* was hailed as the most significant advance in diagnostic medicine since the discovery of x-rays. It combines an advanced x-ray scanning system with a powerful minicomputer and vastly improved imaging quality while making it possible to view parts of the body and abnormalities not previously open to radiography. The CT scanner combines tomography, the process of imaging structures by focusing on a specific body plane and blurring all details from other planes, with a microprocessor that provides high-speed analysis of the tissue variances scanned (Figs. 18–2, 18–3, and 18–4).

Magnetic Resonance Imaging (MRI)

MRI is a technique that offers greater safety, as it does not use x-rays, while providing images and data on body structures such as the heart, large blood vessels, brain, and soft tissue. The MRI is a device that emits FM radiowaves of a certain frequency that are di-

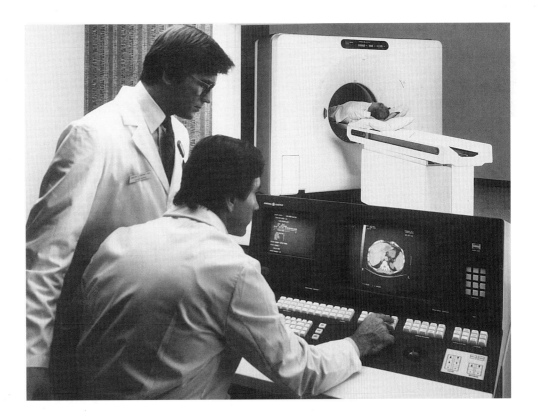

FIGURE 18–2

General Electric CT9800 computed tomography system, a computerized x-ray scanning system. *(Courtesy of General Electric Co., Medical Systems Group, Milwaukee, WI.)*

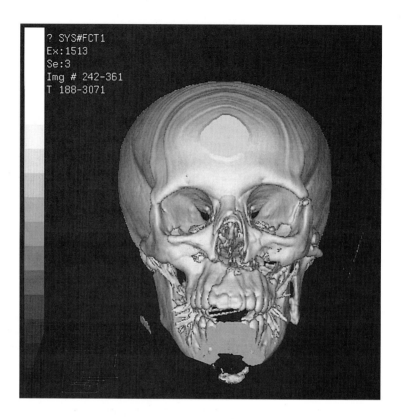

FIGURE 18–3

3D CT scan, multiple facial fractures. *(Courtesy of Teresa Resch.)*

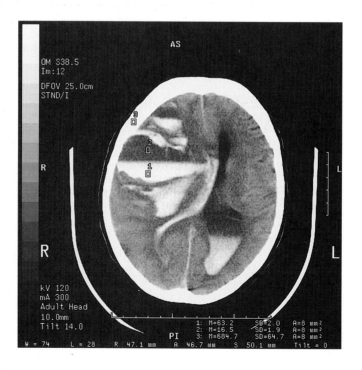

FIGURE 18–4

CT scan of head showing massive bleed with midline shift. *(Courtesy of Teresa Resch.)*

rected at a specific body area that is contained within a magnetic field. After the radiowaves are turned off, hydrogen nuclei in the patient emit weak radiowaves or microwaves that are analyzed by a computer and transformed into cross-sectional pictures (Fig. 18–5).

Ultrasound

Ultrasound literally means "beyond sound." It is sound whose frequency is beyond the range of human hearing. Ultrasound is widely used in diagnostic imaging for evaluation of a patient's internal organs. Its energy is transmitted into the patient and, because various internal organs and structures reflect and scatter sound differently, returning echoes can be used to form an image of a particular structure. These ultrasonic echoes are then recorded as a composite picture of the internal organ and/or structure.

Ultrasonography is the process of using ultrasound to produce a record of ultrasonic echoes as they strike tissues of different densities. The record produced by this process

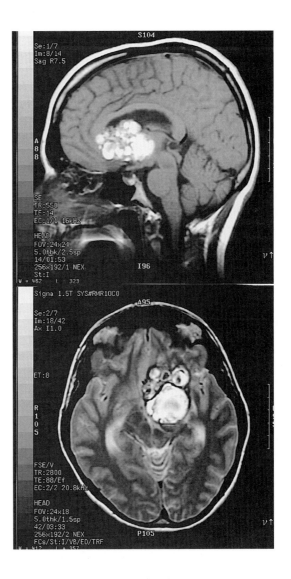

FIGURE 18–5

MRI head showing large hemorrhagic lesion. *(Courtesy of Teresa Resch.)*

is called a *sonogram* or *echogram*. An adaptation of ultrasound technology is *Doppler echocardiography*. It is a noninvasive technique for determining the blood flow velocity in different locations in the heart. This same technique can be used in determining the uterine artery blood flow velocity during pregnancy, as well as to determine the fetal heart rate.

Other Imaging Techniques

Other diagnostic imaging techniques being used include *thermography,* in which detailed images of body parts are developed from data showing the degree of heat and cold present in areas being studied, and *scintigraphy,* which involves the production of two-dimensional images of tissue areas from the scintillations emitted by a radiopharmaceutical, internally administered, that concentrates in a targeted site.

INTERVENTIONAL RADIOLOGY

Interventional radiology is a branch of medicine where certain diseases are treated non-operatively. An interventional radiologist (IR) uses radiologic imaging to guide catheters, balloons, stents, filters, and other tiny instruments through the body's vascular system and/or other systems. An *interventional radiologist* is a physician who has had special training in imaging and who specializes in treating diseases percutaneously.

The procedures and/or surgeries are performed in an interventional suite, generally on an outpatient basis. General anesthesia is usually not necessary, and conscious sedation and/or local anesthesia is more commonly used. These procedures are cost effective and are increasingly replacing traditional surgery.

SOME INTERVENTIONAL PROCEDURES	
Angiography	An x-ray exam of the arteries; a catheter is used to enter the artery and a contrast agent (radiopaque substance) is injected to make the artery visible on x-ray
Balloon Angioplasty	Opens blocked or narrowed blood vessels
Chemoembolization	Delivery of cancer-fighting agents directly to the tumor site
Embolization	Delivery of clotting agents directly to an area that is bleeding or to block blood flow to a problem area, such as a fibroid tumor
Fallopian Tube Catheterization	Opens blocked fallopian tubes, a cause of infertility in women
Needle Biopsy	Diagnostic test for breast or other cancers that is an alternative to surgical biopsy
Stent-graft	A procedure that reinforces a ruptured or ballooning section of an artery with a fabric-wrapped stent, a small cage-like tube to patch the vessel
Thrombolysis	Dissolves blood clots
Transjugular Intrahepatic Portosystemic Shunt (TIPS)	Improves blood flow for patients with severe liver dysfunction
Varicocele Occlusion	A treatment for varicose veins in the testicles, a cause of infertility in men
Vena Cava Filters	Prevent blood clots from reaching the heart

► NUCLEAR MEDICINE

Nuclear medicine uses atomic particles that emit electromagnetic radiation on disintegration. The radiant energy thus released is used for diagnostic, investigative, and therapeutic purposes. It may be administered externally from radiation machines such as the betatron and the linear accelerator or internally from small radionuclides implanted within the body near the site to be irradiated.

RADIATION THERAPY

The treatment of disease by the use of ionizing radiation may be called *radiotherapy, x-ray therapy, cobalt treatment,* or simply *radiation therapy.* In all cases, the aim of this treatment is to deliver a precise, calculated dose of radiation to diseased tissue, such as a tumor, while causing the least possible damage to surrounding normal tissue. *Radiation* can be defined as the process whereby energy is beamed from its source through space and matter to a selected target area. Substances that emit radiation are said to be radioactive. In radiation therapy, the radioactive substances used emit three types of rays: *alpha, beta,* and *gamma.*

Alpha Rays
Alpha rays are the least penetrating of the three types and can be absorbed by a thin sheet of material. They consist of *positively* charged helium particles released by atomic disintegration of radioactive material.

Beta Rays
Beta rays are able to penetrate body tissues for a few millimeters and consist of *negatively* charged electrons released when atoms of radioactive substances undergo disintegration.

Gamma Rays
Gamma rays are electromagnetic waves emitted by atoms of radioactive elements as they undergo disintegration. They are similar to x-rays but originate from the element's nucleus, whereas x-rays derive from the element's orbit. Gamma rays are without mass or electrical charge and have great penetrating power. They can pass through most substances, including the body, but are absorbed by lead.

RADIOTHERAPY AND CANCER

Malignant cells are more sensitive to radiation than are normal cells. They seem less able to repair themselves; therefore, *radiation* is frequently used in the treatment of patients with cancer, as either a *curative* or a *palliative* mode of therapy. Certain types of cancer cells can be destroyed by radiation therapy, thus preventing the unrestrained growth of such tumors. In other cancers, radiation has only a palliative effect, preventing cell growth, reducing pain, pressure, and bleeding, but not providing complete tumor destruction. Important factors that must be considered when determining the use of radiotherapy for the cancer patient include the following:

- The tumor must be surrounded by normal tissue that can tolerate the radiation and then repair itself.
- The tumor must not be widely spread. If the tumor has metastasized, radiation may be used as a palliative form of treatment.
- The tumor must be moderately sensitive to radiation (a radiosensitive tumor).

Radiotherapy is often the treatment of choice for cancers of the skin, uterus, cervix, or larynx or those located within the oral cavity. With other types of cancer, radiotherapy is frequently used in combination with other forms of treatment, including surgery and chemotherapy (Figs. 18–6 and 18–7).

TECHNIQUES OF RADIOTHERAPY

There are two methods for the administration of radiation: *external radiation therapy* (ERT) and *internal radiation therapy* (IRT). The following is an overview of these two methods.

External Radiation Therapy (ERT)

With the *ERT method,* the patient receives calculated doses of radiation from a machine located at some distance from the site of the tumor. The patient is carefully prepared for treatment by a radiation therapist, sometimes assisted by the *dosimetrist* or a radiation physicist. The precise size and location of the tumor are determined, and the *port,* or point of entry for the radiation, is marked using a dye or tattoo. In formulating the treatment plan, a computer is used to calculate the radiation dosage that will be needed to effect maximal destruction of malignant cells and minimal damage to surrounding normal tissue. Special lead blockers or shields may be constructed by a radiation physicist to protect surrounding normal tissue from the harmful effects of radiation.

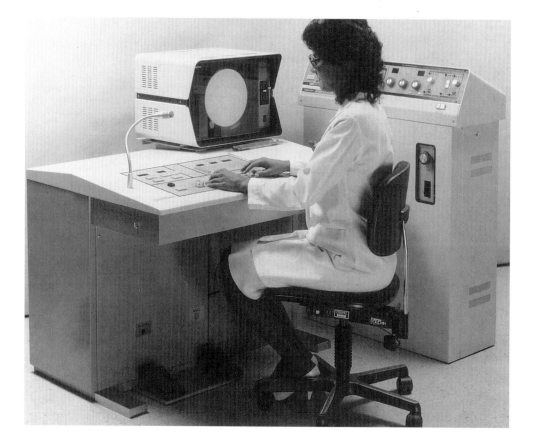

FIGURE 18–6

Toshiba diagnostic imaging system, LX-30A-AA-1. *(Courtesy of Toshiba Medical Systems, Tustin, CA.)*

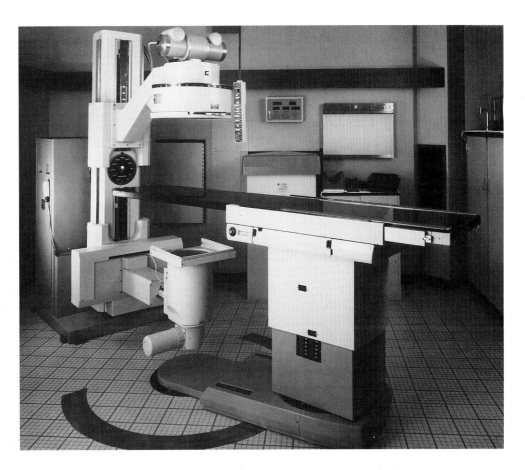

FIGURE 18–7

Toshiba diagnostic imaging system, LX-30A-AA-1. *(Courtesy of Toshiba Medical Systems, Tustin, CA.)*

Internal Radiation Therapy (IRT)

The *IRT method* of treatment can have two forms of administration known as *sealed* and *unsealed radiation therapy.* Sealed radiation therapy involves the implantation of sealed containers of radioactive material near the tumor site within the body. Unsealed radiation therapy involves the introduction of a liquid containing a radioactive substance into the patient through the mouth, via the bloodstream, or by instillation into a body cavity.

Sealed Radiation Therapy.   Radioactive material such as *radium, cesium-137, cobalt-60,* and *iridium-192* is sealed in small gold containers called seeds or within molds, plaques, needles, or other devices designed to hold the radioactive substance near the malignancy. In some cases, the radiation source may be implanted within the diseased tissue. In other cases, special devices or applicators have been designed to hold the implant in position for the desired period of treatment.

Unsealed Radiation Therapy.   *Radioactive iodine-131, radioactive phosphorus-32,* and *radioactive gold-198* are some of the substances used in the unsealed form of internal radiation therapy. *Phosphorus-32* may be intravenously administered for use in the treatment of leukemia or lymphoma. *Gold-198* and/or *phosphorus-32* may be placed in colloidal suspension and instilled in a body cavity for the palliative treatment of certain malignancies. *Iodine-131* may be orally administered, usually in conjunction with a thyroidectomy.

SIDE EFFECTS OF RADIATION

Because radiotherapy unavoidably affects normal tissue while destroying malignant cells, patients usually experience some unpleasant *side effects*. The degree of severity associated with the side effects will depend on the individual, the cancer, its location, and the amount of radiation. The following is a listing of some side effects that may occur as a result of radiation therapy:

1. Anorexia
2. Nausea
3. Vomiting
4. Diarrhea
5. Malaise
6. Mild erythema
7. Edema
8. Ulcers
9. Alopecia
10. Taste blindness
11. Stomatitis
12. Mucositis
13. Xerostomia

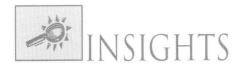

INSIGHTS

MAMMOGRAPHY

Mammography is the process of obtaining x-ray pictures of the breast. It is used as a screening tool for breast cancer and as a means to diagnose early breast cancer. It can detect a cancer the size of a grain of salt, 5 to 7 years before it can be detected by hand, and is also capable of detecting 85 to 90% of existing breast cancers. See Figures 18–8 and 18–9.

A mammogram is the actual x-ray record (film) of the breast. A mammographer is an individual who is responsible for taking the x-ray and a radiologist is an individual who is responsible for making an accurate assessment of the film. It is recommended that the mammographer and radiologist be specifically trained in mammography and breast evaluation and be certified by the American College of Radiology. To ensure quality performance, the x-ray machine, processor, screens, and cassettes must be state-of-the-art equipment and should be properly evaluated on a regular basis.

Screening Guidelines

The American Cancer Society and the National Cancer Institute endorse the following breast-cancer screening guidelines:

- Practice monthly breast self-examination (BSE).

- Between the ages 40 and 49, have your breasts examined by a health professional every year and get a mammogram every 1 or 2 years.

- After age 49, have a mammogram (along with a manual breast examination) every year.

Guidelines to Help You Prepare for a Mammogram

It is best to have a mammogram right after your menstrual cycle, as the breast will be less tender and less swollen. On the day of the test, do not use any deodorant, perfume, powders, oils, or ointments of any sort in the underarm area or on the breasts. These may cause shadows to appear on the mammogram.

Wear a skirt or slacks and a blouse that can be easily removed. You will have to remove all clothing from the waist up and put on a x-ray gown. Do not wear any jewelry around the neck.

If this is your first mammogram, ask your physician to explain the procedure of mammography to you before you go to the health care facility where you will have the mammogram. More knowledge about what is going to happen will generally lessen your fear and you will be better prepared for the procedure.

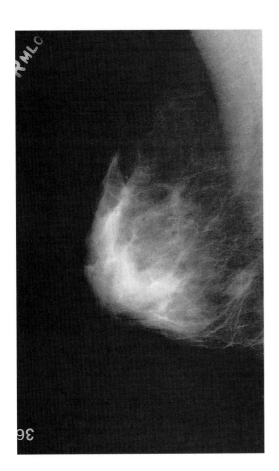

FIGURE 18–8

Normal mammogram. *(Courtesy of Teresa Resch.)*

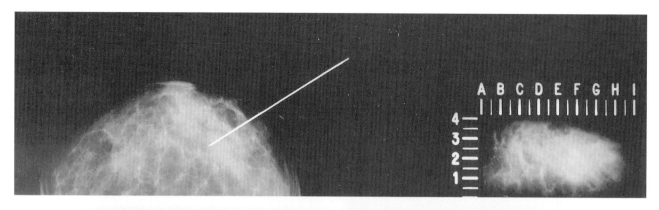

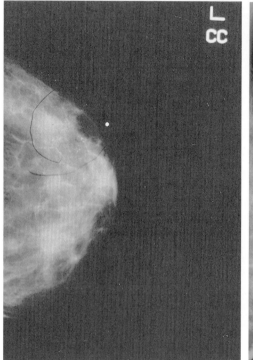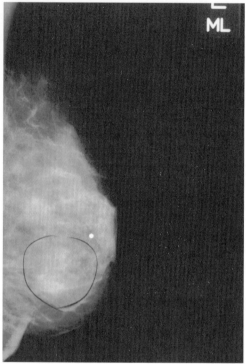

FIGURE 18–9

Mammogram showing cancer with microcalcifications. *(Courtesy of Teresa Resch.)*

The Procedure

Once you reach the x-ray suite, you will be taken to a dressing area, where you are given an x-ray gown and instructed to remove all clothing and jewelry from the waist up. You should put the gown on so that it opens in the front.

You will then be taken to a room where the mammographer explains the procedure. If possible you will stand and remove one breast and place it on the x-ray device. The mammographer will position you by lifting your breast to a 90 degree angle to the chest wall. Your breast will be pulled forward onto the film

holder, centrally with the nipple in profile. Your arm on the side being imaged should be relaxed and your shoulder is back out of the way. You will be asked to turn your head away from the side being imaged. Next, your breast will be compressed. Compression is used in combination with a specific shaped x-ray cone so that the more intense central portion of the x-ray beam penetrates the thicker base of the breast. You will be asked to take a deep breath and to hold it and to be still, while the mammographer goes behind a lead screen and takes the picture. Two images of each breast will be made, one from above and one from the side.

You will be asked to wait while the x-rays are being processed, and if the pictures are satisfactory, then you may dress and leave. A radiologist will read the x-rays and send your physician a report, and then your physician will notify you of the findings.

The Male Patient Having a Mammogram

Approximately 1000 men a year are diagnosed with breast cancer. When a male is scheduled for a mammogram, he is most embarrassed, as breast cancer is a female disease, and not a man's. The male breast generally does not contain as much adipose tissue as the female; therefore, it may be difficult to place the man's breast onto the film holder and obtain the proper amount of compression.

TERMINOLOGY

WITH SURGICAL PROCEDURES & PATHOLOGY

TERM	WORD PARTS			DEFINITION
angiocardiogram (ăn″ jĭ-ō-kăr′ dĭ-ō-grăm)	angio cardio gram	CF CF S	vessel heart record	An x-ray record of the heart and great vessels that is made visible through the use of a radiopaque contrast medium
angiogram (ăn′ jĭ-ō-grăm)	angio gram	CF S	vessel record	An x-ray record of the blood vessels made visible through the use of an injected radiopaque contrast medium
angiography (ăn″ jĭ-ŏg′ ră-fē)	angio graphy	CF S	vessel recording	The process of making an x-ray record of blood vessels
aortogram (ā-ōr′ tō-grăm)	aorto gram	CF S	aorta record	An x-ray record of the aorta that is made visible through the use of an injected radiopaque contrast medium
arteriography (ăr″ tē- rĭ-ŏg′ ră-fē)	arterio graphy	CF S	artery recording	The process of making an x-ray record of the arteries
arthrography (ăr-thrŏg′ ră-fē)	arthro graphy	CF S	joint recording	The process of making an x-ray record of a joint
brachytherapy (brăk″ ĭ thĕr′ ă-pē)	brachy therapy	P S	short treatment	Radiation therapy in which the radioactive substance is inserted into a body cavity or organ. The source of radiation is located a short distance from the body area being treated
bronchogram (brŏng′ kō-grăm)	broncho gram	CF S	bronchi record	An x-ray record of the bronchial tree that is made visible through the use of a radiopaque contrast medium
cholangiogram (kō-lăn′ jĭ-ō-grăm)	chol angio gram	R CF S	gall, bile vessel record	An x-ray record of the bile ducts that is made visible through the use of a radiopaque contrast medium
cholecystogram (kō″ lē- sĭs′ tō-grăm)	chole cysto gram	R CF S	gall bladder record	An x-ray record of the gallbladder that is made visible through the use of a radiopaque contrast medium

Terminology - continued

TERM	WORD PARTS			DEFINITION
cinematoradio-graphy (sĭn″ ĭ-măt″ ō-rā″ dĭ-ŏg′ ră-fē)	cinemato radio graphy	CF CF S	motion ray recording	The process of making an x-ray record of an organ in motion
cineradiography (sĭn″ ē- rā″ dē-ŏg′ ră-fē)	cine radio graphy	R CF S	motion ray recording	The process of making a motion picture record of successive x-ray images appearing on a fluoroscopic screen
cisternography (sĭs″ tĕr-nŏg′ ră-fē)	cisterno graphy	CF S	cistern recording	The process of making an x-ray record of the basal cistern of the brain
dosimetrist (dō-sĭm′ ĕt-rĭst)	dosi metr ist	CF R S	a giving to measure one who specializes	One who specializes in the planning and calculating of radiation dosage
echoencephalo-graphy (ĕk″ ō-ĕn-sĕf″ ă-lŏg′ ră-fē)	echo encephalo graphy	CF CF S	echo brain recording	The process of using ultrasound to determine the presence of a centrally located mass in the brain
echography (ĕk-ŏg′ ră-fē)	echo graphy	CF S	echo recording	The process of using ultrasound as a diagnostic tool. A record is made of the echo produced when sound waves are reflected back through tissues of different density
electrokymogram (ə-lĕk″ trō-kĭ′ mō-grăm)	electro kymo gram	CF CF S	electricity motion record	An x-ray record of the motion of the heart or other moving structures
fluoroscopy (floo-räs′ kə-pē)	fluoro scopy	CF S	fluorescence to view	The process of examining internal structures by viewing the shadows cast on a fluores-cent screen after the x-ray has passed through the body
holography (hŏl-ŏg′ ră-fē)	holo graphy	CF S	whole recording	The making of a picture in which the original object appears in three dimensions
hysterosalpingo-gram (hĭs″ tĕr-ō-săl-pĭn′ gō-grăm)	hystero salpingo gram	CF CF S	uterus fallopian tube record	An x-ray record of the uterus and fallopian tubes that is made visible through the use of a radiopaque contrast medium

continued

Terminology - continued

TERM	WORD PARTS			DEFINITION
intracavitary (ĭn″ tră-kăv′ ĭt-ă-rē)	intra cavit ary	P R S	within cavity pertaining to	Pertaining to within a cavity
intravenous pyelogram (ĭn″ tră-vē′ nŭs pī′ ĕ-lō-grăm)	intra ven ous pyelo gram	P R S CF S	within vein pertaining to renal pelvis record	An x-ray record of the kidney and renal pelvis that is made visible through the use of an injected radiopaque contrast medium
ionometer (ĭŏn′ ō-mē- tĕr)	iono meter	CF S	ion instrument to measure	An instrument used to measure the amount of radiation used by x-rays or radioactive substances
ionotherapy (ī″ŏn-ō-thĕr′ ă-pē)	iono therapy	CF S	ion treatment	Treatment by introducing ions into the body
iontoradiometer (ī-ŏn″ tō-rā″ dĭ-ŏm′ ĭ-tĕr)	ionto radio meter	CF CF S	ion ray instrument to measure	An instrument used to measure the amount and intensity of x-rays
kilovolt (kĭl′ ō-vōlt)	kilo volt	CF R	one thousand volt	1000 V
kilowatt (kĭl′ ō-wătt)	kilo watt	CF R	one thousand watt	1000 W
lymphangiogram (lĭm-făn″ jē- ō-grăm)	lymph angio gram	R CF S	lymph vessel record	An x-ray record of the lymph vessels that is made visible through the use of radiopaque contrast medium
lymphangio-graphy (lĭm-făn″ jē-ŏg′ ră-fē)	lymph angio graphy	R CF S	lymph vessel recording	The process of making an x-ray record of the lymph vessels
mammography (măm-ŏg′ ră-fē)	mammo graphy	CF S	breast recording	The process of obtaining pictures of the breast through the use of x-rays
milliampere (mĭl″ ĭ-ăm′ pēr)	milli ampere	P R	one-thousandth ampere	0.001 A
millicurie (mĭl″ ĭ-kū′ rē)	milli curie	P R	one-thousandth curie	0.001 Ci

Terminology - continued

TERM	WORD PARTS			DEFINITION
myelogram (mī′ ĕ-lō-grăm)	myelo gram	CF S	spinal cord record	An x-ray record of the spinal cord that is made visible through the use of a radiopaque contrast medium
oscilloscope (ŏ-sĭl′ ō-skōp)	oscillo scope	CF S	to swing instrument	An instrument used to record an electrical wave visually on a fluorescent screen of a cathode-ray tube
photofluorogram (fō″ tō-floo′ ĕr-ō-grăm)	photo fluro gram	CF CF S	light fluorescence record	An x-ray record of images seen during fluoroscopic examination
physicist (fĭz′ ĭ-sĭst)	physic ist	R S	nature one who specializes	One who specializes in the science of physics
radiation (rā-dĭ-ā′ shŭn)	radiat ion	R S	radiant process	The process whereby radiant energy is propagated through space or matter
radioactive (rā″ dĭ-ō-ăk′ tĭv)	radio act ive	CF R S	ray acting nature of	Characterized by emitting radiant energy
radiodermatitis (rā″ dĭ-ō-dur′ mă-tī′ tĭs)	radio dermat itis	CF R S	ray skin inflammation	Inflammation of the skin caused by exposure to x-rays or radioactive substances
radiodiagnosis (rā″ dĭ-ō-dī″ ăg-nō′ sĭs)	radio dia gnosis	CF P S	ray through knowledge	To determine a diagnosis through the use of x-rays
radiogenic (rā″ dĭ-ō-jĕn′ ĭk)	radio genic	CF S	ray formation, to produce	Caused or produced by radioactivity
radiograph (rā′ dĭ-ō-grăf)	radio graph	CF S	ray record	A picture produced on a sensitized film or plate by rays; *an x-ray record*
radiographer (rā″ dĭ-ŏg′ ră-fĕr)	radio graph er	CF S S	ray record one who	One who is skilled in making x-ray records
radiography (rā″ dĭ-ŏg′ ră-fē)	radio graphy	CF S	ray recording	The process of making an x-ray record

continued

Terminology - continued

TERM	WORD PARTS			DEFINITION
radiologist (rā″ dĭ-ŏl′ ō-jĭst	radio log ist	CF R S	ray study of one who specializes	One who specializes in radiology
radiology (rā″ dĭ-ŏl′ ō-jē)	radio logy	CF S	ray study of	The study of x-rays, radioactive substances, radioactive isotopes, and ionizing radiation
radiolucent (rā″ dĭ-ō-lū′ sĕnt)	radio lucent	CF R	ray to shine	Property of permitting the passage of radiant energy
radionecrosis (rā″ dĭ-ō-nē- krō′ sĭs)	radio necr osis	CF R S	ray death condition of	Death of tissue caused by exposure to radiant energy
radiopaque (rā″ dĭ-ō-pāk′)	radio paque	CF R	ray dark	Property of obstructing the passage of radiant energy
radioscopy (rā″ dĭ-ŏs′ kō-pē)	radio scopy	CF S	ray to view, examine	The process of viewing and examining the inner structures of the body through the process of x-rays
radiotherapy (rā″ dĭ-ō-thĕr′ ă-pē)	radio therapy	CF S	ray treatment	The treatment of disease by the use of x-rays, radium, and other radioactive substances
roentgenologist (rĕnt″ gĕn-ŏl′ ō-jĭst)	roent geno log ist	R CF R S	roentgen kind study of one who specializes	One who specializes in roentgen diagnosis, therapy, or both
roentgenology (rĕnt″ gĕn-ŏl′ ō-jē)	roent geno logy	R CF S	roentgen kind study of	The study of roentgen rays for diagnostic and therapeutic purposes
sialography (sī″ ă-lŏg′ ră-fē)	sialo graphy	CF S	salivary recording	The process of making an x-ray record of the salivary ducts and glands
sonogram (sōn′ ō-grăm)	sono gram	CF S	sound record	A record produced by ultrasonography
teletherapy (tĕl″ ĕ-thĕr′ ă-pē)	tele therapy	R S	distant treatment	Radiation therapy in which the radioactive substance is at a distance from the body area being treated

Terminology - continued

TERM	WORD PARTS			DEFINITION
thermography (thĕr-mŏg′ ră-fē)	thermo graphy	CF S	heat recording	The process of recording heat patterns of the body's surface; useful in the detection of cancer of the breast
tomography (tō-mŏg′ ră-fē)	tomo graphy	CF S	to cut recording	The process of cutting across and producing images of single tissue planes
ultrasonic (ŭl″ tră-sŏn′ ĭk)	ultra son ic	P R S	beyond sound pertaining to	Pertaining to sounds beyond 20,000 cycles/sec
ultrasonography (ŭl″ tră-sŏn-ŏg′ ră-fē)	ultra sono graphy	P CF S	beyond sound recording	The process of using ultrasound to produce a record of ultrasonic echoes as they strike tissues of different densities. See Figures 18–10 and 18–11.
venography (vē- nŏg′ ră-fē)	veno graphy	CF S	vein recording	The process of making an x-ray record of veins
xeroradiography (zē″ rō-rā″ dē-ŏg′ ră-fē)	xero radio graphy	CF CF S	dry ray recording	The process of making an x-ray record by a dry, totally photoelectric process

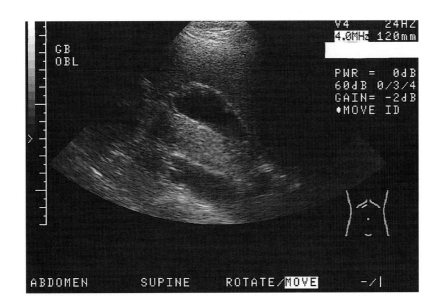

FIGURE 18–10

Ultrasound, abdomen supine. *(Courtesy of Teresa Resch.)*

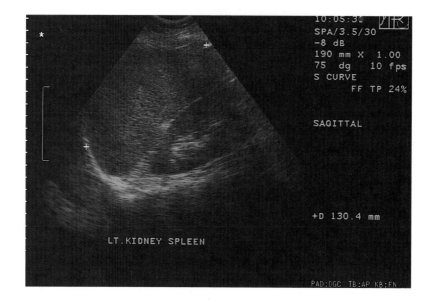

FIGURE 18–11

Ultrasound, left kidney and spleen. *(Courtesy of Teresa Resch.)*

 VOCABULARY WORDS

Vocabulary words are terms that have not been divided into component parts. They are common words or specialized terms associated with the subject of this chapter. These words are provided to enhance your medical vocabulary.

WORD	DEFINITION
alopecia (ăl″ ō-pē′ shĭ-ă)	Pertaining to hair loss
alpha ray (ăl′ fə rā)	A ray of positively charged particles of helium moving at a high speed. It is the least penetrating ray and is stopped by skin or a single sheet of paper.
ampere (ăm′ pēr)	The unit of strength of electricity
anion (ăn′ ī-ŏn)	An ion that carries a negative charge and is attracted to the positive pole *(anode)*
anode (ăn′ ōd)	The positive pole of an electrical current
anorexia (ăn″ ō-rĕks′ ĭ-ă)	A condition in which there is a loss of appetite

Vocabulary - continued

WORD	DEFINITION
aplastic anemia (ă-plăs′ tĭk ăn-nē′ mĭ-ă)	A type of anemia in which there is aplasia or destruction of the bone marrow; may be caused by chemotherapeutic agents, x-rays, or other sources of ionizing radiation
artifact (ăr′ tĭ-făkt)	An artificially produced structure or feature
atom (ăd-əm)	The smallest part of an element; consists of a nucleus that contains protons and neutrons and is surrounded by electrons
barium sulfate (bā′ rĭ-ŭm sŭl′ fāt)	A radiopaque barium compound used as a contrast medium in x-ray examination of the digestive tract
beam (bēm)	A ray of light; In radiology and nuclear medicine, a beam is radiant energy emitted by a group of atomic particles traveling a parallel course
beta ray (bā′ tă rā)	A ray of negatively charged electrons moving at a high speed. It penetrates only a few millimeters of body tissue.
betatron (bā′ tă-trŏn)	A megavoltage machine used in administering external radiation therapy
bombardment (bŏm-bărd′ mənt)	The process of irradiating an atom
cassette (kă-sĕt′)	A light-proof case or holder for x-ray film
cathode (kăth′ ōd)	The negative pole of an electrical current
cesium-137 (sĕ′ zĭ-ŭm)	A radionuclide that is the radioactive substance of choice for the treatment of cervical, uterine, and vaginal cancer
cobalt-60 (kō′ balt)	A radionuclide that serves as the radioactive substance in teletherapy machines. It is also used for implantation (interstitial) in the treatment of some malignancies.
collimator (kŏl″ ĭ-madər)	A device on an x-ray machine that makes rays parallel and not diffuse
cone (kōn)	An object on an x-ray or radiation machine that regulates the beam of radiant energy
contrast medium (kōn′ trăst mēd′ ĭ-ŭm)	A radiopaque substance used in certain x-ray procedures to permit visualization of organs or structures
curie (Ci) (kūr′ ē)	A unit of radioactivity

continued

Vocabulary - continued

WORD	DEFINITION
cyclotron (sī' klō-trŏn)	A megavoltage machine used in administering external radiation therapy
decontamination (dē" kŏn-tăm" ĭ-nā' shŭn)	The process of freeing an object, area, or person of some contaminating substance *(bacteria, poisonous gas, or radioactive substances)*
diaphanography (dĭ"ă-făn-ŏg' ră-fē)	The process of taking infrared photographs of the breast while a white light is being shone through the breast
digital subtraction angiography (dĭj' ĭ-tăl sŭb-trăk' shŭn ăn" jĭ-ŏg' ră-fē)	A method by which the computer performs instantaneous subtraction of the x-ray images, giving high-quality x-ray images of blood vessels with less x-ray dye
dose (dōs)	The amount of medication or radiation that is to be administered
electron (ē- lĕk' trŏn)	A charge or unit of negative electricity that revolves around the nucleus of an atom
enema (ĕn' ĕ-mă)	The process of introducing a substance or solution into the rectum and colon
energy (ĕn' ĕr-jē)	The power or capacity to do work
external radiation (ĕk-stur' năl rā-dĭ-ā' shŭn)	The process of administering radiation to the patient via a radiation machine that is located outside the body
film (film)	A thin, cellulose-coated, light-sensitive sheet or slip of material used in taking pictures
film badge (film badj)	A device that is sensitive to ionizing radiation. It is worn by one who is around x-rays to monitor the degree of exposure to beta and gamma rays.
fluorescence (floo" ō-rĕs' ĕnts)	The property of certain substances to emit light as a result of exposure to and absorption of radiant energy
fractionation (frăk" shŭn-ā' shŭn)	The process of delivering a fraction or portion of a dose of radiation over time to minimize untoward radiation effects on normal tissue
gamma ray (găm' ăh rā)	An electromagnetic wave without mass or electrical charge. It is the most penetrating ray and can pass through the whole body. It can be stopped by lead.
Geiger counter (gī' gĕr kown' tĕr)	An instrument used to detect, measure, and record ionizing radiation; also called a Geiger-Müler counter

Vocabulary - continued

WORD	DEFINITION
half-life (haf′ līf)	The time required for half of the radioactivity of a substance to be reduced by radioactive decay
implant (ĭm-plănt′)	To place within a body cavity or organ; also means to transfer, to graft, or to insert
in vitro (ĭn vē′ trō)	Within a glass
ion (ī-ən)	An atomic particle consisting of an atom or a group of atoms that carry an electrical charge, either negative or positive
ionization (ī″ŏn-ĭ-zā′ shŭn)	The process of breaking up molecules into their component parts
ionizing radiation (ī′ŏn-ī-zĭng rā″ dĭ-ā′ shŭn)	A powerful invisible energy capable of producing ions
iridium-192 (ī-rĭd′ ĭ-ŭm)	A radionuclide used to deliver sealed dosages by internal radiotherapy to certain malignancies
irradiation (i-rā″ dē- ā′ shŭn)	A process of using x-rays, radium rays, ultraviolet rays, gamma rays, or infrared rays in the diagnosis or therapeutic treatment of a patient
isotope (ī′ sō-tōp)	One of a series of nuclides that are chemically identical yet differ in atomic weight and electrical charge. Radioactive isotopes are composed of unstable atoms, and most are artificially produced. Example: cobalt-60 is a radioactive isotope artificially produced from naturally occurring cobalt-59.
lead (lĕd)	A metallic chemical element
linear accelerator (lĭn′ ē-ar ăk-sĕl′ ĕr-ā″ tŏr)	A megavoltage machine used in administering external radiation therapy
megavoltage (mĕg′ ă-vōl″ tĭj)	Pertains to 1,000,000 V
neutron (nū′ trŏn)	An electrically uncharged particle existing in the nuclei of atoms
magnetic resonance imaging (MRI) (măg-nĕt′ ĭk rĕz′ ŏ-năns)	A technique that uses radiowaves and a magnet. A device emits FM radiowaves of a certain frequency that are directed at a specific body area contained within an external magnetic field. After the radiowaves are turned off, hydrogen nuclei in the patient emit weak radiowaves or microwaves that are analyzed by a computer and transformed into cross-sectional pictures.

continued

Vocabulary - continued

WORD	DEFINITION
orthovoltage (or″ thō-vōl′ tĭj)	Pertains to a voltage range of 140 to 400 kV. In radiation therapy, it is used in administering low-energy radiation for palliative treatment of cancer
port (pôrt)	In radiation therapy, refers to the skin area of entry for the radiation
proton (prō′ tŏn)	An electrically positive-charged particle existing in the nuclei of atoms
rad (răd)	Refers to the amount of radiation absorbed. The letters stand for **r**adiation **a**bsorbed **d**ose.
radionuclide (rā″ dĭ-ō-nū′ klĭd)	A radioactive species of an atomic nucleus identified by its atomic number, mass, and energy state
radiotherapist (rā″ dĭ-ō-thĕr′ ă-pĭst)	One who specializes in the use of radiant energy for therapeutic purposes
radium (rā′ dĭ-ŭm)	A radioactive isotope used in the treatment of certain malignant diseases
roentgen (R) (rĕnt′ gĕn)	The international unit for describing exposure dose of x-ray or γ-radiation
scan (skăn)	A process of using a moving device or a sweeping beam of radiation to produce images of organs or structures of the body. See Figure 18–12.
shield (shĕld)	A protective structure used to prevent or reduce the passage of particles or radiation
tagging (tag′ ing)	The process of tracing a radioactive isotope that has become involved in metabolic or chemical actions
volt (V) (vōlt)	The electromotive force or unit of pressure for the flow of electricity
watt (W) (wătt)	The unit of electrical power. One watt is equal to a current of 1 A under 1 V of pressure.
x-ray (x′ rā)	An electromagnetic wave of high energy produced by the collision of a beam of electrons with a target in a vacuum tube (x-ray tube)

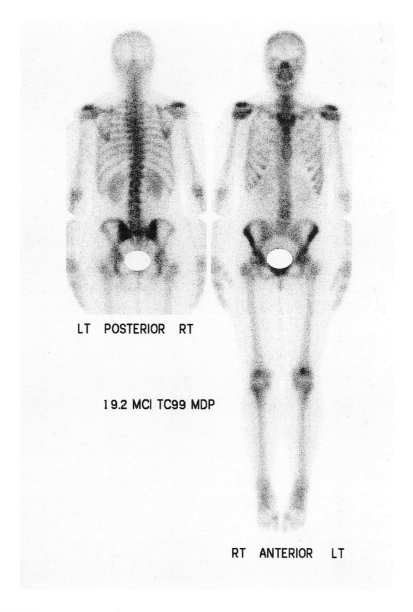

LT   POSTERIOR   RT

1 9.2 MCI TC99 MDP

RT   ANTERIOR   LT

FIGURE 18–12

Nuclear medicine bone scan. *(Courtesy of Teresa Resch.)*

ABBREVIATIONS

AP	anteroposterior	**mAs**	milliampere second
Ba	barium	**mCi**	millicurie
BE	barium enema	**MRI**	magnetic resonance imaging
Ci	curie	**Ra**	radium
CT	computed tomography	**rad**	radiation absorbed dose
ERT	external radiation therapy	**PA**	posteroanterior
IR	interventional radiologist	**PET**	positron emission tomography
IRT	internal radiation therapy	**SBFT**	small-bowel follow-through
kV	kilovolt	**TIPS**	transjugular intrahepatic
kW	kilowatt		portosystemic shunt
lat	lateral	**US**	ultrasound
mA	milliampere		

COMMUNICATION ENRICHMENT

This segment is provided for those who wish to enhance their ability to communicate in either English or Spanish.

▶ Related Terms

English	Spanish	English	Spanish
x-ray	radiografia (rā-dē- ō-grǎ-fē- ǎ)	dark	oscuro (ō s-*cŭ*-rō)
record	registro (rě-*hĭs*-trō)	treatment	tratamiento (trǎ-tǎ-mǐ-*ěn*-tō)
motion	mocion (mō-sǐ-*ō n*)	ampere	amperio (ǎm-*pě*-rǐ-ō)
electricity	electricidad (ě-lěc-*trǐ*-cǐ-dǎd)	atomic	atomico (ǎ-*tō*-mǐ-cō)
measure	medida (mě-*dǐ*-dǎ)	cassette	cartucho (cǎr-*tŭ*-chō)
light	ligero; luz (lǐ-*hě*-rō ; lŭz)	cone	cono (*cō*-nō)
radiant	radiante (rǎ-dǐ-*ǎn*-tě)	curie	curie (cǔ-*rě*)

English	Spanish	English	Spanish
dose	dosis (*dō*-sĭs)	lead	plomo (*plō*-mō)
electron	electrón (ĕ-*lĕc*-trōn)	scan	hojear (ō-hĕ-*ăr*)
energy	energia (ĕ-nĕr-*hĭ*-ă)	shield	escudo (ĕs-*cŭ*-dō)
implant	implantar (ĭm-plăn-*tăr*)		

STUDY AND REVIEW SECTION

LEARNING EXERCISES

▶ **An Overview of Radiology and Nuclear Medicine**

Write your answers to the following questions. Do not refer back to the text.

1. Define radiology. _____

    _____

2. Name three characteristics of x-rays.

    a. _____ b. _____

    c. _____

3. Name two dangers of x-rays.

    a. _____ b. _____

4. List five safety precautions designed to prevent unnecessary exposure to x-rays.

    a. _____ b. _____

    c. _____ d. _____

    e. _____

5. Name four diagnostic tools used in diagnostic radiology.

    a. _____ b. _____

    c. _____ d. _____

6. Define radiation therapy. _____

    _____

▶ Word Parts

1. In the spaces provided, write the definition of these prefixes, roots, combining forms, and suffixes. Do not refer to the listings of terminology words. Leave blank those terms you cannot define.

2. After completing as many as you can, refer back to the terminology word listings to check your work. For each word missed or left blank, write the term and its definition several times on the margins of these pages or on a separate sheet of paper.

3. To maximize the learning process, it is to your advantage to do the following exercises as directed. To refer to the terminology listings before completing these exercises invalidates the learning process.

Prefixes

Give the definitions of the following prefixes:

1. brachy- _____   2. dia- _____

3. intra- _____   4. milli- _____

5. ultra- _____

Roots and Combining Forms

Give the definitions of the following roots and combining forms:

1. act _____   2. ampere _____

3. angio _____   4. aorto _____

5. arterio _____   6. arthro _____

7. broncho _____   8. cardio _____

9. cavit _____   10. chol _____

11. chole _____   12. cine _____

13. cinemato _____   14. cisterno _____

15. curie _____   16. cysto _____

17. dermat _____   18. dosi _____

19. echo _____   20. electro _____

21. encephalo _____   22. fluoro _____

23. geno _____   24. holo _____

25. hystero _____   26. iono _____

27. ionto _____   28. kilo _____

29. kymo _____   30. log _____

31. lucent _____   32. lymph _____

33. mammo _____   34. metr _____

35. myelo _____   36. necr _____

37. oscillo _____   38. paque _____

39. photo _____   40. physic _____

41. pyelo _____   42. radiat _____

43. radio _____   44. roent _____

45. salpingo _____   46. sialo _____

47. son _____   48. sono _____

49. tele _____   50. thermo _____

51. tomo _____   52. ven _____

53. veno _____   54. volt _____

55. watt _____   56. xero _____

Suffixes

Give the definitions of the following suffixes:

1. -ary _____   2. -er _____

3. -genic _____   4. -gnosis _____

5. -gram _____   6. -graph _____

7. -graphy _____   8. -ic _____

9. -ion _____   10. -ist _____

11. -itis _____   12. -ive _____

13. -logy _____   14. -meter _____

15. -osis _____   16. -ous _____

17. -scope _____   18. -scopy _____

19. -therapy _____

▶ Identifying Medical Terms

In the spaces provided, write the medical terms for the following meanings:

1. _____ The process of making an x-ray record of blood vessels

2. _____ The process of making an x-ray record of a joint

3. _____ An x-ray record of the gallbladder that is made visible through the use of a radiopaque contrast medium

4. _____ The process of making an x-ray record of the basal cistern of the brain

5. _____ One who specializes in the planning and calculating of radiation dosage

6. _____ The making of a picture in which the original object appears in three dimensions

7. _____ Pertaining to within a cavity

8. _____ Treatment by introducing ions into the body

9. _____ 1000 V

10. _____ 1000 W

11. _____ The process of obtaining pictures of the breast through the use of x-rays

12. _____ 0.001 Ci

13. _____ One who specializes in the science of physics

14. _____ The process whereby radiant energy is propagated through space or matter

15. _____ Caused or produced by radioactivity

16. _____ One who is skilled in making x-ray records

17. _____ Property of permitting the passage of radiant energy

18. _____ Property of obstructing the passage of radiant energy

19. _____ One who specializes in roentgen diagnosis, therapy, or both

20. _____ A record produced by ultrasonography

▶ **Spelling**

In the spaces provided, write the correct spelling of these misspelled terms:

1. hystersalpingram _____
2. echgraphy _____
3. lymphangogography _____
4. myleogram _____
5. tovl _____
6. radiactive _____
7. radigraphy _____
8. silography _____
9. tomgraphy _____
10. vengraphy _____

WORD PARTS STUDY SHEET

Word Parts	Give the Meaning
brady-	_____
dia-	_____
intra-	_____
milli-	_____
ultra-	_____
act-	_____
ampere-	_____
cavit-	_____
cine-, cinemato-	_____
cisterno-	_____
curie-	_____
dosi-	_____
echo-	_____
electro-	_____
fluoro-	_____
holo-	_____
iono-, ionto-	_____
kymo-	_____
lucent-	_____

mammo-   _____

metr-   _____

oscillo-   _____

paque-   _____

photo-   _____

physic-   _____

radiat-   _____

radio-   _____

roent-   _____

son-   _____

tele-   _____

thermo-   _____

volt-   _____

watt-   _____

-gram   _____

-graph   _____

-graphy   _____

-meter   _____

-scope   _____

-scopy   _____

-therapy   _____

REVIEW QUESTIONS

▶ Matching

Select the appropriate lettered meaning for each numbered line.

_____ 1. alopecia   a. A protective structure used to prevent or reduce
                               the passage of particles or radiation

_____ 2. anorexia   b. A radioactive isotope used in the treatment of
                               certain malignant diseases

_____ 3. beam   c. A ray of light

                            d. Loss of hair

_____ 4. cassette

_____ 5. energy

_____ 6. lead

_____ 7. radium

_____ 8. scan

_____ 9. shield

_____ 10. tagging

e. Loss of appetite

f. Loss of energy

g. A light-proof case or holder for x-ray film

h. The process of tracing a radioactive isotope that has become involved in metabolic or chemical reactions

i. A process of using a moving device or a sweeping beam of radiation to produce images of organs or structures of the body

j. The power or capacity to do work

k. A metallic chemical element

▶ ## Abbreviations

Place the correct word, phrase, or abbreviation in the space provided.

1. anteroposterior _____

2. barium _____

3. computed tomography _____

4. kV _____

5. lat _____

6. Ra _____

7. magnetic resonance imaging _____

8. PA _____

9. curie _____

10. PET _____

ANSWER KEY

▶ CHAPTER 1

WORD PARTS

Prefixes

1. without
2. away from
3. against
4. self
5. bad
6. a hundred
7. through
8. different
9. bad
10. small
11. one thousandth
12. many, much
13. new
14. beside
15. before
16. together
17. three

Roots and Combining Forms

1. stuck to
2. armpit
3. center
4. chemical
5. a shaping
6. formation, produce
7. a thousand
8. large
9. death
10. law
11. rule
12. tumor
13. organ
14. fever
15. heat, fire
16. ray
17. to examine
18. putrefaction
19. hot, heat
20. place
21. cough

Suffixes

1. related to
2. pertaining to
3. pertaining to
4. surgical puncture
5. a key
6. a course
7. shape
8. to flee
9. formation, produce
10. knowledge
11. a step
12. a weight
13. recording
14. condition
15. pertaining to
16. process
17. condition of
18. nature of, quality of
19. liter
20. study of
21. instrument to measure
22. condition of
23. pertaining to
24. disease
25. to carry
26. instrument
27. decay
28. treatment
29. heat
30. condition

IDENTIFYING MEDICAL TERMS

1. adhesion
2. asepsis
3. axillary
4. chemotherapy
5. heterogeneous
6. malformation
7. microscope
8. multiform
9. neopathy
10. oncology

SPELLING

1. antiseptic
2. autonomy
3. centimeter
4. diaphoresis
5. milligram
6. necrosis
7. paracentesis
8. radiology

MATCHING

1. f	6. k
2. d	7. b
3. j	8. i
4. g	9. c
5. a	10. e

ABBREVIATIONS

1. abnormal
2. axillary
3. Bx
4. cardiovascular disease
5. diagnosis-related groups
6. ENT
7. FP
8. g, gm
9. gynecology
10. pediatrics

▶ CHAPTER 2

ANATOMY AND PHYSIOLOGY

1. body . . . cells . . . sustain
2. cell membrane
3. protoplasm . . . cytoplasm . . . karyoplasm
4. karyoplasm
5. cell reproduction . . . . control over activity within the cell's cyto-plasm
6. a. protection
   b. absorption
   c. secretion
   d. excretion
7. connective
8. a. striated (voluntary)
   b. cardiac
   c. smooth (involuntary)
9. excitability . . . conductivity
10. A tissue serving a common purpose
11. A group of organs function-ing together for a common purpose
12. a. integumentary
    b. skeletal
    c. muscular
    d. digestive
    e. cardiovascular
    f. blood and lymphatic
    g. respiratory
    h. urinary
    i. endocrine
    j. nervous
    k. reproductive

13. a. above, in an upward direction
    b. in front of, before
    c. toward the back
    d. toward the head
    e. nearest the middle
    f. to the side
    g. nearest the point of attachment
    h. away from the point of attachment
    i. the front side
    j. the back side
14. midsagittal plane
15. transverse or horizontal
16. coronal or frontal
17. a. thoracic   b. abdominal
    c. pelvic
18. a. cranial   b. spinal

WORD PARTS

Prefixes

1. both
2. up
3. two
4. color
5. down, away from
6. apart
7. outside
8. within
9. similar, same
10. middle
11. through
12. first
13. one

Roots and Combining Forms

1. fat
2. man
3. life
4. tail
5. cell
6. cell
7. to pour
8. formation, produce
9. tissue
10. water
11. cell's nucleus
12. side
13. disease
14. nature

15. to drink
16. body
17. place
18. a turning
19. body organs

Suffixes

1. pertaining to
2. use, action
3. formation, produce
4. pertaining to
5. process
6. study of
7. form, shape
8. resemble
9. like
10. condition of
11. pertaining to
12. a thing formed, plasma
13. body
14. control, stopping
15. incision

IDENTIFYING MEDICAL TERMS

1. adroid
2. bilateral
3. cytology
4. ectomorph
5. karyogenesis
6. somatotrophic
7. unilateral

SPELLING

1. adipose
2. caudal
3. cytology
4. diffusion
5. histology
6. mesomorph
7. perfusion
8. pinocytosis
9. somatotrophic
10. unilateral

MATCHING

1. c   6. i
2. d   7. g
3. e   8. h
4. f   9. j
5. a   10. b

ABBREVIATIONS

1. abd
2. anatomy and physiology
3. central nervous system
4. CV
5. GI
6. lateral
7. respiratory
8. endoplasmic reticulum
9. anterior–posterior
10. posterior–anterior

▶ CHAPTER 3

ANATOMY AND PHYSIOLOGY

1. The skin
2. a. hair
   b. nails
   c. sebaceous glands
   d. sweat glands
3. a. protection
   b. regulation
   c. sensory reception
   d. secretion
4. epidermis . . . dermis
5. a. stratum corneum
   b. stratum lucidum
   c. stratum granulosum
   d. stratum germinativum
6. Keratin
7. Melanin
8. dermis
9. a. papillary layer
   b. reticular layer
10. lunula

WORD PARTS

Prefixes

1. without, lack of
2. self
3. out
4. upon
5. out
6. excessive
7. under
8. within
9. around
10. below

Roots and Combining Forms

1. a thorn
2. ray
3. gland
4. white
5. cancer
6. heat
7. juice
8. corium
9. skin
10. skin
11. skin
12. skin
13. skin
14. skin
15. red
16. red
17. sweat
18. jaundice
19. tumor
20. horn
21. white
22. study of
23. black
24. black
25. fungus
26. nail
27. nail
28. nail
29. thick
30. a louse
31. wrinkle
32. wrinkle
33. hard
34. oil
35. old
36. hot, heat
37. hair
38. hair
39. nail
40. yellow
41. dry

Suffixes

1. pertaining to
2. pain
3. immature cell, germ cell
4. injection
5. skin
6. excision
7. sensation
8. pencil
9. condition
10. pertaining to
11. process
12. condition of
13. one who specializes
14. inflammation
15. study of
16. softening
17. resemble
18. tumor
19. condition of
20. pertaining to
21. disease
22. skin
23. to eat
24. surgical repair
25. flow, discharge
26. instrument to cut
27. tissue

IDENTIFYING MEDICAL TERMS

1. actinic dermatitis
2. cutaneous
3. dermatitis
4. dermatology
5. dermatopathy
6. hyperhidrosis
7. hypodermic
8. icteric
9. onychectomy
10. pachyderma
11. thermanesthesia
12. xanthoderma

SPELLING

1. causalgia
2. dermomycosis
3. ecchymosis
4. erysipelas
5. hypodermoclysis
6. melanoma
7. onychophagia
8. rhytidectomy
9. scleroderma
10 seborrhea

MATCHING

1. d	4. h
2. f	5. j
3. e	6. i

7. b   9. a
8. g   10. c

ABBREVIATIONS

1. FUO
2. TTS
3. hypodermic
4. I & D
5. SG
6. intradermal
7. T
8. UV
9. foreign body
10. psoralen-ultraviolet light

DIAGNOSTIC AND LABORATORY TESTS

1. c
2. d
3. a
4. b
5. a

► CHAPTER 4

ANATOMY AND PHYSIOLOGY

1. 206
2. a. axial   b. appendicular
3. a. flat . . . ribs, scapula, parts of the pelvic girdle, bones of the skull
   b. long . . . tibia, femur, humerus, radius
   c. short . . . carpal, tarsal
   d. irregular . . . vertebrae, ossicles of the ear
   e. sesamoid . . . patella
4. a. shape, support
   b. protection
   c. storage
   d. formation of blood cells
   e. attachment of skeletal muscles
   f. movement, through articulation

5. a. the ends of a developing bone
   b. the shaft of a long bone
   c. the membrane that forms the covering of bones, except at their articular surfaces
   d. the dense, hard layer of bone tissue
   e. a narrow space or cavity throughout the length of the diaphysis
   f. a tough connective tissue membrane lining the medullary canal and containing the bone marrow
   g. the reticular tissue that makes up most of the volume of bone
6. Numbers of the matching answers:
   a. 6   h. 14
   b. 11   i. 1
   c. 4   j. 12
   d. 13   k. 2
   e. 8   l. 3
   f. 10   m. 7
   g. 9   n. 5
7. a. synarthrosis
   b. amphiarthrosis
   c. diarthrosis
8. Abduction
9. the process of moving a body part toward the midline
10. Circumduction
11. the process of bending a body part backward
12. Eversion
13. the process of straightening a flexed limb
14. Flexion
15. the process of turning inward
16. Pronation
17. the process of moving a body part forward
18. Retraction
19. the process of moving a body part around a central axis
20. Supination

WORD PARTS

Prefixes

1. without
2. upon, above
3. water
4. between
5. beyond
6. around
7. many, much
8. under, beneath
9. together
10. together

Roots and Combing Forms

1. vinegar cup
2. achilles, heel
3. extremity, point
4. extremity
5. stiffening, crooked
6. joint
7. joint
8. a pouch
9. heel bone
10. heel bone
11. cancer
12. wrist
13. wrist
14. cartilage
15. cartilage
16. little key
17. clavicle
18. tail bone
19. tail bone
20. glue
21. knuckle
22. to bind together
23. rib
24. rib
25. hip
26. hip
27. skull
28. skull
29. finger or toe
30. finger or toe
31. femur
32. fibrous
33. fibula
34. curve
35. humerus
36. ilium
37. ilium

38. ischium
39. a hum
40. lamina (thin plate)
41. bending
42. loin
43. loin
44. lower jawbone
45. jawbone
46. jaw
47. marrow
48. marrow
49. death
50. elbow
51. bone
52. kneecap
53. kneecap
54. disease
55. foot
56. closely knit row
57. a passage
58. pus
59. spine
60. spine
61. radius
62. sacrum
63. flesh
64. shoulder blade
65. hardening
66. curvature
67. curvature
68. spine
69. vertebra
70. sternum
71. sternum
72. tendon
73. tendon
74. tibia
75. elbow
76. elbow
77. vertebra
78. vertebra
79. sword

Suffixes

1. pertaining to
2. pertaining to
3. pain
4. pertaining to
5. pertaining to
6. immature cell, germ cell
7. surgical puncture
8. a breaking
9. binding
10. pain
11. excision
12. swelling
13. formation, produce
14. formation, produce
15. mark, record
16. to write
17. pertaining to
18. inflammation
19. nature of
20. study of
21. softening
22. enlargement, large
23. resemble
24. tumor
25. shoulder
26. condition of
27. disease
28. lack of
29. fixation
30. growth
31. formation
32. surgical repair
33. formation
34. drooping
35. to burst forth
36. suture
37. rupture
38. instrument to cut
39. incision
40. tension

IDENTIFYING MEDICAL TERMS

1. acroarthritis
2. ankylosis
3. arthrectomy
4. arthritis
5. arthropathy
6. calcaneal
7. carpoptosis
8. chondral
9. chondropathology
10. coccygodynia
11. costal
12. craniectomy
13. dactylic
14. hydrarthrosis
15. intercostal
16. ischialgia; coxalgia
17. lumbar
18. myeloma
19. osteoarthritis
20. osteodynia
21. osteomyelitis or myelitis
22. osteopenia
23. pedal
24. sternalgia
25. xiphoid

SPELLING

1. acromion
2. arthredema
3. bursitis
4. chrondroblast
5. connective
6. cranioplasty
7. dactylomegaly
8. ischial
9. myelitis
10. osteochondritis
11. osteonecrosis
12. patellar
13. phalangeal
14. rachigraph
15. scoliosis
16. spondylitis
17. symphysis
18. tenonitis
19. ulnocarpal
20. vertebral

MATCHING

1. i   6. h
2. j   7. g
3. e   8. a
4. c   9. d
5. b   10. f

ABBREVIATIONS

1. CDH
2. DJD
3. long leg cast
4. osteoarthritis
5. PEMFs
6. rheumatoid arthritis
7. SPECT
8. thoracic vertebra, first
9. temporomandibular joint
10. Tx

DIAGNOSTIC AND LABORATORY TESTS

1. c
2. d
3. c
4. b
5. b

▶ CHAPTER 5

ANATOMY AND PHYSIOLOGY

1. a. skeletal   b. smooth
   c. cardiac
2. 42
3. a. nutrition   b. oxygen
4. a. origin   b. insertion
5. voluntary or striated
6. aponeurosis
7. a. body   b. origin
   c. insertion
8. a. A muscle that counteracts the action of another muscle.
   b. A muscle that is primary in a given movement.
   c. A muscle that acts with another muscle to produce movement.
9. involuntary, visceral, or unstriated
10. a. digestive tract
    b. respiratory tract
    c. urinary tract
    d. eye
    e. skin
11. Cardiac
12. a. movement
    b. maintain posture
    c. produce heat

WORD PARTS

Prefixes

1. lack of
2. away from
3. toward
4. against
5. separation
6. two
7. slow
8. with
9. through
10. difficult
11. into
12. within
13. many
14. four
15. with, together
16. three

Roots and Combining Forms

1. agony
2. arm
3. clavicle
4. turmoil
5. neck
6. finger or toe
7. to lead
8. work
9. a band
10. a band
11. a band
12. fiber
13. fiber
14. equal
15. a rind
16. lifter
17. bending
18. breast
19. black
20. to measure
21. muscle
22. muscle
23. muscle
24. muscle
25. nerve
26. nerve
27. disease
28. to loosen
29. rod
30. to turn
31. flesh
32. flesh
33. hardening
34. to gain
35. convulsive
36. sternum
37. tendon
38. tendon
39. tone, tension
40. twisted
41. to draw
42. will

Suffixes

1. pain
2. pertaining to
3. pertaining to
4. weakness
5. immature cell, germ cell
6. head
7. binding
8. pain
9. excision
10. formation, produce
11. to write, record
12. condition
13. pertaining to
14. process
15. agent
16. inflammation
17. condition
18. motion
19. motion
20. study of
21. destruction
22. softening
23. resemble
24. tumor
25. a doer
26. condition of
27. weakness
28. disease
29. a fence
30. surgical repair
31. stroke, paralysis
32. suture
33. rupture
34. tension, spasm
35. order
36. instrument to cut
37. incision
38. nourishment, development
39. pertaining to

IDENTIFYING MEDICAL TERMS

1. aponeurorrhaphy
2. atonic
3. bradykinesia
4. dactylospasm
5. dystrophy
6. fascioplasty

7. intramuscular
8. levator
9. myasthenia
10. myogenesis
11. myology
12. myoparesis
13. myoplasty
14. myosarcoma
15. myotenositis
16. myotomy
17. neuromyositis
18. polyplegia
19. tenodesis
20. synergetic
21. triceps

SPELLING

1. fascia
2. myokinesis
3. polymyoclonus
4. rhabdomyoma
5. sarcolemma
6. sternocleidomastoid
7. tenotomy
8. torticollis

MATCHING

1. d   6. a
2. i   7. h
3. g   8. c
4. e   9. b
5. j   10. f

ABBREVIATIONS

1. above elbow
2. aspartate transaminase
3. Ca
4. EMG
5. full range of motion
6. musculoskeletal
7. ROM
8. sh
9. total body weight
10. triceps jerk

DIAGNOSTIC AND LABORATORY TESTS

1. b   4. c
2. d   5. a
3. b

► CHAPTER 6

ANATOMY AND PHYSIOLOGY

1. a. mouth
   b. pharynx
   c. esophagus
   d. stomach
   e. small intestine
   f. large intestine
2. a. salivary glands
   b. liver
   c. gallbladder
   d. pancreas
3. a. digestion
   b. absorption
   c. elimination
4. A small mass of masticated food ready to be swallowed
5. A series of wave-like muscular contractions that are involuntary
6. Hydrochloric acid and gastric juices
7. duodenum
8. chyme
9. circulatory system
10. cecum, colon, rectum, and the anal canal
11. liver
12. Stores and concentrates bile
13. Produces digestive enzymes
14. a. It plays an important role in metabolism.
    b. It manufactures bile.
    c. It stores iron, vitamins B_{12}, A, D, E, and K
15. small intestine
16. parotid, sublingual, submandibular
17. a. insulin
    b. glucagon

WORD PARTS

Prefixes

1. lack of
2. up
3. down
4. difficult
5. above
6. excessive, above
7. deficient, below
8. bad
9. large, great
10. around
11. after
12. backward
13. below

Roots and Combining Forms

1. to suck in
2. gland
3. starch
4. anus
5. appendix
6. appendix
7. gall, bile
8. to cast, throw
9. cheek
10. abdomen, belly
11. lip
12. gall, bile
13. common bile duct
14. colon
15. colon
16. colon
17. colon
18. bladder
19. tooth
20. tooth
21. diverticula
22. duodenum
23. intestine
24. intestine
25. esophagus
26. esophaqus
27. stomach
28. stomach
29. gums
30. tongue
31. sweet, sugar
32. blood
33. liver
34. liver
35. hernia
36. ileum
37. ileum
38. lip
39. flank, abdomen
40. to loosen
41. tongue
42. fat
43. study of

44. middle
45. pancreas
46. to digest
47. pharynx
48. meal
49. rectum, anus
50. rectum, anus
51. pylorus, gate keeper
52. rectum
53. saliva
54. sigmoid
55. spleen
56. mouth
57. poison
58. vagus
59. worm

Suffixes

1. pertaining to
2. pertaining to
3. pain
4. pertaining to
5. enzyme
6. hernia
7. injection
8. pain
9. excision
10. vomiting
11. shape
12. formation, produce
13. pertaining to
14. pertaining to
15. process
16. condition of
17. one who specializes
18. inflammation
19. nature of, quality of
20. study of
21. destruction, to separate
22. enlargement, large
23. tumor
24. appetite
25. condition of
26. disease
27. to digest
28. fixation
29. to eat
30. surgical repair
31. suture
32. instrument
33. to view, examine
34. contraction
35. new opening

36. incision
37. pertaining to

IDENTIFYING MEDICAL TERMS

1. amylase
2. anabolism
3. anorexia
4. appendectomy
5. appendicitis
6. biliary
7. celiac
8. colorrhaphy
9. dysphagia
10. hepatitis
11. herniotomy
12. postprandial
13. proctalgia
14. splenomegaly
15. sigmoidoscope

SPELLING

1. biliary
2. colonoscopy
3. enteroclysis
4. gastroenterology
5. hepatotoxin
6. laxative
7. peristalsis
8. sialadenitis
9. vagotomy
10. vermiform

MATCHING

1. e   6. h
2. f   7. j
3. d   8. a
4. b   9. g
5. i   10. c

ABBREVIATIONS

1. a.c.
2. bowel movement
3. bowel sounds
4. cib
5. GB
6. HAV
7. nasogastric
8. nothing by mouth

9. p.c.
10. TPN

DIAGNOSTIC AND LABORATORY TESTS

1. a
2. c
3. d
4. c
5. c

► CHAPTER 7

ANATOMY AND PHYSIOLOGY

1. a. heart   c. veins
   b. arteries   d. capillaries
2. a. endocardium
   b. myocardium
   c. pericardium
3. 300
4. atria . . . interatrial
5. ventricles . . . interventricular
6. a. superior and inferior vena cavae
   b. right atrium
   c. tricuspid valve
   d. right ventricle
   e. pulmonary semilunar valve
   f. left and right pulmonary arteries
   g. lungs
   h. left and right pulmonary veins
   i. left atrium
   j. bicuspid or mitral valve
   k. left ventricle
   l. aortic valve
   m. aorta
   n. capillaries
7. autonomic nervous system
8. sinoatrial node
9. Purkinje system
10. a. radial . . . on the radial side of the wrist
    b. brachial . . . in the antecubital space of the elbow
    c. carotid . . . in the neck

11. a. the pressure exerted by the blood on the walls of the vessels
    b. the difference between the systolic and diastolic readings
12. man's fist . . . 60 to 100
13. 100 and 140 . . . 60 and 90
14. transport blood from the right and left ventricles of the heart to all body parts
15. transport blood from peripheral tissues to the heart

WORD PARTS

Prefixes

1. lack of
2. two
3. slow
4. together
5. within
6. within
7. outside
8. excessive, above
9. deficient, below
10. around
11. before
12. half
13. fast
14. three

Roots and Combining Forms

1. vessel
2. to choke, quinsy
3. vessel
4. aorta
5. aorta
6. artery
7. artery
8. artery
9. fatty substance, porridge
10. fatty substance, porridge
11. atrium
12. atrium
13. heart
14. heart
15. heart
16. dark blue
17. to the right
18. to widen
19. electricity
20. a throwing in
21. sweet, sugar
22. blood
23. to hold back
24. motion
25. study of
26. moon
27. thin
28. mitral valve
29. muscle
30. death
31. sour, sharp, acid
32. vein
33. vein
34. sound
35. lung
36. rhythm
37. hardening
38. a curve
39. pulse
40. narrowing
41. chest
42. to draw, to bind
43. contraction
44. pressure
45. clot of blood
46. tone
47. small vessel
48. vessel
49. a carrier
50. vein
51. vein
52. ventricle

Suffixes

1. pertaining to
2. pertaining to
3. pertaining to
4. immature cell, germ cell
5. surgical puncture
6. injection
7. point
8. pain
9. dilatation
10. excision
11. blood condition
12. relating to
13. formation, produce
14. a mark, record
15. to write
16. recording
17. condition
18. pertaining to
19. having a particular quality
20. process
21. condition of
22. one who specializes
23. inflammation
24. nature of, quality of
25. stone
26. study of
27. softening
28. enlargement, large
29. instrument to measure
30. tumor
31. one who
32. condition of
33. disease
34. surgical repair
35. stroke, paralysis
36. prolapse, drooping
37. to pierce
38. suture
39. instrument
40. contraction, spasm
41. contraction
42. instrument to cut
43. incision
44. crushing
45. tissue
46. pertaining to

IDENTIFYING MEDICAL TERMS

1. angioma
2. angioblast
3. angioplasty
4. angiostenosis
5. arterectomy
6. arteriolith
7. arteriotomy
8. arteritis
9. bicuspid
10. cardiodynia
11. cardiologist
12. cardiomegaly
13. cardiopulmonary
14. constriction
15. embolism
16. phlebitis
17. phlebolith
18. tachycardia
19. vasodilator

SPELLING

1. arterectomy
2. atherosclerosis
3. atrioventricular
4. endocarditis
5. extrasystole
6. ischemia
7. myocardial
8. oxygen
9. phlebitis
10. presystolic

MATCHING

1. d	6. c
2. e	7. a
3. f	8. i
4. g	9. j
5. b	10. h

ABBREVIATIONS

1. AMI
2. A-V, AV
3. blood pressure
4. coronary artery disease
5. CC
6. electrocardiogram
7. high-density lipoproteins
8. H & L
9. myocardial infarction
10. tissue plasminogen activator

DIAGNOSTIC AND LABORATORY TESTS

1. c	4. c
2. a	5. b
3. b	

▶ CHAPTER 8

ANATOMY AND PHYSIOLOGY

1. a. erythrocytes
   b. thrombocytes
   c. leukocytes
2. transport oxygen and carbon dioxide
3. 5
4. 80 to 120 days
5. body's main defense against the invasion of pathogens
6. 8000
7. a. neutrophils
   b. eosinophils
   c. basophils
   d. lymphocytes
   e. monocytes
8. play an important role in the clotting process
9. 200,000 to 500,000
10. a. A.   b. B   c. AB
    d. O
11. a. It transports proteins and fluids
    b. It protects the body against pathogens
    c. It serves as a pathway for the absorption of fats
12. a. spleen
    b. tonsils
    c. thymus

WORD PARTS

Prefixes

1. lack of
2. against
3. self
4. through
5. bad
6. excessive
7. deficient
8. one
9. all
10. many
11. before

Roots and Combining Forms

1. gland
2. gland
3. clumping
4. other
5. vessel
6. unequal
7. base
8. lime, calcium
9. smoke
10. destruction
11. clots, to clot
12. flesh, creatine
13. cell
14. cell
15. cell
16. rose-colored
17. red
18. sweet, sugar
19. little grain, granular
20. blood
21. blood
22. blood
23. white
24. white
25. fat
26. study of
27. lymph
28. lymph
29. large
30. neither
31. kernel, nucleus
32. eat, engulf
33. a thing formed, plasma
34. net
35. putrefying
36. whey, serum
37. iron
38. spleen
39. spleen
40. sea
41. clot
42. clot
43. thymus
44. thymus
45. tonsil

Suffixes

1. capable
2. forming
3. immature cell, germ cell
4. body
5. hernia
6. to separate
7. cultivation
8. cell
9. excision
10. blood condition
11. work
12. formation, produce
13. formation, produce
14. protein
15. knowledge
16. condition
17. pertaining to
18. chemical
19. process

20. one who specializes
21. inflammation
22. study of
23. destruction
24. enlargement
25. tumor
26. condition of
27. disease
28. lack of
29. fixation
30. removal
31. attraction
32. attraction
33. fear
34. formation
35. bursting forth
36. bursting forth
37. control, stopping
38. treatment
39. incision

IDENTIFYING MEDICAL TERMS

1. agglutination
2. allergy
3. antibody
4. anticoagulant
5. antigen
6. antihermorrhagic
7. basocyte
8. coagulable
9. creatinemia
10. eosinophil
11. erythroclastic
12. granulocyte
13. hematologist
14. hemoglobin
15. hyperglycemia
16. hyperlipemia
17. leukocyte
18. lymphostasis
19. mononucleosis
20. prothrombin
21. splenopexy
22. thrombocyte
23. thrombogenic
24. thymitis

SPELLING

1. allergy
2. creatinemia
3. dysglycemia

4. erythrocytosis
5. hematocele
6. hematocrit
7. hemorrhage
8. leukemia
9. lymphadenotomy
10. serology

MATCHING

1. h   6. c
2. d   7. b
3. e   8. a
4. g   9. j
5. f   10. i

ABBREVIATIONS

1. AIDS
2. BSI
3. chronic myelogenous leukemia
4. Hb, Hgb
5. hematocrit
6. HIV
7. pneumocystis carinii pneumonia
8. prothrombin time
9. red blood cell (count)
10. RIA

DIAGNOSTIC AND LABORATORY TESTS

1. d
2. c
3. c
4. b
5. a

▶ CHAPTER 9

ANATOMY AND PHYSIOLOGY

1. a. nose   d. trachea
   b. pharynx   e. bronchi
   c. larynx   f. lungs
2. To furnish oxygen for use by individual cells and to take away their gaseous waste product, carbon dioxide
3. The process whereby the lungs are ventilated and oxygen and carbon dioxide are exchanged between the air in the lungs and the blood within capillaries of the alveoli
4. The process whereby oxygen and carbon dixodide are exchanged between the bloodstream and the cells of the body
5. a. Serves as an air passage way
   b. Warms and moistens inhaled air
   c. Its cilia and mucous membrane trap dust, pollen, bacteria, and foreign matter
   d. It contains olfactory receptors that sort out odors
   e. It aids in phonation and the quality of voice
6. a. nasopharynx
   b. oropharynx
   c. laryngopharynx
7. a. Serves as a passageway for air
   b. Serves as a passageway for food
   c. Aids in phonation by changing its shape
8. Acts as a lid to prevent aspiration of food into the trachea
9. A narrow slit at the opening between the true vocal folds
10. The production of vocal sounds
11. Serves as a passageway for air
12. right bronchus . . . left bronchus
13. Provide a passageway for air to and from the lungs
14. Cone-shaped, spongy organs of respiration lying on either side of the heart
15. A serous membrane composed of several layers
16. diaphragm
17. mediastinum
18. 3 . . . 2
19. alveoli

20. To bring air into intimate contact with blood so that oxygen and carbon dioxide can be exchanged in the alveoli
21. temperature, pulse, respiration, and blood pressure
22. a. The amount of air in a single inspiration or expiration
    b. The amount of air remaining in the lungs after maximal expiration
    c. The volume of air that can be exhaled after a maximal inspiration
23. medulla oblongata . . . pons
24. 30 to 80
25. 15 to 20

WORD PARTS

Prefixes

1. lack of
2. lack of
3. through
4. difficult
5. within
6. good
7. out
8. below, deficient
9. excessive
10. in
11. fast

Roots and Combining Forms

1. air
2. small, hollow air sac
3. coal
4. imperfect
5. bronchi
6. bronchi
7. bronchiole
8. bronchi
9. dust
10. dark blue
11. breathe
12. blood
13. larynx
14. larynx
15. larynx
16. lobe

17. chin
18. fungus
19. nose
20. straight
21. smell
22. oxygen
23. palate
24. breast
25. pharynx
26. voice
27. partition
28. partition
29. speech
30. pleura
31. pleura
32. pleura
33. lung, air
34. lung
35. lung
36. lung
37. pus
38. nose
39. a curve, hollow
40. breath
41. narrowing
42. chest
43. chest
44. almond, tonsil
45. trachea
46. trachea

Suffixes

1. pertaining to
2. pain
3. hernia
4. surgical puncture
5. pain
6. dilation
7. excision
8. a mark, record
9. condition
10. process
11. inflammation
12. instrument to measure
13. condition of
14. disease
15. bearing
16. surgical repair
17. stroke, paralysis
18. breathing
19. to spit
20. bursting forth
21. flow, discharge

22. instrument
23. new opening
24. incision
25. pertaining to

IDENTIFYING MEDICAL TERMS

1. aeropleura
2. alveolus
3. aphonia
4. bronchiectasis
5. bronchitis
6. bronchoplasty
7. dysphonia
8. eupnea
9. hemoptysis
10. inhalation
11. laryngitis
12. laryngostenosis
13. nasomental
14. pharyngalgia
15. pneumothorax
16. rhinoplasty
17. rhinorrhea
18. sinusitis
19. thoracopathy

SPELLING

1. bronchoscope
2. diaphragmatocele
3. expectoration
4. laryngeal
5. orthopnea
6. pleuritis
7. pulmonectomy
8. rhinotomy
9. tachypnea
10. tracheal

MATCHING

1. h		6. b
2. i		7. d
3. k		8. a
4. f		9. e
5. c		10. g

ABBREVIATIONS

1. AFB
2. cystic fibrosis
3. CXR

4. COLD
5. endotracheal
6. postnasal drip
7. R
8. sudden infant death syndrome
9. SOB
10. tuberculosis

DIAGNOSTIC AND LABORATORY TESTS

1. b
2. c
3. c
4. d
5. a

▶ CHAPTER 10

ANATOMY AND PHYSIOLOGY

1. a. kidneys   c. bladder
   b. ureters   d. urethra
2. Extraction of certain wastes from the bloodstream, conversion of these materials to urine, and transport of the urine from the kidney, via the ureters, to the bladder for elimination
3. a. true capsule
   b. perirenal fat
   c. renal fascia
4. A notch
5. Sac-like collecting portion of the kidney
6. arteries, veins, convoluted tubules, and glomerular capsules
7. inner
8. The structural and functional unit of the kidney
9. renal corpuscle . . . tubule
10. glomerulus . . . Bowman's capsule
11. To remove the waste products of metabolism from the blood plasma
12. filtration . . . reabsorption
13. 95 5
14. 1000 to 1500

15. Narrow, muscular tubes that transport urine from the kidneys to the bladder
16. Muscular, membranous sac that serves as a reservoir for urine
17. Small, triangular area near the base of the bladder
18. Convey urine and semen
19. Convey urine
20. urinary meatus
21. Physical, chemical, and microscopic examination of urine
22. a. yellow to amber
    b. clear
    c. 5.0 to 7.0
    d. 1.015 to 1.025
    e. aromatic
    f. 1000 to 1500 mL/day
23. a. renal
    b. transitional
    c. squamous
24. diabetes mellitus
25. renal disease, acute glomerulonephritis, pyelonephritis

WORD PARTS

Prefixes

1. not, apart, lack of
2. without
3. against
4. through
5. through
6. difficult, painful
7. within
8. water
9. excessive
10. not
11. scanty
12. beside
13. around
14. excessive

Roots and Combining Forms

1. gland
2. protein
3. bacteria
4. bile
5. calcium
6. colon

7. to hold
8. bladder
9. bladder
10. bladder
11. producing
12. glomerulus, little ball
13. glomerulus, little ball
14. sweet, sugar
15. blood
16. ketone
17. stone
18. study of
19. passage
20. passage
21. to urinate
22. kidney
23. kidney
24. night
25. penis
26. perineum
27. to fold
28. purple
29. pus
30. renal pelvis
31. renal pelvis
32. kidney
33. hardening
34. narrowing
35. mouth
36. trigone
37. urine
38. urinate
39. urea
40. urine
41. ureter
42. ureter
43. urethra
44. urethra
45. urine
46. urine
47. urine
48. urine
49. vagina
50. bladder

Suffixes

1. pertaining to
2. pain
3. pertaining to
4. hernia
5. pain
6. distention
7. dilation

8. excision
9. blood condition
10. a mark, record
11. pertaining to
12. chemical
13. process
14. one who specializes
15. inflammation
16. stone
17. study of
18. destruction, to separate
19. softening
20. enlargement
21. instrument to measure
22. tumor
23. condition of
24. disease
25. fixation
26. to obstruct
27. surgical repair
28. paralysis
29. formation
30. prolapse, drooping
31. bursting forth
32. suture
33. instrument
34. to view, examine
35. condition
36. tension, spasm
37. dripping, trickling
38. new opening
39. instrument to cut
40. incision
41. tension
42. nourishment, development
43. urine

IDENTIFYING MEDICAL TERMS

1. antidiuretic
2. cystectomy
3. cystitis
4. cystopexy
5. cystorrhaphy
6. dysuria
7. glomerulitis
8. hypercalciuria
9. meatal
10. micturition
11. nephratony
12. nephrolith
13. nephromegaly

14. periurethral
15. pyuria
16. ureteropathy
17. ureterorrhaphy
18. urethralgia
19. urethrospasm
20. urologist

SPELLING

1. cystoplasty
2. cystorrhagia
3. enuresis
4. glycosuria
5. hematuria
6. incontinence
7. nephremia
8. nephrocystitis
9. nephromalacia
10. nephroptosis
11. nocturia
12. ureteroplasty
13. urethrophraxis
14. urinalysis
15. urobilin
16. uropoiesis

MATCHING

1. d	6. g
2. e	7. j
3. b	8. c
4. f	9. h
5. a	10. i

ABBREVIATIONS

1. ADH
2. blood urea nitrogen
3. CRF
4. cystoscopic examination
5. genitourinary
6. hemodialysis
7. IVP
8. peritoneal dialysis
9. potential of hydrogen
10. UA

DIAGNOSTIC AND LABORATORY TESTS

1. c	4. c
2. c	5. b
3. b	

▶ CHAPTER 11

ANATOMY AND PHYSIOLOGY

1. a. pituitary
   b. pineal
   c. thyroid
   d. parathyroid
   e. islets of Langerhans
   f. adrenals
   g. ovaries
   h. testes
2. a. thymus
   b. placenta during pregnancy
   c. gastrointestinal mucosa
3. It involves the production and regulation of chemical substances (hormones) that play an essential role in maintaining homeostasis
4. A chemical transmitter that is released in small amounts and transported via the bloodstream to a targeted organ or other cells.
5. It synthesizes and secretes releasing hormones, releasing factors, release-inhibiting hormones, and release inhibiting factors
6. Because of its regulatory effects on the other endocrine glands
7. a. growth hormone (GH)
   b. adrenocorticotropin (ACTH)
   c. thyroid-stimulating hormone (TSH)
   d. follicle-stimulating hormone (FSH)
   e. luteinizing hormone (LH)
   f. prolactin (PRL)
   g. melanocyte-stimulating hormone (MSH)
8. a. antidiuretic hormone (ADH)
   b. oxytocin
9. melatonin . . . serotonin
10. It plays a vital role in metabolism and regulates the body's metabolic processes.

11. a. thyroxine (T_4)
    b. triiodothyronine (T_3)
    c. calcitonin
12. serum calcium . . .
    phosphorus
13. blood sugar
14. glucocorticoids, mineralocorticoids, and the androgens
15. a. Regulates carbohydrate, protein, and fat metabolism
    b. Stimulates output of glucose from the liver
    c. Increases the blood sugar level
    d. Regulates other physiologic body processes
    *Optional answers to question 15:
    e. Promotes the transport of amino acids into extracellular tissue
    f. Influences the effectiveness of catecholamines such as dopamine, epinephrine, and norepinephrine
    g. Has an anti-inflammatory effect
    h. Helps the body cope during times of stress
16. a. use of carbohydrates
    b. absorption of glucose
    c. gluconeogenesis
    d. potassium and sodium metabolism
17. Aldosterone
18. A substance or hormone that promotes the development of male characteristics
19. a. dopamine
    b. epinephrine
    c. norepinephrine
20. a. It elevates the systolic blood pressure.
    b. It increases the heart rate and cardiac output.
    c. It increases glycogenolysis, thereby hastening release of glucose from the liver. This action elevates the blood sugar level and provides the body

with a spurt of
energy.
*Optional answers to question 20:
    d. It dilates the bronchial tubes.
    e. It dilates the pupils
21. estrogen . . . progesterone
22. testosterone
23. a. thymosin
    b. thymopoietin
24. a. gastrin
    b. secretin
    c. pancreozymin-cholecystokinin
    d. enterogastrone

WORD PARTS

Prefixes
1. toward
2. through
3. within
4. good, normal
5. out, away from
6. out, away from
7. excessive
8. deficient, under
9. all
10. beside
11. before

Roots and Combining Forms
1. acid
2. extremity
3. gland
4. gland
5. cortex
6. flesh
7. cretin
8. to secrete
9. to secrete
10. to secrete
11. small
12. milk
13. old age
14. giant
15. little acorn
16. sweet, sugar

17. seed
18. hairy
19. insulin
20. insulin
21. insulin
22. potassium
23. drowsiness
24. study of
25. mucus
26. eye
27. pine cone
28. pineal body
29. phlegm
30. kidney
31. kidney
32. hardening
33. thymus
34. thymus
35. thyroid, shield
36. thyroid, shield
37. poison
38. nourishment
39. masculine

Suffixes
1. pertaining to
2. pain
3. pertaining to
4. to go
5. excision
6. swelling
7. blood condition
8. formation, produce
9. condition
10. pertaining to
11. condition of
12. one who specializes
13. inflammation
14. study of
15. softening
16. enlargement, large
17. resemble
18. tumor
19. condition of
20. disease
21. fixation
22. growth
23. drooping
24. flow, discharge
25. treatment
26. instrument to cut
27. pertaining to

IDENTIFYING MEDICAL TERMS

1. adenosis
2. cretinism
3. diabetes
4. endocrinology
5. euthyroid
6. exocrine
7. gigantism
8. glucocorticoid
9. hyperkalemia
10. hypocrinism
11. hypogonadism
12. lethargic
13. pinealoma
14. thymitis

SPELLING

1. adenosclerosis
2. cretinism
3. exophthalmic
4. hypothyroidism
5. myxedema
6. pineal
7. pituitary
8. thyroid
9. thyrotome
10. virilism

MATCHING

1. e   6. i
2. f   7. c
3. b   8. j
4. g   9. d
5. h   10. a

ABBREVIATIONS

1. BMR
2. DM
3. fasting blood sugar
4. glucose tolerance tests
5. PBI
6. parathormone
7. radioimmunoassay
8. STH
9. thyroid function studies
10. vasopressin

DIAGNOSTIC AND LABORATORY TESTS

1. a
2. c
3. c
4. b
5. c

▶ **CHAPTER 12**

ANATOMY AND PHYSIOLOGY

1. a. central   b. peripheral
2. neurons
3. a. cause contractions in muscles
   b. cause secretions from glands and organs
   c. inhibit the actions of glands and organs
4. An axon is a long process reaching from the cell body to the area to be activated.
5. A dendrite resembles the branches of a tree and has short, unsheathed processes that transmit impulses to the cell body.
6. Sensory nerves transmit impulses to the central nervous system.
7. interneurons
8. a. a single elongated process
   b. a bundle of nerve fibers
   c. groups of nerve fibers
9. brain . . . spinal cord
10. a. receives impulses
    b. processes information
    c. responds with appropriate action
11. a. dura mater
    b. arachnoid
    c. pia mater
12. a. cerebrum
    b. diencephalon
    c. midbrain
    d. cerebellum
    e. pons
    f. medulla oblongata
    g. reticular formation
13. frontal lobe
14. somesthetic area
15. auditory . . . language
16. vision
17. a. is relay center for all sensory impulses
    b. relays motor impulses from the cerebellum to the cortex
18. a. is a regulator
    b. produces neurosecretions
    c. produces hormones
19. coordination of voluntary movement
20. a. regulates and controls breathing
    b. regulates and controls swallowing
    c. regulates and controls coughing
    d. regulates and controls sneezing
    e. regulates and controls vomiting
21. a. conducts sensory impulses
    b. conducts motor impulses
    c. is a reflex center
22. 120 . . . 150
23. a. olfactory
    b. optic
    c. oculomotor
    d. trochlear
    e. trigeminal
    f. abducens
    g. facial
    h. acoustic
    i. glossopharyngeal
    j. vagus
    k. accessory
    l. hypoglossal
24. a. cervical   c. lumbar
    b. brachial   d. sacral
25. a. controls sweating
    b. controls the secretions of glands
    c. controls arterial blood pressure
    d. controls smooth muscle tissue

26. a. sympathetic
    b. parasympathetic

WORD PARTS

Prefixes
1. lack of
2. lack of
3. star-shaped
4. slow
5. two
6. difficult
7. upon
8. half
9. water
10. excessive
11. below
12. within
13. small
14. little
15. beside
16. beside
17. many
18. fire
19. four
20. below
21. above
22. together

Roots and Combining Forms
1. extremity
2. to walk
3. spider
4. imperfect
5. imperfect
6. center
7. head
8. head
9. little brain
10. little brain
11. cerebrum
12. color
13. reservoir, cavity
14. cord
15. skull
16. skull
17. cell
18. tree
19. a disk
20. dura, hard
21. I, self

22. electricity
23. brain
24. brain
25. feeling
26. foramen
27. knot
28. glue
29. blood
30. sleep
31. sleep
32. thin plate
33. lobe
34. study of
35. word
36. large
37. membrane
38. membrane
39. membrane
40. mind
41. memory
42. spinal cord
43. spinal cord
44. muscle
45. nerve
46. nerve
47. nerve
48. papilla
49. to engulf, eat
50. dusky
51. gray
52. mind
53. mind
54. spine
55. root
56. root
57. hardening
58. a thorn
59. vertebra
60. body
61. sleep
62. sympathy
63. sympathy
64. tentorium, tent
65. mind, emotion
66. a bore, a hole
67. vagus, wandering
68. little belly

Suffixes
1. pertaining to
2. pain
3. pain

4. pertaining to
5. weakness
6. germ cell
7. hernia
8. cell
9. binding
10. excision
11. swelling
12. feeling
13. glue
14. mark, record
15. to write
16. recording
17. condition
18. pertaining to
19. process
20. condition
21. one who specializes
22. inflammation
23. motion
24. motion
25. to talk
26. a sheath, husk
27. diction
28. study of
29. destruction
30. softening
31. madness
32. instrument to measure
33. measurement
34. imitating
35. memory
36. mind
37. tumor
38. eye, vision
39. condition of
40. weakness
41. disease
42. to eat
43. speak
44. fear
45. a wasting
46. formation
47. surgical repair
48. stroke, paralysis
49. action
50. suture
51. strength
52. new opening
53. order
54. instrument to cut
55. incision
56. crushing

IDENTIFYING MEDICAL TERMS

1. amnesia
2. analgesia
3. aphagia
4. arachnitis
5. ataxia
6. cephalalgia
7. cerebellar
8. craniectomy
9. dyslexia
10. encephalitis
11. epidural
12. hemiparesis
13. hypnology
14. macrocephalia
15. meningitis
16. meningopathy
17. myelotome
18. neuralgia
19. neuritis
20. neurocyte
21. neurology
22. neuroma
23. neuroplasty
24. neurosis
25. phagomania
26. polyneuritis
27. psychology
28. radiculitis
29. vagotomy
30. ventriculometry

SPELLING

1. anesthesia
2. atelomyelia
3. cerebrospinal
4. craniotomy
5. encephalocele
6. meningioma
7. meningomyelocele
8. neuropathy
9. poliomyelitis
10. ventriculometry

MATCHING

1. g   4. b
2. d   5. e
3. c   6. h
7. j   9. a
8. f   10. i

ABBREVIATIONS

1. AD
2. ALS
3. central nervous system
4. cerebral palsy
5. CT
6. HDS
7. intracranial pressure
8. lumbar puncture
9. multiple sclerosis
10. PET

DIAGNOSTIC AND LABORATORY TESTS

1. a
2. b
3. c
4. d
5. c

► CHAPTER 13

ANATOMY AND PHYSIOLOGY

1. hearing . . . equilibrium
2. a. external   c. inner
   b. middle
3. a. auricle
   b. external acoustic meatus
   c. tympanic membrane
4. auricle
5. a. lubrication
   b. protection
6. a. malleus   c. stapes
   b. incus
7. to transmit sound vibrations
8. a. transmitting sound vibrations
   b. equalizing air pressure
   c. control of loud sounds
9. cochlea, vestibule, and the semicircular canals
10. a. cochlear duct
    b. semicircular ducts
    c. utricle and saccule
11. organ of Corti
12. vestibule
13. eighth cranial nerve
14. the position of the hear
15. a. endolymph
    b. perilymph

WORD PARTS

Prefixes

1. within
2. within
3. around

Roots and Combining Forms

1. hearing
2. to hear
3. to hear
4. hearing
5. the ear
6. gall, bile
7. land snail
8. electricity
9. maze
10. maze
11. larynx
12. study of
13. breast
14. fungus
15. drum membrane
16. drum membrane
17. nerve
18. ear
19. ear
20. pharynx
21. voice
22. old
23. pus
24. nose
25. hardening
26. stirrup
27. fat
28. a jingling
29. drum

Suffixes

1. pertaining to
2. pain
3. hearing
4. pain
5. excision
6. a mark, record
7. recording
8. pertaining to

9. one who specializes
10. inflammation
11. stone
12. study of
13. serum, clear fluid
14. instrument to measure
15. measurement
16. form
17. tumor
18. condition of
19. surgical repair
20. flow
21. instrument
22. instrument to cut
23. incision
24. pertaining to
25. pertaining to

IDENTIFYING MEDICAL TERMS

1. audiologist
2. audiometry
3. auditory
4. endaural
5. labyrinthitis
6. myringoplasty
7. myringotome
8. otodynia
9. otolaryngology
10. otopharyngeal
11. otoscope
12. perilymph
13. stapedectomy
14. tympanectomy
15. tinnitus

SPELLING

1. acoustic
2. audiology
3. cholesteatoma
4. electrocochleography
5. labyrinthitis
6. myringoplasty
7. otomycosis
8. otosclerosis
9. tympanic
10. tympanitis

MATCHING

1. h   3. i
2. e   4. a

5. g   8. c
6. b   9. d
7. j   10. f

ABBREVIATIONS

1. AC
2. AD
3. left ear
4. AU
5. ear, nose, throat
6. eyes, ears, nose, throat
7. HD
8. Oto
9. serous otitis media
10. UCHD

DIAGNOSTIC AND LABORATORY TESTS

1. a
2. b
3. c
4. d
5. b

▶ CHAPTER 14

ANATOMY AND PHYSIOLOGY

1. orbit, muscles, eyelids, conjunctiva, and the lacrimal apparatus
2. fatty tissue
3. optic nerve . . . ophthalmic artery
4. a. support
   b. rotaty movement
5. intense light, foreign particles, . . . impact
6. A mucous membrane that acts as a protective covering for the exposed surface of the eyeball
7. Structures that produce, store, and remove the tears that cleanse and lubricate the eye
8. eyeball, its structures, and the nerve fibers
9. vision
10. optic disk

11. The process of sharpening the focus of light on the retina
12. Answers to the matching question:
    1. c
    2. e
    3. b
    4. a
    5. f
    6. d
    7. h
    8. i
    9. j
    10. g

WORD PARTS
Prefixes

1. lack of, without
2. two
3. double
4. out
5. in
6. inward
7. beyond
8. within
9. three

Roots and Combining Forms

1. dull
2. disproportionate
3. unequal
4. eyelid
5. eyelid
6. choroid
7. choroid
8. pupil
9. cornea
10. ciliary body
11. ciliary body
12. sac
13. tear
14. tear
15. electricity
16. focus
17. angle
18. iris
19. iris
20. cornea
21. cornea
22. tear

23. study of
24. measure
25. to shut
26. muscle
27. blind
28. eye
29. eye
30. eye
31. eye
32. eye
33. lens
34. lentil, lens
35. light
36. old
37. pupil
38. retina
39. retina
40. sclera
41. point
42. tone
43. turn
44. uvea
45. foreign material
46. dry

Suffixes

1. pertaining to
2. pertaining to
3. pertaining to
4. germ cell
5. binding
6. excision
7. mark, record
8. recording
9. condition
10. pertaining to
11. process
12. condition of
13. one who specializes
14. inflammation
15. study of
16. destruction, to separate
17. softening
18. instrument to measure
19. tumor
20. eye, vision
21. condition of
22. disease
23. fear
24. surgical repair
25. stroke, paralysis
26. prolapse, drooping
27. instrument
28. stretching

IDENTIFYING MEDICAL TERMS

1. amblyopia
2. bifocal
3. blepharoptosis
4. corneal
5. dacryoma
6. diplopia
7. emmetropia
8. intraocular
9. iridomalacia
10. keratitis
11. keratoplasty
12. lacrimal
13. ocular
14. ophthalmopathy
15. photophobia

SPELLING

1. astigmatism
2. cycloplegia
3. iridectomy
4. ophthalmologist
5. phacosclerosis
6. pupillary
7. retinoblastoma
8. scleritis
9. tonometer
10. uveal

MATCHING

1. e   6. d
2. f   7. g
3. j   8. b
4. h   9. a
5. c   10. i

ABBREVIATIONS

1. DVA
2. emmetropia
3. hypermetropia (hyperopia)
4. IOL
5. L & A
6. myopia
7. right eye
8. OS
9. OU
10. exotropia

DIAGNOSTIC AND LABORATORY TESTS

1. c
2. b
3. c
4. d
5. d

▶ CHAPTER 15

ANATOMY AND PHYSIOLOGY

1. a. ovaries
   b. fallopian tubes
   c. uterus
   d. vagina
   e. vulva
   f. breasts
2. To perpetuate the species through sexual or germ cell reproduction
3. a. body   b. isthmus
   c. cervix
4. The bulging surface of the body of the uterus extending from the internal os of the cervix upward above the fallopian tubes
5. a. broad ligaments
   b. round ligaments
   c. uterosacral ligaments
   d. ligaments that attach to the bladder
6. a. peritoneum
   b. endometrium
   c. myometrium
7. a. menstruation
   b. functions as a place for the protection and nourishment of the fetus during pregnancy
   c. uterine wall contracts rhythmically and powerfully to expel the fetus from the uterus
8. a. The process of bending forward of the uterus at its body and neck
   b. The process of bending the body of the uterus backward at an angle,

with the cervix usually unchanged from its normal position

c. The process of turning the fundus forward toward the pubis, with the cervix tilted up toward the sacrum

d. The process of turning the uterus backward, with the cervix pointing forward toward the symphysis pubis

9. uterine tubes or oviducts
10. a. serosa   c. mucosa
    b. muscular
11. Finger-like processes that work to propel the discharged ovum into the fallopian tube
12. fertilization
13. a. Serves as a duct for the conveyance of the ovum from the ovary to the uterus
    b. Serve as ducts for the conveyance of spermatozoa from the uterus toward each ovary
14. Almond-shaped organs attached to the uterus by the ovarian ligament
15. a. primary   c. graafian
    b. growing
16. pituitary gland (anterior lobe)
17. a. production of ova
    b. production of hormones
18. musculomembranous . . . vestibule
19. a. female organ of copulation
    b. passageway for discharge of menstruation
    c. passageway for birth of the fetus
20. a. mons pubis
    b. labia major
    c. labia minora
    d. vestibule
    e. clitoris
21. perineum
22. A surgical procedure to prevent tearing of the perineum

and to facilitate delivery of the fetus
23. mammary glands
24. areola . . . nipple
25. a. prolactin
    b. insulin
    c. glucocorticoids
26. A thin yellowish secretion containing mainly serum and white blood cells; the "first milk"
27. a. menstruation
    b. proliferation
    c. luteal or secretory
    d. premenstrual or ischemic
28. A condition that affects certain women and may cause distressful symptoms such as nausea, constipation, diarrhea, anorexia, headache, appetite cravings, backache, muscular aches, edema, insomnia, clumsiness, malaise, irritability, indecisiveness, mental confusion, and depression

WORD PARTS

Prefixes
1. lack of
2. lack of
3. before
4. down
5. together
6. against
7. difficult, painful
8. within
9. good, normal
10. within
11. many
12. new
13. none
14. scanty
15. all
16. beside
17. around
18. after
19. before
20. first
21. false
22. backward
23. three

Roots and Combining Forms
1. to miscarry
2. lamb
3. Bartholin's glands
4. receive
5. cervix
6. a coming together
7. vagina
8. cul-de-sac
9. bladder
10. vulva
11. a bed
12. fibrous tissue
13. belonging to birth
14. female
15. blood
16. hymen
17. womb, uterus
18. womb, uterus
19. study of
20. breast
21. breast
22. month
23. month
24. month
25. womb, uterus
26. uterus
27. muscle
28. birth
29. birth
30. ovum, egg
31. ovary
32. ovary
33. to bear
34. labor
35. cessation
36. pelvis
37. perineum
38. pus
39. rectum
40. tube
41. tube
42. tube
43. birth
44. uterus
45. vagina
46. sexual intercourse
47. turning

Suffixes
1. pertaining to
2. pertaining to
3. hernia

4. surgical puncture
5. pregnancy
6. excision
7. formation, produce
8. recording
9. condition
10. pertaining to
11. process
12. one who specializes
13. inflammation
14. study of
15. measurement
16. tumor
17. condition of
18. surgical repair
19. to burst forth
20. suture
21. flow
22. instrument
23. instrument to cut
24. incision

IDENTIFYING MEDICAL TERMS

1. abortion
2. amniotome
3. antepartum
4. cervicitis
5. colporrhaphy
6. dysmenorrhea
7. eutocia
8. fibroma
9. gynecology
10. hymenectomy
11. mammoplasty
12. menorrhea
13. neonatal
14. oogenesis
15. postpartum

SPELLING

1. amniocentesis
2. bartholinitis
3. dystocia
4. episiotomy
5. hysterotomy
6. menorrhagia
7. oophoritis
8. salpingitis
9. vaginitis
10. venereal

MATCHING

1. f   6. a
2. j   7. g
3. d   8. h
4. c   9. b
5. e   10. i

ABBREVIATIONS

1. abortion
2. AFP
3. abdominal hysterectomy
4. CS; C-section
5. diethylstilbestrol
6. EDC
7. pregnancy one
8. gynecology
9. IUD
10. PID

DIAGNOSTIC AND LABORATORY TESTS

1. b
2. c
3. a
4. c
5. d

▶ CHAPTER 16

ANATOMY AND PHYSIOLOGY

1. a. testes
   b. various ducts
   c. urethra
   d. bulbourethral gland
   e. prostate gland
   f. seminal vesicles
2. a. sacrotum   b. penis
3. To provide the sperm cells necessary to fertilize the ovum, thereby perpetuating the species
4. A pouch-like structure located behind the penis
5. corpora cavernosa penis and the corpus spongiosum
6. 15 to 20

7. glans penis
8. The loose skin folds that cover the penis
9. A lubricating fluid
10. a. It is the male organ of copulation
    b. It is the site of the orifice for the elimination of urine and semen from the body.
11. They are two ovoid-shaped organs located in the scrotum. Each testis is about 4 cm long and 2.5 cm wide.
12. Seminiferous tubules
13. a. It is responsible for the development of secondary male characteristics during puberty.
    b. It is essential for normal growth and development of the male accessory sex organs.
    c. It plays a vital role in the erection process of the penis.
    d. It affects the growth of hair on the face.
    e. It affects muscular development and vocal timbre.
14. rete testis
15. A coiled tube lying on the posterior aspect of the testis
16. a. It is a storage site for sperm.
    b. It is a duct for the passage of sperm.
17. ductus deferens or the vas deferens
18. a. ductus deferens
    b. arteries
    c. veins
    d. lymphatic vessels
    e. nerves
19. Production of a slightly alkaline fluid
20. It is about 4 cm wide and weighs about 20 g. It is composed of glandular, connective, and muscular tissues and lies behind the urinary bladder.

21. Enlargement of the prostate that sometimes occurs in older men
22. bulbourethral . . . Cowper's
23. a. prostatic
    b. membranous
    c. penile
24. It transmits urine and semen out of the body.
25. 20

WORD PARTS

Prefixes

1. lack of
2. lack of
3. around
4. upon
5. water
6. under
7. scanty
8. beside

Roots and Combining Forms

1. glans
2. to cut
3. hidden
4. bladder
5. testis
6. to pour
7. testicle
8. testicle
9. testicle
10. penis
11. a muzzle
12. prostate
13. prostate
14. a rent (opening)
15. seed
16. seed
17. seed, sperm
18. sperm
19. testicle
20. twisted vein
21. vessel
22. vesicle
23. animal
24. life

Suffixes

1. pain
2. pertaining to
3. immature cell, germ cell
4. hernia
5. to kill
6. excision
7. formation, produce
8. condition
9. process
10. condition of
11. inflammation
12. enlargement
13. condition of
14. fixation
15. surgical repair
16. incision
17. urine

IDENTIFYING MEDICAL TERMS

1. balanitis
2. epididymectomy
3. orchidectomy
4. orchidoplasty
5. prostatalgia
6. prostatocystitis
7. spermatoblast
8. spermatozoon
9. spermicide
10. testicular

SPELLING

1. cryptorchism
2. hypospadias
3. orchidotomy
4. prostatomegaly
5. spermaturia

MATCHING

1. e		6. i
2. c		7. h
3. f		8. k
4. b		9. a
5. g		10. d

ABBREVIATIONS

1. BPH
2. gonorrhea
3. HPV
4. herpes simplex virus-2
5. sexually transmitted diseases
6. TPA
7. transurethral resection
8. urogenital
9. VD
10. WR

DIAGNOSTIC AND LABORATORY TESTS

1. c
2. a
3. b
4. c
5. c

► CHAPTER 17

AN OVERVIEW OF CANCER

1. a. carcinomas
   b. sarcomas
   c. mixed cancers
2. The process whereby normal cells have a distinct appearance and specialized function
3. The process whereby normal cells lose their specialization and become malignant
4. a. active migration
   b. direct extension
   c. metastasis
5. a. Change in bowel or bladder habits
   b. A sore that does not heal
   c. Unusual bleeding or discharge
   d. Thickening or lump in breast or elsewhere
   e. Indigestion or difficulty in swallowing
   f. Obvious change in a wart or mole
   g. Nagging cough or hoarseness
6. a. surgery
   b. chemotherapy
   c. radiation therapy
   d. immunotherapy

WORD PARTS

Prefixes

1. up
2. star-shaped
3. excessive
4. new
5. little
6. before

Roots and Combining Forms

1. gland
2. vessel
3. crab
4. cancer
5. cancer
6. cartilage
7. chorion
8. cell
9. tree
10. fiber
11. glue
12. glue
13. blood
14. safe
15. smooth
16. white
17. white
18. fat
19. lymph
20. lymph
21. marrow
22. black
23. membrane
24. mucus
25. fungus
26. marrow
27. muscle
28. kidney
29. kidney
30. nerve
31. tumor
32. bone
33. net
34. retina
35. rod
36. flesh
37. flesh
38. seed
39. mouth
40. monster
41. thymus
42. poison
43. grating
44. dry

Suffixes

1. immature cell
2. blood condition
3. formation
4. produce
5. formation, produce
6. condition
7. pertaining to
8. inflammation
9. tumor
10. pertaining to
11. plate
12. formation
13. a thing formed
14. formation
15. treatment
16. pertaining to

IDENTIFYING MEDICAL TERMS

1. carcinogen
2. chondrosarcoma
3. glioma
4. hypernephroma
5. leukemia
6. lymphoma
7. melanoma
8. myosarcoma
9. osteogenic sarcoma
10. sarcoma

SPELLING

1. anaplasia
2. fibrosarcoma
3. lymphosarcoma
4. myeloma
5. oncogenic
6. seminoma

MATCHING

1. e
2. i
3. d
4. g
5. c
6. f
7. j
8. b
9. h
10. a

ABBREVIATIONS

1. Adeno-Ca
2. Bx
3. cancer
4. chemotherapy
5. DNA
6. interleukin-2
7. LAK
8. metastases
9. tumor necrosis factor
10. TNM

▶ CHAPTER 18

AN OVERVIEW OF RADIOLOGY AND NUCLEAR MEDICINE

1. The study of x-rays, radioactive substances, radioactive isotopes, and ionizing radiation
2. a. invisible
   b. cause ionization
   c. cause fluorescence
   *Alternate characteristics to those listed:
   d. travel in a straight line
   e. able to penetrate substances
   f. destroy cells
3. a. Can depress the hematopoietic system, cause leukopenia, leukemia
   b. Can damage the gonads
4. a. wearing a film badge
   b. lead screens
   c. lead-lined room
   d. protective clothing
   e. gonad shield
5. a. computed tomography
   b. magnetic resonance imaging
   c. thermography
   d. scintigraphy
6. Treatment of disease by the use of ionizing radiation

WORD PARTS

Prefixes

1. short
2. through
2. within
4. one-thousandth
5. beyond

Roots and Combining Forms

1. acting
2. ampere
3. vessel
4. aorta
5. artery
6. joint
7. bronchi
8. heart
9. cavity
10. gall, bile
11. gall
12. motion
13. motion
14. cistern
15. curie
16. bladder
17. skin
18. a giving
19. echo
20. electricity
21. brain
22. fluorescence
23. kind
24. whole
25. uterus
26. ion
27. ion
28. one thousand
29. motion
30. study of
31. to shine
32. lymph
33. breast
34. to measure
35. spinal cord
36. death
37. to swing
38. dark
39. light
40. nature
41. renal pelvis
42. radiant
43. ray
44. roentgen
45. fallopian tube
46. salivary
47. sound
48. sound
49. distant
50. heat
51. to cut
52. vein
53. vein
54. volt
55. watt
56. dry

SUFFIXES

1. pertaining to
2. one who
3. formation, produce
4. knowledge
5. record
6. record
7. recording
8. pertaining to
9. process
10. one who specializes
11. inflammation
12. nature of
13. study of
14. instrument to measure
15. condition of
16. pertaining to
17. instrument
18. to view, examine
19. treatment

IDENTIFYING MEDICAL TERMS

1. angiography
2. arthrography
3. cholecystogram
4. cisternography
5. dosimetrist
6. holography
7. intracavitary
8. ionotherapy
9. kilovolt
10. kilowatt
11. mammography
12. millicurie
13. physicist
14. radiation
15. radioactive
16. radiographer
17. radiolucent
18. radiopaque
19. roentgenologist
20. sonogram

SPELLING

1. hysterosalpingogram
2. echography
3. lymphangiography
4. myelogram
5. volt
6. radioactive
7. radiography
8. sialography
9. tomography
10. venography

MATCHING

1. d
2. e
3. c
4. g
5. j
6. k
7. b
8. i
9. a
10. h

ABBREVIATIONS

1. AP
2. Ba
3. CT
4. kilovolt
5. lateral
6. radium
7. MRI
8. posteroanterior
9. Ci
10. positron emission tomography

CRITICAL THINKING ANSWERS

▶ **CHAPTER 3**

1. pruritus
2. vesicle
3. contact dermatitis
4. itching
5. corticosteroid
6. a. stay away from poison oak and/or poison ivy
   b. when working outside, wear clothing that covers arms and legs
   c. after working in the yard, immediately take a bath or shower to remove any possible contamination of skin with poison oak or poison ivy
7. erythroderma
8. edema

▶ **CHAPTER 4**

1. kyphosis
2. ESTRADERM
3. animal liver
4. nuts

▶ **CHAPTER 5**

1. waddling
2. electromyography
3. splints

▶ **CHAPTER 6**

1. pyrosis
2. gastrointestinal

3. acidity
4. Mylanta
5. 300

▶ **CHAPTER 7**

1. dyspnea
2. electrocardiogram
3. nitroglycerin
4. seek medical attention without delay

▶ **CHAPTER 8**

1. diarrhea
2. immune
3. AZT and/or zidovudine

▶ **CHAPTER 9**

1. anorexia
2. *Mycobacterium tuberculosis*
3. isoniazid

▶ **CHAPTER 10**

1. sensation
2. urinalysis
3. sulfonamide

▶ **CHAPTER 11**

1. polydipsia
2. glucose
3. diet

▶ **CHAPTER 12**

1. memory
2. electroencephalogram
3. assistance

▶ **CHAPTER 13**

1. tinnitus
2. otoscopy
3. antibiotic

▶ **CHAPTER 14**

1. photophobia
2. complete
3. ultrasonic

▶ **CHAPTER 15**

1. dyspareunia
2. gynecologic
3. Prempro
4. HRT

▶ **CHAPTER 16**

1. urgency
2. Proscar
3. impotence
4. prostate

GLOSSARY OF COMPONENT PARTS

▶ PREFIXES

a-,	no, not, without, lack of, apart
ab-,	away from
ad-,	toward, near, to
ambi-,	both
an-,	no, not, without, lack of
ana-,	up
ant-,	against
ante-,	before
anti-,	against
apo-,	separation
astro-,	star-shaped
auto-,	self

bi-,	two, double
brachy-,	short
brady-,	slow

cac-,	bad
cata-,	down
centi,-,	a hundred
chromo-,	color
circum-,	around
con-,	with, together
contra-,	against

de-,	down, away from
di(a)-,	through
dia-,	through, between
dif-,	apart, free from, separate
dipl-,	double

di(s)-,	two
dys-,	bad, difficult, painful

ec-,	out, outside, outer
ecto-,	outside, outer, out
em-,	in
en-,	within
end-,	within, inner
endo-,	within, inner
ep-,	upon, over, above
epi-,	upon, over, above
eso-,	inward
eu-,	good, normal
ex-,	out, away from
exo,-	out, away from
extra,-	outside, beyond

hemi-,	half
hetero-,	different
homeo-,	similar, same, likeness
hydr-,	water
hydro-,	water
hyp-,	below, deficient
hyper-,	above, beyond, excessive
hypo-,	below, under, deficient

in-,	in, into, not
infra-,	below
inter-,	between
intra-,	within

mal-,	bad
mega-,	large, great

meso-,	middle
meta-,	beyond, over, between, change
micro-,	small
milli-,	one thousandth
mono-,	one
multi-,	many, much

neo-.	new
nulli-,	none

olig-,	little, scanty
oligo-,	little, scanty

pan-,	all
par-,	around, beside
para-,	beside, alongside, abnormal
per-,	through
peri-,	around
poly-,	many, much, excessive
post-,	after, behind
pre-,	before, in front of
primi-,	first
pro-,	before, in front of
proto-,	first
pseudo-,	false
pyro-,	fire

quadri-,	four

retro-,	backward

semi-,	half
sub-,	below, under, beneath
supra-,	above, beyond
sym-,	together
syn-,	together, with

tachy-,	fast-
tri-,	three-

ultra-,	beyond
uni-,	one

▶ ROOTS AND COMBINING FORMS

abort,	to miscarry
absorpt,	to such in
acanth,	a thorn
aceta-bul,	vinegar cup
achillo,	Achilles, heel
acid,	acid
acoust,	hearing
acr,	extremity, point
acro,	extremity
act,	acting
actin,	ray
aden,	gland
adeno,	gland
adhes,	stuck to
adip,	fat
aero,	air
agglu-tinat,	clumping
agon,	agony
albin,	white
albumin,	protein
all,	other
alveol,	small, hollow air sac
ambly,	dull
ambul,	to walk
ametr,	disproportionate
amnio,	lamb
ampere,	ampere
amyl,	starch
andr,	man
angi,	vessel
angin,	to choke, quinsy
angio,	vessel
aniso,	unequal

ankyl,	stiffening, crooked
ano,	anus
anthrac,	coal
append,	appendix
appen-dic,	appendix
aort,	aorta
aorto,	aorta
arachn,	spider
arter,	artery
arteri,	artery
arterio,	artery
arthr,	joint
arthro,	joint
atel,	imperfect
atelo,	imperfect
ather,	fatty substance, porridge
athero,	fatty substance, porridge
atri,	atrium
atrio,	atrium
audio,	to hear
auditor,	hearing
aur,	the ear
axill,	armpit

bacteri,	bacteria
balan,	glans
barth-olin,	Bartholin's glands
baso,	base
bil,	bile
bili,	gall, bile
bio,	life
blephar,	eyelid
ble-pharo,	eyelid
bol,	to cast, throw
brachi,	arm
bronch,	bronchi
bronchi,	bronchi
bron-chiol,	bronchiole
broncho,	bronchi
bucc,	cheek
burs,	a pouch

calc,	lime, calcium
calcane,	heel bone
cal-caneo,	heel bone

calci,	calcium
cancer,	crab
capn,	smoke
carcin,	cancer
carcino,	cancer
card,	heart
cardi,	heart
cardio,	heart
carp,	wrist
carpo,	wrist
caud,	tail
caus,	heat
cavit,	cavity
celi,	abdomen, belly
centr,	center
centri,	center
cephal,	head
cephalo,	head
cept,	receive
cere-bell,	little brain
cere-bello,	little brain
cerebro,	cerebrum
cervic,	cervix
cheil,	lip
chemo,	chemical
chol,	gall, bile
chole,	gall, bile
chole docho,	common bile duct
chondr,	cartilage
chondro,	cartilage
chorio,	chorion
choroid,	choroid
chor-oido,	choroid
chromo,	color
chym,	juice
cine,	motion
cinem-ato,	motion
cis,	to cut
cister-no,	reservoir, cavity, cistern
clast,	destruction
clavicul,	little key
cleido,	clavicle
clon,	turmoil
coagul,	clots, to clot
coccyge,	tail bone
coccygo,	tail bone
cochleo,	land snail

coit,	a coming together
col,	colon
colla,	glue
collis,	neck
colo,	colon
colon,	colon
colono,	colon
colpo,	vagina
condyle,	knuckle
coni,	dust
connect,	to bind together
contin-ence,	to hold
cor,	pupil
cordo,	cord
coriat,	corium
corne,	cornea
cortic,	cortex
cost,	rib
costo,	rib
cox,	hip
coxo,	hip
crani,	skull
cranio,	skull
creat,	flesh
creatin,	flesh, creatine
cretin,	cretin
crin,	to secrete
crine,	to secrete
crino,	to secrete
crypt,	hidden
culdo,	cul-de-sac
curie,	curie
cutane,	skin
cyan,	dark blue
cycl,	ciliary body
cyclo,	ciliary body
cyst,	bladder, sac
cysti,	bladder, sac
cysto,	bladder, sac
cyt,	cell
cyth,	cell
cyto,	cell

dacry,	tear
dacryo,	tear
dactyl,	finger or toe
dactylo,	finger or toe
dendro,	tree
dent,	tooth
denti,	tooth
derm,	skin
derma,	skin

dermat,	skin
dermato,	skin
dermo,	skin
dextro,	to the right
didym,	testis
dilat,	to widen
disk,	a disc, disk
diverti-culi,	diverticula
dosi,	a giving
duct,	to lead
duoden,	duodenum
dur,	dura, hard
dwarf,	small

echo,	echo
ego,	I, self
electro,	electricity
embol,	a throwing in
encep-phal,	brain
ence-phalo,	brain
enchy-ma,	to pour
enter,	intestine
entero,	intestine
eosino,	rose-colored
episio,	vulva, pudenda
erget,	work
erysi,	red
erythro,	red
eso-phage,	esophagus
eso-phago,	esophagus
esthesio,	feeling
eunia,	a bed

fasc,	a band
fasci,	a band
fascio,	a band
femor,	femur
fibr,	fibrous tissue, fiber
fibro,	fiber
fibul,	fibula
fluoro,	fluorescence
foc,	focus
fora-mino,	foramen
format,	a shaping
fus,	to pour

galacto,	milk
gan-glion,	knot
gastr,	stomach
gastro,	stomach
gen,	formation, produce
gene,	formation, produce
genet,	producing
genital,	belonging to birth
geno,	kind
ger,	old age
gigant,	giant
gingiv,	gums
glandul,	little acorn
gli,	glue
glio,	glue
glomer-ul,	glomerulus, little ball
glomer-ulo,	glomerulus, little ball
glosso,	tongue
gluco,	sweet, sugar
glyc,	sweet, sugar
glyco,	sweet, sugar
glycos,	sweet, sugar
gonad,	seed
gonio,	angle
granulo,	little grain, granular
gryp,	curve
gyneco,	female

halat,	breathe
hem,	blood
hemat,	blood
hemato,	blood
hemo,	blood
hepat,	liver
hepato,	liver
hernio,	hernia
hidr,	sweat
hirsut,	hairy
histo,	tissue
holo,	whole
humer,	humerus
hydr,	water
hymen,	hymen
hypn,	sleep
hypno,	sleep
hyster,	womb, uterus
hystero,	womb, uterus

iatr,	treatment	litho,	stone	myringo,	drum, membrane
icter,	jaundice	lob,	lobe	myx,	mucus
ile,	ileum	lobo,	lobe		
ileo,	ileum	log,	study of	naso,	nose
ili,	ilium	logo,	word	nat,	birth
ilio,	ilium	lord,	bending	nata,	birth
immuno,	safe	lucent,	to shine	necr,	death
insul,	insulin	lumb,	loin	nephr,	kidney
insulin,	insulin	lumbo,	loin	nephro,	kidney
insu-		lun,	moon	neur,	nerve
lino,	insulin	lymph,	lymph	neuri,	nerve
iono,	ion	lympho,	lymph	neuro,	nerve
ionto,	ion			neutro,	neither
irid,	iris			noct,	night
irido,	iris	macro,	large	nom,	law
isch,	to hold back	mammo,	breast	norm,	rule
ischi,	ischium	mandi-		nucle,	kernel, nucleus
iso,	equal	bul,	lower jawbone	nyctal,	blind
		mano,	thin		
		mast,	breast		
kal,	potassium	maxill,	jawbone	ocul,	eye
karyo,	cell's nucleus	maxilla,	jawbone	olecran,	elbow
kel,	tumor	meat,	passage	onco,	tumor
kerat,	horn, cornea	meato,	passage	onych,	nail
kerato,	cornea	medullo,	marrow	onychi,	nail
keton,	ketone	melan,	black	onycho,	nail
kilo,	a thousand	melano,	black	oo,	ovum, egg
kinet,	motion	men,	month	oophor,	ovary
kymo,	motion	mening,	membrane	oph-	
kyph,	a hump	meninge,	membrane	thalm,	eye
		meningi,	membrane	ophthal-	
		meningo,	membrane	mo,	eye
labi,	lip	meno,	month	opt,	eye
laby-		ment,	chin, mind	opto,	eye
rinth,	maze	mes,	middle	orch,	testicle
laby-		mester,	month	orchido,	testicle
rintho,	maze	metr,	to measure	organ,	organ
lacrim,	tear	metr,	womb, uterus	ortho,	straight
lamin,	lamina, thin plate	metri,	uterus	oscillo,	to swing
laparo,	flank, abdomen	mic-		osm,	smell
laryng,	larynx	turit,	to urinate	osteo,	bone
larynge,	larynx	mitr,	mitral valve	oto,	ear
laryngo,	larynx	mnes,	memory	ot,	ear
later,	side	mucos,	mucus	ovul,	ovary
laxat,	to loosen	muscul,	muscle	ox,	oxygen
leio,	smooth	my,	muscle	oxy,	sour, sharp, acid
lemma,	a rind	my,	to shut		
letharg,	drowsiness	myc,	fungus		
leuk,	white	myco,	fungus	pachy,	thick
leuko,	white	myel,	marrow, spinal cord	palato,	palate
levat,	lifter	myelo,	marrow, spinal cord	pan-	
lingu,	tongue	myo,	muscle	creat,	pancreas
lip,	fat	myos,	muscle	papill,	papilla
lipo,	fat	myring,	drum, membrane		

paque,	dark	por,	a passage	sarco,	flesh
para,	to bear	porphyr,	purple	scapul,	shoulder blade
partum,	labor	prandi,	meal	scler,	hardening, sclera
patell,	kneecap	presby,	old	sclero,	hard
patella,	kneecap	proct,	rectum, anus	scoli,	curvature
path,	disease	procto,	rectum, anus	scolio,	curvature
patho,	disease	prostat,	prostate	scop,	to examine
pause,	cessation	prostato,	prostate	sebo,	oil
pec-		psych,	mind	semin,	seed
torat,	breast	psycho,	mind	senil,	old
ped,	foot	pulmo,	lung	sept,	putrefaction
pedicul,	a louse	pulmon,	lung	septic,	putrefying
pelvi,	pelvis	pul-		sero,	whey, serum
pen,	penis	monar,	lung	sert,	to gain
penile,	penis	pupill,	pupil	sial,	saliva
pept,	to digest	py,	pus	sialo,	salivary
perine,	perineum	pyel,	renal pelvis	sidero,	iron
perineo,	perineum	pyelo,	renal pelvis	sig-	
phaco,	lens	pyo,	pus	moido,	sigmoid
phago,	to eat, engulf	pylor,	pylorus, gate keeper	sino,	a curve
phak,	lentil, lens	pyret,	fever	sinus,	a curve, hollow
phalange,	closely knit row	pyro,	heat, fire	somat,	body
pharyng,	pharynx			somato,	body
phar-				somn,	sleep
ynge,	pharynx	rachi,	spine	son,	sound
pheo,	dusky	rachio,	spine	sono,	sound
phim,	a muzzle	radi,	radius	spadias,	a rent, an opening
phleb,	vein	radiat,	radiant	spastic,	convulsive
phlebo,	vein	radico,	root	sperm,	seed
phon,	voice	radicul,	root	spermat,	seed
phone,	voice	radio,	ray	spermi,	sperm
phono,	sound	recto,	rectum	sphygmo,	pulse
photo,	light	relaxat,	to loosen	spin,	spine, a thorn
phragm,	partition	ren,	kidney	spiro,	breath
phrag-		reno,	kidney	splen,	spleen
mato,	partition	reti-		spleno,	spleen
phras,	speech	culo,	net	spondyl,	vertebra
physic,	nature	retin,	retina	spon-	
physio,	nature	retino,	retina	dylo,	vertebra
pine,	pine cone	rhabdo,	rod	staped,	stirrup
pineal,	pineal body	rhino,	nose	steat,	fat
pino,	to drink	rhytid,	wrinkle	sten,	narrowing
pitui-		rhytido,	wrinkle	stern,	sternum
tar,	phlegm	roent,	roentgen	sterno,	sternum
plasma,	a thing formed,	rotat,	to turn	stetho,	chest
	plasma	rrhythm,	rhythm	stigmat,	point
pleur,	pleura			stom,	mouth
pleura,	pleura			stomat,	mouth
pleuro,	pleura	sacr,	sacrum	strict,	to draw, to bind
plicat,	to fold	salping,	tube	sym-	
pneumo,	lung, air	sal-		path,	sympathy
pneu-		pingo,	tube	sym-	
mon,	lung	salpinx,	tube, fallopian tube	patho,	sympathy
polio,	gray	sarc,	flesh	systol,	contraction

tele,	distant
tendo,	tendon
teno,	tendon
tenon,	tendon
tenos,	tendon
tens,	pressure
tentori,	tentorium, tent
terat,	monster
testi-	
cul,	testicle
thalass,	sea
thermo,	hot, heat
thoraco,	chest
thorax,	chest
thromb,	clot of blood
thrombo,	clot
thym,	thymus, mind, emotion
thymo,	thymus
thyr,	thyroid, shield
thyro,	thyroid, shield
tibi,	tibia
tinnit,	a jingling
toc,	birth
tomo,	to cut
ton,	tone, tension
tono,	tone
tonsill,	almond, tonsil
topic,	place
topo,	place
tort,	twisted
tox,	poison
toxic,	poison
trache,	trachea
tracheo,	trachea
tract,	to draw
tre-	
phinat,	a bore
trich,	hair
tricho,	hair
trigon,	trigone
trism,	grating
trop,	turn
troph,	a turning
tuss,	cough
tympan,	drum

uln,	elbow
ulno,	elbow
ungu,	nail
ur,	urine
ure,	urinate

urea,	urea
uret,	urine
ureter,	ureter
uretero,	ureter
urethr,	urethra
urethro,	urethra
urin,	urine
urinat,	urine
urino,	urine
uro,	urine
uter,	uterus
uve,	uvea

vagin,	vagina
vago,	vagus, wandering
varico,	twisted vein
vas,	vessel
vascul,	small vessel
vaso,	vessel
vector,	a carrier
ven,	vein
venere,	sexual intercourse
veni,	vein
veno,	vein
ventri-	
cul,	ventricle
ventri-	
culo,	little belly
vermi,	worm
vers,	turning
vertebr,	vertebra
vertebro,	vertebra
vesic,	bladder
vesicul,	vesicle
viril,	masculine
viscer,	body organs
volt,	volt
volunt,	will

watt,	watt

xantho,	yellow
xen,	foreign material
xer,	dry
xero,	dry
xiph,	sword

zoo,	animal
zoon,	life

► SUFFIXES

-able,	capable
-ac,	pertaining to
-age,	related to
-al,	pertaining to
-algesia,	pain
-algia,	pain
-ant,	forming
-ar,	pertaining to
-ary,	pertaining to
-ase,	enzyme
-asthenia,	weakness
-ate,	use, action

-betes,	to go
-blast,	immature cell, germ cell
-body,	body

-cele,	hernia
-cen-	
tesis,	surgical puncture
-ceps,	head
-cide,	to kill
-clasia,	a breaking
-clave,	a key
-clysis,	injection
-colon,	colon
-crit,	to separate
-cul-	
ture,	cultivation
-cusis,	hearing
-cuspid,	point
-cyesis,	pregnancy
-cyte,	cell

-derma,	skin
-desis,	binding
-drome,	a course
-dynia,	pain

-ectasia,	distention
-ectasis,	dilatation, dilation, distention
-ectasy,	dilation
-ectomy,	excision
-edema,	swelling
-emesis,	vomiting
-emia,	blood condition

-er,	relating to, one who	-lymph,	serum, clear fluid	-plasty,	surgical repair
-ergy,	work	-lysis,	destruction, to	-plegia,	stroke, paralysis
-esthesia,	feeling		separate	-pnea,	breathing
				-poiesis,	formation
				-poietic,	formation
-form,	shape	-malacia,	softening	-praxia,	action
-fuge,	to flee	-mania,	madness	-ptosis,	prolapse, drooping
		-megaly,	enlargement, large	-ptysis,	to spit
		-meter,	instrument to	-punc-	
-gen,	formation, produce		measure, measure	ture,	to pierce
-genes,	produce	-metry,	measurement		
-genesis,	formation, produce	-mine-			
-genic,	formation, produce	tic,	imitating	-rrhage,	to burst forth,
-glia,	glue	-mnesia,	memory		bursting forth
-globin,	protein	-morph,	form, shape	-rrhagia,	to burst forth,
-gnosis,	knowledge				bursting forth
-grade,	a step			-rrhaphy,	suture
-graft,	pencil	-noia,	mind	-rrhea,	flow, discharge
-gram,	a weight, mark,			-rrhexis,	rupture
	record				
-graph,	to write, record	-oid,	resemble, form		
-graphy,	recording	-oma,	tumor	-scope,	instrument
		-omion,	shoulder	-scopy,	to view, examine
		-opia,	eye, vision	-sepsis,	decay
-hexia,	condition	-opsia,	eye, vision	-sis,	condition
		-or,	one who, a doer	-some,	body
		-orexia,	appetite	-spasm,	tension, spasm,
-ia,	condition	-ose,	like		contraction
-ic,	pertaining to	-osis,	condition of	-stalsis,	contraction
-ician,	physician	-ous,	pertaining to	-stasis,	control, stopping
-ide,	having a particular			-staxis,	dripping, trickling
	quality			-sthenia,	strength
-in,	chemical, pertaining	-paresis,	weakness	-stomy,	new opening
	to	-pathy,	disease	-systole,	contraction
-ine,	pertaining to	-pelas,	skin		
-ion,	process	-penia,	lack of, deficiency		
-ism,	condition of	-pepsia,	to digest	-tasis,	stretching
-ist,	one who specializes,	-pexy,	fixation	-taxia,	order
	agent	-phagia,	to eat	-therapy,	treatment
-itis,	inflammation	-phasia,	speak	-thermy,	heat
-ity,	condition	-pheresis,	removal	-tome,	instrument to cut
-ive,	nature of, quality of	-phil,	attraction	-tomy,	incision
		-philia,	attraction	-tone,	tension
		-phobia,	fear	-tony,	tension
-kinesia,	motion	-phore,	bearing	-tripsy,	crushing
-kinesis,	motion	-phoresis,	to carry	-trophy,	nourishment,
		-phragm,	a fence		development
		-phraxis,	to obstruct		
-lalia,	to talk	-phthisis,	a wasting		
-lemma,	a sheath, husk, rind	-physis,	growth	-um,	tissue
-lexia,	diction	-plakia,	plate	-uria,	urine
-liter,	liter	-plasia,	formation	-us,	pertaining to
-lith,	stone	-plasm,	a thing formed,		
-logy,	study of		plasma		

-y,   condition, pertaining
               to, process

Suffixes that mean pertaining to
are:
-ac
-al
-ar
-ary
-ic
-in
-ine
-ous
-us
-y

Suffixes that mean condition of
are:
-hexia
-ia
-ism
-ity
-osis
-sis
-y

GENERAL INDEX

Page numbers followed by f and t indicate figures and tables, respectively.

Superior vena cava vein, 224t
Supernatant, 341
Supination, 108, 109f
Supine position, 160, 590
Supplemental air, 297
Suprapubic prostatectomy (SPP), 542
Suprarenals, 359f, 360t–361t, 365
Supratentorial, 417
Suprax, 452
Surfactant, 299
Surgery, cancer, 564
Surgical and medical specialties, 15, 15t–17t
Surgicel, 278
Surrogate mother, 512
Suspensory ligaments, 498
Sweat, 63, 66
Sweat glands, 64f, 66
Sweat test, 92
Symmetrel, 423
Sympathectomy, 417
Sympathetic ganglia, 405
Sympathetic nervous system, 405–406, 406f
Sympathetic trunk, 405
Sympathomimetics, 417, 480
Symphysis, 124
Synapse, 396
Synaptic cleft, 396
Synarthrosis, 108
Syncope, 421
Syndesis, 124
Syndrome, 12
Synergetic, 156
Synergist, 147
Synovectomy, 161
Synovia, 126
Synthroid, 377
Syphilis, 542, 545–546, 546f
Systemic, 48
Systemic lupus erythematosus (SLE), 90
Systole, 241

T

T cell lymphoma, 277f
T lymphocytes, 259t, 260, 263, 264, 264t
TACE, 513
Tachycardia, 233
Tachypnea, 305
Tactile, 421
Tagamet, 198
Tagging, 612
Tambocor, 244
Tamponade (cardiac), 578
Tapazole, 377
Taste buds, 178

Taut, 80
Tay-Sachs disease, 421
Tedral SA, 310
Telangiectasia, 80
Telangiectasis, 241, 242f
Teletherapy, 606
Temazepam, 423
Temovate, 91
Temperature (T), 90
Temporal arteritis, 235f
Temporal artery, 219, 223f
Temporal lobe, 397, 399f
Temporomandibular joint (TMJ), 128
Tendon, 144, 145f, 161
Tendon sheath, giant cell tumor of, 161, 163f
Tendoplasty, 124
Tennis elbow, 127
Tenodesis, 156
Tenodynia, 156
Tenonitis, 124
Tenorrhaphy, 156
Tenotomy, 156
Tensilon, 163
Teratoma, 575
Terpin hydrate, 310
Terramycin, 452
Tessalon, 310
Testex, 543
Testicular, 540
Testis(es), 359f, 361t, 367, 530, 531f, 532, 533f
Testosterone, 360t, 361t, 366, 367, 376, 532, 543
    abuse, 543
    replacement therapy, 543
    toxicology, 544
Test-tube baby, 512
Tetany, 364
Tetracy, 452
Tetracycline, 452, 480, 545
Tetrahydrozoline, 480
Thalamus, 397f, 398, 398t
Thalassemia, 271
Theelin, 513
Theophylline, 310
Thermanesthesia, 72
Thermography, 130, 594, 607
Thermometer, 12
Thermoscan Instant Thermometer, 451f
Thermotherapy, 159
Thiazide diuretics, 342
Thiethylperazine, 452
Thioguanine, 565
Thiopental, 424
Thiosulfil, 343
Thiotepa, 564

Thoracic cavity, 39, 41f, 296
Thoracic curve, 108, 109f
Thoracic spinal nerves, 405
Thoracic surgery specialty, 17t
Thoracic vertebra
    first (T-1), 128
    second (T-2), 128
    third (T-3), 128
Thoracocentesis, 305
Thoracopathy, 305
Thoracoplasty, 305
Thoracotomy, 305
Three-day measles, 80
Throat culture, 311
Thrombectomy, 272
Thrombin, 260, 275
Thrombocytes, 259f, 259t, 260, 272, 280
Thrombogenic, 272
Thrombokinase, 260
Thrombolysis, 272, 594
Thrombolytic agents, 278
Thrombophlebitis, 241, 242f
Thromboplastin, 275
Thrombosis, 233, 272
Thymectomy, 373
Thymitis, 272, 373
Thymocyte, 272
Thymoma, 272, 575
Thymopexy, 373
Thymopoietin, 361t, 367
Thymosin, 361t, 367
Thymus, 262, 263f, 265, 359f, 361t, 367, 367f
Thyroid, 373
Thyroid cartilage, 295
Thyroid function studies (TFS), 377
Thyroid gland, 359f, 360t, 364
Thyroid hormones, 377
Thyroid scan, 379
Thyroidectomy, 373
Thyroiditis, 373
Thyroid-stimulating hormone (TSH), 360t, 362f, 363, 377
Thyrolar, 377
Thyroptosis, 373
Thyrosis, 373
Thyrotherapy, 374
Thyrotome, 374
Thyrotoxicosis, 364, 374
Thyrotropin-releasing hormone (TRH), 358, 362f
Thyroxine (T$_4$), 360t, 364, 376, 377, 379
Tibial, 125
Tibial artery
    anterior, 221t
    posterior, 223f
Tibial vein, anterior, 224t

Tibialis anterior muscle, 146t, 148f

Tick bite, 82f

Tidal volume (TV), 296, 310, 311

Tigan, 198

Time, Spanish terminology, 22

Tine test, 91

Tinea, 80, 87f–88f

Tinnitus, 448

Tissue plasminogen activator (tPA), 241, 243

Tissues, 34, 36

Tobacco, 566–567

Tocainide, 244

Toenails, 65–66

Tolazamide, 378

Tolbutamide, 378

Tolinase, 378

Tomography, 607
  computed. *See* Computed tomography
  positron emission, 423, 425, 614

Tongue, 178, 180f

Tonic, 157

Tonocard, 244

Tonography, 475

Tonometer, 475

Tonometry, 481

Tonsil(s), 180f, 263f
  faucial or palatine, 179, 180f, 262, 293
  lingual, 262, 293
  pharyngeal (adenoids), 262, 293

Tonsillectomy, 272, 305

Tonsillectomy and adenoidectomy (T & A), 309

Tonsillitis, 305

Topical, 46

Topography, 12

Torecan, 452

Torsion, 161

Torticollis, 157

Toshiba diagnostic imaging system, 596f–597f

Total body weight (TBW), 163

Total lung capacity (TLC), 286, 298, 310, 311

Total parenteral nutrition (TPN), 197

Toxic goiter, 364

Toxic shock syndrome (TSS), 512, 513

Trabeculoplasty, laser, 477, 479

Trachea, 293f, 295, 297f

Tracheal, 305

Trachealgia, 305

Tracheitis, 305

Tracheolaryngotomy, 305

Tracheostomy, 305

Trachoma, 478

Tracrium, 164

Traction (Tx), 127, 128

Tracts, nerve, 395

Transcutaneous electrical nerve stimulations (TENS), 421, 423

Transcutaneous nerve stimulation (TNS), 423

Transderm Scop, 198

Transdermal therapeutic system (TTS), 90

Transesophageal echocardiography (TEE), 243

Transfusion, 275

Transient ischemic attack (TIA), 423

Transjugular intrahepatic portosystemic shunt (TIPS), 594, 614

Transluminal coronary angioplasty, percutaneous, 240, 243

Transurethral resection (TUR), 542

Transurethral resection of prostate (TURP or TUR), 539

Transverse fracture, 113, 113f, 114

Transverse plane, 39, 40f

Trapezius muscle, 146t, 147t, 148f, 149f

Trauma surgery specialty, 17t

Trendelenburg position, 161

Trephination, 417

Treponema pallidum, 545

Treponema pallidum agglutination (TPA), 542

Tretinoin, 91

Triage, 12

Triamcinolone, 129

Triamcinolone acetonide, 310

Triamterene, 343

Triazolam, 423

Triceps, 157

Triceps jerk (TJ), 163

Triceps muscle, 147t, 149f

Trichiasis, 478

Trichomoniasis, 546

Trichomycosis, 73

Tricuspid, 233

Tricuspid valve, 215

Tridione, 423

Trifluridine, 481

Trifocal, 475

Trigeminal nerve (V), 402, 403f, 404t

Triglycerides, 233, 245

Trigonitis, 337

Trihexyphenidyl, 423

Triiodothyronine (T₃), 360t, 364, 377, 379

Triiodothyronine resin uptake (T₃RU), 360t, 377

Trimester, 509

Trimethadione, 423

Trimethobenzamide, 198

Trimethoprim, 343

Triphasil, 513

Trismus, 575

Trisomy, 542

Trochanter, 107

Trochlear nerve (IV), 402, 403f, 404t

Tronothane, 424

Tropicamide, 480

True skin, 64

Tubercle, 107

Tuberculosis (TB), 309, 310

Tuberculosis skin tests, 91–92

Tuberosity, 107

Tubule, 326

Tumor, 561–562, 574, 578

Tumor, node, metastasis (TNM), 579

Tumor grading systems, 560

Tumor necrosis factor (TNF), 566, 579

Tums, 197

Tuning fork test, 453

Tylenol, 129, 423

Tympanectomy, 448

Tympanic, 449

Tympanic membrane, 440, 441f

Tympanic thermometer, 450, 451f

Tympanitis, 449

Tympanometry, 453

Tympanoplasty, 450

Tzanck test, 92

U

Ulcer, 67f, 80, 88f, 194

Ulcerative colitis
  chronic, 197

Ulnar, 125

Ulnar artery, 221t

Ulnocarpal, 125

Ulnoradial, 125

Ultrasonic, 607

Ultrasonography, 245, 379, 593–594, 607, 607f–608f
  brain, 425
  diagnostic, 510
  Doppler, 510
  fetal, 503f
  gallbladder, 200, 201f
  kidney, 202f, 344
  liver, 200–201, 202f
  ocular, 481

Ultrasound (US), 593, 614

Ultrasound diathermy, 158

Ultraviolet (UV), 90

Ultraviolet radiation, 567

Umbilical region, 42, 43f

Ung (ointment), 90

SPANISH INDEX

▶ **INSTALLATION INSTRUCTIONS FOR THE COMPUTERIZED STUDY GUIDE FOR STUDENTS**

REQUIREMENTS

- Microsoft® Windows95™ or higher
- CD-ROM drive
- Printer recommended

PURPOSE AND OBJECTIVES

This self-assessment program consists of a test section and a study plan section. The student is tested on material in a given chapter of the textbook. A study plan is then generated from test items that were missed or items that the student indicated he or she did not know. The study plan includes page references to assist the student with review of the accompanying textbook.

SOFTWARE INSTALLATION

1. Start your computer, and insert the CD into your CD-ROM drive.
2. Click on **START,** and select **RUN.** In the box that appears, type **x:\setup.exe** and **replace x** with your CD-ROM drive letter, then click the **OK** button. An install message box will appear, giving you the option to install your study guide or abort the operation.
3. Proceed with installation by clicking the **OK** button.
4. You will then be asked to select a destination directory. The study guide will install to the following directory (C:/alsg4) unless you place it elsewhere. Select directory and click the **OK** button.
5. An installation status box will appear. You will still have the opportunity to abort the operation by clicking the **CANCEL** button.
6. After installation is complete, you will be asked to select a Group for your study guide icon. Select or type in a new Group name and click **OK** when finished.
7. To open your study guide after installation, click on the icon you chose in Step 6, then double click on the program to begin.

PROGRAM INSTRUCTIONS

1. Select the chapter you wish to study. Use the arrow buttons to browse through the list of chapters. When you have found the number and name of the chapter you wish to study, click on the **BEGIN** button to start the test.
2. To select an answer, use your mouse and click on the button next to the appropriate option.
3. For the fill-in questions, type your response, then press the **ENTER** key.
4. Using the SKIP button. It is very important not to guess. If you are not sure of the answer to a question, click the **SKIP** button. The correct answer will then be displayed. The personal study plan helps you find the answers to each of the questions that you answered incorrectly or skipped.
5. You may interrupt a chapter test and finish it at a later time. You will only receive a score and study plan upon completion of an entire chapter test. To save your position, click the **EXIT** button. The Save Bookmark button is checked by default.

6. Print/View Study Plan. After completing a chapter test, you can view and/or print your individualized study plan. Click on the **PRINT YOUR PLAN** button to print the study plan. If you do not print the plan at this time, you will not be able to retrieve it later for viewing or printing. If you wish to retake a chapter test, your previous study plan for that chapter will be deleted. A chapter test can be taken as many times as you wish.

7. A performance report is shown at the end of each test. This report will appear on each completed chapter.

Customer Support

Please call or fax us at:
1-800-748-7734 or (913)441-2881
FAX # (913)441-2119
Email: escinc@concentric.net

Or write to:

Educational Software Concepts, Inc.
660 South 4th Street • PO Box 13267
Edwardsville, Kansas 66113

LICENSE AGREEMENT AND LIMITED WARRANTY

READ THE FOLLOWING TERMS AND CONDITIONS CAREFULLY BEFORE OPENING THIS DISK PACKAGE. THIS IS AN AGREEMENT BETWEEN YOU AND APPLETON & LANGE (THE "COMPANY"). BY OPENING THIS SEALED PACKAGE, YOU ARE AGREEING TO BE BOUND BY THESE TERMS AND CONDITIONS. IF YOU DO NOT AGREE WITH THESE TERMS AND CONDITIONS, DO NOT OPEN THE DISK PACKAGE. PROMPTLY RETURN THE DISK PACKAGE AND ALL ACCOMPANYING ITEMS TO THE COMPANY.

1. GRANT OF LICENSE: In consideration of your adoption of textbooks and/or other materials published by the Company, and your agreement to abide by the terms and conditions of this Agreement, the Company grants to you a nonexclusive right to use and display the copy of the enclosed software program (hereinafter the "SOFTWARE") so long as you comply with the terms of this Agreement. The Company reserves all rights not expressly granted to you under this Agreement. This license is *not* a sale of the original SOFTWARE or any copy to you.

2. USE RESTRICTIONS: You may *not* sell, license, transfer or distribute copies of the SOFTWARE or Documentation to others. You may *not* reverse engineer, disassemble, decompile, modify, adapt, translate or otherwise reproduce the SOFTWARE or any part of it, or create derivative works based on the SOFTWARE or the Documentation without the prior written consent of the Company.

3. MISCELLANEOUS: This Agreement shall be construed in accordance with the laws of the United States of America and the State of New York, except for that body of law dealing with conflicts of law, and shall benefit the Company, its affiliates and assignees. If any provision of this Agreement is found void or unenforceable, the remainder will remain valid and enforceable according to its terms. Use, duplication or disclosure of the SOFTWARE by the U.S. Government is subject to the restricted rights applicable to commercial computer software under FAR 52.227.19 and DFARS 252.277-7013.

4. LIMITED WARRANTY AND DISCLAIMER OF WARRANTY: Because this SOFTWARE is being given to you without charge, the Company makes no warranties about the SOFTWARE, which is provided "AS-IS". **THE COMPANY DISCLAIMS ALL WARRANTIES, EXPRESS OR IMPLIED, INCLUDING WITHOUT LIMITATION, THE IMPLIED WARRANTIES OF MERCHANTABILITY AND FITNESS FOR A PARTICULAR PURPOSE. THE COMPANY DOES NOT WARRANT, GUARANTEE OR MAKE ANY REPRESENTATION REGARDING THE USE OR THE RESULTS OF THE USE OF THE SOFTWARE. IN NO EVENT, SHALL THE COMPANY, ITS PARENTS, SUBSIDIARIES, AFFILIATES, LICENSORS, DIRECTORS, OFFICERS, EMPLOYEES, AGENTS, SUPPLIERS OR CONTRACTORS BE LIABLE FOR ANY INCIDENTAL, INDIRECT, SPECIAL OR CONSEQUENTIAL DAMAGES ARISING OUT OF OR IN CONNECTION WITH THE LICENSE GRANTED UNDER THIS AGREEMENT INCLUDING, WITHOUT LIMITATION, LOSS OF USE, LOSS OF DATA, LOSS OF INCOME OR PROFIT, OR OTHER LOSSES SUSTAINED AS A RESULT OF INJURY TO ANY PERSON, OR LOSS OF OR DAMAGE TO PROPERTY, OR CLAIMS OF THIRD PARTIES, EVEN IF THE COMPANY OR AN AUTHORIZED REPRESENTATIVE OF THE COMPANY HAS BEEN ADVISED OF THE POSSIBILITY OF SUCH DAMAGES.**

SOME JURISDICTIONS DO NOT ALLOW THE EXCLUSION OF IMPLIED WARRANTIES OR THE LIMITATION ON LIABILITY FOR INCIDENTAL, INDIRECT, SPECIAL OR CONSEQUENTIAL DAMAGES, SO THE ABOVE LIMITATIONS MAY NOT ALWAYS APPLY. THE WARRANTIES IN THIS AGREEMENT GIVE YOU SPECIFIC LEGAL RIGHTS AND YOU MAY ALSO HAVE OTHER RIGHTS WHICH VARY IN ACCORDANCE WITH LOCAL LAW.

No sales personnel or other representative of any party involved in the distribution of the software is authorized by the company to make any warranties with respect to the software beyond what is contained in this agreement. Oral statements do not constitute warranties, shall not be relied upon by you and are not part of this agreement. The entire agreement between you and the Company is embodied herein.

ACKNOWLEDGMENT

YOU ACKNOWLEDGE THAT YOU HAVE READ THIS AGREEMENT, UNDERSTAND IT AND AGREE TO BE BOUND BY ITS TERMS AND CONDITIONS. YOU ALSO AGREE THAT THIS AGREEMENT IS THE COMPLETE AND EXCLUSIVE AGREEMENT BETWEEN YOU AND THE COMPANY.

Should you have any questions concerning this agreement or if you wish to contact the Company for any reason, please contact in writing: Appleton & Lange/Simon & Schuster, c/o Starpak, 237 22nd Street, Greeley, CO 80631. (800)991-0077

a-, an-	bi-
prefix	prefix
ab-	brachy-
prefix	prefix
ad-	brady-
prefix	prefix
ambi-	cac-, mal-
prefix	prefix
ante-	centi-
prefix	prefix
anti-	con-
prefix	prefix
auto-	contra-
prefix	prefix

two, double	no, not, without, lack of
meaning	meaning
short	away from
meaning	meaning
slow	toward, near, to
meaning	meaning
bad	both
meaning	meaning
a hundred	before
meaning	meaning
with, together	against
meaning	meaning
against	self
meaning	meaning

de-	ep-, epi-
prefix	prefix
dia-	eu-
prefix	prefix
dif-	ex-, exo-
prefix	prefix
dipl-	extra-
prefix	prefix
dys-	hemi-, semi-
prefix	prefix
ec-, ecto-	hetero-
prefix	prefix
end-, endo-	homeo-
prefix	prefix

upon, over, above	down, away from
meaning	meaning
good, normal	through, between
meaning	meaning
out, away from	apart, free from, separate
meaning	meaning
outside, beyond	double
meaning	meaning
half	bad, difficult, painful
meaning	meaning
different	out, outside, outer
meaning	meaning
similar, same	within, inner
meaning	meaning

hydro-	mega-
prefix	prefix
hyper-	meso-
prefix	prefix
hypo-	meta-
prefix	prefix
in-	micro-
prefix	prefix
infra-	milli-
prefix	prefix
inter-	mono-
prefix	prefix
intra-	multi-
prefix	prefix

large, great	water
meaning	meaning

middle	above, beyond, excessive
meaning	meaning

beyond, over, between, change	below, under, deficient
meaning	meaning

small	in, into, not
meaning	meaning

one thousandth	below
meaning	meaning

one	between
meaning	meaning

many, much	within
meaning	meaning

neo-	post-
prefix	prefix
olig-, oligo-	pre-, pro-
prefix	prefix
pan-	pseudo-
prefix	prefix
para-	retro-
prefix	prefix
per-	sub-
prefix	prefix
peri-	supra-
prefix	prefix
poly-	sym-, syn-
prefix	prefix

after, behind	new
meaning	meaning

before, in front of	little, scanty
meaning	meaning

false	all
meaning	meaning

backward	beside, alongside, abnormal
meaning	meaning

below, under, beneath	through
meaning	meaning

above, beyond	around
meaning	meaning

with, together	many, much, excessive
meaning	meaning

tachy-	-blast
prefix	suffix
tri-	-centesis
prefix	suffix
ultra-	-cyte
prefix	suffix
uni-	-ectasis
prefix	suffix
-ac, -al, -ar, -ary, -ic, -in, -ine, -ous, -us, -y	-ectomy
suffix	suffix
-algesia, -algia, -dynia	-emesis
suffix	suffix
-ate	-gen, -genesis, -genic
suffix	suffix

immature cell, germ cell	fast
meaning	meaning
surgical puncture	three
meaning	meaning
cell	beyond
meaning	meaning
dilatation, dilation, distention	one
meaning	meaning
excision	pertaining to
meaning	meaning
vomiting	pain
meaning	meaning
formation, produce	use, action
meaning	meaning

-gram	-megaly
suffix	suffix
-hexia, -ia, -ism, -ity, -osis, -sis, -y	-oma
suffix	suffix
-itis	-pathy
suffix	suffix
-ive	-penia
suffix	suffix
-logy	-plasm
suffix	suffix
-lymph	-plegia
suffix	suffix
-lysis	-ptosis
suffix	suffix

enlargement, large	weight, mark, record
meaning	meaning
tumor	condition of
meaning	meaning
disease	inflammation
meaning	meaning
lack of, deficiency	nature of, quality of
meaning	meaning
a thing formed, plasma	study of
meaning	meaning
stroke, paralysis	serum, clear fluid
meaning	meaning
prolapse, drooping	destruction, to separate
meaning	meaning

-rrhea	-tome
suffix	suffix
-rrhaphy	-tomy
suffix	suffix
-rrhexis	-trophy
suffix	suffix
-scopy	adeno
suffix	combining form
-spasm	arterio
suffix	combining form
-stasis	arthro
suffix	combining form
-staxis	cardio
suffix	combining form

instrument to cut	flow, discharge
meaning	meaning
incision	suture
meaning	meaning
nourishment, development	rupture
meaning	meaning
gland	to view, examine
meaning	meaning
artery	tension, spasm
meaning	meaning
joint	control, stopping
meaning	meaning
heart	dripping, trickling
meaning	meaning

chondro	hepato
combining form	combining form

costo	myo
combining form	combining form

cranio	naso rhino
combining form	combining form

dermato	nephro reno
combining form	combining form

erythro	neuro
combining form	combining form

gastro	patho
combining form	combining form

hemato	thoraco
combining form	combining form

liver	cartilage
meaning	meaning
muscle	rib
meaning	meaning
nose	skull
meaning	meaning
kidney	skin
meaning	meaning
nerve	red
meaning	meaning
disease	stomach
meaning	meaning
chest	blood
meaning	meaning